Medical Coding in the Real World
Second Edition

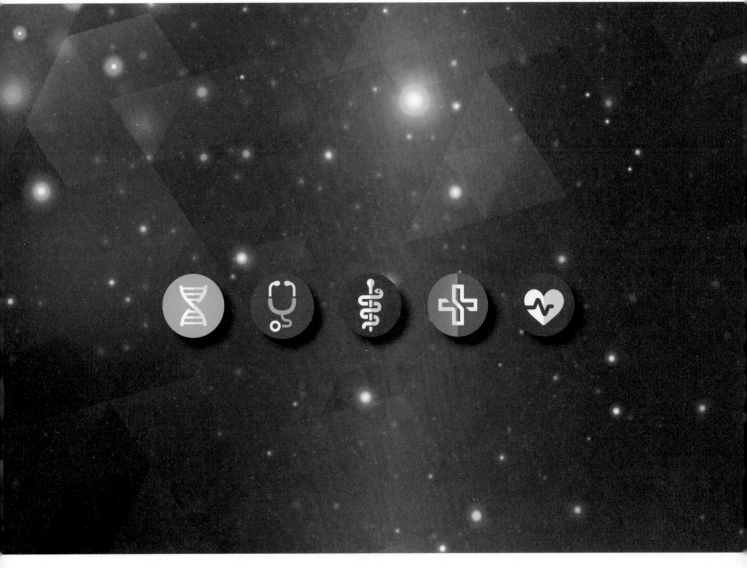

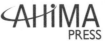
AHIMA
PRESS

Medical Coding in the Real World

Second Edition

Elizabeth Roberts

MA Ed, CCS, CPC

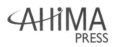

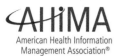

ISBN: **978-1-58426-759-1**
AHIMA Product No.: AC234019

AHIMA Staff:
Colton Gigot, MA, Production Development Editor
Megan Grennan, Managing Editor
Rachel Schratz, MA, Assistant Editor

Cover image: © filo, iStockphoto

For more information, including updates, about AHIMA Press publications, visit http://www.ahima.org/education/press.

American Health Information Management Association
233 North Michigan Avenue, 21st Floor
Chicago, Illinois 60601-5809
ahima.org

Brief Table of Contents

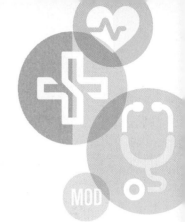

Detailed Table of Contents

Part II   Coding in the Real World   179

About the Author

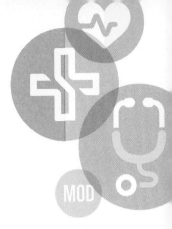

Elizabeth Roberts, MA Ed, CCS, CPC, has worked in the healthcare industry for nearly 20 years and is an experienced coding educator. Mrs. Roberts has a master's degree in education and extensive experience in healthcare coding and reimbursement. In addition to serving as the program director for the allied health department at Vista College and lead instructor for the medical billing and coding department for Virginia College in Austin, Texas, she also spent three years as the senior director of content for ImplementHIT, a healthcare information technology company that specializes in bite-sized educational modules for medical providers and clinical staff. She now educates providers and clinical staff as the physician coding educator for Optum in Colorado Springs, CO. An experienced consultant in healthcare coding and reimbursement, including practice management, HIPAA, compliance, insurance regulations, and healthcare coding (CPT, ICD-10, HCPCS), Mrs. Roberts enjoys helping billers, coders, clinical staff, and providers unweave the complicated tangle of coding and billing in order to optimize healthcare reimbursement.

Preface

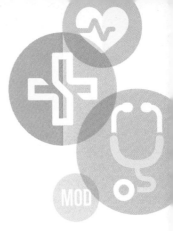

Job opportunities within the fields of medical billing, coding, and health information management (HIM) are growing. According to the Bureau of Labor Statistics (BLS), one of the sectors with the fastest annual employment growth is healthcare and social assistance, with 1.6 percent annual employment growth, amounting to an anticipated 3.4 million new jobs within this sector by 2028. Out of the 30 fastest growing occupations, 18 are in healthcare and related occupations. This continued demand and growth of the healthcare industry is due to many factors, including an aging population, increased life expectancy, and the growth of chronic conditions that require ongoing medical care (BLS 2019).

Although many healthcare jobs are held by healthcare professionals such as doctors, nurse practitioners, physician assistants, and other healthcare clinical support personnel such as physical therapists and medical assistants, any growth in the field of healthcare clinical workers leads to a concurrent growth of healthcare administrative support workers such as billers, coders, and healthcare information management specialists (among others).

This is great news for us, as growth in the healthcare sector over the next ten years represents potentially millions of new jobs requiring educated, certified professionals. This text will help you learn the basics of these administrative professions, and train you for the real world of healthcare coding.

One of the major advantages of the professions within health information management, which includes healthcare coding, is that there is no ceiling. You can go virtually as far as your motivation takes you! As you start out in the field, keep in mind that there are additional certifications and educational programs that can help you advance in your field of interest, and allow you to increase your earning potential through promotions or career transitions. The American Health Information Management Association (AHIMA), the premier association of health information management (HIM) professionals worldwide, offers an interactive career map, which includes dozens of job descriptions and possible career pathways at https://my.ahima.org/careermap (see figure I.1).

Major coding and HIM organizations, such as AHIMA, typically conduct a periodic salary or coding survey to evaluate the world of coding from the coder's perspective, and to see how job responsibilities, salaries, and career expectations are changing.

As you go through this text and associated workbook, keep certifications and continuing education in mind, as they are the key to your success in a coding career. It is important to begin your coding education with an open mind. You might find coding tedious and difficult at first, but try to have fun with it! Once you have a solid coding education, the possibilities for your future are endless. This textbook is the first step in your goal toward a rewarding and exciting career. It contextualizes all learning within that "real-world" setting, and presents instructions on how to correctly identify, select, and apply healthcare codes from each of the major code sets (ICD-10-CM, ICD-10-PCS, CPT, and HCPCS), thus preparing you for *medical coding in the real world.*

Figure I.1.   AHIMA Career Map

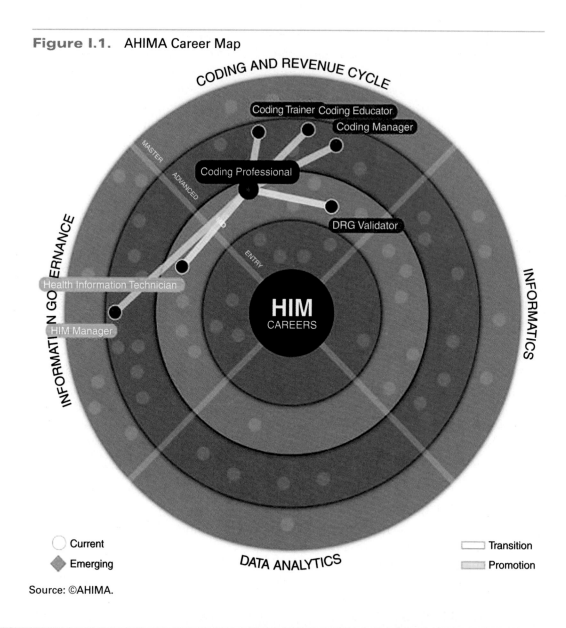

Source: ©AHIMA.

How to Use This Textbook

Hands-on medical coding in the real world is the basis for this coding textbook. It is organized into coding systems within medical specialties, as they are encountered in the real world, and teaches all necessary code sets as necessitated in a real-world setting. For example, healthcare codes pertaining to orthopedic conditions and services to treat those conditions are discussed within the context of an orthopedic healthcare practice. This means identifying and assigning all codes on the claim, not just those found in a certain section in the CPT coding manual, and includes diagnoses codes, supply codes, and various other necessary procedural codes, as necessary, per service.

Medical Coding in the Real World, Second Edition, emphasizes the real world of coding, and contextualizes codes so that students see their role in a healthcare practice. In this way, students learn what it is like to code in a real-world context. For example, instead of learning how to code labor and delivery services based on reading the labor and delivery chapter in the CPT coding manual, you will learn labor and delivery as if you were working in an actual obstetrician's office.

The chapters in this text are organized into medical specialties or settings, and students learn how to code within this contextualized space. Each chapter focuses on all of the various types of codes that are utilized within each specialty, including all procedural, diagnosis, and supply or service codes.

Chapters are organized in such a way as to build upon each other, so that more complicated specialties, or more complicated coding and application of coding guidelines, are discussed after the basic components of coding and coding guidelines are mastered. The basics of all outpatient professional coding is presented first, followed by chapters that are centered around a medical specialty or healthcare setting, and the ICD-10-CM, CPT, or HCPCS codes used within that specialty or setting. Inpatient facility coding (ICD-10-PCS) is presented at the end of the text. Evaluation and Management coding is taught early on in the text so that students can utilize their knowledge of E&M codes throughout the text and apply them as necessary throughout the chapters.

When using this text, it is imperative for the student to have a paper copy of all of the code books discussed herein, including ICD-10-CM, CPT, HCPCS, and ICD-10-PCS. This text is designed to help the student learn how to accurately locate and apply healthcare codes from each of these code books.

Part I of this text discusses the basics of medical billing and coding. Chapter 1, Your Coding Career, discusses the many aspects of a job as a medical coder, including coding certifications. Chapter 2, Healthcare Billing Basics, includes a high overview of the basic principles of healthcare billing, such as the Health Insurance Portability and Accountability Act (HIPAA) and performance measures. Chapter 3, Basics of Coding, defines medical coding and medical code sets. Chapter 4, Learning the ICD-10-CM Code Book, defines and examines the organization of the ICD-10-CM code book, the structure of ICD-10-CM diagnosis codes, and basics on how to select ICD-10-CM codes from a diagnostic statement. Chapter 5, Learning the CPT and HCPCS Code Books, examines the CPT and HCPCS code sets and books.

Part II of this text discusses specific code sets, coding guidelines, and presents practice coding scenarios organized within healthcare-specialty-specific chapters. Chapter 6, Supplies and Services, discusses the HCPCS code set within the context of an ambulance supplier and durable medical equipment supplier. This chapter also includes a section on coding for medications administered in the healthcare setting. Chapter 7, Behavioral Health Services, examines the medical codes used within the specialty of behavioral health. This chapter also provides a preliminary discussion of evaluation and management coding. Chapter 8, Primary Care Services, examines the medical codes used within the specialty of primary care. This chapter provides a more thorough examination of evaluation and management coding and auditing. Chapter 9, Eye and Vision Services, examines the medical codes used in ophthalmology and optometry services. Chapter 10, Urgent Care and Emergency Department Services, examines the medical codes used within both the urgent care and emergency department setting. Chapter 11, Surgical Services, examines the medical codes used to identify and report surgical services performed by professionals within the inpatient and outpatient hospital settings. Chapter 12, Anesthesia and Pain Management Services, examines the codes used to identify services performed by anesthesiologists and interventional pain management specialists. Chapter 13, Radiology and Imaging Services, examines the codes used to identify radiology and imaging services, excluding radiation oncology. Chapter 14, Laboratory and Pathology Services, examines the codes used to report laboratory and pathology services. Chapter 15, Orthopedic Services, examines the medical codes used to report conditions and services performed within the specialty of orthopedics. Chapter 16, Physical, Occupational, and Speech Therapy Services, examines the codes used to report services provided by physical therapists, occupational therapists, and speech-language pathologists. Chapter 17, Obstetrics and Gynecology Services, examines the codes reported to identify services performed in both obstetrics (such as labor and delivery) and gynecology. Chapter 18, Healthcare Specialist Services, Part I, examines the codes used within three medical specialties, including hematology and oncology, neurology, and urology and nephrology. Chapter 19, Healthcare Specialist Services, Part II, examines the codes used within the specialties of gastroenterology and cardiology. Chapter 20, Inpatient Hospital Services, defines and examines the ICD-10-PCS code set and coding used to report facility services.

This text is thus best used in a linear fashion, from the earliest chapters, progressing to subsequent chapters, to ensure understanding of all materials presented. The following pedagogical items are included to enhance the learning process.

- Learning objectives to identify actionable outcomes after reading each chapter.
- Key terms to solidify healthcare and coding terminology.
- Figures and tables provide visual references for complex concepts and guidelines.
- **Key to Success** boxes call out insightful information from the perspective of a professional coder.
- **HCC Coding Corner** boxes provide detailed information about applying hierarchal condition category (HCC) coding. HCC icons also appear in the margin of applicable text.
- **MOD** boxes address additional details about appending modifiers to codes.
- **There's a Code for That** exercises appear throughout each chapter and provide practice to the immediate concepts.
- Codes and code descriptions are highlighted throughout the text.
- **Putting It All Together** is a section at the end of relevant chapters to tie key concepts together within a real-world coding scenario.
- End-of-chapter content provides an opportunity to practice the concepts presented in the chapter. Exercises range from true/false, matching, and multiple-choice questions to fill-in-the-blank coding questions.
- End-of-chapter case studies present an opportunity for students to abstract and code a real medical record to determine all applicable codes (ICD-10-CM, CPT, HCPCS, ICD-10-PCS), in a guided manner.

This book refers to the 2020 version of the Healthcare Common Procedure Coding System (HCPCS) and the 2020 versions of the following code sets.

- International Classification of Diseases, Tenth Revision, Clinical Modification (ICD-10-CM)
- International Classification of Diseases, Tenth Revision, Procedure Coding System (ICD-10-PCS)
- Current Procedural Terminology (CPT)

Student Workbook

This text is accompanied by a comprehensive student workbook designed to enhance important information addressed in each chapter, and to reinforce learning through practice. The *Medical Coding in the Real World Student Workbook*, Second Edition, includes 20 chapters, each of which corresponds to the information presented in the textbook. Each workbook chapter includes a number of exercises that range from true/false, multiple choice, matching, and coding questions, to short answer questions, case studies, and practice focused on correctly completing insurance claim forms and other related paperwork.

The student workbook is meant to be a companion to the textbook, and should be used in conjunction with the textbook, chapter by chapter. In this manner, the workbook should be used to reinforce the information learned in each chapter of the text, and to provide practice selecting, sequencing, and reporting the appropriate ICD-10-CM, CPT, HCPCS, and ICD-10-PCS codes, as necessary.

References

American Health Information Management Association (AHIMA). 2019. Career Map. https://my.ahima.org/careermap.

Bureau of Labor Statistics (BLS). September 4, 2019. *Employment Projections 2018-2028*. http://www.bls.gov/news.release/pdf/ecopro.pdf.

Health Information Careers. 2017. *Coding Professional*. http://hicareers.com/CareerMap/FullDescription.aspx?ID=46.

Acknowledgments

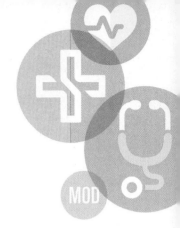

This text would not have been possible without the love and support of my family, especially my husband. And to all of my past, present, and future students of medical coding—this is for you!

AHIMA Press would like to thank Gloria Anderson, MEd, RHIA, CCS, and Linda Hyde, RHIA, for their contributions to this edition of *Medical Coding in the Real World*.

Part I

Medical Billing and Coding Basics

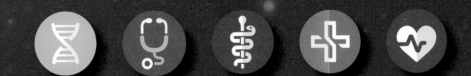

Your Coding Career

Learning Objectives

- Identify the different types of healthcare facilities and practices and how coding practices differ within each setting
- Identify professional organizations that support health information management, and the benefits of coding certifications

- Recognize the different types of healthcare providers, including different types of healthcare specialists

Key Terms

Administrative personnel
Ambulatory surgical center (ASC)
American Health Information
    Management Association
    (AHIMA)
Certified Coding Specialist (CCS)
Classification system
Clinical personnel
Coding certification
Continuing education unit (CEU)
Date of service
Diagnosis

Emergency department
Encounter
Healthcare billing
Healthcare coding
Healthcare provider
Healthcare specialty
Hospital
Inpatient
Internal medicine provider
Large group practice
Mid-level provider

Outpatient
Physician
Primary care provider (PCP)
Procedure
Professional organization
Remote coding
Small group practice
Solo practice
Surgical specialist
Urgent care facility

There are so many career options in healthcare billing and coding that it may seem a little overwhelming to students entering the field. Essentially every health service that is provided must be coded and billed appropriately, so there are thousands of different career options on the administrative side of medicine. A coder's job and the codes that he or she bills will depend largely on the type of healthcare setting and healthcare practice in which they work. This could range from an endocrinologist's office, to a long-term care facility, or a healthcare billing company. On the other hand, a coder might choose to work in the inpatient hospital setting, an ambulatory surgical center, or chemotherapy infusion center. The career options for coders are endless.

This chapter discusses possibilities in the profession of coding, the importance of professional organizations, and the different types of healthcare settings and healthcare specialties in order to help incoming coders understand what to expect once they find themselves in the real world of healthcare billing and coding. This chapter also briefly discusses the differences between healthcare facility (inpatient) coding versus professional (physician) coding. It is also important to note that the main part of this textbook focuses on professional physician coding and billing, which differs from facility coding in the inpatient setting. Professional coding is discussed from chapter 6 through chapter 19, and facility coding is specifically addressed in chapter 20.

This textbook covers the four major healthcare code sets related to procedure coding, diagnosis coding, and coding for supplies and services. These code sets include the *International Classification of Diseases, Tenth Revision, Procedure Coding System* (ICD-10-PCS) and *International Classification of Diseases, Tenth Revision, Clinical Modification* (ICD-10-CM) as well as *Current Procedural Terminology* (CPT) and the *Healthcare Common Procedure Coding System* (HCPCS).

Where Could You Work?

The type of coding in which you specialize will depend on where you work, so it is important to understand these different settings. In the world of healthcare billing and coding, there are two main work settings—a billing and coding company, or an actual healthcare practice or facility. A billing or coding company handles the billing or coding for a healthcare practice or facility; the only contact you might have with patients would be communication regarding healthcare bills. A healthcare practice or facility sees and treats patients on a daily basis. A coder in a healthcare practice or facility may have job duties that require interaction with patients, such as answering phone calls, scheduling appointments, checking patients in and out, communication with patients regarding bills, or in performing other administrative duties. Your job description and daily responsibilities will change significantly, depending on in which of these settings you work.

The following sections introduce healthcare coding and discuss the differences in healthcare settings, including billing and coding companies, different types of healthcare practices, and inpatient and outpatient coding.

What Is Healthcare Coding?

Healthcare coding is the practice of assigning numeric or alphanumeric codes to identify the treatment, services, or supplies provided to a patient during a healthcare encounter, also known as the *procedure*. A **procedure** is an action of diagnosing or treating a condition by a healthcare professional. Codes are also assigned to identify the reason why the patient was provided with healthcare services, otherwise known as the *diagnosis*. A **diagnosis** is a word or phrase used by a physician to identify a medical condition from which an individual patient suffers or a reason for which the patient needs, seeks, or receives healthcare. Healthcare codes are assigned based on the healthcare provider's documentation for each **date of service**, or each specific day that the patient received healthcare services or care.

Codes are a type of classification system that translates healthcare procedures or diagnoses into a set of numeric or alphanumeric codes. A **classification system** is a clinical vocabulary, terminology, or nomenclature that lists words or phrases with their meanings, provides for the proper use of clinical words as names or symbols, and facilitates mapping standardized terms to broader classifications for administrative, regulatory, oversight, and fiscal requirements.

Individual codes are compiled and organized into a number of different code books, and it is the coding professional's job to read through the documentation from the date of service, determine which procedures, services, or supplies were provided to the patient and the reason(s) they were provided, and then determine which code(s) appropriately identify those components of the patient visit. The coding professional must also be aware of the setting in which the services were provided, as codes may change depending on the healthcare setting. For example, providers in one healthcare setting may report codes for the supplies and services provided to the patient during an encounter, whereas those in another setting may not.

Once the codes are selected, they are listed on a claim. A claim, used for payment for the services rendered, is a specialized form that contains information regarding:

- The patient,
- Responsible party for the services,
- Healthcare provider,
- Date of service,
- Procedures,
- Diagnoses,
- Any supplies used, and
- Additional details (such as date of injury or last menstrual period, if applicable).

The claim may be in a paper format, which is printed and then mailed to the responsible party, or in an electronic format, which is sent directly to the responsible party via an electronic data interchange system that transmits data between computer systems. The responsible party for the claim is usually a health insurance company, also called the third-party payer. The codes sent on a claim are used for both payment and reporting purposes. For example, when an insurance company receives a claim, it is analyzed and then paid as a bill would be. In this sense, coders are an inherent part of the billing process. Without coders to analyze documentation, select, and report the appropriate codes for services, healthcare services would not be paid for by insurance companies. See figure 1.1 for a simplified illustration of the medical claims process.

Figure 1.1. Medical claims process

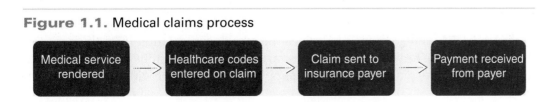

Healthcare billing is different than healthcare coding. **Healthcare billing** is the practice of sending a coded healthcare claim to a third-party payer or insurance company for payment, as described in chapter 2 (Healthcare Billing Basics), and then following that claim until it is paid in full. This can include billing patients for any remaining balance, sending appeals to insurance companies for underpaid or unpaid claims, and sending patient accounts to outside collections agencies for nonpayment.

A correctly coded healthcare claim is required for healthcare providers to collect the correct payment for the services provided to a patient. In this sense, healthcare billers and coders work together to ensure that the healthcare services are reported accurately and then billed correctly to the payer, to ensure appropriate payment for services rendered to each patient for each date of service. This textbook introduces the billing concepts for each healthcare specialty before discussing the coding process for each specialty. This helps student coders understand the close connection between billing and coding and ensuring correct payment for healthcare services.

Billing and Coding Companies

A billing or coding company does just that—billing and coding of insurance claims for healthcare practitioners and healthcare facilities. Many healthcare practices, ranging from single-physician healthcare offices to large inpatient hospitals, outsource their billing and coding to a company that performs these functions for them. They choose not to code health records and send healthcare claims directly but instead send the billing information and healthcare documentation to an outside company that will complete their billing and coding of healthcare insurance claims.

Outsourcing to a billing and coding company has its advantages. For example, the provider's office or healthcare facility does not have to use internal resources to code and send claims but still maintains access to a highly trained or certified staff capable of coding and billing expertly for their services. However, there are also some disadvantages to outsourcing to a billing company. When using a billing company, the provider's office or healthcare facility has no control over the billing processes or the training of the employees at the billing company, which can lead to misunderstandings. Furthermore, there might be hidden costs or contractual misunderstandings with the billing company, causing frustration or heavy expenses.

The agreement between healthcare facilities and billing and coding companies varies greatly depending on the company. For example, some billing companies perform just the billing of the claims; the encounters are submitted to the company pre-coded by staff members within the healthcare practice. In this case, the codes for the encounter (procedures, supplies and services, and diagnosis codes, all of which are addressed in chapters 6 through 20 of this textbook), are identified and entered by staff such as the doctor, nursing or healthcare assisting staff, or coder within the healthcare practice. An **encounter** is the contact between a patient and a provider who has primary responsibility for assessing and treating the condition of the patient at a given time and who exercises independent judgment in the care of the patient. The codes from this encounter are then sent to the billing company that enters those codes on a claim form, sends the claim to the patient's insurance company, and then follows up on the claim until it is paid in full.

Other billing and coding companies provide services that are more comprehensive. In this case, the billing company receives the raw documentation from the patient's encounter from the healthcare practice or inpatient facility; identifies the correct codes for each procedure, diagnosis, or other supplies or services provided to the patient;

enters these codes correctly on the insurance claim; sends the claim to the insurance company or third-party payer; and follows up with it until it is paid in full.

The specific job responsibilities of working in a billing and coding company thus depend on the type of service the company provides. As a coder, you may have opportunities to work in a billing and coding company. As an expert in the codes that represent medical necessity (ICD-10-CM) and the procedures, services, and supplies provided to the patient (CPT, HCPCS, ICD-10-PCS), you can decipher the complicated healthcare documentation used to support the codes selected. You may also choose to learn more about the billing side of coding and the complex world of billing regulations surrounding the correct coding and payment of healthcare claims. Either way, working in a billing or coding company is an exciting possibility. (Note that although this textbook does discuss billing in specific scenarios, it does not cover all billing procedures, rules, and regulations.)

Furthermore, although many billing companies are located within physical offices, other billing and coding practices are online. Coders have the opportunity to work on-site with a team of billing and coding specialists in an administrative setting, or in a virtual setting from a personal computer.

Virtual coding positions are often referred to as remote coding positions. A remote coding position is one in which the coder is not required to be physically present in the office or facility setting while completing his or her work. A remote coder can work from home, a coffee shop, or anywhere else with Internet access. Coding remotely requires an in-depth understanding of coding, reliable access to the proper equipment, and the ability to stay on-task without getting distracted. Because of the possibility of additional confidentiality and security risks in remote coding, working remotely also requires knowledge of Health Insurance Portability and Accountability Act (HIPAA) privacy and security rules and regulations that govern patient privacy and access to confidential patient health information (discussed more in depth in chapter 2) to ensure secure access to patient information. Many online coding positions require completion of a face-to-face training, short term of on-site coding, or trial period before allowing a coder to work remotely, while others may require the successful completion of a coding test and a coding certification. This ensures that the coder has a complete understanding of coding processes before he or she works off-site without direct supervision or assistance.

Remote coding positions are becoming more numerous in the world of healthcare, as employers realize the cost savings involved. Because the employee is not actually on-site, less business overhead in terms of space, equipment, and materials is required. Large facilities, such as hospital systems, are more likely to employ remote coders who are expected to maintain a certain percentage of coding accuracy. Coding accuracy is the percentage of codes that are identified correctly for either diagnoses or procedures (or both) from health record documentation. As a remote coder for a healthcare facility, a coding accuracy of 90 to 95 percent is typically required, although some healthcare facilities may require a coding accuracy percentage of up to 98 percent!

Key to Success

Working in a virtual setting might sound convenient, but it is not for everyone. Working in a remote environment requires a great deal of self-discipline, time management skills, organization, diligence, and motivation. The remote environment also comes with plenty of distractions, both online (that is, social media, email, and other websites) and at home (for example, housework, family, and pets). If you are considering a remote coding position in the future, it is a good idea to compare its pros and cons with those of an on-site position, including all potential distractions and how you will overcome them to ensure success in your coding position.

Types of Healthcare Practices

If you choose to work at a healthcare practice, your job functions may vary, and you may have more interaction among patients or healthcare practitioners. For example, you might have to assist the administrative staff, answer phones with the receptionist, schedule appointments, and interact directly with the healthcare practitioners and clinical staff daily. In the inpatient setting, it is more likely that you would have less contact with patients, as the coding and billing office is usually separate from other administrative offices.

Not all healthcare practices are alike, however. The type of practice and the exact job functions that you are required to perform depend largely on the type of healthcare practice in which you work. A **solo practice** is a healthcare office that has one doctor who typically owns the practice and sees all of the patients that come into the office each day. A **small group practice** has from two to five healthcare providers, all of whom see patients each day. These doctors work together and may see each other's patients when needed; they may also rotate their schedules to share responsibilities. Typically, in any type of healthcare group practice, one or more of the doctors will own the business, as well as see patients, all within the same healthcare specialty. A **large group practice** may have anywhere from six to dozens of providers. Many times, a large group practice is made up of healthcare providers from many different healthcare specialties. For example, a large group practice in an inner-city area may provide family practice, pediatric, and obstetrics and gynecology services. Healthcare providers in any of these types of practices may also complete rounds at inpatient facilities, such as hospitals or long-term care facilities—leaving the office throughout the day, at a certain time each day, or on certain days of the week to treat patients who are in the inpatient setting. For example, an obstetrician working in a small group practice may have to leave the office if he or she is called to perform a delivery at the hospital, and then return to the office to see the rest of his or her patients once the delivery is done.

When a healthcare provider treats or performs a procedure on a patient in a facility such as a hospital, skilled nursing facility, or emergency room, he or she bills for the service for reimbursement. The facility itself also bills to obtain reimbursement for the supplies, treatments, or other resources used during the patient's stay. For example, if the patient delivered a baby at the hospital, the hospital would bill for the labor and delivery suite, room and board provided to the patient during her stay, and any other supplies or hospital resources used during the delivery, such as the use of an operating suite to perform a cesarean section. Therefore, the delivery of the infant in the hospital setting would require at least two claims: one for the professional physician services (the delivery procedure) and another for the hospital facility charge (the facility resources used during the patient's stay). If the patient received any other services, such as an anesthesia service by an anesthesiologist for pain management, then the anesthesiologist would report his or her services separately as well. Keep in mind the division between facility (inpatient) and professional (outpatient) billing and coding, as facility and professional services are often reported with different codes depending on who is reporting the service (facility or professional). See figure 1.2 for an example of these differences.

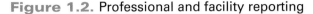

Figure 1.2. Professional and facility reporting

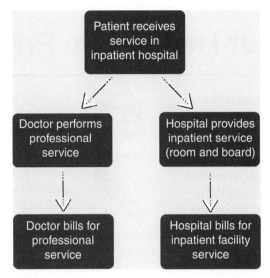

A **hospital** is a large facility that provides specialized healthcare treatments and has a large staff of healthcare providers and nurses on hand at all times. Hospitals may range from smaller, locally owned hospitals with a hundred staff members, to extensive hospital systems maintained throughout a large geographic area that employ thousands of staff members. An **ambulatory surgical center (ASC)** is a healthcare facility that provides same-day surgical services to patients on an outpatient basis. ASC procedures are minor or less invasive than surgeries performed in the inpatient hospital setting, and patients are discharged home on the same day of the surgery. An **emergency department (ED)** or **urgent care facility** may be either a standalone facility or attached to a larger facility, such as a hospital. Emergency departments and urgent care facilities provide same-day care for patients with healthcare emergencies or urgent healthcare needs. Healthcare may also be provided in other settings as needed, such as long-term care facilities, nursing homes, hospice, or even in the patient's home. Study figure 1.3 to learn more about the differences between healthcare practices.

As a general rule, the smaller the practice in which you work, the more likely you will be responsible for performing many different tasks, not just those of a biller or coder. For example, in a small single physician practice, you may have to perform all of the administrative duties in the office. On the other hand, in a larger practice you will be a smaller cog in the machine and have less varied responsibilities. For example, you may be responsible only for entering the codes on a claim or entering insurance payments using company software.

Either way, it is important to be flexible, especially as you are starting your career. This may require working in several different positions in the healthcare office. A student entering the field, would usually begin at an entry-level position and then progress into a full-time coder position. For example, you may begin your coding career as a healthcare receptionist, appointment scheduler, or health record technician. There are many different job responsibilities within the field of health information management (HIM), and it helps to learn as much as you can about every aspect of the healthcare office or facility. As you become more skilled in the field of healthcare administration and coding, you may work as a biller or coder, or in any number of other administrative positions in the healthcare office. Working in different positions can help you determine exactly where you fit best within the organization, ultimately

Figure 1.3. Types of healthcare practices

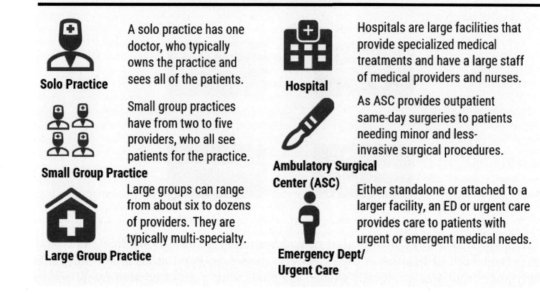

Types of Healthcare Practices

Solo Practice
A solo practice has one doctor, who typically owns the practice and sees all of the patients.

Small Group Practice
Small group practices have from two to five providers, who all see patients for the practice.

Large Group Practice
Large groups can range from about six to dozens of providers. They are typically multi-specialty.

Hospital
Hospitals are large facilities that provide specialized medical treatments and have a large staff of medical providers and nurses.

Ambulatory Surgical Center (ASC)
As ASC provides outpatient same-day surgeries to patients needing minor and less-invasive surgical procedures.

Emergency Dept/ Urgent Care
Either standalone or attached to a larger facility, an ED or urgent care provides care to patients with urgent or emergent medical needs.

increasing your career success in the long run. For instance, an expert-level coder in the field of HIM may become an auditor, a coding educator of a large healthcare facility or practice, or an independent coding consultant.

Key to Success

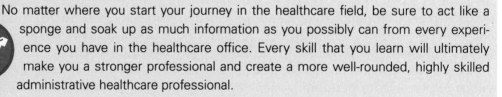

No matter where you start your journey in the healthcare field, be sure to act like a sponge and soak up as much information as you possibly can from every experience you have in the healthcare office. Every skill that you learn will ultimately make you a stronger professional and create a more well-rounded, highly skilled administrative healthcare professional.

Inpatient and Outpatient Billing

It is key to note the difference between inpatient and outpatient healthcare settings. This is an important distinction, as not only do the job functions differ, but the codes and billing practices differ vastly between the settings.

An **inpatient** healthcare facility is also referred to as an acute-care setting. An inpatient facility is one in which the patient stays overnight or, if necessary, for several days or more. These facilities include inpatient hospitals, long-term care facilities such as skilled nursing facilities, and inpatient mental health facilities. Many inpatient hospitals are large facilities with several departments or units based upon the type of care provided, such as labor and delivery, orthopedics, or pediatrics. Furthermore, inpatient hospitals are staffed by hundreds of clinical personnel such as physicians, nurses, and various clinical assistants in areas such as digital laboratory, imaging services, and pharmacy. **Clinical personnel** are those who are trained as healthcare providers or practitioners—such as doctors, nurse practitioners, and physician assistants—as well as personnel like registered nurses, healthcare assistants, and clinical nursing assistants who are trained and qualified to provide assistive healthcare services. Clinical personnel are qualified to provide healthcare services, advice, and treatments.

Administrative staff within an inpatient hospital are also numerous and include staff members with the responsibilities of ensuring that the facility runs efficiently, such as registration and management staff, and staff that ensures the correct coding and prompt payment for healthcare services. Administrative personnel handle the daily functions of the business side of the healthcare practice, such as sending claims and billing patients. They also handle nonclinical patient services like handling healthcare records requests, registering patients, scheduling appointments, and verifying patient insurance coverage.

By contrast, an outpatient setting is one in which patients are not admitted to the healthcare facility, even though they may stay at the facility overnight. Also referred to as ambulatory care, outpatient services are provided to a patient who presents for the treatment and then returns home. Outpatient services can range from vaccinations to diagnostic screenings, mental health services, and complex surgical procedures. The main difference between inpatient and outpatient services is the fact that an outpatient is typically treated and discharged on the same date of service, although he or she may stay overnight in certain circumstances.

It is important to understand the difference between inpatient and outpatient healthcare settings because the codes used in each setting differ. Even though the patient may have received the same service in an inpatient facility that could have been done in an outpatient facility, it is billed differently depending on where the service was performed and which healthcare entity is reporting the service. As previously described, healthcare providers who perform services in the hospital setting still bill with outpatient codes, as they are billing for services independently of the inpatient facility (see figure 1.2). Figure 1.4 illustrates the different codes that may be used, depending on the healthcare setting.

Figure 1.4. Inpatient and outpatient code sets

Billing Type	Inpatient Setting		Outpatient Setting	
	Diagnosis	Procedure/Supplies	Diagnosis	Procedure/Supplies
Professional Reporting (doctor)	ICD-10-CM	CPT & HCPCS	ICD-10-CM	CPT & HCPCS
Facility Reporting (hospital)	ICD-10-CM	ICD-10-PCS	ICD-10-CM	CPT & HCPCS ICD-10-PCS

Keep in mind that because the codes used in each setting differ, it may be necessary to specialize in a certain type of coding. For example, a coder working in an inpatient facility setting should focus on ICD-10-PCS and ICD-10-CM coding as well as CPT and HCPCS coding, which may also be used in some facilities; a coder working in the professional setting should focus on ICD-10-CM, CPT, and HCPCS coding. This textbook provides training on all of these code sets.

Notice that inpatient and outpatient settings both use the ICD-10-CM code set to report diagnoses. The main differences between the codes used in these two settings are for procedures and supplies and services. Inpatient hospital services are billed using ICD-10-PCS codes, with the occasional use of CPT and HCPCS codes. In the outpatient setting, CPT and HCPCS codes are used to bill for services provided to the patient during the outpatient encounter, and ICD-10-PCS codes are not utilized at all.

As shown in figure 1.4, outpatient facilities (such as those provided by an outpatient hospital) may also use ICD-10-PCS codes for reporting purposes.

Key to Success

The majority of chapters in this textbook are centered around outpatient healthcare practices because most healthcare services are provided in an outpatient setting, which utilizes three main code sets: ICD-10-CM, CPT, and HCPCS. Inpatient coding is discussed in chapter 20 (Inpatient Hospital Services), which covers ICD-10-PCS coding used in the inpatient setting and for facility reporting.

Types of Healthcare Providers

In addition to understanding the various types of healthcare practices, it is important to understand the different types of healthcare providers. This includes the differences between physicians and mid-level providers, as well as the differences between healthcare specialists and primary care physicians.

Healthcare Provider Types

A **healthcare provider** is a "physician or other qualified healthcare professional," and includes any individual "who is qualified by education, training, licensure/ regulation (when applicable), and facility privileging (when applicable) who performs a professional service within his/her scope of practice and independently reports that professional service" (AMA 2019, xiii). The term *healthcare practitioner* may also be used in lieu of *healthcare provider*, and the two may be used interchangeably.

The term *healthcare provider* is important to understand because it is more all-encompassing than *physician* or *doctor*. A **physician** is a medical doctor who has completed post-doctoral medical training in his or her chosen specialty. However, physicians are not the only healthcare professionals who are qualified to provide services. There are additional healthcare providers who are also trained, qualified, and licensed to provide healthcare services. These individuals are often referred to as **mid-level providers**, although they may prefer to be called "advanced practitioners" (Bishop 2012). Thus, a healthcare provider may be any of the provider types listed in table 1.1.

Table 1.1. Healthcare provider types

Physicians	Mid-Level Providers
Medical Doctor (MD)	Anesthesiologist Assistant (AA)
Doctor of Osteopathy (DO)	Certified Nurse Midwife (CNM)
Doctor of Podiatric Medicine (DPM)	Certified Registered Nurse Anesthetist (CRNA)
Doctor of Optometry (OD)	Clinical Nurse Specialist (CNS)
Doctor of Dental Surgery (DDS)	Clinical Social Worker (CSW)
	Nurse Practitioner (NP)
	Physician Assistant (PA)
	Physical Therapist (PT)

As the healthcare industry changes, the number of mid-level providers is increasing. As such, the healthcare clinic in which you work is likely to bill for services provided by many provider types. For example, a small group practice may be comprised of two medical doctors (MDs), two nurse practitioners (NPs), and a certified nurse midwife (CNM).

Healthcare Specialists

Not only are there several types of providers and various workplace settings, but there are also a great deal of different provider specialties. A **healthcare specialty** is a branch of healthcare practice in which a provider specializes after completing his or her residency after medical school. Healthcare specialties are typically divided among four possible areas: surgical or internal technique, body or organ system, diagnostic or therapeutic services, or the age of patients treated.

The first major division is between surgical versus internal medicine specialties. **Surgical specialists** treat and diagnose patients through major surgical techniques—for instance, exploratory abdominal surgery or nephrectomy (removal of a kidney). The major service performed by **internal medicine providers** is the establishment of a diagnosis and subsequent treatment without using surgical techniques, such as diagnosing strep throat and treating with antibiotics, or monitoring a patient's chronic health conditions.

Some specialties are organ- or body system–based, as many healthcare conditions involve a specific organ or body system (for example, endocrinologists specialize in disorders of the endocrine system). Yet other specialties are centered around obtaining diagnostic information or a specific treatment method, such as physical therapy or radiation oncology. Additional specialties are determined by the patient's age—typically pediatrics (patients from birth to age 18) or geriatrics (treating elderly patients). Within specialties, you will also find subspecialties that combine two more general specialties; for example, a pediatric endocrinologist is a specialist who sees pediatric patients with disorders of the endocrine system.

This does not, however, mean that a patient can only be seen by one type of specialist. It is common for a patient to see a number of different specialists, depending on his or her healthcare needs. For instance, a patient with end-stage renal disease (ESRD) who requires a kidney transplant might be managed by an internal medicine doctor, but the actual kidney transplant procedure will be completed by a surgical specialist.

Healthcare specialists are experts in their area of medicine but may not be experts in all areas of medicine—which is why there is a distinction between healthcare specialists and general practitioners, also referred to as a **primary care provider (PCP)**. These healthcare providers are skilled in treating and diagnosing ailments of the entire body, as well as educated about parameters necessary to maintain health and procedures that measure health, such as mammograms and colonoscopies. PCPs provide preventive care and advice to patients in the form of annual physical examinations and health guidance, maintain the patient's comprehensive health record and history, and refer patients to specialists when necessary. Types of general practitioners include family practice providers, pediatricians (although these individuals treat a specific age group, they are regarded as PCPs because they treat the whole patient), and internal medicine providers. Obstetrics and gynecology (OBGYN) providers may also be considered primary care practitioners when they perform primary care services, although others may perform only specialist services. Table 1.2 provides additional information about different specialty types.

Table 1.2. Types of healthcare specialties

	Provider Type	Description
Primary Care Providers: Provide whole healthcare, maintain patient health history, and perform preventive examinations and services	Pediatrician	Treats patients ages 0–18
	Family Practice	Treats patients from birth to elderly
	General Practitioner Adult Medicine Provider	Treats adult patients
	Internal Medicine	Specializes in the prevention and treatment of adult diseases
	Obstetrics and Gynecology Women's Health	Can act as a PCP for female patients
Specialty Providers: Specialize in a particular area of healthcare expertise, including diagnosis, management, and treatment	Holistic and Integrative Specialists	Specializes in whole-body health with an emphasis on holistic techniques, such as acupuncture
	Behavioral Health	Specializes in the mental health of patients, includes psychiatric services and addiction medicine
	Allergy/Immunology	Specializes in disorders of the immune system
	Anesthesiology and Pain Management	Specializes in anesthesia services and the treatment and management of pain
	Cardiology	Specializes in the diagnosis and treatment of the cardiovascular system; can be surgical, invasive, non-invasive, or specialize in treatment strategies
	Bariatric Surgery Burn-Trauma Surgery Cardiothoracic Surgery Colorectal Surgery General Surgery Hand Surgery Maxillofacial Surgery OB/GYN Surgery Orthopedic Surgery Orthopedics Foot and Ankle Surgery Orthopedics Hand Surgery Orthopedics Hip Surgery Orthopedics Knee Surgery Orthopedics Shoulder Surgery Orthopedics Spine Surgery Pediatric Surgery Plastic and Reconstructive Surgery Surgical Oncology Thoracic Surgery Transplant Surgery Vascular Surgery	Specializes in performing and developing surgical techniques for each respective body system or organ
	Therapy and Rehabilitation	Specializes in performing and developing therapeutic and rehabilitative services for patients and includes physical and occupational therapists and speech language pathologists
	Laboratory and Pathology	Specializes in the testing or pathology and laboratory specimens
	Obstetrics and Gynecology	Specializes in women's health, pregnancy, and childbirth and includes labor and delivery, maternal fetal medicine, fertility services, and midwife services

Neurology	Specializes in diagnosis and treatment of conditions affecting the neurological system
Orthopedics	Specializes in diagnosis and treatment of orthopedic conditions, such as fractures and osteoporosis
Dermatology	Specializes in the dermatological system (skin)
Geriatric Medicine	Specializes in geriatric medicine for elderly patients
Hematology and Oncology	Specializes in the detection, management, and treatment of blood conditions and malignancies; specialists within this field can sub-specialize in certain types of cancers and cancer treatments
Gastroenterology	Specialized in conditions affecting the gastrointestinal system
Radiology and Imaging	Specializes in the performance of either diagnostic or therapeutic radiology services, in addition to other types of imaging services such as ultrasounds or MRIs
Endocrinology	Specializes in ailments of the endocrine system, such as diabetes mellitus
Hospice and Palliative Care	Provides end-of life treatment for terminally ill patients
Infectious Disease	Specializes in the detection, treatment, and management of infectious diseases, such as HIV
Nephrology	Specializes in conditions affecting the kidneys
Ophthalmology Optometry	Specializes in the detection and treatment of eye conditions as well as vision services
Otolaryngology	Specializes in the ears, nose, and throat
Podiatry	Specializes in conditions affecting the feet
Rheumatology	Specializes in rheumatism, arthritis, and other disorders of the joints
Urology	Specializes in the urological system as well as the male reproductive system

If all healthcare providers can bill for services rendered, then why does it matter to discuss the differences between specialties and the distinction between specialists and primary care providers? The reasons are twofold. First, there are billing differences between PCPs and specialists, and a patient's insurance company may require a referral or a prior authorization from a PCP to a specialist before a patient can see the specialist (figure 1.5). The exact nature of this process depends on the patient's insurance company and plan, but it is important to understand this process because it will impact the ability to bill for services if you work in a healthcare specialist's office.

Figure 1.5. Healthcare referral process

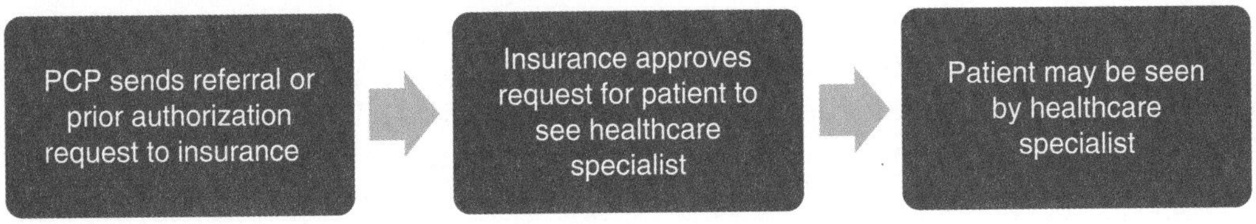

PCP sends referral or prior authorization request to insurance → Insurance approves request for patient to see healthcare specialist → Patient may be seen by healthcare specialist

The second reason why it is important to understand this difference is because a healthcare specialist only sees a certain set of healthcare conditions or only performs certain types of procedures, and the codes used in specialty offices are specific to that field. For example, a pediatrician sees a great number of sick patients and performs many well-check examinations and vaccinations, so coders in that pediatric office will be skilled at coding for sick visits, well-check examinations, and vaccinations. On the other hand, a cardiothoracic surgeon performs complex surgical procedures on the cardiothoracic system—such as a heart and lung transplants—so coders working in this specialty are skilled with those particular codes.

Taking this into account, this textbook contextualizes all coding training within a healthcare specialty. This helps beginning coders to consider a small selection of codes and begin to understand the connections between the procedure performed or service provided, as well as the reason(s) why the procedure was performed or the service was provided. For example, chapter 7 (Behavioral Health) presents the codes that are commonly reported for behavioral health services, such as psychotherapy and depression. Coding in the real world involves understanding the specific codes that are used in each specialty, understanding the unique billing circumstances or requirements for that specialty, and accurately reporting procedures and diagnoses on the same claim, according to coding guidelines. Subsequent chapters discuss the details of coding and billing for many specialty types, including primary care, durable medical equipment suppliers, ambulance suppliers, imaging centers, and laboratories.

As a healthcare coder, it is important to be aware of the many professional organizations that help professionals in this field become further educated, maintain networking relationships, keep up to date in the field, and earn coding certifications.

Professional Organizations and Coding Certifications

A **professional organization** is an association of individuals that is committed to furthering the interests of a particular profession. These organizations are an important part of the community of HIM professionals, as they not only offer educational training and resources but also help define specific industry standards and job descriptions, communicate changes within the industry, and provide networking opportunities and professional advice.

The **American Health Information Management Association (AHIMA)** is the premier worldwide association for HIM professionals. It is considered the leading source of knowledge within HIM and is a respected source of education and training for those in the profession (AHIMA 2019a). Belonging to a professional organization like AHIMA allows a coder to be on the cutting edge of developments in the profession and stay up to date with constantly changing code sets, coding guidelines, and important regulations that may impact the coding profession.

Becoming a member of any professional organization typically involves paying an annual or biannual membership fee, which allows access to the organization's many professional resources. For example, becoming a member of AHIMA allows access to the AHIMA Body of Knowledge (BoK), the *Journal of AHIMA* monthly publication, and discounts on AHIMA products such as books and certification exams. Membership also includes access to the AHIMA Engage community, an online forum where professionals can share advice, opinions, and expertise on HIM topics (AHIMA 2019b).

Certification is another important benefit offered by many professional organizations in HIM, healthcare coding, and medical billing. A **coding certification** is a professional document of achievement given only to those individuals who can demonstrate proficiency on a coding examination. Coding examinations range in scope, length, expense, and difficulty, but they all focus on the ability of an individual to identify and assign the correct diagnosis and procedure codes for coding and billing. For example, the **Certified Coding Specialist (CCS)** certification, offered by AHIMA, demonstrates a coder's ability to assign diagnosis and procedure codes as well as their knowledge of coding systems, medical terminology, disease processes, and pharmacology. Many employers require certification for a coder to be eligible for certain coding positions.

Once a credential is attained, a coder must stay up to date in his or her field of coding by attaining **continuing education units (CEUs)**. A CEU is a unit of measurement used in continuing education programs, and a certified coder must attain a certain number of CEUs each year to maintain his or her certification. For example, a coder with a CCS certification must attain 20 CEUs every two years (AHIMA 2019c). A continuing education program is any type of industry-specific training that offers specific instruction on a topic in the professional's field of expertise. It can be in the form of a short (one-hour) webinar, a day- or weekend-long professional training conference, or even in the form of an industry newsletter or online training course. If the CEUs are not completed within the given time frame, the coder faces the risk of losing the certification. The means of obtaining a CEU can vary—from attending the annual AHIMA conference and seminars, to watching webinars online, or completing quizzes on educational material. Each one of these learning experiences carries a specific amount of CEUs; for example, one CEU is achieved for a watching a coding webinar and answering a small quiz on the content. Once a CEU is earned, the learner gets a CEU certificate proving that he or she has earned the CEU.

Not all certifications offered by professional HIM and billing and coding organizations are aimed specifically at coding. For example, AHIMA also offers certifications on healthcare administration, health data analysis, healthcare privacy and security, documentation improvement, healthcare technology, and healthcare informatics. The opportunities in the field of healthcare are endless. Learning coding might just be one small step in the pathway to career success.

See appendix A (Coding Certifications and Professional Coding Organizations) for a more comprehensive list of coding certifications and professional organizations.

End-of-Chapter Content

Instructions: Indicate whether the following statements are true or false (T or F). For false statements, rewrite the statement on the line below to make the statement true.

1. Working in different positions can help a beginning coder determine where he or she best fits within a healthcare organization.

   _____

   _____

(Continued on next page)

(Continued)

2. An outpatient healthcare facility is also referred to as an acute-care setting.

_____

_____

3. An inpatient healthcare facility is also referred to as an ambulatory care setting.

_____

_____

4. Inpatient facilities include hospice, skilled nursing facilities, and rehabilitation hospitals.

_____

_____

5. Mid-level providers can bill for their services without being under the supervision of a licensed physician.

_____

_____

6. A nurse practitioner is one type of mid-level provider.

_____

_____

7. A surgical specialist treats the whole patient, including preventative medicine.

_____

_____

8. A pediatrician treats patients of all ages.

_____

_____

9. A dermatologist specializes in treating conditions of the skin.

_____

_____

10. An otolaryngologist may be referred to as an ENT (ear, nose, and throat) doctor.

_____

_____

Instructions: Choose the best answer.

1. Which of the following is an advantage of outsourcing to a billing or coding company?
   a. The provider's office must spend more money to get their claims paid.
   b. The provider's office has access to expert billers and coders.
   c. The billing and coding office is less skilled in coding than the provider's office.
   d. The provider's office must pay to have the billing company process their claims.

2. Which of the following might be one of your job responsibilities if you worked in a billing and coding company?
   a. Coding claims
   b. Taking vital signs
   c. Administering immunizations
   d. Prescribing medications

3. Which of the following types of practices has only one provider?
   a. Large group practice
   b. Ambulatory surgical center
   c. Solo practice
   d. Small group practice

4. Which of the following types of healthcare practices specializes in providing outpatient surgeries to patients?
   a. Emergency department
   b. Urgent care
   c. Inpatient hospital
   d. Ambulatory surgical center

5. Andres works in a group practice in which one third of the providers are pediatricians, one third are internal medicine doctors, and one third are cardiologists. In what type of healthcare practice does Andres work?
   a. Large single-specialty group practice
   b. Hospital
   c. Ambulatory surgical center
   d. Large multi-specialty group practice

6. Which of the following services would be provided by an outpatient healthcare practice?
   a. Vaccinations
   b. Open heart surgery
   c. Kidney transplant surgery
   d. Provider education and training

7. Which of the following codes sets is used to bill for inpatient facility procedures?
   a. ICD-10-CM
   b. ICD-10-PCS
   c. Hospital service codes
   d. CPT

8. Which of the following code sets is used to report diagnoses in both the inpatient and outpatient settings?
   a. ICD-10-CM
   b. ICD-10-PCS
   c. Hospital services codes
   d. CPT

9. Which of the following healthcare provider types is a mid-level provider?
   a. DO
   b. PA
   c. DDS
   d. DPM

10. What type of healthcare specialist would treat the patient's entire body, including providing health maintenance measures?
    a. An endocrinologist
    b. A primary care practitioner
    c. A healthcare specialist
    d. A mid-level provider

References

American Health Information Management Association (AHIMA). 2019a. Who We Are. http://www.ahima.org/about/aboutahima.

American Health Information Management Association (AHIMA). 2019b. AHIMA Engage. https://engage.ahima.org/home.

American Health Information Management Association (AHIMA). 2019c. Recertification. http://www.ahima.org/certification/Recertification.

American Medical Association (AMA). 2019. *CPT 2020 Professional Edition*. Chicago: AMA.

Bishop, C. S. 2012. Advanced Practitioners Are Not Mid-Level Providers. https://www.ncbi.nlm.nih.gov/pmc/articles/PMC4093350/.

CHAPTER

Healthcare Billing Basics

Learning Objectives

- Examine the basic components of the Health Insurance Portability and Accountability Act (HIPAA) and their impact on healthcare operations
- Examine the billing considerations for codes used in the healthcare setting, including different insurance and payer types and evaluate their billing rules and guidelines

- Understand Hierarchical Condition Category (HCC) coding and its importance to the healthcare office
- Understand performance measures and quality improvement and their importance to the healthcare office

Key Terms

Accountable care organization
Accreditation
Administrative safeguards
Advance beneficiary notice (ABN)
Allowable amount
Business associates (BAs)
Capitation
Centers for Medicare and Medicaid Services (CMS)
Charge amount
Children's Health Insurance Program (CHIP)
CMS-1500
Coinsurance
Commercial insurance
Comorbidity
Complication
Computerized physician order entry (CPOE)

Confidentiality agreement
Copayment
Coverage limitations
Covered entities (CEs)
Data analytics
Deductible
De-identified documentation
Electronic protected health information (e-PHI)
Employer-sponsored insurance
Encryption
Enforcement Rule
Entitlement health insurance
Fee schedule
Fee-for-service
Government-sponsored insurance
HCC coding
Health insurance exchange

Health Insurance Marketplace
Health Insurance Portability and Accountability Act (HIPAA)
Healthcare operations
Hierarchical Condition Category (HCC)
Individual insurance
Insurance policy
Insured party
Medicaid
Medical necessity
Medicare
Medigap
Minimum necessary
Noncovered services
Notice of Privacy Practices
Out-of-pocket expense
Patient Centered Medical Home (PCMH)

Payment	Protected health information (PHI)	Technical safeguards
Performance measures		Third-party payer
Per member per month (PMPM)	Provider contracting	Treatment
	Quality improvement (QI)	Treatment, payment, and healthcare operations (TPO)
Physical safeguards	Referral	
Premium	Reimbursement	
Prior authorization (PA)	Risk adjustment	TRICARE
Privacy Rule	Risk analysis	UB-04
Prospective payment system (PPS)	Security Rule	Workers' compensation insurance
	Supplemental insurance	

In the healthcare industry, there are many regulations and guidelines that must be followed to ensure patient confidentiality, maintain compliancy, optimize insurance reimbursement, and confirm all services are documented and coded correctly. These rules and regulations are a fundamental part of ensuring that healthcare coders and billers are doing their job properly and legally. Some of these rules are governmental regulations, such as the Health Insurance Portability and Accountability Act (HIPAA); others are specific to certain insurance carriers or third-party payers, such as the requirement to provide a Medicare patient with a written notice for a noncovered procedure. Yet other guidelines are an integral component of each of the healthcare code sets and correct healthcare coding, such as ICD-10-CM guidelines that impact risk adjustment, which determines the cumulative health risk of a patient population. Performance measures and quality improvement guidelines, set by public health and other organizations, focus on a more health-centered model of patient care, rather than focusing on only the financial side of healthcare insurance reimbursement.

This chapter focuses on the regulations and guidelines that impact daily job functions and are a necessary part of understanding important concepts and practices in healthcare. These guidelines may outline the differences between how insurance claims are billed, identify nuances in coding for third-party payers, and determine the impact of national and organizational programs in billing and coding, such as Hierarchical Condition Category (HCC) coding.

HIPAA and Confidentiality

In 1996, Congress passed the **Health Insurance Portability and Accountability Act,** otherwise known as HIPAA. HIPAA is the federal legislation enacted to provide continuity of health coverage, control fraud and abuse in healthcare, reduce healthcare costs, and guarantee the security and privacy of health information. It limits exclusion for pre-existing healthcare conditions, prohibits discrimination against employees and dependents based on health status, guarantees availability of health insurance to small employers, and guarantees renewability of insurance to all employees regardless of company size. HIPAA requires covered entities (most healthcare providers and organizations) to transmit healthcare claims in a specific format and develop, implement, and comply with the standards of the Privacy Rule and the Security Rule; it also mandates that covered entities apply for and utilize national identifiers in HIPAA transactions (HIPAA 1996).

HIPAA made sweeping changes throughout the US healthcare system. Although there was always a precedent of patient confidentiality within healthcare, HIPAA took this further by creating and enforcing strict guidelines regarding patient confidentiality.

Before HIPAA was enacted, there was no federal law aimed at protecting the privacy of patients, and most confidentiality regulations were handled at a company- or state-wide level. After the implementation of HIPAA, privacy breaches or lack of patient confidentiality became punishable at the federal level, placing a great deal of emphasis on maintaining the privacy and integrity of patient information, including all healthcare and demographic information and claim data. Healthcare practices must now proactively protect the confidentiality of their patients by following the guidelines set forth by HIPAA.

However, not everyone is subject to HIPAA guidelines. Only covered entities and their business associates are held to HIPAA standards of confidentiality. These standards include the HIPAA Privacy, Security, and Enforcement Rules, as well as HIPAA confidentiality agreements.

Covered Entities and Business Associates

Before going into the specifics of HIPAA, it is important to understand what is protected under the provisions of HIPAA, as well as who is required to comply with HIPAA regulations.

HIPAA regulations specifically cover protected health information. **Protected health information (PHI)** is any health information that is individually identifiable, such as health records, laboratory reports, and patient healthcare history forms. PHI can be stored or transmitted on paper or electronic media; it can also be transmitted orally. The Privacy Rule governs the confidentiality for all PHI that is handled in the office, which includes:

- Patient demographic data
- Information related to the patient's past, present, or future physical or mental health
- Information related to the provision of healthcare to the patient
- Information related to the payment (past, present, or future) for the provision of healthcare to the patient (OCR 2013a)

There are two main groups that deal with PHI, and thus must comply with HIPAA regulations—covered entities and business associates. HIPAA covered entities (CEs) deal directly with patient PHI and are thus accountable for the integrity of the privacy afforded. Covered entities include healthcare plans, healthcare clearinghouses, and any healthcare provider who transmits patient health information in an electronic format.

On the other hand, business associates (BAs) provide services to or perform functions and activities on behalf of a covered entity, and have access to PHI. These BAs include billing companies and entities that provide claims processing, data analysis, or utilization review. If a person or organization does *not* have access to PHI, then they are not considered BAs and as such are not subject to HIPAA regulations.

HIPAA is composed of three rules that together keep all aspects of patient care confidential and must be followed by CEs and BAs. These three rules are the Privacy Rule, Security Rule, and Enforcement Rule.

HIPAA Privacy Rule

Published in December 2000, the HIPAA Privacy Rule—also known as the Standards for Privacy of Individually Identifiable Health Information—sets national standards for the protection of personal health information by CEs, such as health plans and healthcare providers. This rule also enacted standards that allow individuals to understand and control how their personal health information is used. The main goal of the Privacy Rule is to secure the protection of patient health information while at the same time allowing that information to be utilized appropriately by covered entities and for public health services. In order to understand the Privacy Rule, it is essential to know what is included in PHI (listed previously), such as individually identifiable health information like patient healthcare conditions, procedures performed or services provided, or patient insurance information. Privacy rules impact all staff members in the healthcare office or facility, including coders. For example, a coder working in a healthcare office accesses electronic health records via a username and individual password and cannot discuss patient information with anyone except other staff members in the healthcare office who are also involved in the patient's care.

Many components of the HIPAA Privacy Rule work together to safeguard the privacy of patient information. They include PHI; treatment, payment, and healthcare operations (TPO); the minimum necessary standard; and the HIPAA Notice of Privacy Practices (OCR 2013a).

Protected Health Information

PHI includes common personal identifiers such as patient name, address, birth date, and Social Security number, which are all pieces of individually identifiable information. However, records that have been properly de-identified may not be subject to strict Privacy Rule standards. In **de-identified documentation** all the aforementioned identifying characteristics have been removed. For example, an employment record with the employee's personal information—name, Social Security number, and date of birth—removed would be a de-identified employment record. A de-identified health record note containing patient health information but no identifying information (such as name or date of birth), is no longer considered PHI.

PHI may be released to the person who is the subject of the information, but release of this information to any other parties is strictly regulated. Included in these regulations is the treatment, payment, and healthcare operations (TPO) standard, which helps identify appropriate releases of PHI.

Treatment, Payment, and Healthcare Operations Standard

An integral component of the Privacy Rule is that some PHI must be used for certain purposes in the healthcare office and between certain parties. For example, how could an insurance company process a claim for a healthcare service if the healthcare provider were unable to release key information from the healthcare visit to them? Because of this need for specific information, the Privacy Rule allows for the use of PHI in treatment, payment, and healthcare operations.

The **treatment, payment, and healthcare operations (TPO)** standard of the Privacy Rule allows the use of PHI for the following:

- **Treatment** refers to the provision, coordination, and management of a patient's healthcare and related services by that patient's healthcare providers. This includes consultation between providers regarding a patient and referral of the patient from one healthcare provider to another.
- **Payment** refers to the activities of the patient's health insurance plan to obtain premiums for health insurance, to determine coverage benefits, and to furnish payment for healthcare services delivered to a covered beneficiary. This also refers to the healthcare provider's activities related to obtaining payment for services rendered to the patient.

- **Healthcare operations** includes various services provided by healthcare practitioners during which patient PHI may be accessed and used. This includes case management and coordination of care among multiple healthcare providers, participation in a heath record audit or healthcare review, evaluations of healthcare provider performance, and business planning and development.

TPO standards regulate when and to whom PHI may be shared or released but fail to specify exactly what and how much of the health record can be released. The amount of records released is governed by the minimum necessary standard (OCR 2013a).

Minimum Necessary Standard

Under the **minimum necessary** standard, when a release of PHI is warranted and allowed, only the *minimum necessary* amount of PHI needed for the TPO should be released. Any information that is not directly related to the TPO may not be released. For example, if a general practitioner refers a patient to a plastic surgeon to revise a keloid scar, only the parts of the health record pertaining to that scar and how it was caused (such as records pertaining to the location, severity, and healing status of the keloid scar) should be released to the plastic surgeon. In this case, the plastic surgeon does not need to know the patient's entire health history; therefore, that information would not be released to the surgeon's office.

When releasing PHI, an effective standard is to first evaluate each portion of the PHI and determine if it is necessary for inclusion in the release, and to then justify the reasons why the information should be included. For example, if a health records technician is releasing the vaccination records for a patient to attend public school, only the portion of the health record that tabulates vaccinations given to the patient should be provided. In this case, the health records technician has received a request to prove that the patient has been fully vaccinated. After searching through the health record and locating the vaccination records, she evaluates each part of the vaccination record to ensure the requested information is located on the record, such as the patient's identifying information (name and date of birth), and a list of vaccinations given to the patient and the date they were given. Any portions of this record that were not directly related to the vaccinations that the patient had been given (such as prior illness, injuries, or health encounters) would not be released. Instead of sending the entire health record, only the minimum necessary amount of information is given—in this example, *only* the one or two pages that list the vaccines the patient has received.

There are some exceptions to the minimum necessary standard, however. The minimum necessary requirement does not have to be met in the following circumstances:

- When requested by an authorized healthcare provider
- When requested by the individual who is the subject of the information, or their representative
- When disclosed to the Department of Health and Human Services for an investigation or complaint
- When required by law
- When required for compliance with HIPAA regulations (OCR 2013a)

Patients should be educated and informed regarding HIPAA regulations and when their PHI may or may not be used or released. This is accomplished using a Notice of Privacy Practices.

Notice of Privacy Practices

As a way of informing patients and other individuals about their privacy rights under HIPAA regulations, each CE must provide a **Notice of Privacy Practices** to each patient. This is a written description of the CE's privacy practices and must be signed and kept on record for each patient. Although individual CEs are able to create their own notices, each Notice of Privacy Practices must contain certain elements as required by the Privacy Rule. Some of these items are listed as follows:

- It must inform patients of the ways in which the CE may use or disclose PHI.
- It must state the CE's duty to protect patient privacy.
- It must inform patients how to complain to the Department of Health and Human Services (HHS) if they believe that their privacy rights have been violated.
- It must include additional contact information for obtaining further information, as well as for making privacy complaints to the CE. (OCR 2013a)

In addition to the Privacy Rule, HIPAA also enforces two other important rules—the Security Rule and the Enforcement Rule.

Security Rule

The HIPAA **Security Rule**, also known as the Security Standards for the Protection of Electronic Health Information, regulates both the technical and nontechnical safeguards that organizations must put in place to keep electronic protected health information secure (OCR 2013b). **Electronic protected health information (e-PHI)** is essentially the same as PHI, except that it is stored or transferred in an electronic format, such as electronic health records (EHRs), rather than a paper format. The Security Rule is a direct response to the transition from paper health records to electronic health records and covers the numerous ways that e-PHI is put at risk. For example, healthcare providers use electronic health applications for **computerized physician order entry (CPOE)**—when a healthcare provider uses an electronic device to record medication or treatment orders and access EHR and radiology, laboratory, and pharmacy applications. Healthcare insurance plans, on the other hand, provide electronic access to claims and eligibility information among other applications. While these electronic applications have the possibility to make the entire workforce more efficient, they present a number of potential security risks.

The main goal of the Security Rule is to protect e-PHI and to reduce the possibility of breaches of the information stored in e-PHI systems by creating and maintaining appropriate administrative, technical, and physical safeguards. Because healthcare organizations differ greatly in size, the Security Rule is designed to be flexible and scalable from the smallest one-physician office to a large, multispecialty hospital or healthcare insurance plan. Covered entities can thus design security standards that are appropriate for their specific businesses, depending on their size and resources, as long as they:

- Ensure the integrity, confidentiality, and availability of all their e-PHI
- Identify and protect their e-PHI against security threats
- Protect their e-PHI from unauthorized use or disclosure
- Ensure that their workforce is educated in and complies with all security standards regarding their e-PHI (OCR 2013b)

The Security Rule has three main components—administrative, physical, and technical safeguards—each of which are designed to protect the privacy and integrity of e-PHI.

These safeguards require a number of different security standards, which affect coders in a number of different ways.

Administrative Safeguards

Administrative safeguards refer to the activities that a CE must perform in relation to the risks to e-PHI from an administrative perspective. Under HIPAA, administrative safeguards are administrative actions, policies, and procedures that manage the selection, development, implementation, and maintenance of security measures to protect e-PHI and to manage the conduct of the CE's or BA's workforce in relation to the protection of that information (45 CFR 164.304). This includes risk analysis, which evaluates the likelihood of a security breach happening, and the impact that such a breach would have on the CE's e-PHI. Once all risks are identified and evaluated, appropriate security measures should be taken to address those risks and documentation should clearly identify all chosen security measures as well as the rationale for those measures. Furthermore, the CE must maintain all of its security precautions and review records on a regular basis to track and detect any e-PHI incidents, including identifying any new threats.

Physical Safeguards

Physical safeguards refer to physical restrictions created by the CE, which ensure the integrity of e-PHI. Under HIPAA, physical safeguards are Security Rule measures such as locking doors, facility access controls, workstation use, workstation security, and device and media controls to safeguard data and various media from unauthorized access and exposure. The main provision of the Security Rule is that a CE must limit physical access to its facility while at the same time allowing access only to authorized persons (45 CFR 164.304). For example, if the healthcare facility has an in-house server that holds all e-PHI, then this server should be located within a secure area that is accessible only to authorized persons. CEs should also implement policies and procedures for individual workstations to ensure that only authorized personnel can access and view the electronic media. These policies should also specify how e-PHI should be transferred, removed, disposed of, and reused.

Technical Safeguards

Technical safeguards refer to the policies and procedures that relate to ensuring the privacy and integrity of e-PHI from the technical side. Under HIPAA, technical safeguards are the technology and the policies and procedures for its use that protect e-PHI and control access so that only authorized persons can access the information (45 CFR 164.304). For example, a coder working in an online environment would have to log on to the company's secure system using a unique personal identifier or login name and password. Audit controls designed to record and examine access and other electronic activities within the e-PHI system must also be implemented. Integrity controls refer to policies and procedures employed to ensure that e-PHI is not improperly altered or destroyed. Finally, the CE must also ensure transmission security that guards against unauthorized access to e-PHI transferred over an electronic network. This is typically accomplished by using encryption, or data that has been transformed into unintelligible information that is unrecognizable without the correct key to translate the data.

The last HIPAA rule is the Enforcement Rule, which ensures that CEs and BAs are held accountable for the provisions of HIPAA.

Enforcement Rule

The HIPAA Enforcement Rule contains provisions regarding compliance to HIPAA rules and regulations, investigations into breaches in privacy, and the imposition of monetary penalties for HIPAA violations. It also includes procedures for HIPAA violation hearings and the appeal process. The Enforcement Rule governs the activities of CEs with respect to their cooperation in the enforcement process and the actions that parties can take during compliance investigations and civil hearings and appeals (OCR 2017). In other words, the Enforcement Rule specifies the fines and penalties that a CE would have to pay if a breach were to happen and defines the legal process regarding investigations into HIPAA breaches.

HIPAA Confidentiality Agreement

Under the strict regulations put forth by HIPAA, patient confidentiality and the integrity of PHI is a prominent concern for many healthcare practices. It is important to understand all of the regulations as set forth by HIPAA, as well as the administrative, physical, and technical safeguards that are implemented by individual healthcare organizations. Coders must access the health records and documentation of patient encounters with healthcare providers, as well as secured patient demographic and insurance information. As such, they are also required to be knowledgeable about HIPAA and to follow its many guidelines.

Many healthcare organizations provide HIPAA training to their employees and have all employees sign a HIPAA confidentiality agreement—a legal document signed by the employee after HIPAA training that indicates the employee has been trained in aspects of HIPAA compliance and agrees to abide by the healthcare facility's measures taken to ensure HIPAA compliance. This agreement is kept on file to demonstrate HIPAA compliance and the facility's good faith measures to certify that all employees are educated in HIPAA compliance and specific measures are taken by the facility to guarantee compliance.

Billing Considerations

There are more billing considerations than can be discussed in a single chapter, so this chapter includes a general overview of health insurance and discusses the basic components of how to bill a healthcare claim, including entering codes on a claim form, different types of third-party payers, varying methods of reimbursement, authorizations for services rendered, and advance beneficiary notices. Billing considerations go hand-in-hand with coding considerations, so it is important to understand the different guidelines. Being a proficient coder is not just about selecting the right code; it is about understanding the many intricacies between the codes entered and the end goal of the claim, which is usually payment. Effective coding is about entering codes correctly on claims to optimize the reimbursement that the practice or facility may receive from the healthcare claim. Keep in mind, however, that healthcare codes are used for purposes other than payment. These additional purposes are discussed in chapter 3 (Basics of Coding).

Reimbursement, sometimes called payment, is the money that a healthcare practice or facility receives in return for providing a healthcare service to a patient. For example, reimbursement is the payment that a doctor's office receives for performing a routine physical examination, administering vaccinations, or performing a surgery.

Reimbursement is also the money that a hospital receives for providing supplies and services, such as room and board, for a hospital patient. If a patient has healthcare insurance and the healthcare service provided was a covered service, then the insurance company will provide reimbursement for that service, minus any fees for which the patient is responsible. If the patient does not have health insurance, then he or she is responsible for all of the charges for the doctor's services and must pay the doctor's fees out of pocket (refer to chapter 1 for a discussion of health insurance).

In a real-world setting, new coders are typically trained on specific best practices when abstracting and selecting codes for different insurance companies, insurance plans, and services rendered. These best practices may be printed out in the office's employee handbook, billing handbook, or simply on notes throughout the office, which are introduced to the new coder as necessary.

The first part of understanding how to correctly select codes and enter them on a claim is to learn the basics of the claim form itself. The following sections discuss healthcare claim forms as well as third-party payers; types of reimbursement for healthcare services; and authorizations, certifications, and referrals.

Healthcare Claim Forms

All codes are entered on a healthcare claim, which is then sent to the payer for reimbursement. The payer of a healthcare claim is most commonly the patient's health insurance coverage, although in some instances the patient may be directly responsible for payment of all healthcare services received. A **third-party payer** is a company or organization other than the patient that is liable for payment of the healthcare claim. The healthcare provider is the first party, and the patient is the second party. The most common third-party payer is a health insurance company. The type of claim that is used depends on where the patient was seen, either in the inpatient or the outpatient setting, as well as how the claim is billed. Although many insurance claims are now sent electronically, it is important to recognize the many different pieces of information that are included on a healthcare claim, which is best done by examining the CMS-1500 and UB-04 claim forms.

The **CMS-1500** form (figure 2.1) is the standard paper claim form used to bill third-party payers in the professional, or physician outpatient, setting. The CMS-1500 form was developed by CMS and is maintained by the National Uniform Claim Committee (NUCC). It was most recently updated in 2012 to include enough space for up to 12 diagnosis codes. Previously, the form only allowed enough room for four diagnosis codes. This allows healthcare offices to provide a greater amount of detail regarding the patient's diagnosis and why the patient required treatment.

The **UB-04** form, also known as the CMS-1450 form (figure 2.2), is the standard paper claim form maintained by the National Uniform Billing Committee (NUBC) used to bill third-party payers in the facility inpatient setting. It may also be used to report services performed in the facility outpatient setting. This chapter focuses on entering codes on the CMS-1500 claim form, as the majority of this textbook discusses professional practitioner, supplier, and ambulance coding. Instructions on entering codes on the UB-04 claim form used for inpatient or facility billing are found in chapter 20 (Inpatient Hospital Services).

There are three sections of the CMS-1500 claim form, which are designated by vertical arrows on the right side of the page (figure 2.3). The top section is for "Carrier" information, including the name of the third-party payer and the billing or claims address. The second section, labeled "Patient and Insured Information,"

Figure 2.1. Sample CMS-1500 claim form

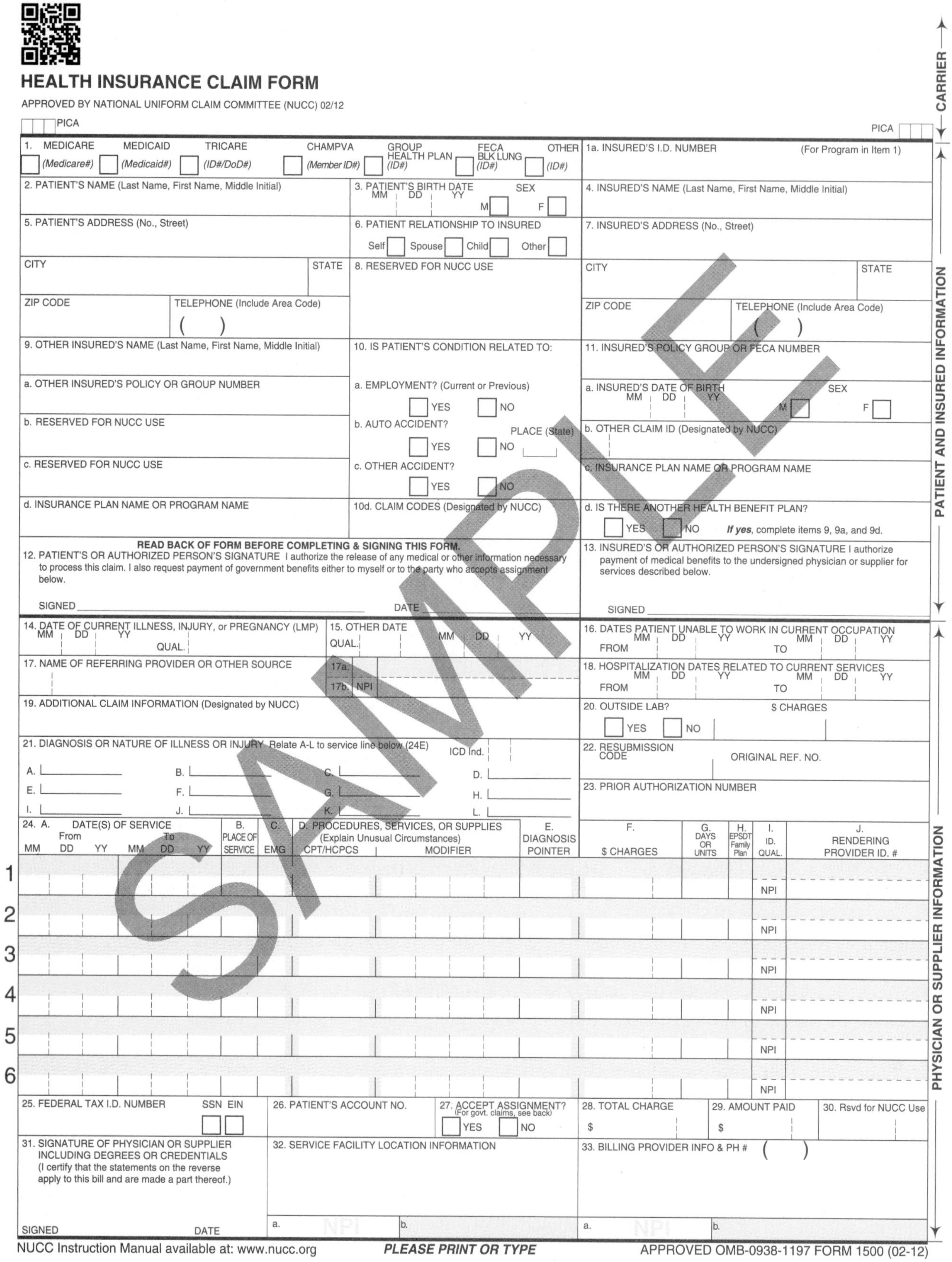

HEALTH INSURANCE CLAIM FORM

APPROVED BY NATIONAL UNIFORM CLAIM COMMITTEE (NUCC) 02/12

PICA | PICA

1. MEDICARE (Medicare#) | MEDICAID (Medicaid#) | TRICARE (ID#/DoD#) | CHAMPVA (Member ID#) | GROUP HEALTH PLAN (ID#) | FECA BLK LUNG (ID#) | OTHER (ID#) | 1a. INSURED'S I.D. NUMBER (For Program in Item 1)

2. PATIENT'S NAME (Last Name, First Name, Middle Initial)

3. PATIENT'S BIRTH DATE MM DD YY SEX M F

4. INSURED'S NAME (Last Name, First Name, Middle Initial)

5. PATIENT'S ADDRESS (No., Street)

6. PATIENT RELATIONSHIP TO INSURED — Self Spouse Child Other

7. INSURED'S ADDRESS (No., Street)

CITY | STATE

8. RESERVED FOR NUCC USE

CITY | STATE

ZIP CODE | TELEPHONE (Include Area Code) ( )

ZIP CODE | TELEPHONE (Include Area Code) ( )

9. OTHER INSURED'S NAME (Last Name, First Name, Middle Initial)

10. IS PATIENT'S CONDITION RELATED TO:

11. INSURED'S POLICY GROUP OR FECA NUMBER

a. OTHER INSURED'S POLICY OR GROUP NUMBER

a. EMPLOYMENT? (Current or Previous) YES NO

a. INSURED'S DATE OF BIRTH MM DD YY SEX M F

b. RESERVED FOR NUCC USE

b. AUTO ACCIDENT? YES NO PLACE (State)

b. OTHER CLAIM ID (Designated by NUCC)

c. RESERVED FOR NUCC USE

c. OTHER ACCIDENT? YES NO

c. INSURANCE PLAN NAME OR PROGRAM NAME

d. INSURANCE PLAN NAME OR PROGRAM NAME

10d. CLAIM CODES (Designated by NUCC)

d. IS THERE ANOTHER HEALTH BENEFIT PLAN? YES NO *If yes,* complete items 9, 9a, and 9d.

READ BACK OF FORM BEFORE COMPLETING & SIGNING THIS FORM.

12. PATIENT'S OR AUTHORIZED PERSON'S SIGNATURE I authorize the release of any medical or other information necessary to process this claim. I also request payment of government benefits either to myself or to the party who accepts assignment below.

SIGNED _____ DATE _____

13. INSURED'S OR AUTHORIZED PERSON'S SIGNATURE I authorize payment of medical benefits to the undersigned physician or supplier for services described below.

SIGNED _____

14. DATE OF CURRENT ILLNESS, INJURY, or PREGNANCY (LMP) MM DD YY QUAL.

15. OTHER DATE QUAL. MM DD YY

16. DATES PATIENT UNABLE TO WORK IN CURRENT OCCUPATION FROM MM DD YY TO MM DD YY

17. NAME OF REFERRING PROVIDER OR OTHER SOURCE

17a. 17b. NPI

18. HOSPITALIZATION DATES RELATED TO CURRENT SERVICES FROM MM DD YY TO MM DD YY

19. ADDITIONAL CLAIM INFORMATION (Designated by NUCC)

20. OUTSIDE LAB? YES NO $ CHARGES

21. DIAGNOSIS OR NATURE OF ILLNESS OR INJURY Relate A-L to service line below (24E) ICD Ind.

A. B. C. D. E. F. G. H. I. J. K. L.

22. RESUBMISSION CODE ORIGINAL REF. NO.

23. PRIOR AUTHORIZATION NUMBER

24. A. DATE(S) OF SERVICE From MM DD YY To MM DD YY | B. PLACE OF SERVICE | C. EMG | D. PROCEDURES, SERVICES, OR SUPPLIES (Explain Unusual Circumstances) CPT/HCPCS MODIFIER | E. DIAGNOSIS POINTER | F. $ CHARGES | G. DAYS OR UNITS | H. EPSDT Family Plan | I. ID. QUAL. | J. RENDERING PROVIDER ID. #

1 — NPI
2 — NPI
3 — NPI
4 — NPI
5 — NPI
6 — NPI

25. FEDERAL TAX I.D. NUMBER SSN EIN

26. PATIENT'S ACCOUNT NO.

27. ACCEPT ASSIGNMENT? (For govt. claims, see back) YES NO

28. TOTAL CHARGE $

29. AMOUNT PAID $

30. Rsvd for NUCC Use

31. SIGNATURE OF PHYSICIAN OR SUPPLIER INCLUDING DEGREES OR CREDENTIALS (I certify that the statements on the reverse apply to this bill and are made a part thereof.)

SIGNED _____ DATE _____

32. SERVICE FACILITY LOCATION INFORMATION

a. NPI b.

33. BILLING PROVIDER INFO & PH # ( )

a. NPI b.

NUCC Instruction Manual available at: www.nucc.org | *PLEASE PRINT OR TYPE* | APPROVED OMB-0938-1197 FORM 1500 (02-12)

CARRIER — PATIENT AND INSURED INFORMATION — PHYSICIAN OR SUPPLIER INFORMATION

Source: CMS 2019a.

Figure 2.2. Sample UB-04 claim form

			3a PAT. CNTL #		4 TYPE OF BILL
1	2		b. MED. REC. #		
			5 FED. TAX NO.	6 STATEMENT COVERS PERIOD FROM THROUGH	7

8 PATIENT NAME	a		9 PATIENT ADDRESS	a		c	d	e
b								

| 10 BIRTHDATE | 11 SEX | 12 DATE | ADMISSION 13 HR | 14 TYPE | 15 SRC | 16 DHR | 17 STAT | 18 | 19 | 20 | CONDITION CODES 21 22 23 24 25 26 27 28 | 29 ACDT STATE | 30 |

31 OCCURRENCE CODE DATE	32 OCCURRENCE CODE DATE	33 OCCURRENCE CODE DATE	34 OCCURRENCE CODE DATE	35 OCCURRENCE SPAN CODE FROM THROUGH	36 OCCURRENCE SPAN CODE FROM THROUGH	37
a						
b						

38		39 VALUE CODES CODE AMOUNT	40 VALUE CODES CODE AMOUNT	41 VALUE CODES CODE AMOUNT
	a			
	b			
	c			
	d			

42 REV. CD.	43 DESCRIPTION	44 HCPCS / RATE / HIPPS CODE	45 SERV. DATE	46 SERV. UNITS	47 TOTAL CHARGES	48 NON-COVERED CHARGES	49
1							
2							
3							
4							
5							
6							
7							
8							
9							
10							
11							
12							
13							
14							
15							
16							
17							
18							
19							
20							
21							
22							
23	PAGE ____ OF ____	CREATION DATE		TOTALS ➡			

50 PAYER NAME	51 HEALTH PLAN ID	52 REL INFO	53 ASG. BEN.	54 PRIOR PAYMENTS	55 EST. AMOUNT DUE	56 NPI	
A							57 OTHER PRV ID
B							
C							

58 INSURED'S NAME	59 P.REL	60 INSURED'S UNIQUE ID	61 GROUP NAME	62 INSURANCE GROUP NO.
A				
B				
C				

63 TREATMENT AUTHORIZATION CODES	64 DOCUMENT CONTROL NUMBER	65 EMPLOYER NAME
A		
B		
C		

66 DX	67 A B C D E F G H								68
	I J K L M N O P Q								

69 ADMIT DX	70 PATIENT REASON DX a b c	71 PPS CODE	72 ECI a b c	73

74 PRINCIPAL PROCEDURE CODE DATE	a. OTHER PROCEDURE CODE DATE	b. OTHER PROCEDURE CODE DATE	75	76 ATTENDING NPI QUAL
				LAST FIRST
c. OTHER PROCEDURE CODE DATE	d. OTHER PROCEDURE CODE DATE	e. OTHER PROCEDURE CODE DATE		77 OPERATING NPI QUAL
				LAST FIRST

80 REMARKS	81CC a		78 OTHER NPI QUAL
	b		LAST FIRST
	c		79 OTHER NPI QUAL
	d		LAST FIRST

UB-04 CMS-1450   APPROVED OMB NO.   **NUBC**™ National Uniform Billing Committee LIC9213257   THE CERTIFICATIONS ON THE REVERSE APPLY TO THIS BILL AND ARE MADE A PART HEREOF.

Source: CMS 2019b.

Figure 2.3. Sections of the CMS-1500 form

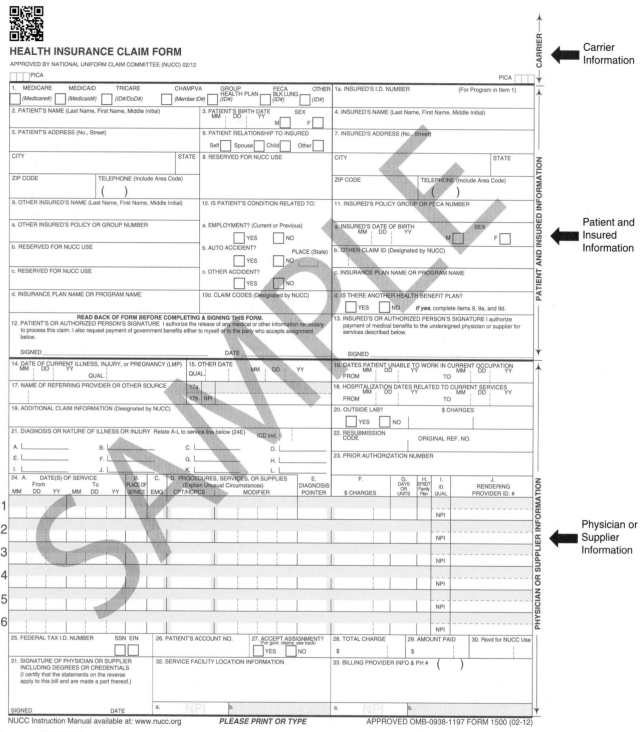

Source: CMS 2019a.

contains identifying information for the patient and insured, including his or her basic demographics as well as information about the insurance policy and coverage details, such as insurance identification number, group number, and employer name. Other fields in this section are used to identify secondary insurance coverage and details about the claim.

For coding purposes, the most important section of the CMS-1500 claim form occupies the second half of the page and is designated by the arrows that read "Physician or Supplier Information." This section of the claim form includes information that is specific to the services provided to the patient on the claim, such as:

- Where the service was provided
- Important dates, such as hospitalization dates or dates unable to work
- ICD-10-CM diagnosis codes to represent medical necessity for the service provided
- Dates of service for the claim
- CPT and HCPCS codes to identify the actual service, procedure, or supply provided
- Modifiers to provide more information regarding the service provided
- Charges for individual services, and the number of units per service
- Provider identifying information, such as rendering provider and billing provider
- Additional service information

Figure 2.4. Box 21: Diagnosis or nature of illness or injury

21. DIAGNOSIS OR NATURE OF ILLNESS OR INJURY Relate A-L to service line below (24E)			ICD Ind.
A.	B.	C.	D.
E.	F.	G.	H.
I.	J.	K.	L.

Source: CMS 2019a.

Each box of the CMS-1500 claim form is numbered so that individual areas may be easily referenced. Box 21 (figure 2.4) is where diagnosis codes are entered; lines A through L provide enough space for 12 individual diagnosis codes. These diagnosis codes identify the medical necessity for the services provided. **Medical necessity** relates to the reason why a healthcare service or treatment is performed. The standards of medical necessity must be met in order for an insurance company to cover a healthcare service, so in order to be medically necessary a service must meet the accepted standards of medicine, and it must be used to prevent, treat, or diagnose an illness or injury, condition, or disease (or the symptoms thereof). In other words, a service or procedure must be medically necessary, or it will not be paid for by the patient's insurance company.

Medical necessity is identified by reporting up to 12 diagnosis codes on the healthcare claim. One diagnosis code is entered per line. If there are more than 12 diagnoses for the claim, then either they may be entered on additional claims forms or only the 12 most important diagnoses may be entered on the claim (with the additional diagnoses being left off of the claim). Some electronic billing systems will allow additional diagnoses, over 12, to be entered on a claim by using a special code. The specific diagnoses that should always be reported on the claim are the ones that are primarily responsible for the services provided, in addition to those that are required per ICD-10-CM guidelines. These 12 diagnoses should clearly identify the medical necessity for the procedures performed or the services provided. Chapter 3 (Basics of Coding) and chapter 4 (Learning the ICD-10-CM Code Book) of this textbook provide additional information on how to select, assign, and sequence diagnosis codes to identify the medical necessity for a service. Throughout the remaining chapters of this textbook, diagnosis coding is discussed within the context of specific healthcare specialties.

In addition to diagnosis codes, the CMS-1500 claim form also includes fields for procedure codes. Procedure codes are entered in box 24.D (see figure 2.5). This box is where procedures, services, or supplies are reported using the appropriate CPT/ HCPCS procedure codes and up to four modifiers. Procedure, service, and supply codes and modifiers are discussed in additional detail in chapter 5 (Learning the CPT and HCPCS Code Books). Within the physician or supplier information section of the CMS-1500 claim form, there are six lines, on which six individual procedures may be included on an individual claim form. If more than six procedures were performed, then additional claim forms may be added. This is usually done automatically by the billing system that is utilized to bill claims. When entering codes in the system, coders simply have to report all applicable procedure and diagnosis codes, and the system determines if an additional form is needed or not.

Figure 2.5. Boxes 24.A through 24.D

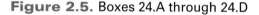

Source: CMS 2019a.

Figure 2.6. Boxes 21 through 30

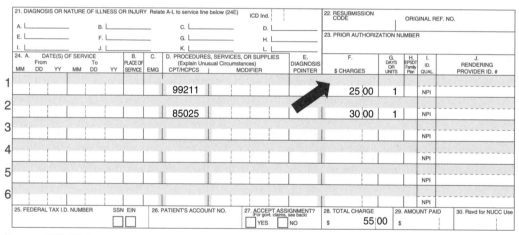

Source: CMS 2019a.

Each procedure code is attached to a charge, entered as a dollar amount, for the service rendered. On the CMS-1500 claim form, charges are entered in box 24.F. When multiple procedure codes are entered, the total charge amount for all services is entered at the bottom of the claim, in box 28—this is the total claim amount. Figure 2.6 shows two procedure codes with charges: CPT code 99211 is attached to a $25.00 charge, and CPT code 85025 is attached to a $30.00 charge. The total for these charges together (the total claim amount) is $55.00, as listed in box 28, below the individually listed charges.

Unlike procedure codes, diagnosis codes are not attached to charges, so entering additional diagnoses on the claim will not increase the charge amount for that claim. However, this does not mean that diagnosis codes are less important than procedure codes. Remember that diagnosis codes identify the medical necessity for the service performed; if the service is not considered medically necessary, the third-party payer will likely deny payment for the service. Diagnosis codes are an essential component of determining the risk factor for healthcare services for each patient, which is used to estimate the future cost of healthcare needs for the patient.

Another important component of the CMS-1500 form is found in box 24.G, which identifies how many units of a specific procedure were performed. The example in figure 2.6 lists one unit of each procedure performed, meaning that each procedure was performed only once and is being billed only once (with one unit). When an individual procedure code is billed more than once, the number of units should correspond to the number of times the procedure is being billed. For example, if the procedure identified by CPT code 85025 had been performed twice, then the number of units would be changed to two units.

Chapter 6 (Supplies and Services), chapter 7 (Behavioral Health), and chapter 10 (Urgent Care and Emergency Department Services) discuss additional areas of the CMS-1500 claim form that are relevant to coders, such as box 24.B Place of Service, which identifies where the service was performed. As you read through this textbook, pay attention to these areas of the CMS-1500 form, as it is a necessary part of learning how to code. Coding is more than simply selecting the correct diagnosis and procedure codes; it is knowing how to place these codes correctly on a CMS-1500 (or UB-04) form and including all other necessary elements appropriate to bill a third-party payer.

Key to Success

As the healthcare industry changes, so does the CMS-1500 form, so do not be surprised if it changes again in the future. For example, the form used to only have enough room for four diagnosis codes—now it can hold 12! To keep abreast of changes and updates to the form, you can reference the NUCC website at http://www.nucc.org.

Third-Party Payers

A third-party payer is the party that pays for the healthcare claim when a patient has a health insurance policy. For example, if a patient who subscribes to a commercial insurance company presents to the office for treatment, any charges for treating the patient will be sent on a healthcare claim to his or her third-party payer, the commercial insurance company. However, if the patient does not have any healthcare insurance coverage, then the claim will be paid directly by the patient. Any payments that come directly from the patient are referred to as **out-of-pocket expenses**, or patient responsibility amounts.

In its most basic form, health insurance protects against high out-of-pocket costs to the patient, who pays a **premium**—a monthly charge to keep the insurance policy active for coverage—in return for the insurance company paying for any healthcare services that the patient receives. This is similar to automobile insurance—an individual pays a monthly amount (premium) to an auto insurance company that covers any costs incurred in the case of an accident or other expense (barring mechanical expenses). In the same way that car insurance pays to fix a person's car if he or she gets in an accident, health insurance pays for the healthcare expenses when a patient goes to the doctor.

It is not quite this simple, however. There are many different aspects of this relationship that govern to which healthcare practitioners and facilities the patient must go, what healthcare services will be covered by the insurance, and how much the patient must also pay for the healthcare service. These differences depend on the patient's type of insurance plan, and the policy and coverage limitations. **Coverage limitations** refer to the services that an insurance plan will pay for (cover) when they are provided by a healthcare practitioner, as well as what services will not be covered and classified as the patient's out-of-pocket expense.

There are hundreds of different insurance plans, both commercial and government-sponsored, so it is impossible to address features of all policies here, but it is important to understand the basic types of insurance plans and the relationship between insurance plans and reimbursement. There are two main divisions in insurance plans—commercial and government-sponsored. Nontraditional insurance is an additional insurance type, which may be used to cover healthcare expenses.

Commercial Insurance

Commercial insurance plans are run by for-profit companies, which are not government entities, and require a monthly premium in return for healthcare coverage. Examples of commercial health insurance companies include Blue Cross Blue Shield Association, United Healthcare, Kaiser Permanente, and Cigna.

Each health insurance company offers different insurance policies. An **insurance policy** is a formal contract between an individual and the insurance company. The **insured party**, otherwise known as the policy holder, is the individual who is the primary benefit holder on the insurance policy. This policy defines many things, including:

- Covered healthcare expenses for which the insurance company will pay
- The exact terms under which the insurance will pay for a healthcare expense
- The duration of coverage
- The premium amount
- Patient out-of-pocket expenses
- Plan maximums and any other limitations

If more than just one individual is covered by the insurance policy, this contract will also identify all others covered by the policy, as well as specific coverage and patient responsibility amounts. For example, if the insured party pays premiums for additional family members—such as his or her spouse and children—then the health insurance policy will identify these additional benefit holders and specify how they are covered by the policy.

Premiums for commercial plans are paid in several different ways, but the two most common are employer-sponsored or individual plans. **Employer-sponsored insurance** plans are those offered by an employer to eligible employees within the organization. This results in many people signing up for the same plan, so the premiums are typically lower and there are fewer coverage limitations such as noncovered services or high out-of-pocket amounts (addressed in the following sections). The employer traditionally pays a portion of the health insurance premiums, which reduces the premium amount the individual must pay for coverage.

Individual insurance plans are purchased by an individual who does not go through an employer to attain coverage. In today's changing world of health insurance coverage, in addition to purchasing coverage through an employer-sponsored plan, individuals may now purchase an individual plan through a government-run health insurance exchange. A **health insurance exchange** allows insurance companies to offer health insurance plans to individuals who must pay premiums for coverage. However, if the patient does purchase health insurance coverage through an exchange, and if he or she qualifies financially, the government may provide the patient with a subsidy to help pay for the premiums. It is important to understand that even though this healthcare exchange was created and is overseen by a government agency (either by the federal or state government), it is not government-sponsored insurance. The insurance companies offering coverage on the exchanges are for-profit commercial entities, and the policies offered require patient out-of-pocket expenses and premiums paid for coverage.

Commercial insurance plans typically share costs with the patient by requiring certain out-of-pocket expenses depending on the service provided, as specified by the insurance policy. This means that they require the patient to pay for an amount of services provided, depending on the patient's policy. Usually if the patient has a plan with higher premiums, he or she gets the benefit of lower out-of-pocket expenses. There are four main types of patient responsibility: copayments, deductible, coinsurance, and noncovered services.

Copayment

A **copayment**, or copay, is an amount of money that the patient is responsible for paying to the healthcare provider before he or she may be seen. For example, if a patient has a $30 copayment on his or her policy for office services, then the patient must pay $30 to the doctor's office before being seen. Copayment amounts depend on the healthcare setting as well as the type of service provided. For example, emergency department copays are typically much larger (such as $150) because the service is expected to be more expensive. The type of service also affects the copayment amount. For example, according to federal regulations, insurance companies must cover preventive services such as routine examinations and specific vaccinations at 100 percent, meaning patients do not have to pay anything out of pocket for these services (Healthcare.gov 2019). In this case, if the patient presented to his doctor's office for a routine examination, he would not have to pay any copay amount.

Deductible

A **deductible** is a preset amount that must be paid in full before insurance benefits will begin. Deductibles can range from a few hundred to many thousands of dollars, depending on the insurance policy. For example, Patient A may have an employer-sponsored group insurance plan with a $750 deductible, whereas Patient B has an individual health insurance plan through a healthcare exchange with a $6,000 deductible. No matter what the amount is, no insurance benefits will be paid until the patient pays the full deductible amount (out of the patient's pocket). If Patient A is seen for any type of healthcare services, she will have to pay $750 out of her own pocket before any additional charges will be paid by her insurance company. The same goes for Patient B—even though his deductible is much larger, it still works in the same manner. He will have to pay $6,000 out of his own pocket before his insurance plan will pay for any additional charges.

Deductibles are reset at the end of each benefit year, and the amount paid into the deductible each year also resets. For example, if Patient A had met her $750 deductible (meaning she had paid $750 out of pocket for services provided) in the benefit year 2020 (January 1, 2020 to December 31, 2020), then this amount would reset to $750 for the new benefit year (January 1, 2021 to December 31, 2021). She would have to pay another $750 in 2021 before any benefits would be paid by her insurance company.

Coinsurance

Coinsurance refers to a category of patient responsibility that is based on a percentage of allowed amount. An **allowable amount** is the maximum amount of money that an insurance policy will agree to pay for a specific CPT (procedure) or HCPCS code. The allowable amount and the actual charge sent by the healthcare office for the procedure (as indicated in box 24.F of the CMS-1500 form) often do not correspond. For example, a healthcare office may charge $200.00 for procedure code 10021, Fine needle aspiration; without imaging guidance, but the allowable amount is only $170.23. This means that the insurance only *allows* $170.23 to be paid for procedure code 10021, no matter how much the healthcare office charges for it. The difference between the allowable amount and the charge amount is usually written off, or adjusted off of the account, and not billed to the patient (note that there are some exceptions and some insurance plans will allow the patient to be billed for the difference).

Coinsurance amounts kick in after any copayments or deductibles have been paid and do not have a limit nor do they reset at the end of each benefit year. They are usually referred to as a percentage amount (a percentage of the allowable amount that the patient is required to pay). For example, if a patient has an 80/20 coinsurance, the insurance company will pay for 80 percent of the allowable amount, and the patient will be responsible to pay for 20 percent of the allowable amount. If Patient A has an 80/20 coinsurance on her plan, and the allowed amount of the doctor's charges equal $100, then her insurance will pay $80 and she will have to pay $20 for the service. As previously mentioned, coinsurance amounts do not reset and there is no limit to the coinsurance like the deductible, so the amount paid will greatly depend on the charge for the service provided. If Patient A was seen in the hospital and the allowed amount added up to $10,000, then her insurance would pay $8,000 and she would pay $2,000.

It is important to understand that patients may have all three types of patient responsibility amounts on their coverage. Patient A might have a copayment for services rendered, a deductible, and a coinsurance. This means that she must pay a copay before being seen by a healthcare provider. If she has not met her deductible for that benefit year, then she must pay for all of the doctor's charges before her insurance will pay anything. Furthermore, even after she has met her deductible and paid her copay, she will still have to pay her coinsurance amount.

Noncovered Services

There is one more category of charges that falls onto patient responsibility, or out-of-pocket expenses—noncovered services. **Noncovered services** are services that are specifically excluded from coverage per the insurance policy. This means that the service will not be covered (paid for) by the patient's health insurance. For example, if Patient A is seen at her physician's office and receives a vision screening, but vision services are not covered on her policy, then the insurance will not pay for the vision screening charge. This noncovered service will be transferred to the patient's responsibility, meaning that Patient A will have to pay for the entire cost of the vision screening. Figure 2.7 illustrates the four types of patient responsibility.

Government-Sponsored Insurance

Government-sponsored insurance is a type of entitlement health insurance coverage that is provided by the government. Government-sponsored insurance is managed at either the state or federal level or a combination of both, depending on the type of insurance. Entitlement health insurance is a type of coverage for which individuals must be eligible based on certain criteria. In other words, government health insurance plans are not offered to everyone; rather they are provided only to individuals who meet the eligibility criteria for coverage. Some of these plans are offered free of charge, so the insured does not have to pay premiums or out-of-pocket expenses. Others are offered with smaller premiums than commercial plans and with a varying level of patient out-of-pocket expenses.

Figure 2.7. Types of patient responsibility

 # Types of Patient Responsibility

Copayment: A set amount of money that a patient must pay the healthcare provider before he or she may be seen

Deductible: An amount that must be paid in full before insurance benefits will begin.

Coinsurance: A category of patient responsibility that is based on a percentage of allowed charges

Noncovered Service: A service that is specifically excluded from coverage per the insurance policy

The federal and individual state governments also run a variety of health programs including health insurance plans. These include the Veterans Health Administration (VHA) and Indian Health Services (IHS), among others. The three main types of government-sponsored entitlement health insurance plans are Medicare, Medicaid, and TRICARE.

Medicare

Medicare is a federal health insurance plan for individuals who are age 65 or older, individuals with disabilities, and those with end-stage renal disease (ESRD). Medicare is unique because it is funded by federal funds and individual plan premiums that are paid by plan enrollees. In return, Medicare health insurance plans share costs with enrollees by requiring copayments, deductibles, and coinsurance amounts that differ depending on the type of coverage the patient has. Medicare is also strict about covered versus noncovered services, as there are many healthcare supplies and services that are not covered by Medicare. These include long-term (or custodial) care, dentures and most dental care, eye examinations, and certain supplies or products such as hearing aids (Medicare.gov 2019a). When a service is likely noncovered by Medicare, it may be necessary to complete an advance beneficiary notice, as described later in this chapter. Remember that noncovered services are the patient's direct responsibility, so the patient will have to pay the full amount for the noncovered service.

Medicare is managed by the Centers for Medicare and Medicaid Services (CMS), a federal organization that administers Medicare, Medicaid, the Children's Health

Insurance Program (CHIP), and the Health Insurance Marketplace (the federal online health insurance exchange that allows individuals to purchase insurance plans offered by commercial companies). CMS is an important organization, as it administers both Medicare and Medicaid and, in doing so, sets the standard for what many health insurance companies cover and consider medically necessary. The CMS website is a great resource for coders, billers, and healthcare information management professionals, as it also provides official information and education on topics that are important to the healthcare industry, such as HIPAA training (CMS 2019c).

Advance Beneficiary Notices

It is important to understand the difference between insurance companies in terms of what each will or will not cover, as the majority of all payments in the healthcare office come from health insurance payments on claims for covered services. A coding professional needs to know what specific services a person's health insurance may or may not cover and ensure payment for that service. This is especially important in the case of Medicare, which may or may not cover specific services depending on coverage determinations and medical necessity.

In some circumstances, it may be necessary to issue an advance beneficiary notice (ABN), a form issued to Medicare patients to inform them that a service might not be covered (that is, paid) by Medicare (see figure 2.8). An ABN is used only when a healthcare provider is furnishing an item or providing a service that is usually paid for by Medicare but might *not* be covered in this specific instance. For example, a provider performs a procedure that Medicare may not consider medically necessary, in which case they will not cover the service. It also gives the patient the option of either refusing the service or agreeing to pay for the service if Medicare does not pay. An ABN should be issued include when:

- Medicare may not pay for an item or service
- Medicare usually pays for the item or service
- Medicare is expected to deny the payment because the service or item is not considered medically reasonable and necessary

The ABN allows patients to make an informed decision on their healthcare and the costs that may be incurred due to services performed. In other words, it is a way of protecting the patient from unknown healthcare expenses, as well as giving patients transparent information about their healthcare costs.

An ABN is an important part of understanding the link between properly documented, reported, and coded services and the payment for such services, because it shows how the services reported with procedure codes must match the reason why those services were rendered (as identified by the diagnosis codes). This is just one example of how coding cannot be removed from billing, as it is integral to ensuring payment of claims. As such, many sections of this textbook discuss the billing implications of coding (such as ABNs), to create a more comprehensive view of coding in the real world.

Medicaid

Not to be confused with Medicare, Medicaid is a government-sponsored entitlement health insurance program for individuals and families with little or no resources. This means that, for example, a family of four living at the poverty line can qualify for Medicaid for the entire family, which will cover healthcare expenses for all eligible individuals within the family (Medicaid.gov 2019). Medicaid eligibility requirements and specific income amounts are set by each individual state, so they vary from state

Figure 2.8. Advance beneficiary notice (ABN)

A. Notifier:

B. Patient Name: **C. Identification Number:**

Advance Beneficiary Notice of Noncoverage (ABN)

NOTE: If Medicare doesn't pay for **D.**＿＿＿＿＿＿below, you may have to pay.
Medicare does not pay for everything, even some care that you or your health care provider have good reason to think you need. We expect Medicare may not pay for the **D.**＿＿＿＿＿＿below.

D.	E. Reason Medicare May Not Pay:	F. Estimated Cost

WHAT YOU NEED TO DO NOW:
- Read this notice, so you can make an informed decision about your care.
- Ask us any questions that you may have after you finish reading.
- Choose an option below about whether to receive the **D.**＿＿＿＿＿＿listed above.
  Note: If you choose Option 1 or 2, we may help you to use any other insurance that you might have, but Medicare cannot require us to do this.

G. OPTIONS: Check only one box. We cannot choose a box for you.
☐ **OPTION 1.** I want the **D.**＿＿＿＿＿＿listed above. You may ask to be paid now, but I also want Medicare billed for an official decision on payment, which is sent to me on a Medicare Summary Notice (MSN). I understand that if Medicare doesn't pay, I am responsible for payment, but **I can appeal to Medicare** by following the directions on the MSN. If Medicare does pay, you will refund any payments I made to you, less co-pays or deductibles.
☐ **OPTION 2.** I want the **D.**＿＿＿＿＿＿listed above, but do not bill Medicare. You may ask to be paid now as I am responsible for payment. **I cannot appeal if Medicare is not billed.**
☐ **OPTION 3.** I don't want the **D.**＿＿＿＿＿＿listed above. I understand with this choice I am **not** responsible for payment, and **I cannot appeal to see if Medicare would pay.**

H. Additional Information:

This notice gives our opinion, not an official Medicare decision. If you have other questions on this notice or Medicare billing, call **1-800-MEDICARE** (1-800-633-4227/**TTY:** 1-877-486-2048).
Signing below means that you have received and understand this notice. You also receive a copy.

I. Signature:	J. Date:

CMS does not discriminate in its programs and activities. To request this publication in an alternative format, please call: 1-800-MEDICARE or email: AltFormatRequest@cms.hhs.gov.

According to the Paperwork Reduction Act of 1995, no persons are required to respond to a collection of information unless it displays a valid OMB control number. The valid OMB control number for this information collection is 0938-0566. The time required to complete this information collection is estimated to average 7 minutes per response, including the time to review instructions, search existing data resources, gather the data needed, and complete and review the information collection. If you have comments concerning the accuracy of the time estimate or suggestions for improving this form, please write to: CMS, 7500 Security Boulevard, Attn: PRA Reports Clearance Officer, Baltimore, Maryland 21244-1850.

Form CMS-R-131 (Exp. 03/2020)   Form Approved OMB No. 0938-0566

Source: CMS 2019d.

to state depending on the amount of resources allocated to the Medicaid program. Therefore, a family of four living in New Mexico may find that they are eligible for Medicaid for the entire family, including the adults, whereas that same family living in Texas may find that only the children are eligible for Medicaid coverage.

The Medicaid program is unique in that it is not necessary to pay insurance premiums in return for health insurance coverage, and there are no patient out-of-pocket expenses. It is also unique in that it is jointly funded and run by both the federal and state governments, although coverage and eligibility requirements may vary from state-to-state.

The **Children's Health Insurance Program (CHIP)** is a program that is similar to Medicaid but covers children in low-income families who do not qualify for Medicaid benefits. For example, if a family's income is low, but not low enough for the entire family to qualify for Medicaid, then only the children may be eligible for coverage under CHIP. Depending on a family's resources and income level and the state in which the individuals live, the CHIP program may require a modest premium as well as low patient out-of-pocket expenses. For example, the annual CHIP premium may be less than $50, and copayments of $5 to $35 may be required at the time services are rendered (Texas HHS 2017).

Key to Success

Although they sound alike, do not confuse Medic*are* with Medic*aid*. They are both government-sponsored health insurance programs administered by CMS, but Medicare is for the elderly, disabled, and those with ESRD, and Medicaid is for those with low income and few resources.

TRICARE

TRICARE is a government-sponsored entitlement health insurance plan administered by the United States Defense Health Agency (DHA). It is a federally run health insurance plan, separate from both Medicare and Medicaid. TRICARE provides health insurance coverage for individuals who are part of the US armed forces and their dependents. This includes uniformed members of the Army, Navy, Marines, Air Force, Coast Guard, Public Health Service, and the National Oceanic and Atmospheric Administration (NOAA). Recipients of TRICARE insurance may or may not have to pay premiums for coverage and out-of-pocket expenses, depending on the member's type of service, status, and enrollment plan. Those in active status typically do not have to pay premiums for coverage nor out-of-pocket expenses, whereas their dependents on the insurance coverage may have to pay modest amounts for services, such as a $12 copayment. TRICARE also covers retirees of the US Armed Forces, who must pay an inexpensive annual premium as well as modest out-of-pocket expenses. For example, the annual TRICARE health insurance premium for a family of four may be less than $1,000 (TRICARE 2017).

Nontraditional Insurance

In addition to commercial and government-sponsored insurance plans, there are a few different types of insurance coverage that will cover healthcare expenses. In order to be covered by one of these plans, patients have to either pay a premium or meet some other type of eligibility requirement. Coverage for claims under the following policies varies depending on the reason for treatment and the type of coverage the patient has, as well as other factors. For example, an automobile insurance plan may cover up to $25,000 of eligible healthcare expenses. So, if a car accident resulted in an injury, the automobile insurance would cover up to $25,000 of the healthcare expenses related to that injury.

It is important to be aware of these nontraditional insurance types, as the biller needs to send the claim for healthcare services to a different insurance company (not the patient's usual health insurance) and may also require additional codes on the healthcare claim to identify the extenuating circumstances surrounding the accident or injury. These extenuating circumstances are reported using external cause codes, which identify the manner in which the injury occurred, place of occurrence, activity in which the patient was engaged when the injury occurred, and the patient's status when the injury occurred (such as work, volunteer, or leisure activity status). External cause codes are diagnosis codes and are introduced in chapter 4.

Types of nontraditional insurance include workers' compensation, automobile and homeowner's insurance, and supplemental insurance policies.

Workers' Compensation

Workers' compensation insurance is a type of insurance that covers injuries and illnesses that were suffered by a patient while on the job. Workers' compensation differs from both commercial and government-sponsored insurance plans because the patient neither pays an insurance premium nor has to meet some sort of eligibility criteria. Workers' compensation insurance is provided to the patient by his or her employer. In this case, the employer pays the premiums to the insurance company, to cover any healthcare expenses for his or her employees.

Although workers' compensation requirements vary from state to state and based on company size and number of employees, employers are required to cover the healthcare expenses for any employee who suffers a work-related illness or injury. For example, if an employee working as a construction worker were injured by a forklift while doing his job, the healthcare expenses incurred by this injury would be covered by workers' compensation insurance. In addition to healthcare expenses, workers' compensation may also provide the patient with money to help cover the costs of being out of work because of the injury or due to any disability that may result from the injury. Furthermore, if the employee suffers a fatal accident, workers' compensation may provide financial compensation to his or her survivors. These additional disability or survivor benefits may be funded by the state in which the patient lives.

There are many required forms, healthcare examinations, and updates that are required in workers' compensation claims. Also, the type of workers' compensation coverage greatly depends on the state in which the injury occurred, the type of employer, and specifics surrounding the way in which the injury or illness occurred. Because of these complicated details, workers' compensation claims are usually managed by agencies that deal specifically with workers' compensation, and they sometimes employ healthcare providers solely to provide workers' compensation examinations and evaluations.

Automobile and Homeowner's Insurance

Most people are familiar with automobile insurance, which covers damage to your vehicle or another's vehicle in the case of a motor vehicle accident. As with health insurance, policy holders pay a premium in return for coverage, and the insurance company shares the expenses with the individual through deductibles. Homeowner's insurance is also a familiar type of insurance, except this insurance covers damage to an individual's home. For example, if a person's home is damaged by a fire, the homeowner's insurance will pay the owner of the policy a pre-determined amount to help cover the costs of lost or damaged personal items, to repair the structure, or to purchase new appliances.

Both auto and homeowner's insurance will also cover the costs of healthcare claims in certain circumstances. For example, Patient A was driving her vehicle and texting on her cell phone when she collided with Patient B's car, resulting in a whiplash injury for Patient B and damage to both vehicles. In this case, the motor vehicle accident (MVA) was caused by Patient A, so her auto insurance will pay for the claims to repair both vehicles, and she will have to share some of these costs by paying her deductible amount. Furthermore, the healthcare provided to Patient B will also be covered by Patient A's auto insurance. In this case, her car insurance is paying for a healthcare claim.

Homeowner's insurance may also pay for healthcare services in certain circumstances. For example, Patient A was spending time at Patient B's house when she slipped on the stairs exiting the residence and fractured her ankle. Patient A may choose to file a claim for her injuries through Patient B's homeowner's insurance, which will pay for her healthcare claims.

Supplemental Insurance

Supplemental insurance plans are also important to understand, as they may impact the patient's ability to pay for healthcare services. Healthcare administrative personnel may need to help patients by providing CMS-1500 forms for healthcare services or other proof of healthcare services rendered.

Supplemental insurance policies help patients pay the out-of-pocket expenses related to healthcare. For example, if a patient with a high-deductible health insurance plan is injured in a recreational football game accident, his healthcare expenses are covered by his regular health insurance company; however, he is still responsible for the charge amount sent to his deductible. In this case, if the patient had a supplemental accident insurance policy, the supplemental insurance could help him pay for his deductible.

Supplemental insurance policies differ depending on the type of insurance coverage and the specifics of coverage. They range from accident coverage (as in the previous example) to coverage for cancer treatments, coverage for disabilities only, or for coverage of a specific set of healthcare services or treatments. Supplemental insurance plans are typically low cost, and patients can pick and choose which type of coverage they prefer and tailor coverage to their specific needs. These plans act as an umbrella in that they help cover the patient from the financial burdens for which he or she may be responsible in the case of a healthcare emergency or unplanned treatment.

One example of a commercial supplemental accident insurance policy is that offered by Aflac. An individual must subscribe to an Aflac policy by paying monthly premiums and, in return, Aflac reimburses the patient a specified amount of money if he or she suffers a certain type of accidental injury. For example, Patient A has an Aflac policy that covers accidental injuries, including fractures. Patient A just suffered a fractured ankle, for which Aflac will pay the patient $500. The patient sends in a claim to Aflac with information regarding the injury, and Aflac sends the patient the funds that correspond to each specific injury (or service performed to treat the injury). This money can be used to cover the cost of the healthcare service as well as any other financial obligations that Patient A may have incurred due to the injury, such as out-of-pocket expenses, income lost from time out of work, or costs spent traveling to and from healthcare appointments (Aflac 2017).

Another common supplemental insurance is Medigap, a policy that is specifically for Medicare beneficiaries. It is designed to "fill the gap" left by patient out-of-pocket expenses such as copayments, deductibles, and coinsurance amounts. Unlike Medicare, Medigap policies are not run by the government. Instead, they are offered by commercial insurance companies specifically to cover the gaps in Medicare coverage, which result in patient balances that are not payable by Medicare. In order to obtain Medigap coverage, individuals must pay a monthly premium to the commercial insurance company for coverage. Like all supplemental insurance plans, Medigap will not cover all fees, but only those fees and remaining amounts as specified in the Medigap policy.

Medigap differs from traditional supplemental insurance policies (like Aflac) in that it is administered by an actual health insurance company. After the primary insurance has paid its share, healthcare claims are sent directly to Medigap policies for payment just like a regular health insurance claim. Aflac, on the other hand, requires proof only of the patient's diagnosis or treatment. In the case of an Aflac claim, the healthcare office may have to provide a CMS-1500 claim form or complete an Aflac form so the patient can submit this proof to his or her supplemental insurance plan for payment. Review examples of the different types of third-party payers in figure 2.9.

Figure 2.9. Third-party payers

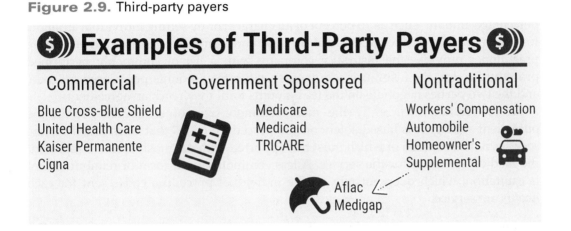

In addition to the varying kinds of insurance plans, there are also different forms of reimbursement for healthcare services. The three most common reimbursement types are fee-for-service, capitation, and prospective payment.

Reimbursement Types

As previously discussed, reimbursement for healthcare services occurs when an insurance company pays a healthcare provider for a service rendered. Forms of reimbursement vary depending on the healthcare setting, provider type, and ways in which the healthcare provider has contracted with the insurance company. In order for a doctor to be able to send a healthcare claim for payment to any insurance company, he or she must be fully contracted with the patient's insurance company. For example, if Dr. Alameda sees a patient with Effective Eagle Insurance, then in order for Dr. Alameda to send a claim to Effective Eagle and get paid for any healthcare services rendered to the patient, she must be contracted with Effective Eagle. **Provider contracting** is when the insurance company and the healthcare provider come into an agreement so that when the healthcare provider delivers healthcare services to patients, the insurance company will provide reimbursement for the healthcare services provided. The contract signed by both parties defines important terms, informs each party of their rights and responsibilities to each other and to the patient, and defines the payment for services performed.

In the outpatient setting, the two most common ways in which the payment can be made are either by fee-for-service or through capitation. In the inpatient or facility settings, prospective payment systems are used to determine the amount of payment before the patient receives healthcare services.

Fee-for-Service

Fee-for-service reimbursement is separately reporting and billing each procedure, treatment, or item performed by the healthcare provider (namely, one fee for each service) on the claim for the healthcare service. For example, if a primary care provider performs a sick visit examination, then he reports the sick visit examination and may choose to set the fee for that particular service at $75. On the other hand, the fee for a wart removal may be $110. Each service has a different fee, as determined by the work, risk, overhead, and skill involved in that service. The dollar amount charged for each service is referred to as the charge amount.

Typically, insurance companies do not pay the full charge amount. Rather, they pay the amount that is pre-determined in the fee schedule agreed upon during provider contracting. A fee schedule is a list of dollar amounts that the insurance company will pay for services performed by the healthcare provider. This is done either with a percentage amount (such as 70 percent of all charges) or by setting individual amounts for each particular service performed. In this more common scenario, the healthcare practitioner provides the insurance company with a list of commonly performed procedure codes, the insurance company specifies fee amounts per procedure code, and the two parties negotiate on the fee amounts until they reach an agreement.

Fee-for-service is currently the most common type of reimbursement in the outpatient setting. It is based solely on the procedure codes that were billed for the services rendered, each of which must be supported with diagnosis codes to represent the medical necessity for the service. A less commonly used form of reimbursement is capitation, which does not rely on the individual procedure codes sent for each healthcare service.

Capitation

Capitation is a reimbursement type in which an insurance company pays a healthcare provider a set dollar amount each month for each patient. This per member per month payment (PMPM)—the amount paid per patient each month—is defined in the provider contract along with other stipulations regarding payments and claims requirements. Capitation plans also require that the patients select and see their primary care physician, who is the recipient of the capitation plan payment.

In capitation, the insurance company makes the monthly payment to the healthcare provider whether or not the patient is seen by the provider. When the patient does present for treatment, the provider cannot bill this service for reimbursement (because he or she already has been paid via the monthly capitation payment). This creates problems when the patient is seen an inordinate number of times throughout the month, which might require the provider to spend more resources treating the patient than the monthly capitation payment covers. On the other hand, there typically will be months in which patients are not seen at all. Capitation plans thus put the focus less on the actual procedures performed, and more on efforts to keep the patient well, thereby not requiring health treatments or other services and containing healthcare costs overall.

Even though providers are not paid for particular services performed, it does not mean that a healthcare claim is not coded and sent to the insurance company. This claim is still sent to prove the medical necessity of the service and to describe any procedures that were performed on the patient; however, the claim is not reimbursed.

In the changing era of healthcare insurance, capitation contracts are becoming more common. The PMPM payment may be linked to the patient's overall risk score, as determined by HCC codes, discussed later in this chapter.

The final type of reimbursement is called prospective payment, which reimburses provided services with a pre-determined, fixed amount, based on the patient's diagnosis and the services performed.

Prospective Payment Systems

A **prospective payment system (PPS)** is a type of reimbursement system based on preset payment levels rather than actual charges billed after the service has been provided. It is founded on pre-determined payment rates or periods and linked to the anticipated intensity of services delivered as well as the patient's condition. PPS is used for inpatient services (Inpatient Prospective Payment System, or IPPS), outpatient facility services (Outpatient Prospective Payment System, or OPPS), home healthcare services, and skilled nursing facility services. This does not mean that the facility must see into the future to predict the patient's health needs; instead, the PPS groups the factors surrounding the patient's admission into a category of payment. For example, if an otherwise healthy patient with appendicitis was seen in the inpatient setting and received an appendectomy, then the payment for the inpatient services would be based on the diagnosis of appendicitis, as well as the procedure performed (appendectomy). On the other hand, if the patient had a diagnosis of appendicitis along with diabetes mellitus, hypertension, and chronic kidney disease, as well as advanced age, then the payment for this patient would be higher for the same procedure, because the additional diagnoses would categorize the patient's service into a higher payment category. These additional diagnoses are called comorbidities and complications. More about prospective payment systems is discussed in chapter 20.

A **comorbidity** is either a medical condition that coexists with the primary cause for hospitalization and affects the patient's treatment and length of stay, or a pre-existing condition (like diabetes mellitus or hypertension) that, because of its presence with a specific diagnosis (like appendicitis), causes an increase in length of stay by at least one day in approximately 75 percent of cases. A **complication** is a medical condition that arises during an inpatient hospitalization (for example, a postoperative wound infection), or a condition that arises during the hospital stay that prolongs the length of stay at least one day in approximately 75 percent of the cases. The more complications or comorbidities that a patient has, the more likely the facility will have to expend greater resources on treating the patient, requiring a higher level of payment than for the same service rendered on an otherwise healthy patient.

In certain instances, before a service can be rendered, that service must be authorized by the insurance company. These are called prior authorizations, prior certifications, or referrals.

Authorizations, Certifications, and Referrals

Just because a patient has health insurance and is seen by a doctor does not mean that the patient's insurance company will pay for anything that the healthcare provider does. Furthermore, this does not mean that the patient can see whichever doctor he or she prefers. Because healthcare services can be costly, health insurance plans have many stipulations that must be followed for patients to be seen by doctors other than their primary care physicians or to receive specialized treatments such as magnetic resonance imaging (MRIs) or physical therapy services. These specialized services and treatments must be pre-authorized before health insurance will pay for them.

A **prior authorization (PA)** (sometimes called a prior certification), is permission from an insurance company for a patient to receive a healthcare service from a provider. Consider the following example.

Dr. Alameda sees a teenage boy in her office following an accident at his school in which he sustained a head injury during a soccer game. She would like to order a CT scan to rule out any serious injuries. Before she can send the patient to the hospital to receive the service, she must contact the patient's health insurance company and provide specific details about the incident and the patient's diagnosis, as well as her justification for sending the patient for the scan. This is the prior authorization request. If the insurance company agrees, then it will authorize the service and Dr. Alameda can then call the hospital to schedule the boy for the service. If the patient's insurance does not authorize the service, then it will not pay for it.

In this example, if the CT scan were denied, the doctor might have to determine if a different imaging service should be performed. It may be necessary to send the request to a utilization review professional who can determine if the service requested is indeed medically necessary and should be authorized by the insurance company. Typically, when a request is sent for a utilization review, it is handled by either the clinical staff or the healthcare provider. Once the service has been approved, the insurance company will issue an authorization number, which must be included on the claim in order to receive payment for the service. The prior authorization number should be entered in box 23 of the paper CMS-1500 claim form (see figure 2.10).

Figure 2.10. Box 23

23. PRIOR AUTHORIZATION NUMBER

Source: CMS 2019a.

A **referral** is similar to a prior authorization. A referral is a request from one doctor—usually the patient's primary care provider—who sends (refers) the patient to another doctor, or for a service from another provider. The requirement for a referral depends on the patient's insurance policy. Some plans require referrals whenever the patient is seen by a provider other than his or her PCP, whereas other policies require referrals only for out-of-network providers (providers that are not contracted with the patient's insurance company).

Dr. Alameda sees a patient with high anxiety and feelings of depression. She wants this patient to see a psychiatrist. This patient's insurance requires a referral in order to authorize any service provided by any doctor other than the patient's primary care physician, Dr. Alameda. Because of this, Dr. Alameda must send a referral request to the insurance company, who will examine the patient's diagnoses and treatment requested and either authorize or deny the referral. Furthermore, in order for the psychiatrist to see the patient, a referral number is needed to confirm that the insurance has authorized the service and psychiatrist will get reimbursed for any authorized services that he or she performs.

As with prior authorizations, if the insurance company does not authorize the referral to the psychiatrist, then it will not pay for any of the fees charged by the psychiatrist. The patient still has the option to go see the psychiatrist, but if she does, she must pay out of pocket for any services received. Therefore, it is especially important for coders and billers to understand the varying health insurance types, as each health insurance has different requirements regarding authorizations.

Key to Success

Prior authorizations, prior certifications, and referrals are like permission slips for patients to see another doctor or to receive a healthcare service. The request is to the insurance company, who then provides permission for the service and agrees to pay for it. Without the permission, insurance will not reimburse the healthcare providers for the nonauthorized service. The patient can still receive the service but is responsible for paying for it out of his or her own pocket.

In addition to reimbursement, there are other factors that impact the financial side of medicine, some of which can provide either lucrative incentive bonuses or damaging penalties for providers and healthcare clinics. These include Hierarchical Condition Category coding and risk adjustment, as well as performance measures and quality improvement.

Risk Adjustment and HCC Coding

As a way of predicting their budget for the upcoming year, insurance plans analyze their patient pool (all of the patients that are covered by each specific insurance plan), in terms of how healthy they are and how likely they are to incur expensive treatments in the following year. This is called **risk adjustment** and is performed by insurance companies as a part of their financial analysis. In many cases, patient risk scores, as determined by the risk adjustment process, are compiled for a certain patient population and used to determine the amount of PMPM payment for capitated contracts. Risk adjustment is a complex methodology that takes into account all known health elements of each patient that is a member of that particular health plan. Risk adjustment uses a multifaceted approach to analyze patient risk, which includes:

- Patient diagnosis
- Age
- Gender
- Socioeconomic status
- Insurance type
- Specific claims data (AHIP 2016)

These components add up to a single risk score per patient, which is then used to calculate the total risk score for the group. For example, if health plan A risk adjusts its patient base and finds that 50 percent of patients have diabetes mellitus along with another chronic condition, then it can safely assume treatments will be more common and more expensive than if only 25 percent of its patient base had diabetes mellitus with another chronic condition.

Because most risk adjustment data are calculated based on patient diagnosis codes and claims data, it makes sense that coders are at the forefront of risk analysis. As risk analysis becomes more important for health plans to manage their bottom lines, job opportunities are only set to increase.

The majority of risk analysis comes into play in what are called Hierarchical Condition Categories (HCC), based on individual patient diagnosis codes and correct documentation techniques. Additionally, it is important to understand accountable care organizations and their role in risk analysis.

Hierarchical Condition Categories (HCCs)

The bulk of risk analysis data are in the form of patient diagnosis codes, which are taken from the claims submitted by healthcare providers for services rendered to a health plan's patients. These codes are tabulated into what is called a **Hierarchical Condition Category (HCC)**. Otherwise known as HCC coding, this is the practice of categorizing all patient diagnosis claims within groups of conditions, which are positioned strategically in order of least to greatest risk. For example, diabetes mellitus is included within HCCs, as it is a chronic condition that has a long-term impact on the patient's health. When a patient with diabetes mellitus presents for treatment and the provider's office reports the diagnosis code for the patient's diabetes, this code is captured by the patient's health insurance company and placed into a HCC. Some categories (or conditions) are considered riskier than others, and thus result in a higher risk adjustment. Ultimately, the more diagnoses that fit into HCCs, the higher the risk for the patient population. This results in additional funding to the insurance plan, which uses risk adjustment (by utilizing HCCs) to calculate how much money they may have to pay each year for patient healthcare services.

HCCs result in risk adjustment scores for each patient that are tallied up to complete the risk adjustment score for the entire patient population, as previously described. Usually only conditions that are costlier to manage medically are found in HCCs, and some patients can have different conditions that will place them in multiple HCCs. For example, a patient may have a liver condition as well as a personal history that includes substance abuse and an amputation. Because these three conditions are all tabulated in HCC adjustments, they would add up to a higher risk adjustment score than if the patient only had one of these conditions. Additional diagnoses calculated in HCCs include infections, disability status, transplant status, disease interactions, cerebrovascular diseases, psychiatric conditions, and diabetes, among others.

Therefore, HCCs are completely reliant on the diagnosis codes included on claims. In turn, diagnosis codes are completely reliant on the provider's documentation of the patient's healthcare condition and the services performed. Coders are uniquely suited to engage in HCC coding and ensure that all HCC codes are captured on all claims and supported by documentation in the health record.

HCC coding is specially focused on capturing all patient conditions that impact the HCC and are fully supported by documentation in the health record. HCC coding is a growing field of healthcare coding due in part to the growth of Medicare Advantage plans, which base their payments on the relative health of the patient as identified by the HCC within which the patient falls (Optum360 2017). This is different than fee-for-service coding that generally focuses on CPT and HCPCS codes and charges reported for reimbursement purposes. In fee-for-service coding, the focus is on diagnoses that impact reimbursement by indicating the medical necessity for the service provided. The diagnosis code identifies the medical necessity for the service provided, and the insurance company pays for the service. HCC coding is more inclusive, however, and requires reporting of all reportable diagnosis codes in order to present a complete picture of the patient's health. Consider the following example.

Wanda presented to her PCP's office for a sick visit, with a bad cough and a fever that has persisted for the last few days. Wanda has a significant healthcare history, including a past history of breast cancer, diabetes mellitus type 2, and she is status post an amputation of her left foot following a gangrenous foot ulcer. At her visit today, her PCP performs a basic medical examination and diagnoses Wanda with acute bronchitis, prescribes an antibiotic, and schedules a follow-up examination for her in two days to see how she is doing.

Key to Success

Note that in the given example, Wanda, the patient, is "status post" amputation of her left foot following a gangrenous foot ulcer. This means that she has had a recent amputation of the left foot. The term *status post*, sometimes abbreviated as S/P, is a common phrase in healthcare and is used to indicate that a patient has had a significant event or procedure happen in the recent past. For example, a patient who had a motor vehicle accident (MVA) one week ago may be identified in the health record as status post MVA.

In coding for reimbursement purposes only, the only diagnosis that would be required would be that of bronchitis. However, this diagnosis would be insufficient for HCC coding purposes. Because acute bronchitis is not a chronic or long-lasting condition expected to impact the patient health for a long period, it is not included in HCC calculations. Therefore, if only the acute bronchitis code were included in the healthcare claim, it would be a misrepresentation of the patient's overall health status and would not impact the risk score for the patient. HCC coding would require the reporting of all additional conditions of the patient, including the history of cancer, diabetes, and amputation status. These additional codes do impact the HCC and therefore would allow a more accurate representation of the patient's risk than if only the acute bronchitis code were reported. In other words, HCC coding is not only about reimbursement for healthcare services; it recognizes that diagnosis codes are used for more than just medical necessity and, in this case, help to create a better picture of the patient's overall health.

HCC coding requires coders who are skilled at understanding coding rules and HCCs and who can correctly identify and assign all diagnosis codes from health record documentation. Because only certain diagnosis codes for healthcare conditions impact the HCC, it is important to understand these particular conditions and how they should be accurately documented in the health record in order to substantiate code selection. Throughout the rest of this textbook you will find HCC Coding Corners, which discuss conditions that impact HCC coding and how they should be supported by documentation in the health record.

HCC Coding Corner

HCC Coding Corners discuss conditions that impact HCC coding and how they should be supported by documentation in the health record.

Accountable Care Organizations

An **accountable care organization (ACO)** is a group of healthcare providers that coordinate to provide high-quality care to their patients. This group of providers can be comprised of many different healthcare offices such as individual providers, large healthcare groups, hospitals, and other healthcare clinics. The ACO focuses on providing high-quality care, especially to patients with chronic conditions (such as those who fall into HCCs), and ensuring that these patients have access to quality care when needed.

There are three main goals of an ACO:

- Providing better care for patients, which results in
- Better health for the Medicare advantage population, as indicated by the
- Lower cost of providing care to these patients. (CMS 2019e)

ACOs that meet these goals have the opportunity to participate in the Medicare Shared Savings Program, which allows all of the providers grouped into the ACO to report their data for each performance year together and share in any savings accrued by participation in the ACO. This shared savings is what makes participation in an ACO especially important to the bottom line for the participating healthcare providers. As part of this process, claims for a healthcare office are paid regularly for a period of time, often called the performance year. After the year is over, the claims are reviewed to see if the ACO generated losses or savings for the Medicare plan for the performance year (CMS 2019e).

This review is a complicated process initiated by the insurance company or companies; it includes an analysis to ensure that all diagnosis codes that impact HCCs were captured at least once per patient per year. If the review shows that the ACO generated savings for the Medicare program (by correctly reporting all necessary HCC codes and providing high-quality care to patients as indicated by other factors), then these savings are shared with the ACO. The healthcare offices involved in the ACO receive an additional payment, sometimes called an incentive payment, based on their performance throughout the year.

One of the last major components to understanding the basics of billing for healthcare services is knowing how healthcare providers are increasingly held accountable for the *quality* of the service that they provide to patients. These initiatives are called performance measures or quality improvement initiatives, and they serve to quantify the quality of care provided by healthcare providers.

Performance Measurement

Historically, it has been difficult to measure the effectiveness of a healthcare provider outside of, perhaps, a patient questionnaire. However, in today's world of data analytics, all the data generated from a healthcare office can be used to measure the performance of a healthcare service. **Data analytics** refers to the act of quantifying qualitative data and analyzing it to categorize it and extract patterns. In other words, it is the quantitative analysis of the quality of care provided to patients. The data analyzed can be from a single medical doctor or from hospitals comprised of as many as thousands of healthcare providers. This data is then used to create a measure of the quality that a healthcare practitioner provides his or her patients.

This data is used to determine the level of care provided to patients, as represented by a quality score, such as a star rating. This level of care is identified with special performance measures that rate specific desired outcomes, or procedure codes that identify extra steps the healthcare practice has taken to improve the quality of care. The process of analyzing this data and determining the quality of care provided is called *performance measurement*.

Key to Success

If you are interested in data analytics, AHIMA offers a specialty Certified Health Data Analyst (CHDA®) certification. For more information on this and other certifications, refer to the appendix, Coding Certifications and Professional Coding Organizations.

Performance measures are a set of predefined quality outcomes that are used to determine the quality of care provided to patients. Performance measurement analyzes the success of a healthcare practice, facility, or other group, in meeting its pre-determined performance measures. Results from the performance measurement help the healthcare practice identify opportunities for improvement or areas of success, which can be shared with other providers to learn from that success.

These measures can be internally created by each specific healthcare entity. For example, if a healthcare office has the goal to reduce incidence of undiagnosed postpartum depression, it may choose to create a measure that identifies all mothers who receive a postpartum depression evaluation. Measuring how many mothers receive the evaluation in terms of a percentage indicates how well the practice is accomplishing its goal of reducing undiagnosed postpartum depression. If the percentage is 50 percent, this means only half of women received the evaluation and that the practice needs to do a better job of administering the evaluation. On the other hand, if the score were 100 percent, it would mean that all postpartum women received the evaluation and the office had met its pre-determined goal. These percentages are the measures of the performance goal.

Performance measures are also set by a number of official organizations and healthcare associations that measure specific outcomes desired for specific settings, specialties, or types of providers. For example, one of the performance measures for pediatric patients is the percentage of all patients who are at least two years of age who have received all age-appropriate vaccines at the time of reporting (CMS 2012). This is a specific measure that pediatricians can use to analyze their success at administering vaccines to their patients.

Many of these measures are compiled into official groups by agencies like CMS or the National Committee for Quality Assurance (NCQA), who endorse a set of measures, all of which combine to create a well-rounded picture of performance. Additionally, certain insurance plans may also endorse a set of measures for their patient population. For example, there are numerous measures used to identify the quality of care provided to diabetic patients through comprehensive diabetes care. This group of measures for comprehensive diabetes care includes measures for blood pressure control, performance of an eye examination, hemoglobin A1c control status and testing, and medical attention for nephropathy (NCQA 2019). These measures combine to form a more inclusive picture of the quality of care provided to diabetes patients.

Performance measures are also used for more than simply determining how good a doctor is at his or her job or how good a healthcare practice is. Performance measurement is important for other reasons, including quality improvement, transparency, accreditation, recognition as a medical home, and financial incentives.

Quality Improvement

Quality improvement (QI) uses the information generated from performance measurement to establish processes or programs that are aimed at improving quality scores. For example, if a healthcare practice's quality score for postpartum depression evaluations is 50 percent, then it is necessary to review the process of how the evaluation is administered, how patients are identified, and how the healthcare practice can improve that score. On the other hand, if the score is already 100 percent, then the healthcare practice can share their best practices with other offices to help them succeed in their performance measures.

Depending on the size of the organization and past performance measures, quality improvement may play a large role in an organization. For example, if a large hospital system has poor scores on surgical site infections or hospital-acquired conditions, it may choose to implement a QI program that employs a number of doctors, nurses, and administrative staff to focus solely on improving performance measures throughout the organization.

Transparency

An important part of creating performance scores is being transparent to stakeholders of the organization, such as patients and organizations that provide funding. This means that all stakeholders can clearly see the quality scores of the organization. Transparency about quality allows patients to make informed decisions regarding their healthcare services. For example, a patient may choose to go to a hospital with high quality scores and avoid a hospital with low quality scores, as these scores indicate the quality of care that the patient may receive at either organization. Scores are publicly available and searchable through Medicare resources such as Medicare Physician Compare, which permits users to search through publicly available provider data to compare performance results (Medicare.gov 2019b), as well as through individual hospital websites.

Accreditation

There are several different organizations in the healthcare industry, many of which provide accreditation of healthcare entities. **Accreditation** is a recognition or certification that an entity meets specific performance standards. For example, accreditation of a vocational college that offers a coding program demonstrates that the program is rigorous, meets all standards, and has positive outcomes in terms of student success. Healthcare practices and facilities can be accredited by organizations such as the Accreditation Association for Ambulatory Health Care (AAAHC), the Joint Commission, or the NCQA. Accreditation of a healthcare facility indicates that the facility meets all standards and has consistently high performance scores.

Recognition as a Medical Home

A medical home is an important recognition for outpatient practices. As the name indicates, a **Patient Centered Medical Home (PCMH)** is centered in the patient's primary care office (such as a primary care physician), and acts as a home for all the healthcare services that the patient needs. This does not mean that it provides all the healthcare services that a patient might need, but instead helps to coordinate care between different healthcare providers and specialists, coordinate medical treatments and prescriptions, and communicate with the patient's insurance company about patient progress, preventive examinations and screenings, and other services. Performance measures are vital to the concept of the medical home, as a medical office attains a PCMH status by maintaining solid performance measurements and implementing office policies aimed at providing quality care to its patients.

Financial Incentives

Finally, performance measurement is important because of the connection between high (or low) performance scores and financial incentives (or penalties). Financial incentive programs provide bonus payments for healthcare entities that have high performance scores. For example, in the professional physician setting, there are two important programs.

- Merit-based Incentive Payment System (MIPS), which is a program that awards a positive payment adjustment (an incentive payment) to healthcare providers who demonstrate high performance in four categories: quality of care delivered, cost of care delivered, improvement activities, and advancing care information (QPP 2019).
- Alternative Payment Model (APM), which is an arrangement between the healthcare provider and insurance, so that practitioners who provide high-quality and cost-effective care can get added incentives for high-quality care provided to patients. APMs can focus on a specific medical condition, an episode of care, or a certain patient population in the healthcare practice (QPP 2017).

In the hospital setting, Medicare employs three separate programs that are designed to pay hospitals for high quality scores.

- The Hospital Readmissions Reduction Program focuses on reducing the number of readmissions for high-cost or high-volume procedures. Hospitals that reduce the number of readmissions for certain identified conditions or procedures (such as hip and knee replacements or coronary artery bypass graft surgery) are eligible for incentive payments (CMS 2019f).
- The Hospital Value-Based Purchasing (VBP) Program compares the performance measures for hospitals across the country and offers incentives on each hospital's performance (CMS 2019g).
- The Hospital-Acquired Condition Reduction Program reduces payments to hospitals with high rates of hospital-acquired conditions (HACs), such as catheter-induced urinary tract infections. This program is designed to encourage hospitals to improve patient safety during hospital stays by reducing the amount of infection or other adverse safety events acquired during the hospitalization period (CMS 2019h).

Some of these incentives can be quite lucrative, ranging in the hundreds of thousands of dollars, depending on the size of the healthcare facility, so they are a huge impetus for engaging in performance measurement and trying to achieve higher performance scores. On the other hand, if the facility engages in performance measurement and the scores are low, the healthcare facility may be penalized and ordered to pay a monetary penalty, or fine, due to their poor performance scores.

Case Study | Healthcare Billing Basics—ABNs

The following case study examines the relationship between a healthcare service and insurance benefits. The patient in this case scenario has traditional Medicare insurance, and the healthcare service provided is debridement of toenails, which is considered routine foot care. Debridement of toenails is a necessary part of healthcare services for patients with systemic conditions, such as diabetes and peripheral vascular disorders, that make it difficult for blood to flow to the lower extremities, especially the feet. In other words, only certain conditions (as identified by the patient's diagnosis codes) identify debridement of toenails by a healthcare provider as being medically necessary.

The patient in this case study has diabetes mellitus as well as onychomycosis of the toenails (toenail fungus), a condition that causes thickening and discoloration of the nails as well as other symptoms that make debridement necessary. Debridement is performed to remove excessive nail tissue and clean off dead debris from the nails. The patient's health insurance, Medicare, is very specific about exactly what signs, symptoms, or systemic conditions a patient must have in order to cover debridement of nails.

In the following case study, carefully review the healthcare encounter documentation as well as the Medicare coverage guidelines for routine foot care, which includes debridement. At the end of the case study, determine whether the foot care described in the healthcare encounter will be covered by Medicare according to the guidelines provided.

PATIENT: Jeff Saunders   **DOB:** 06/23/1932

DATE OF SERVICE: 9/28/20xx

REASON FOR VISIT: Patient complains of thickened, discolored toenails. Requesting foot care.

HISTORY OF PRESENT ILLNESS:
Patient presents with diabetes mellitus, type 2, which he has had for the last 20 years, as well as onychomycosis of the toenails, which he has had for the last 2 years. He is requesting debridement of his toenails at today's clinic.

PHYSICAL EXAMINATION:
General inspection of the skin showed: Dry skin with skin discoloration
Palpation of the skin showed: Decreased skin turgor
Toenail examination: All of the toenails were elongated, hypertrophied (thickened), discolored, and showed to have subungual debris. Both of the first great toenails were ingrown and tender to the touch.
Vascular examination: Posterior tibialis pulse right 1+, left 1+. Dorsalis pedis pulse right 1+, left 1+. Decreased hair growth of the right leg. Decreased hair growth of the left leg.
Mental status: The patient was oriented to person, place, and time.
Sensory examination: Decreased response to light touch, decreased response to vibration.
Coordination: The patient's balance was impaired.
Mobility: Normal gait. Patient noted to have limitations in mobility including the use of a cane. Partial weight-bearing status on the right. Partial weight-bearing status on the left.
Left foot examination: Tenderness upon palpitation of the great toe.
Right foot examination: Tenderness upon palpitation of the left toe.

ASSESSMENT:
Onychomycosis of multiple toenails with type 2 diabetes mellitus

PLAN:
Nail debridement today. The toenails were debrided without incident. Abrasive dremel was used to smooth toenails. Feet and toes were cleansed with alcohol solution. More than 6 nails were debrided. We discussed that his diagnosis will qualify for coverage of routine foot care. I referred him to our nail clinic where he can make an appointment at his earliest convenience.

<u>ABN</u>: Patient signed the advance beneficiary notice of noncoverage. He knows that if Medicare doesn't cover the service then he will be responsible for the charges.

SIGNED: Dr. Ivan Foote, MD

Using the routine foot care coverage information provided, determine whether the patient's care qualifies for coverage under the patient's insurance plan.

Routine Foot Care General Information
Routine foot care is not a covered benefit. Medicare assumes that the patient or caregiver can perform the services related to routine foot care, and therefore these services are excluded from coverage, with certain exceptions. See the following guidelines for coverage of routine foot care.

Routine foot care is defined as:

- Cutting or removing corns and/or calluses
- Trimming, cutting, clipping, or debridement of nails
- Hygienic and preventive maintenance of nails, including:
  o Cleaning and soaking feet
  o Using skin creams or moisturizers
  o Any other routine service performed.

Exceptions
Medicare allows exceptions to this exclusion when medical conditions exist that place the beneficiary at increased risk of infection and/or injury if the service were not performed by a medical professional.

Systemic Conditions
The presence of a systemic condition, such as diabetes mellitus or vascular disease, may result in severe circulatory embarrassment or areas of diminished sensation in the individual's legs and/or feet. In these instances, certain foot care services that would otherwise be considered routine may pose a threat when performed by a non-healthcare practitioner.

Class Findings
Routine foot care may be covered when "class findings" related to one or more of the patient's systemic conditions are documented. Documentation must include clear evidence of one of the following:

- One (1) Class A finding
- Two (2) Class B findings
- One (1) Class B and two (2) Class C findings

Class A Finding
Nontraumatic amputation of foot or integral skeletal portion thereof

Class B Findings

- Absent posterior tibial pulse
- Absent dorsalis pedis pulse
- Advanced trophic changes (at least three of the following):
    - Decrease or absence of hair growth in the extremities
    - Nail thickening (hypertrophy)
    - Skin discoloration
    - Thin and shiny skin texture
    - Rubor or redness of skin

Class C Findings

- Claudication
- Temperature changes (cold feet)
- Edema
- Paresthesia (abnormal spontaneous sensations in feet)
- Burning

Guidelines/Instructions

Submit modifier GA when there is a valid ABN on file for the service. Modifier GA should be used when the service was performed but does not meet class findings. In this case, obtain an ABN from the patient and append modifier GA to the code for the procedure. GA may not be submitted when services are statutorily excluded. Submit modifier GY with items of services that are statutorily excluded or that do not meet the definition of any Medicare benefit. You my offer the beneficiary a CMS ABN.

Use the following steps to review the patient's healthcare encounter and benefits to determine whether Medicare will cover the nail debridement.

1. Read through the healthcare encounter in full. Pay special attention to the Physical Examination and Plan sections, which identify details of the patient's condition and describe the procedure he undergoes.
2. Review the routine foot care guidelines in full. Pay special attention to the Systemic Conditions and Class Findings sections, which identify when routine foot care may be considered a covered benefit.
3. After reading both sections of the case study, determine whether the procedure will be covered by the patient's insurance by comparing the coverage requirements to the healthcare encounter:
    a. The coverage guidelines specify that if the patient has a systemic condition such as diabetes or a vascular condition then routine foot care may be covered. Does the patient have a systemic condition? If yes, what is the condition?
    b. Review the healthcare encounter documentation to determine whether the patient meets any of the class findings:
        i. Does the patient meet any Class A findings?
        ii. Does the patient meet any Class B findings? If so, how many? (The patient must meet at least three of the class findings in order to qualify for coverage.)
        iii. Does the patient meet any Class C findings?
    c. Based on the class findings, does the patient qualify for routine foot care (debridement) in this scenario?

Key to Success

Reviewing the coverage guidelines and the associated healthcare encounter in the case study illustrates how detail-oriented you must be in order to correctly determine benefits. The details explaining coverage requirements, medical conditions, procedures performed, and ultimately whether or not a service may be covered by an insurance plan are often in the fine print. As a medical coder, these details are a vital component of your job! Make it a habit to read the fine print and pay attention to these tiny details for both healthcare billing and healthcare coding scenarios.

4. According to the guidelines for coverage, the patient must meet the two requirements—a systemic condition as well as class findings. Does the patient meet both of these requirements? If so, the service will be covered by Medicare. If not, the service is expected not to be covered by Medicare. Is the service expected to be covered by Medicare based on the above?

5. According to the coverage guidelines, if the service is expected *not* to be covered by Medicare, what should you do?

End-of-Chapter Content

Instructions: Indicate whether the following statements are true or false (T or F). For false statements, rewrite the statement on the line below to make the statement true.

1. HIPAA made sweeping changes to the healthcare industry by introducing performance measurement.

_____

_____

2. PHI stands for private healthcare information.

_____

_____

3. The minimum necessary standard dictates that only the minimum necessary amount of PHI should be shared when a release of PHI is warranted.

_____

_____

4. Risk adjustment evaluates the likelihood that a security breach might happen.

_____

_____

(Continued on next page)

(Continued)

5. Reimbursement, otherwise known as payment, is the money that a provider receives for healthcare services.

_____

_____

6. The CMS-1500 claim form is used for billing services performed in the outpatient setting for professional services.

_____

_____

7. A health insurance company is also referred to as a third-party payer.

_____

_____

8. Insurance premiums are the payments that are sent to healthcare providers for services rendered.

_____

_____

9. Commercial insurance policies are run by for-profit companies.

_____

_____

10. In an employer-sponsored insurance plan, the employers pay the entire premium amount for the patient.

_____

_____

Instructions: Choose the best answer.

1. Which of the following is a covered entity under HIPAA?
   a. Healthcare provider
   b. Healthcare billing company
   c. Patient
   d. Lawyer

2. Which HIPAA rule sets national standards for the protection of PHI?
   a. Security Rule
   b. Privacy Rule
   c. PHI Rule
   d. Encryption Rule

3. What is the name of the document that informs patients about their privacy rights under HIPAA?
   a. HIPAA Confidentiality Agreement
   b. Privacy Agreement
   c. Covered Entity Notice
   d. Notice of Privacy Practices

4. Which HIPAA rule contains provisions that cover compliance to HIPAA rules and regulations, investigations into breaches in privacy, and the imposition of monetary penalties?
   a. Privacy Rule
   b. Security Rule
   c. Enforcement Rule
   d. HIPAA Confidentiality Agreement

5. Which of the following would be used to bill an insurance company for services that were performed in the inpatient facility setting?

    a. CMS-1500 claim form
    b. UB-04 claim form
    c. NUCC claim form
    d. CMS claim form

6. How many individual diagnoses can be entered on a single CMS-1500 claim form?

    a. 12
    b. 16
    c. 4
    d. 8

7. If a service is specifically excluded from coverage in an insurance policy, who must pay for the healthcare service if it is provided?

    a. The healthcare provider
    b. The insurance company
    c. The patient
    d. The service is provided free of charge.

8. Which of the following patient out-of-pocket expenses is a percentage of allowable amount?

    a. Copayment
    b. Deductible
    c. Coinsurance
    d. Noncovered service

9. Which of the following government-sponsored health insurance plans covers individuals who are elderly or disabled?

    a. Medicare
    b. Medicaid
    c. Entitlement health insurance
    d. TRICARE

10. Which of the following is an example of nontraditional insurance?

    a. TRICARE
    b. Commercial Blue Cross Blue Shield policy
    c. Automobile insurance
    d. Medicaid

11. Which of the following types of reimbursement pays a per member per month amount?

    a. Fee-for-service
    b. Capitation
    c. Prospective payment system
    d. Risk adjustment

12. Which of the following is an insurance process that analyzes their patient pool in terms of health risk and how likely those patients are to incur expensive treatments for the coming year?

    a. Risk adjustment
    b. Risk analysis
    c. Performance measurement
    d. Quality improvement

13. What is the process of analyzing data to determine the quality of care that a healthcare practice or facility is delivering?

    a. HCC coding
    b. Performance measurement
    c. Risk adjustment
    d. Risk analysis

14. Which of the following refers to the act of quantifying data and analyzing it to categorize and extract patterns?

    a. Data referrals
    b. Prior authorization requests
    c. Data analytics
    d. Risk analysis

15. If a healthcare practice or facility receives high performance scores, which of the following might happen?

    a. They might receive financial incentives.
    b. They might receive financial penalties or fines.
    c. They may have to increase their efforts at quality improvement.
    d. They might have to begin seeing fewer patients.

References

45 CFR 164.304: Definitions.

Aflac. 2019. Aflac Accident Insurance. https://www.aflac.com/individuals/products/accident-insurance.aspx.

America's Health Insurance Plans (AHIP). 2016. The Medicare Advantage Risk Adjustment System: What It Is and Why It's Important. https://www.ahip.org/wp-content/uploads/2016/04/Risk-Adjustment-Why-is-it-important.pdf.

Centers for Medicare and Medicaid Services (CMS). 2019a. CMS 1500. https://www.cms.gov/Medicare/CMS-Forms/CMS-Forms/CMS-Forms-Items/CMS1188854.html.

Centers for Medicare and Medicaid Services (CMS). 2019b. CMS 1450. https://www.cms.gov/Medicare/CMS-Forms/CMS-Forms/CMS-Forms-Items/CMS1196256.html.

Centers for Medicare and Medicaid Services (CMS). 2019c. Medicare Program-General Information. https://www.cms.gov/Medicare/Medicare-General-Information/MedicareGenInfo/index.html.

Centers for Medicare and Medicaid Services (CMS). 2019d. FFS ABN. https://www.cms.gov/medicare/medicare-general-information/bni/abn.html.

Centers for Medicare and Medicaid Services (CMS). 2019e. Shared Savings Program: For Providers. https://www.cms.gov/Medicare/Medicare-Fee-for-Service-Payment/sharedsavingsprogram/for-providers.

Centers for Medicare and Medicaid Services (CMS). 2019f. Readmissions Reduction Program (HRRP). https://www.cms.gov/Medicare/Medicare-Fee-for-Service-Payment/AcuteInpatientPPS/Readmissions-Reduction-Program.

Centers for Medicare and Medicaid Services (CMS). 2019g. The Hospital Value-Based Purchasing (VBP) Program. https://www.cms.gov/Medicare/Quality-Initiatives-Patient-Assessment-Instruments/Value-Based-Programs/HVBP/Hospital-Value-Based-Purchasing.

Centers for Medicare and Medicaid Services (CMS). 2019h. Hospital-Acquired Condition Reduction Program (HACRP). https://www.cms.gov/Medicare/Medicare-Fee-for-Service-Payment/AcuteInpatientPPS/HAC-Reduction-Program.html.

Centers for Medicare and Medicaid Services (CMS). 2012 (October). 2014 Clinical Quality Measures (CQMs) Pediatric Recommended Core Measures. https://www.cms.gov/Regulations-and-Guidance/Legislation/EHRIncentivePrograms/Downloads/2014_CQM_PrediatricRecommended_CoreSetTable.pdf.

Healthcare.gov. 2019. Preventive Health Services. https://www.healthcare.gov/coverage/preventive-care-benefits/.

Health Insurance Portability and Accountability Act of 1996. Public Law 104-191.

Medicaid.gov. 2019. Eligibility. https://www.medicaid.gov/medicaid/eligibility/index.html.

Medicare.gov. 2019a. What Part A & Part B Doesn't Cover. https://www.medicare.gov/what-medicare-covers/not-covered/item-and-services-not-covered-by-part-a-and-b.html.

Medicare.gov. 2019b. Improving Health Care Quality. https://www.medicare.gov/physiciancompare/#about/improvinghealthcarequality.

National Committee for Quality Assurance (NCQA). 2019. Comprehensive Diabetes Care. http://www.ncqa.org/report-cards/health-plans/state-of-health-care-quality/2016-table-of-contents/diabetes-care.

Office for Civil Rights (OCR). 2017. The HIPAA Enforcement Rule. https://www.hhs.gov/hipaa/for-professionals/special-topics/enforcement-rule/index.html.

Office for Civil Rights (OCR). 2013a. Summary of the HIPAA Privacy Rule. https://www.hhs.gov/hipaa/for-professionals/privacy/laws-regulations/index.html.

Office for Civil Rights (OCR). 2013b. Summary of the HIPAA Security Rule. https://www.hhs.gov/hipaa/for-professionals/security/laws-regulations/index.html.

Optum 360. 2016. The Three Keys to HCCs and Risk Adjustment. https://www.optum360coding.com/CodingCentralArticles/?id=1636.

Quality Payment Program (QPP). 2019. An Introduction to Group Participation in the Merit-based Incentive Payment System (MIPS) in 2019. https://qpp-cm-prod-content.s3.amazonaws.com/uploads/520/2019%20Group%20Participation%20Guide.pdf.

Quality Payment Program (QPP). 2017. Medicaid and the Quality Payment Program. https://qpp.cms.gov/docs/QPP_Medicaid_All_Payer_Fact_Sheet.pdf.

Texas Health and Human Services (Texas HHS). 2017. CHIP Children's Medicaid: Costs. https://chipmedicaid.org/en/Costs.

TRICARE. 2017. Cost and Fees Sheet. https://tricare.mil/~/media/Files/TRICARE/Publications/Misc/Costs_Sheet.pdf.

Resources

Centers for Medicare and Medicaid Services (CMS). 2019. http://www.cms.gov.

Centers for Medicare and Medicaid Services (CMS). 2019. Shared Savings Program. https://www.cms.gov/Medicare/Medicare-Fee-for-Service-Payment/sharedsavingsprogram/index.html?redirect=/sharedsavingsprogram/.

Centers for Medicare and Medicaid Services (CMS). 2018 (October). Medicare Learning Network: Medicare Advance Written Notices of Noncoverage. https://www.cms.gov/Outreach-and-Education/Medicare-Learning-Network-MLN/MLNProducts/downloads/abn_booklet_icn006266.pdf.

Health Resources and Services Administration (HRSA). 2011 (April). Performance Management and https://www.hrsa.gov/sites/default/files/quality/toolbox/508pdfs/performancemanagementandmeasurement.pdf.

Medicare.gov. 2019. What's Medicare Supplement Insurance (Medigap)? https://www.medicare.gov/supplement-other-insurance/medigap/whats-medigap.html.

National Quality Forum (NQF). 2019. Measuring Performance. http://www.qualityforum.org/Measuring_Performance/Measuring_Performance.aspx.

National Uniform Claim Committee (NUCC). 2019. http://www.nucc.org.

Solove, D. J. 2013 (April). HIPAA turns 10: Analyzing the past, present and future impact. *Journal of AHIMA* 84(4): 22–28. http://bok.ahima.org/doc?oid=106325#.WXXeLYgrI2w.

TRICARE. 2019. http://www.tricare.mil.

3

CHAPTER

Basics of Coding

Learning Objectives

- Identify the types of codes, including the history of the ICD, CPT, and HCPCS code sets, and explain their uses in the healthcare setting
- Analyze the additional uses of codes
- Discuss future coding developments
- Analyze the connection between code linkage and medical necessity and understand how to link codes on a healthcare claim
- Discuss healthcare coding guidelines

Key Terms

Clinical modification (CM)

Code linkage

Coding guidelines

Current Procedural Terminology (CPT)

Evaluation and management (E/M) service

HCPCS Level I codes

HCPCS Level II codes

Healthcare codes

Healthcare Common Procedure Coding System (HCPCS)

International Classification of Diseases (ICD)

International Classification of Diseases, Tenth Revision, Clinical Modification (ICD-10-CM)

International Classification of Diseases, Tenth Revision, Procedure Coding System (ICD-10-PCS)

International Classification of Diseases, Eleventh Revision (ICD-11)

International Classification of Diseases, Ninth Revision (ICD-9)

Legacy system

Medical necessity

Modifier

Procedural coding system (PCS)

Reportable diagnoses

Learning healthcare coding begins with learning the different types of codes, the settings in which they are used, and the many uses of codes. But knowing what a code is and what it is used for is not enough to be a proficient healthcare coding professional. Proficient coding involves understanding the guidelines that govern proper coding, and how to use them to correctly select, sequence, and report codes. Furthermore, it is also imperative to understand medical necessity, the connection between medical necessity and codes, and how to link the two together.

This chapter presents the basics of coding—explaining the different code sets, discussing the history and future of coding and the current uses of codes, examining and applying coding guidelines, and analyzing medical necessity and code linkage, including how to link codes on a claim to indicate medical necessity for the service provided.

What Are Healthcare Codes?

The implementation of HIPAA (discussed in chapter 2) required the Department of Health and Human Services (HHS) to adopt national standards for healthcare transactions, security, and code sets. Although healthcare codes had been used prior to the implementation of HIPAA, this requirement further imbedded the use of coding into the world of healthcare and reimbursement.

Healthcare codes are the numeric or alphanumeric translations of all the services, supplies, treatments, diagnoses, conditions, and other reasons for healthcare services. Envision all the different procedures, services, surgeries, therapies, treatments, and supplies that could be provided to a patient in a healthcare setting. Also consider all of the different diagnoses, problems, diseases, healthcare conditions, or other reasons why a patient may need a healthcare service. There are an infinite number of possible scenarios. Now imagine how difficult it would be to report all those scenarios to a third-party payer on a single sheet of paper, or in a single electronic file. This is where codes come into play. For example, instead of describing a patient's condition, the coder translates the condition (strep throat) into an ICD-10-CM diagnosis code (J02.0, Streptococcal pharyngitis), and enters the code on the healthcare claim.

Healthcare code sets are the tabulated listings of the diagnoses, procedures, diagnostic tests, and treatments, equipment, and supplies provided to patients in the healthcare setting. There are five code sets outlined in HIPAA regulations adopted for use by HHS. They include International Classification of Diseases (ICD), Healthcare Common Procedure Coding System (HCPCS), Current Procedural Terminology (CPT), Codes on Dental Procedures and Nomenclature (CDT), and National Drug Codes (NDC). For the purposes of healthcare coding, this textbook focuses on three code sets—ICD, CPT, and HCPCS. These three code sets are used in inpatient, outpatient, facility, and physician settings, as necessary. Each one of these codes are unique; they have a different format, number of characters or digits, and are either numeric (containing only numbers) or alphanumeric (containing both numbers and letters). Furthermore, each of these codes sets is used for a unique purpose.

International Classification of Diseases (ICD) Codes

The origins of tracking patient diagnoses can be traced back to 17th century London with the London Bills of Mortality, compiled by John Graunt, which attempted to classify all the causes of death and track childhood mortality rates. Beginning in 1837, William Farr continued to collect information on, and worked to secure internationally recognized classifications for, the causes of death. In 1893, a statistician named Jacques

Bertillon presented his Bertillon Classification of Causes of Death, which was adopted by the American Public Health Association in 1898 and recommended for use in Canada, Mexico, and the United States, with the additional recommendation that this data set be revised every 10 years (WHO 2017).

Over the next 75 years, this classification system was expanded and formalized to include not just causes of death but also causes of morbidity (sickness), combinations of illnesses and diseases, manifestations of diseases, and other reasons for healthcare encounters. The ninth revision of the International Classification of Diseases (ICD-9) was developed in October 1975 during the International Conference for the Ninth Revision of the International Classification of Diseases, assembled by the World Health Organization (WHO). This revision was divided into three different volumes and included detailed code descriptions with subclassifications and extended code structure. The ICD-9 code set was used in the United States from 1975 until the implementation of ICD-10 on October 1, 2015 (WHO 2017).

International Classification of Diseases (ICD) codes are now in their 10th revision, ICD-10. WHO developed the ICD-10 code set in 1993, which was revised for use in the United States through a development committee composed of CMS, the National Center for Healthcare Statistics (NCHS), the American Hospital Association (AHA), and the American Health Information Management Association (AHIMA). On October 1, 2015, the United States replaced the ICD-9 code set by implementing ICD-10, making it the last industrialized nation in the world to transition from ICD-9 to ICD-10.

The version of ICD-10 that is now used in the United States is different than what is used by other countries and was developed specifically to coordinate with data reporting requirements and to correspond with US clinical practices. It includes two major divisions: Clinical Modification (CM) and Procedural Coding System (PCS). ICD-10 **Clinical Modification (CM)** is the compilation of ICD-10 codes used to report diagnoses. ICD-10 **Procedural Coding System (PCS)** is the compilation of ICD-10 codes that are used to report hospital inpatient procedures. These two divisions are unique to the US version of ICD-10. No other country uses the PCS codes, as these codes are used specifically for billing purposes to identify the procedure(s) performed in the inpatient setting. These two divisions are used for different purposes and are published as two different coding manuals, each with a different organization and format.

The format and structure of the ICD-10-CM and PCS code books are discussed in chapter 4 (Learning the ICD-10-CM Code Book) and chapter 20 (Inpatient Hospital Services), respectively. Furthermore, specific ICD-10-CM diagnosis codes and coding guidelines are discussed throughout chapters 6 through 19. The following sections introduce ICD-10-CM and ICD-10-PCS coding, as well as ICD-9.

International Classification of Diseases, Tenth Revision, Clinical Modification (ICD-10-CM)

International Classification of Diseases, Tenth Revision, Clinical Modification (ICD-10-CM) codes are three- to seven-character alphanumeric codes that are used to identify a patient diagnosis or other reason for a healthcare encounter. For example, if a patient presented to a healthcare office and was diagnosed with a headache, an ICD-10-CM code for headache (R51, Headache) would be assigned on the claim. On the other hand, if the patient was not ill but presented to the office for a flu shot, then the ICD-10-CM code assigned on the claim would indicate that the patient presented for the administration of a vaccine (Z23, Encounter for immunization). It is very common that patients have more than one diagnosis or reason for a visit. In these cases, use of more than one code is allowed. Up to 12 unique ICD-10-CM codes are allowed per outpatient claim form (using the CMS-1500 claim form). If it is necessary to include more than 12 diagnosis codes on a claim, additional codes may be sent on additional claim forms (refer to chapter 2 for the discussion on the CMS-1500 claim form). Electronic billing systems may also have the capability to include additional diagnosis codes. In the hospital setting, over 20 diagnosis codes may be assigned on the UB-04 claim form.

An ICD-10-CM code must be assigned for every single patient for every single healthcare encounter. This is because ICD-10-CM codes represent the medical necessity for the service performed. As discussed in chapter 2 (Healthcare Billing Basics), **medical necessity** refers to the reason why a healthcare service or treatment is performed. The standards of medical necessity must be met in order for an insurance company to cover a healthcare service, so in order to be medically necessary a service must meet the accepted standards of medicine, and it must be used to prevent, treat, or diagnose an illness or injury, condition, or disease (or the symptoms thereof).

The link between ICD-10-CM codes and medical necessity is extremely important to understand, because if the diagnosis codes do not support the medical necessity for a procedure or service, insurance will not pay for it. In other words, the diagnosis code *is* the medical necessity for the service.

Key to Success

The patient's diagnosis should always identify the reason why the patient is receiving healthcare services. Without a diagnosis code to indicate that a service was medically necessary, health insurance will not reimburse the healthcare provider for the procedure.

More about medical necessity and its indications for any procedures performed or supplies given to the patient is discussed later in this chapter. The ICD-10-CM codes and code book are also discussed in detail in chapter 4.

International Classification of Diseases, Tenth Revision, Procedure Coding System (ICD-10-PCS)

The second division of the ICD-10 code set is known as ICD-10-PCS. **International Classification of Diseases, Tenth Revision, Procedure Coding System (ICD-10-PCS)** codes are seven-character alphanumeric codes that are used in hospital reporting to identify procedures that were performed in the hospital inpatient setting. As such, these codes are used only for facility billing. For example, if a patient received an appendectomy (removal of the appendix) in an inpatient hospital, the hospital would use a PCS appendectomy code to report that the patient had an appendectomy procedure performed during his or her stay. PCS codes may also be used in the outpatient hospital (facility) setting for statistical purposes.

Unlike ICD-10-CM codes, PCS codes do not identify any medical necessity for the service performed. PCS codes are used only to report actual procedures that were performed on patients, such as surgeries, deliveries, or radiologic examinations. However, procedures represented by PCS codes must still be supported with medical necessity, which means that both ICD-10-CM and PCS codes may be reported on the same claim. For example, the PCS code for a rhinoplasty (090K0ZZ, Alteration of Nasal Mucosa and Soft Tissue, Open Approach), would be reported in addition to the ICD-10-CM code that represent the medical necessity for the rhinoplasty (M95.0, Acquired deformity of nose).

Keep in mind that PCS codes are used only for inpatient facility billing purposes, such as inpatient hospital services. Because ICD-10-PCS codes are used primarily in the inpatient setting, this textbook focuses on them in chapter 20. The remaining chapters of this textbook discuss outpatient coding, which utilizes ICD-10-CM, CPT, and HCPCS codes.

Key to Success

Do not get confused by the differences between ICD-10-*CM* and ICD-10-*PCS* codes. CM stands for Clinical Modification, which is used for diagnostic coding. PCS stands for Procedural Coding System, which is the section of ICD-10 codes that represent procedures and other services performed. CM = diagnosis; PCS = procedure.

International Classification of Diseases, Ninth Revision (ICD-9)

International Classification of Diseases, Ninth Revision (ICD-9) codes are the International Classification of Diseases codes that were used prior to the implementation of ICD-10 codes. ICD-9 diagnosis codes were three- to five-digit numeric or alphanumeric codes that served essentially the same purpose as ICD-10-CM; they were used to report patient diagnoses or other reasons for a patient encounter. However, they were out of date clinically and allowed little room for critical elements in diagnosis reporting, such as the laterality of a condition (whether a condition occurred on the right, left, or on both sides of the body). Thus, the code set was changed to the more inclusive ICD-10 code set, which allowed for more detail regarding patient conditions. The codes were updated to include relevant clinical and encounter information as well as more functionality for reporting combinations of healthcare conditions.

The ICD-9 code set is no longer maintained by any governing committee, nor is it updated on an annual basis (as the other code sets are). However, even though ICD-9 codes are no longer mandated for use by CMS through HIPAA, this does not mean that they are irrelevant. While HIPAA-covered entities had to switch from the ICD-9 to ICD-10-CM code set on October 1, 2015, there are a few entities that did not have to make the change, such as automobile insurance carriers. In rare instances, ICD-9 codes may still be required to bill a nontraditional insurance claim. More importantly, because all HIPAA-covered entities used ICD-9 before October 1, 2015, old accounts receivable, collected and reported data, and patient records contain codes from ICD-9 rather than ICD-10-CM. Therefore, it is important to understand ICD-9 coding as a **legacy system**—an older and outdated coding system that has been replaced by a more clinically accurate, up-to-date coding system in ICD-10-CM.

Healthcare Common Procedure Coding System (HCPCS) Codes

Healthcare Common Procedure Coding System (HCPCS) codes have a shorter history than either ICD or CPT, but this does not mean that they are any less important. In the early 1980s, CMS developed a code set—HCPCS codes—for the purpose of identifying services, products, or supplies that were not included within the CPT code set. In 1983, CMS required that an HCPCS code be reported for reimbursement on Medicare claims (CMS 2019a). Although this standard set the requirement for Medicare claims only, third-party payers followed suit and HCPCS codes quickly became a standardized code set for all claims.

Figure 3.1. HCPCS code set divisions

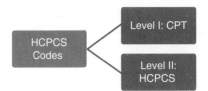

The adoption of HCPCS was due in part to the need for a standard code set to be recognized by all insurance payers, facilitating the submission of claims for reimbursement. The HCPCS code set included additional services and supplies that were not included in the CPT code set, such as durable medical equipment and medicinal agents administered in the health setting. However, HCPCS did not include all surgical and healthcare procedures and treatments that were included in the CPT code set. Because HCPCS is not as extensive as CPT, the CPT code set was adopted as part of HCPCS. Although CPT codes are developed and maintained as a separate code set by the AMA, they are still included within the HCPCS code set as a separated level of codes. This created two levels within the HCPCS code set: Level I and Level II codes (figure 3.1).

- **HCPCS Level I codes** (commonly referred to as CPT) are the CPT codes that are developed, maintained, and copyrighted by the AMA. They represent the healthcare procedure, treatment, or service provided at the healthcare encounter.
- **HCPCS Level II codes** (commonly referred to as HCPCS or Level II codes) are the HCPCS codes that are developed, maintained, and published by CMS. They represent the supply, service, or other treatment provided to the patient and include ambulance services (CMS 2019a).

Both Level I and Level II codes are used for professional reporting and reimbursement purposes. They are published in separate code books but may be used concurrently to bill for services provided. A single claim may include both CPT and HCPCS codes.

Key to Success

Although CPT (Level I) codes are technically part of the HCPCS code set, they are usually referred to simply as CPT codes. HCPCS codes, however, are still sometimes referred to as Level II codes. Remember, Level II codes are the same as HCPCS codes (see figure 3.1).

HCPCS Level I: Current Procedural Terminology (CPT) Codes

In 1965, the Health Care Financing Administration (HCFA), now known as CMS, passed Medicare and Medicaid (discussed in chapter 2), which made it necessary to implement a standardized system of reporting procedures for reimbursement. Before that time, most patients paid out of pocket for healthcare services and were later reimbursed by their insurance company. The passage of Medicaid and Medicare changed this dynamic, and it became necessary to create a standardized set of codes that could be used for billing purposes. HCFA appointed the American Medical Association (AMA) to create a set of codes for use in billing procedures, which became the Current Procedural Terminology code set first published in 1966. These codes have been updated annually since 1970 (Beck 2007). The current version, CPT-4, is still in use today and is referred to simply as CPT.

Current Procedural Terminology (CPT) codes are five-digit numeric or alphanumeric codes used to report procedures, treatments, and diagnostic and therapeutic services that were performed in the outpatient setting. Unlike the other code sets discussed in this textbook, which are in part developed by CMS, the CPT code set is developed, maintained, and copyrighted by the American Medical Association (AMA).

Similar to ICD-10-PCS codes in purpose, CPT codes are used to report the services provided to and the procedures performed on patients and are commonly used for reimbursement purposes. However, whereas ICD-10-PCS codes are used in the hospital inpatient setting, CPT codes are used in all outpatient settings and for reporting inpatient services performed by professional healthcare providers. For example, if a physician treated a fracture and placed a cast on a fractured arm, this service would be reported with a CPT code (24500, Closed treatment of humeral shaft fracture; without manipulation), and there would be a specific dollar amount charged for that specific CPT code (determined by the healthcare provider's office) that corresponds to the work, risk, and skill required to perform the service. In this way, healthcare providers can charge and get paid more for procedures that are riskier or require more skill, more overhead, or more work than they can for other procedures. For example, if a doctor performed a low-level sick visit that required 10 minutes of face-to-face time, he would charge less than if he performed a high-level face-to-face visit that required an hour of his time.

CPT codes encompass any type of procedure, treatment, diagnostic test, or other service that a healthcare provider could perform. These include office visits and evaluations, anesthesia services, surgical procedures, radiologic studies and treatments, laboratory and pathology procedures, and miscellaneous healthcare procedures such as hearing evaluations or chiropractic adjustments. Because they are reimbursed by insurance companies, medical necessity is required and indicated by an ICD-10-CM code placed on the same claim. Without an accompanying ICD-10-CM code to guarantee that the procedure was medically necessary, the service will not be reimbursed. For example, if an orthopedist manipulated a fracture and placed a cast on a patient's arm, he would include the CPT code for the procedure, attached to a charge for that specific procedure. He would also need to identify the medical necessity for the service by including an ICD-10-CM code for the diagnosis (fracture), indicating that the service was medically necessary. See figure 3.2 for an illustration of this example.

CPT codes may also be appended with a **modifier** that identifies any additional information regarding the service provided or modifies the code description. CPT modifiers are developed and maintained by the AMA and are published in an appendix

Figure 3.2. Comparison of medical necessity and medical procedure

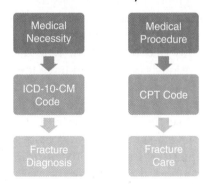

to the CPT code book. This appendix also lists a small number of HCPCS modifiers, published and maintained by CMS, that are also included in the HCPCS code book. Modifiers can alter the code description or provide more information regarding the service, and they typically impact payment of the codes themselves. For instance, modifier -53, Discontinued procedure, indicates that the service was discontinued. If this modifier is appended to (placed at the end of) a procedure code, this indicates that the procedure was discontinued and not completed in full. The payment for the procedure will likely be reduced, because the full procedure was not completed. For example, if a bronchoscopy were discontinued in the middle of the service because the patient went into respiratory distress, the CPT code for the bronchoscopy would be appended with modifier -53 to identify that the procedure was discontinued, and the resulting payment from the insurance company would be less than it would be for a fully completed procedure. On the other hand, modifier -22, Increased procedural services indicates that a procedure required more work, time, or effort to complete than is typically necessary. Returning to the previous example, if the bronchoscopy instead were especially difficult due to obstructions in the bronchi, the same bronchoscopy code would be assigned, but it would be appended with modifier -22 to identify that the procedure required increased work. In this case, the insurance would reimburse the provider at a higher rate than usual because the procedure was increased in terms of difficulty, time, or effort.

HCPCS Level II: HCPCS Codes

HCPCS codes are five-character alphanumeric codes that are used to report supplies, services, and miscellaneous procedures that are performed or provided in the outpatient setting and are not described by CPT codes. HCPCS codes are commonly used in conjunction with CPT codes and are accepted by all third-party payers.

The majority of HCPCS codes represent any additional supplies that may be used in the outpatient setting, or any supplies that may be provided to the patient for take-home use. For example, if a patient presented to the healthcare office and required a nebulizer breathing treatment, and the office provided the patient with a nebulizer machine, oxygen mask, and oxygen tubing, HCPCS codes would be used to identify these items, with an appropriate charge attached to each item. Services such as ambulance transportation, as well as drugs or other medications that are administered in the healthcare setting, are also included in the HCPCS code set. HCPCS codes are not required for every claim, but instead are only used when supplies and certain services are provided to the patient, as medically necessary. More about HCPCS coding and coding for supplies provided to the patient in the office setting is discussed in chapter 6 (Supplies and Services).

Like CPT codes, HCPCS codes must also be supported with a diagnosis code to identify the medical necessity for the service or item supplied to the patient. For example, if a patient were given a nebulizer machine in the office so they could continue breathing treatments at home, the diagnosis code included on the claim would have to indicate the medical necessity for the supply, such as asthma or pneumonia. For an ambulance service provided to a patient who had suffered a laceration in a work-related accident, the diagnosis code would have to identify the patient's injuries that required the ambulance transportation.

There are many codes within the HCPCS code set that are used specifically for Medicare beneficiaries. Because CMS maintains and develops the HCPCS Level II codes, many of these codes have been developed specifically for use on Medicare and Medicaid claims. For example, cervical and prostate cancer screenings provided to Medicare patients would be reported with the appropriate HCPCS codes, rather than the equivalent CPT code(s). Therefore, if services are provided to a Medicare patient, it is always necessary to check for the appropriate HCPCS code before using a CPT code. Refer to the discussion of billing considerations in chapter 2 to review the many ways in which a patient's insurance company impacts the codes that are reported.

Modifiers may also be appended to HCPCS codes to alter the meaning of the HCPCS supply or service. HCPCS modifiers are developed and maintained by CMS and are published in the HCPCS code book. They work in essentially the same way as CPT modifiers, by providing more information regarding a service or supply. For example, modifiers -AE, Registered dietician, and -AH, Clinical psychologist, identify the type of provider that provided the service; modifiers -T6, Right foot, second digit, and -LM, Left main coronary artery, identify the exact anatomical location of the procedure. Modifiers are always two characters, are either numeric or alphanumeric, and are always placed at the end of outpatient procedure codes (CPT or HCPCS). Modifiers are never used in conjunction with diagnosis codes (ICD-10-CM or ICD-9) or inpatient procedure codes (ICD-10-PCS).

Key to Success

Do not confuse ICD-10-PCS codes with CPT or HCPCS codes. PCS codes are used by a facility to identify the procedures that were performed on a patient and in the inpatient setting, and they are not attached to charges on claims. CPT and HCPCS codes, however, are attached to charges for procedures performed by individual healthcare professionals that may have been provided in an inpatient or outpatient setting, such as office or clinic visits, surgical procedures, or diagnostic studies.

Updates to the Code Sets

Each code set is updated at least on an annual basis. Every year it is necessary to purchase new code books, review changes to the codes and code guidelines, and update

Figure 3.3. Code updates schedule

CODE UPDATES

Code Type	Updated on
CPT	January 1st of each year
ICD-10 CM/PCS	October 1st of each year
HCPCS	Periodically, new manuals published on January 1st of each year

any coding strategies as necessary. Updates to the ICD-10 system are implemented on October 1st of every year, and updates to the CPT codes are implemented on January 1st of each year. Changes to the HCPCS code set are made on a quarterly basis (every three months), but new books are published only at the beginning of each year and are effective in January (see figure 3.3). HCPCS code changes are also published through CMS provider bulletins published on the CMS website when available.

Note that usually only a handful of changes are made to code sets each year, as necessitated by advancements in medicine, new clinical treatments, and changes in clinical discourse. Therefore, coding professionals do not have to learn all new codes every year. Instead, it is important to review new codes and code changes to make any necessary changes in daily coding practices and update healthcare practice management and EHR systems.

Putting the Codes Together

There are two categories of codes—diagnosis and procedure—to every claim, whether professional physician (submitted on the CMS-1500 claim form) or facility inpatient (submitted on the UB-04 claim form). The diagnosis codes (ICD-10-CM) identify the medical necessity for the procedure or supply provided (ICD-10-PCS, CPT, HCPCS). Both must be included on every claim sent (see figure 3.2). At minimum, one procedure code (either CPT or HCPCS) must be submitted with one diagnosis code

Figure 3.4. Healthcare codes and their uses

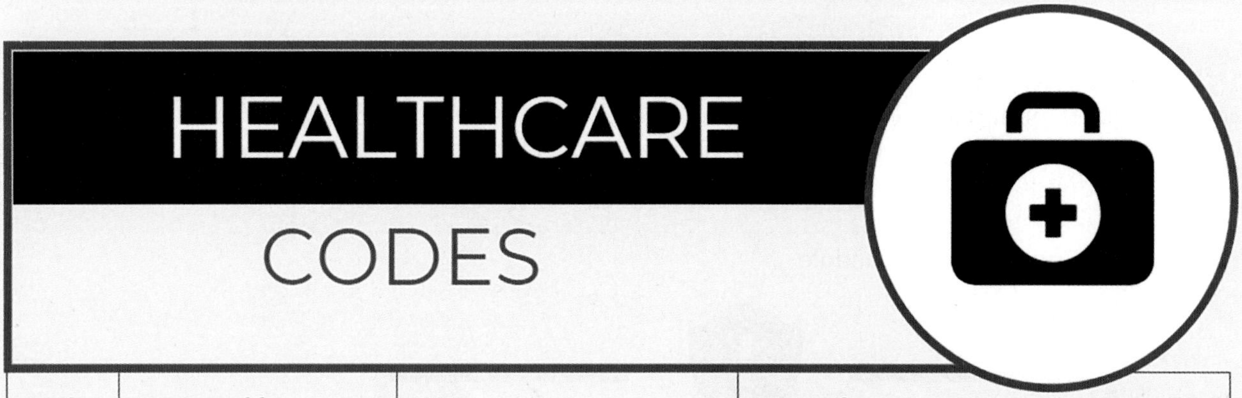

HEALTHCARE
CODES

Code	Reported by	Use	Example
ICD-10-CM	Facility and professional	Medical necessity	J03.90, Acute tonsillitis, unspecified
ICD-10-PCS	Facility (inpatient and outpatient)	Reporting procedures	0BDN0ZX, Extraction of Right Pleura, Open Approach, Diagnostic
CPT	Professional and outpatient facility	Reporting procedures, charging for services	33050, Resection of pericardial cyst or tumor
HCPCS	Professional and outpatient facility	Reporting procedures, charging for services	J1644, Injection, heparin sodium, per 1000 units

(ICD-10-CM) for professional or physician encounters. For facility or inpatient claims, at least one diagnosis code must be reported (ICD-10-CM) on each claim to identify why the patient was present in the inpatient setting. If a procedure was performed, then procedure (ICD-10-PCS) codes would be necessary to identify the service(s) rendered. It is important to understand that all of these codes are used in conjunction with one another and they cannot be separated. Refer to chapter 2 to review the CMS-1500 claim form; the UB-04 claim form is discussed in greater detail in chapter 20.

The majority of this textbook requires the learner to identify both the procedure codes (ICD-10-PCS, CPT, or HCPCS) and the diagnosis codes (ICD-10-CM or ICD-9) for practice exercises, as would be required in a real-world setting. Although this approach is more challenging at first—especially when learning how to use each of the code sets and without having experience in coding—it is ultimately more representative of the actual job of a coder. Examine figure 3.4 to review the types of codes and their uses.

Distinguishing between Diagnoses and Procedures

ICD-10-CM codes are used to identify the reason why a patient received healthcare services, which is usually some sort of medical diagnosis. CPT codes are used to report the procedures, services, or treatments that were performed by the healthcare provider. It is easy for beginning coders to get confused when learning about procedural coding, especially when trying to keep procedural coding and diagnostic coding separate. Procedures are the *verbs*; that is, a procedure is what the healthcare provider *did* to the patient. Diagnoses are the reasons *why* those procedures were performed. If confused, it can be helpful to ask the following questions, especially when coding for complicated procedures.

What did the doctor do? = Procedure code (CPT)

Why did the doctor do it? = Diagnosis code (ICD-10-CM)

It is important to clearly understand this distinction before moving forward with coding. Read the following vignette for help understanding the differences between diagnostic and procedural coding.

Rudy is a beginning coding professional and is having a hard time learning the differences between diagnostic and procedural coding. She knows that diagnosis codes are ICD-10-CM codes and that procedure codes are CPT codes, but she is still having problems understanding the two when she is faced with complicated healthcare documentation. She is currently working on a health record for a patient who came in for a diagnostic colonoscopy. During the colonoscopy, the doctor encountered a number of small polyps in the sigmoid colon. The doctor then did a biopsy of three of the polyps during the colonoscopy.

Before Rudy starts coding for this service, she must have a good understanding of all components of this healthcare service. She first looks up all of the terms that she doesn't understand in her medical dictionary and other resources. For example, although Rudy does know what a colonoscopy is, she isn't sure what a polyp is; she also is unsure if she understands exactly what a biopsy is, so she looks up these two terms in her medical dictionary. As she learns more about the procedure and medical diagnosis, she underlines important terms and took notes in the margins of her books to remember these components.

Now that she fully understands the healthcare service described in the documentation, Rudy must code for both the diagnosis and the procedure on the claim, but she is having difficulty starting. Her coding supervisor suggested that, to help, she ask herself the following questions: What did the doctor do, and why did the doctor do it? The answers to these questions will help her abstract the documentation and differentiate between the diagnosis and the procedure, which she can then look up in her code books.

First, she asks herself: What did the doctor do? Searching through the documentation, she pulls out the word that identifies the procedure—colonoscopy. The doctor also did a biopsy because he found multiple polyps during the colonoscopy, so the procedure was a colonoscopy with biopsy of three polyps. Note that in order to describe the full procedure, Rudy had to read through the entire description and put the two actions together— colonoscopy and biopsy—which came out to be a colonoscopy with biopsy of three polyps.

Now that she has the procedure, Rudy asks herself the next question: Why did the doctor do it? In this case, the patient came in for a diagnostic colonoscopy, during which the doctor found multiple polyps and performed a biopsy. So, in this case, the reason why the doctor did the colonoscopy with the biopsy was because of the polyps.

Now that Rudy has her answers, she can begin to search for the codes in the code books. She knows that the procedure was a colonoscopy with biopsy of three polyps, which she will look up in the CPT code book; and the diagnosis was polyps of the sigmoid colon, which she will look up in the ICD-10-CM code book.

What did the doctor do? **Colonoscopy with biopsy of three polyps**
Why did the doctor do it? **Polyps in the sigmoid colon**

Complete the exercises in There's a Code for That 3.1 to practice asking and answering these two questions.

3.1

There's a Code for That

Determining the procedure versus the diagnosis

Using the two questions *what did the doctor do?* and *why did the doctor do it?*, identify the procedures and diagnoses from the following statements. (Only identify the diagnosis and procedure; do not look up the codes for either.)

1. A patient presented to the office of his psychiatrist to begin treatment for depression. After psychoanalysis and a physical examination, his psychiatrist prescribed an antidepressant.

   Procedure: _____

   Diagnosis: _____

2. A patient presented to the emergency room complaining of severe abdominal pain, fever, and vomiting. After evaluation, it is determined that she has a ruptured appendix. She is rushed into emergency appendectomy surgery to remove the ruptured appendix.

   Procedure: _____

   Diagnosis: _____

3. A 15-year-old male presented to the office of his PCP for a refill of his asthma prescription. After brief evaluation and management service, the physician assistant refilled his asthma prescription.

   Procedure: _____

   Diagnosis: _____

4. A 15-year-old male presented to the office of his PCP with wheezing and trouble breathing due to his asthma. After an extended evaluation and management service and a nebulizer breathing treatment, the physician diagnosed the patient with asthma with acute exacerbation (asthma attack), and prescribed a rescue inhaler.

   Procedure: _____

   Diagnosis: _____

5. A 45-year-old patient with suspected pneumonia received a chest x-ray. X-ray confirms pneumonia in the lower left lobe of the lung.

   Procedure: _____

   Diagnosis: _____

In addition to reporting diagnoses and procedures, codes have multiple other uses. From risk adjustment to performance measures (discussed in chapter 2), as the uses of codes become more varied, job opportunities for coding professionals increase and become more diverse.

Additional Uses of Healthcare Codes

In addition to identifying the medical necessity for a service or identifying the procedure performed or supply provided, there are numerous other uses of codes. These range from simple internal tracking to nationwide (and international) reporting of diseases. They include the following.

- *Public health and tracking of disease.* The billions of diagnoses reported by health providers each year are tracked and analyzed by official organizations, such as the Centers for Disease Control (CDC). This information is used for public health purposes (CDC 2015). For example, if the CDC notes an increase in the incidence of certain sexually transmitted diseases, it might fund more research into effective reduction and treatment strategies, including public health campaigns that inform the public about the dangers of unprotected sex. Healthcare conditions are also tracked in the same way on an international scale. For example, worldwide health issues like pandemics or epidemics are tracked via codes. **Reportable diagnoses** are diseases or medical conditions that are important to public health (MedlinePlus 2019). When a healthcare office receives a positive result for a reportable diagnosis, it must report this positive result to the necessary state or federal agency. For example, a positive tuberculosis result must be reported to the appropriate official agency so that the government can track any potential outbreak of tuberculosis and any other preventable activities (CDC 2010).

- *Internal tracking.* Codes are used internally by both large and small healthcare practices and facilities to evaluate their own patient population and treatment. For example, if a small healthcare practice is about to order their supply of the influenza vaccine for the coming flu shot season, they might analyze how many influenza vaccines were given in the previous year to estimate how many vaccines they may have to administer during this flu shot season. For a large healthcare practice, such as a hospital with thousands of healthcare providers, codes may be used to identify internal facility issues, such as the number of patients who acquire a urinary tract infection due to catheterizations.

- *Performance measurement and quality improvement.* Facilities also use the data generated from codes to track their performance on certain performance measures and implement quality improvement programs when necessary. In the CPT and HCPCS code sets, special codes may also be reported to track a healthcare clinic's performance and quality initiatives. For example, a radiologist may report a special code to identify that a patient receiving a mammogram has already been scheduled for her *next* mammogram, or that a neurologist determined that a head imaging study was not necessary to evaluate a patient's recurring migraines. These codes are tracked internally as well as reported to specific insurance carriers to identify that the healthcare office is providing quality care and engaging in proactive actions regarding the patient's healthcare. Refer to chapter 2 for a refresher on performance measurement and quality improvement.

- *Risk adjustment.* Risk adjustment and HCC coding (also discussed in chapter 2) are important to many practices and facilities, the data for which is calculated from patient diagnosis codes. HCC coding is an increasing area of concern for many healthcare providers and can impact the bottom line for both insurance companies and individual practices.

Key to Success

As the healthcare market evolves from fee-for-service reimbursement to risk adjustment plans, HCC coding is set to become more important for beginning coders. The risk adjustment world is very compliance-oriented. Therefore, coding professionals must be knowledgeable about coding guidelines and insurance rules and regulations. They must also be detail-oriented and proficient in abstracting documentation from health records. Some healthcare clinics have a combination of both risk adjustment and fee-for-service plans, so it is also important that coding professionals be flexible in their coding abilities.

- *Research and funding.* The information compiled from the analysis of codes is also used in research and funding. If a certain type of cancer is becoming more prevalent, for example, additional research or funding may be allocated toward that specific type of cancer, its causes, and its treatment. This is an important use of codes, as it helps identify future public health needs as well as the efficacy of healthcare treatments. Remember also that insurance plans may use previous years' HCC codes and risk adjustment scores to determine the level of funding to allocate to a specific patient population over the course of the coming year.

- *Evaluate the utilization of healthcare facilities.* The use of procedure codes can help support decisions for new healthcare equipment or other utilization of healthcare facilities. For example, procedure codes may be used to track the number of patients whose operations used robotic assistance or those who received care in a pediatric critical care unit. If a large hospital facility purchases a $250,000 full-body x-ray machine, facility leadership can evaluate how many patients are served using that machine to help justify the cost. On the other hand, utilization tracking might result in the closure of a certain area of the hospital or specialized service that costs more to operate than it generates.

Codes have been in use for over 100 years, and their usage has evolved to a multifaceted approach to analyzing, predicting, and tracking healthcare conditions, procedures, and facility usage, as well as charging for services provided and analyzing funding for a year's worth of services from an insurance perspective.

The Future of Healthcare Coding

The healthcare industry changes rapidly, and just as codes have evolved over the last 100 years, they will continue to evolve into new forms with new uses and new meanings. It is therefore important to briefly look into the future of coding to see what may lie on the horizon.

WHO released the ICD-10 code set in 1993, and while the United States transitioned to ICD-10 as recently as 2015, a completely new, updated diagnosis coding system has already been developed. The **International Classification of Diseases, 11th revision (ICD-11)**, was developed and completed by WHO in 2018 (WHO 2019). ICD-11 will be systematically implemented throughout the world just as ICD-10 was; however, the timeframe for adoption and implementation of the ICD-11 code set is dependent on each country adopting it.

As part of the natural progression of diagnosis codes and the conditions they represent, the ICD code set was revised from ICD-10 to ICD-11 to better reflect progress in healthcare practice and clinical study, as well as to be used with electronic practice management systems and health applications. Some of the features included within the ICD-11 codes, which are either completely new or build upon the foundations of ICD-10, are as follows:

- Available in multiple languages
- Enables collaboration and revision by peers and interested parties to ensure accuracy and relevance
- Structured in such a way that definitions, signs, symptoms, and other related information may be recorded more accurately
- Compatible with electronic health record systems (WHO 2015)

It is important to understand that the ICD-11 code set was finalized and released in 2018. However, it is unlikely that the United States will adopt the ICD-11 codes any time soon. It took more than 20 years after its release for the United States to transition from ICD-9 to the ICD-10 code set, so any update to ICD-11 will likely happen years in the future (Butler 2018).

Code Linkage and Medical Necessity

This chapter has previously discussed medical necessity, but it is essential to go one step further and detail how to identify the medical necessity for specific procedures by linking them together. This is called code linkage.

As previously discussed, medical necessity is indicated using ICD-10-CM codes that identify and justify the reason why a procedure was performed. In other words, the diagnosis code must match the procedure and indicate that the procedure was necessary for medical reasons. If the codes do not match (that is, if there is no evidence of medical necessity for the procedure provided), then the procedure performed may be considered not medically necessary, and thus may not be reimbursed by the third-party payer.

Code linkage refers to linking diagnosis and procedure codes together to identify the medical necessity for specific procedures. Note that code linkage is necessary only for reported professional services provided by a qualified healthcare practitioner and reported on the CMS-1500 claim form. Inpatient facility claims billed on the UB-04 form do not utilize the code linkage concept. The concept of code linkage is especially important when claims have more than one procedure or diagnosis code. Consider the following example.

Dr. Alameda has just seen Benjamin for a sick visit encounter. He is an avid swimmer and has been experiencing severe ear pain for the last few days. During the encounter, Dr. Alameda diagnoses Benjamin with otitis externa (swimmer's ear) of the left ear and prescribes an antibiotic. She also notes a small common wart (verruca vulgaris) on the bottom of his left palm that has been causing him some discomfort. After obtaining approval from the patient, she freezes the wart (cryosurgery) and covers it with a bandage and tells Benjamin that the wart should fall off and he should return to the office if he has any further problems with it.

In this example, the patient has two diagnoses: left sided swimmer's ear (H60.332, Swimmer's ear, left ear), and verruca vulgaris (B07.9, Viral wart, unspecified). There were also two procedures performed: an office evaluation and management service to identify the encounter with the doctor (99213, Office or other outpatient visit, established patient, level 3), and the freezing of the wart (17000, Destruction, premalignant lesions; first lesion). An **evaluation and management (E/M)** service is a patient encounter with a healthcare professional in which the patient receives assessment, counseling, or routine health services. In other words, the healthcare provider evaluates the patient's healthcare needs or condition and then manages said needs or condition. E/M services, otherwise known as "patient encounters" or "office visits," are a common component of many healthcare services. Coding for E/M services is discussed in detail in chapter 7 (Behavioral Health Services) and chapter 8 (Primary Care Services) of this textbook.

In the previous example, two unrelated procedures were performed (an E/M service and the freezing of a wart) for two unrelated diagnoses (swimmer's ear and viral wart). Therefore, it is necessary to link each diagnosis code with the procedure code that it supports (code linkage). The diagnosis of swimmer's ear would be linked to the office E/M service, and the diagnosis of the wart would be linked to the cryosurgery for the removal of the wart. The linkage identifies the medical necessity for each service: the cryosurgery was performed because of the wart, and the office evaluation was performed because of the swimmer's ear (see figure 3.5). If the procedures and diagnoses were not linked correctly, the claim may be denied for lack of medical necessity.

A healthcare office links codes together with the same software it uses to report codes and send claims. Code linkage is done in different ways depending on the type of system used, but it typically involves identifying the specific diagnosis code(s) for each procedure. For example, if the swimmer's ear diagnosis were the first diagnosis on the claim, it would be assigned diagnosis number 1 or letter *A* on the CMS-1500 claim form. The wart diagnosis would be assigned as diagnosis number 2 or letter *B* on the CMS-1500 claim form. Because the office evaluation procedure code is listed as the primary procedure on the claim, it is linked to diagnosis A. The secondary procedure, the cryosurgery, would be linked to diagnosis B. Up to 12 individual ICD-10-CM diagnosis codes may be included on a CMS-1500 paper claim, and as many procedure codes as necessary are also included. Therefore, taking great care during the code linkage process is essential to ensuring accurate reimbursement for the procedures performed and all of the charges billed. Figures 3.5 and 3.6 illustrate the properly linked codes from the example.

Figure 3.5. Code linkage example

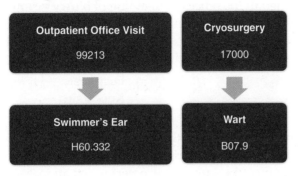

Figure 3.6. Code linkage

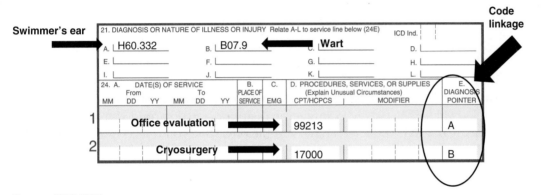

Source: CMS 2019b.

On the CMS-1500 claim form, it is easy to see the code linkage to ensure that all codes are linked properly. There are 12 lines on which to enter individual diagnosis codes (boxes 21.A through 21.L). The letter of the diagnosis corresponds to the procedure code it supports, as indicated in each line (lines 1 and 2). Box 24.E is the Diagnosis Pointer box, in which the letter of the diagnosis code is entered onto the line for the procedure to which it corresponds. In this example, diagnosis A for swimmer's ear is linked to procedure 1 for the E/M service, and diagnosis B for the wart is linked to procedure 2 for the cryosurgery.

Because each procedure provided or item supplied, whether inpatient or outpatient, must be linked to a diagnosis code to identify the medical necessity for the service, CPT and HCPCS codes should all be supported with corresponding ICD-10-CM codes.

Complete the exercises in There's a Code for That 3.2 to practice code linkage.

Code Linkage and Medical Necessity

3.2

There's a Code for That

Review the following scenarios and match the procedure(s) to the appropriate medical necessity for the procedure(s). Link the procedures and diagnoses by drawing a line from the procedure to the matching diagnosis. Note that some diagnoses may be used for multiple procedures, and vice-versa.

(Continued on next page)

3.2
Continued

1. A patient presented to the office complaining of blurry vision, and the provider completed a visual screening examination along with an E/M encounter. During the encounter, the patient also complained of pain in the left knee, and the physician performed an injection of the right knee joint.

Procedure:	Diagnosis:
Visual screening	Knee Pain
Joint injection	Blurry vision

2. A pregnant patient presenting to the office for a routine pregnancy checkup complained of an abscess on her right upper shoulder. The provider completed the routine pregnancy checkup and also performed an incision and drainage of the abscess.

Procedure:	Diagnosis:
Routine pregnancy checkup	Pregnancy
Incision and drainage of cyst	Abscess of right upper shoulder

3. A 15-year-old patient presented to the urgent care clinic after sustaining an injury during after-school football practice. The patient collided with another player on the field and suffered a 5-cm laceration of the right leg, which was sutured by the urgent care physician. The patient also complained of pain in the left ankle. After x-ray examination the physician determined that there was an acute fracture of the left ankle, and the physician completed fracture care with casting of the left ankle.

Procedure:	Diagnosis:
Suture of wound	Fracture of left ankle
X-ray examination	Laceration of right leg
Fracture care with casting	

4. A 78-year-old male with chronic obstructive pulmonary disease (COPD) and emphysema presented to the office of his PCP for a refill of his pulmonary medications. During the encounter, he complained of a quick-growing mole on his left torso. The physician completed an E/M office visit, determined that the mole was suspicious for malignancy, and performed a biopsy of the mole.

Procedure:	Diagnosis:
Evaluation and management office visit	COPD
Skin biopsy	Mole on left torso
	Emphysema

Besides knowing the different types of codes, the history of their development, and how to properly link them to indicate medical necessity, a coder must also know the rules for their usage. Rules that govern coding are called guidelines, and each set of codes has its own guidelines. It is important to be able to accurately locate, read, and use applicable guidelines to be a successful coding professional.

Coding Guidelines

Finding the correct code(s) is only one part of being a skilled coder. Coding professionals must also know how to report identified codes appropriately. There are several rules that help coders locate, select, and sequence codes. These rules, otherwise known as coding guidelines, specify which codes to use in given situations, how to sequence them, which modifiers to use, and how to combine them with other codes. Coding guidelines also may describe how specific details of the healthcare encounter need to be documented in order to warrant selection of specific codes.

Official coding guidelines exist for CPT codes as well as ICD-10-CM and ICD-10-PCS codes. Guidelines are published for reference on an annual basis with the code books. Depending on the publisher and the edition of the code book, official coding guidelines may or may not be included in the code book itself. Whether or not a code book actually contains guidelines or coding advice depends on both the publisher and edition of the code book. For example, the CPT Standard edition does not contain the same coding guidelines and advice as that of the CPT Professional edition, which contains additional guidelines, anatomical drawings, and notations throughout the book. Coding guidelines and where to find them are discussed in chapters 4, 5, and 20 of this textbook, with specific coding guidelines discussed contextually throughout.

Key to Success

Additional coding guidelines and resources to help interpret coding guidelines are available through other publications, such as *CPT Assistant* and the American Hospital Association (AHA) Coding Clinic. Professional organizations, such as AHIMA, also offer coding advice and interpretations of coding guidance for coding professionals.

The Importance of Documentation

The importance of accurate, appropriate documentation cannot be overstated. Not only does it provide the information to help substantiate a code but it is the record of everything that occurs in the healthcare setting. Without documentation to support code selection, it is not only impossible but unethical and illegal to select codes arbitrarily. Remember:

If it's not documented, it never happened!

Even if the patient came into the office with a certain condition and the physician performed several procedures, if that physician failed to document the encounter in the health record, then *it cannot be coded*.

Every code that is selected from a patient encounter must be substantiated by documentation in the health record. Being able to abstract encounter documentation is an important part of being able to code correctly and select diagnosis and procedure codes that are fully supported by documentation in the health record.

Key to Success

This textbook includes case studies from the real world that are designed to help you learn how to abstract documentation from healthcare encounters to identify healthcare codes. Although it may be difficult at first, this is the best way to learn what it takes to code from real healthcare encounters. Read through the instructions for each case study carefully, as they are designed to guide you through the process of abstracting health record documentation and, ultimately, selecting the correct code(s).

Healthcare coding professionals must first review the documentation, extract the necessary information, and select the right code(s), as supported by the documentation. Once the correct code(s) are selected, the coder must review any guidelines or other rules before sequencing the codes on the claim. They may also be required to ensure that the documentation includes the following required characteristics:

- *Complete:* Documentation for each encounter must be complete and signed by the healthcare provider. The healthcare provider's credential must also be clearly noted.

- *Detailed:* Documentation must include sufficient detail to support code selection. This textbook discusses the necessary details for code selection at length, but it is important to remember that all necessary details must be included in the provider's documentation in order to select a code. For example, the detail of laterality (on which side a condition occurred) must be included in the documentation if a coder is to select a diagnosis code that indicates the laterality.

- *Legible:* In the days of paper health records, legibility was a huge documentation burden. Now that the majority of healthcare providers have transitioned to electronic health records, legibility is not as big of an issue. However, if using paper records, all documentation must be fully legible. Illegible handwriting is just as bad as incomplete documentation and makes code selection impossible.

- *Contain all necessary patient identifiers:* Every component of the patient's health record (whether on paper or in electronic format) must contain at least two patient identifiers. Usually, the patient's name and date of birth are the easiest two patient identifiers to include on patient health records.

- *Formatted:* Specific encounter types are typically formatted into the same template. This eases code selection and facilitates understanding when reviewing the documentation of the healthcare encounter. Some examples of formatted records would be problem-oriented visit templates, vaccine administration records, surgical notation templates, anesthesia records, and laboratory results. Many of these templates and formats are illustrated in their respective sections throughout this textbook.

Not only does incomplete documentation cause problems logistically by not allowing for correct code selection, but it can also create problems in the long run in the case of audits or insurance chart reviews. Proper documentation, on the other hand, supports code selection, adheres to documentation standards, and allows a coder to most effectively utilize coding guidelines. For coding professionals interested in documentation improvement, AHIMA offers the certified documentation improvement practitioner (CDIP) certification (see appendix A, Coding Certifications and Professional Coding Organizations, in this textbook).

Guidelines for Code Sets

Each code set has its own unique set of guidelines, or rules, to help identify, select, and sequence the correct codes. In addition to official guidelines, many insurance plans provide specific guidance on how codes should be listed on claims. Coders may find that, even though the official coding guidelines offer one direction, an insurance company requires the coder to code something differently. For example, ICD-10-CM coding guidelines might require the coder to sequence a pain code after the code for the acute condition, whereas the insurance requires the acute condition to be placed before the pain code. This is a very common scenario. Ultimately, coding in the real world is more complicated than simply following the rules in a code book; however, as long as the coder does not code anything fraudulently, unethically, or for something that is not supported by the documentation, the best course of action is usually to code the encounter as indicated by the patient's health insurance. Nevertheless, it is advisable to follow the coding guidelines as best as possible in every situation. This is especially true in coding certification exams, which often specifically test a coding professional's ability to utilize the coding guidelines.

Key to Success

As a new coding professional, it is a good idea to purchase the best code books possible, or even additional specialty coding reference guides. When learning coding for the first time, or in your first position as a coder, purchasing high-quality manuals is a solid investment to help you in your journey to becoming an expert coding professional.

Specific coding guidelines are discussed throughout this textbook, when applicable. Additionally, how to locate and use the coding guidelines is discussed in chapter 4 and chapter 5. When coding throughout the rest of this textbook and in the real world, remember to use the coding guidelines—they are the rules that help you correctly select, sequence, and assign codes.

Key to Success

It is extremely important to understand the components of the code books you use, as each code book may differ or include different components, depending on the publisher. As you learn coding for the first time, remember that these code books are *yours* and should be used to enhance your understanding of coding. Don't be afraid to write, underline, and take notes in your code books, especially if it helps you understand how to use the code sets.

Case Study | Abstracting a Health Record

PATIENT: Eve Jeffers   **DOB:** 07/14/1962

DATE OF SERVICE: 04/07/20xx

TYPE OF SERVICE: OFFICE VISIT WITH X-RAYS

SUBJECTIVE:
Chief Complaint: Fall two days ago, bruise on left chest near pacemaker. Recent chest cold.

History of Present Illness: Patient fell on Saturday night as she was walking the dog. States that she felt lightheaded, grabbed a chair, and then fell, bumping her face and her upper left chest on the chair. She states that she now has a bruise over her left upper chest over the top of her pacemaker. She also states that as she fell she bumped her left pinky toe on the chair and it is now purple and swollen.

Review of Systems:
Constitutional: feeling poorly, no fever, no chills, and not feeling tired
Cardiovascular: no chest pain and no palpitations
Respiratory: no shortness of breath with cough
Gastrointestinal: no abdominal pain, no nausea, no constipation, no diarrhea, no heartburn, and no vomiting
Genitourinary: no dysuria
Musculoskeletal: no arthralgias
Neurological: dizziness, but no headache
Hematologic/lymphatic: a tendency for easy bruising

Past, Family, Social History:
Current medications reviewed. No known drug allergies (NKDA). Family history of diabetes mellitus.

OBJECTIVE:
Physical Examination:
Constitutional: alert and in no acute distress.
Neck: normal in appearance, supple; no jugular-venous distention. The thyroid was not enlarged.
Cardiovascular: edema was present on ankles. Heart rate and rhythm were normal and no acute murmurs. Heart tones are very distant; difficult to hear due to cough/congestion.
Pulmonary: normal respiratory rhythm and effort, no respiratory distress.
Musculoskeletal: normal gait. No apparent limitations in mobility.
Neurologic: motor exam was normal.
Skin: weathered skin.
Psychiatric: a decrease in concentrating ability was observed; but oriented to person, place, and time. Affect was normal and not pleasant.

ASSESSMENT and PLAN:

1. Acute upper respiratory infection (URI). Cough is likely associated with acute URI. Will need to re-evaluate with a spike in temperature or if breathing/cough gets worse. STAT chest x-ray done with no sign of pneumonia or heart failure.

2. Bruising. Bruising on chest over pacemaker site, resolving. Still tender to the touch. Chest x-ray confirms that pacemaker leads are intact and pacemaker battery pack is undamaged.

3. Fracture of 5th toe on right foot, initial encounter. Lower limb x-ray confirms fracture of 5th toe of the right foot. Completed fracture care with buddy strapping of toes.

SIGNED: Dr. D.K. Williams, MD

Determine the procedure(s) and diagnoses from the case study by answering the following questions. After you determine the procedure(s) and diagnoses, identify the medical necessity for the procedure(s) with code linkage.

1. Read through the case study in full. Pay attention to individual details in the documentation. Then answer the following question: *What did the doctor do?* List the procedures individually:

   a. _____

   b. _____

   c. _____

2. Now answer the question: *Why did the doctor do it?* List the diagnoses individually:

   a. _____

   b. _____

   c. _____

3. Now that you have the procedure(s) and all associated diagnoses, identify the medical necessity for the procedures by linking them with the diagnosis code(s). List the individual procedures and diagnoses, and link them by drawing a line from the procedure to the matching diagnosis.

   Procedure: **Diagnosis:**

   _____   _____

   _____   _____

   _____   _____

End-of-Chapter Content

Instructions: Indicate whether the following statements are true or false (T or F). For false statements, rewrite the statement on the line below to make the statement true.

1. HIPAA standardized the use of five different code sets.

   _____

   _____

2. Inpatient and outpatient coding consists of the three main code sets: ICD, CPT, and HCPCS.

   _____

   _____

(Continued on next page)

(Continued)

3. The two divisions of the ICD code set are CM and CPT.

_____

_____

4. The CM at the end of ICD-10-CM stands for classifications of morbidity.

_____

_____

5. For professional claims, medical necessity is identified by code linkage.

_____

_____

6. ICD-9 codes were implemented on October 1, 2015.

_____

_____

7. The CPT code set is published by CMS.

_____

_____

8. Codes may be used to evaluate the utilization of facility resources.

_____

_____

9. Procedural classifications were first developed in the 17th century.

_____

_____

10. HCPCS codes may also be referred to as Level II codes.

_____

_____

Instructions: Choose the best answer.

1. What are the alphanumeric translations of services, supplies, and diagnoses?
   a. Healthcare codes
   b. Healthcare transcriptions
   c. Translations of healthcare diagnoses
   d. International Classification of Diseases

2. Codes are either numeric or:
   a. Seven characters
   b. Alphanumeric
   c. Six digits
   d. They are only numeric

3. Which of the following ICD code set revisions is currently in use?
   a. ICD-9
   b. ICD-10
   c. ICD-11
   d. CPT-4

4. Which of the following code sets is used to report hospital or facility inpatient procedures?
   a. ICD-10-CM
   b. HCPCS
   c. CPT
   d. ICD-10-PCS

5. What is the reason why a healthcare procedure was performed?
   a. Medically unnecessary
   b. CPT codes
   c. Medical necessity
   d. Personal reasons

6. What is code linkage?
   a. Linking diagnosis codes with other diagnosis codes to identify medical necessity for a procedure
   b. Linking HCPCS codes with CPT codes to identify medical necessity for a procedure
   c. Linking ICD-10-PCS codes with HCPCS codes to identify the medical necessity for a procedure
   d. Linking ICD-10-CM codes with a procedure code to identify the medical necessity for the procedure

7. In which of the following situations might you use an ICD-9 code?
   a. For a claim with a date of service before 10/01/2015
   b. For a claim with a date of service after 10/01/2015
   c. For all claims no matter what the date of service
   d. For hospital inpatient claims only

8. Which of the following is a five-digit numeric code that is used to report procedures?
   a. ICD-10
   b. HCPCS
   c. CPT
   d. ICD-9

9. Which of the following code sets is used to report diagnoses or supplies rather than procedures?
   a. CPT
   b. ICD-10-CM
   c. ICD-10-PCS
   d. HCPCS

10. Which of the following code sets evolved over the course of hundreds of years and began as a registry system for the causes of mortality?
    a. ICD
    b. CPT
    c. HCPCS
    d. NDC

11. Which of the following are the two divisions of the ICD-10 code set?
    a. CM and CPT
    b. PCS and HCPCS
    c. PCS and CM
    d. CPT and PCS

12. The HCPCS code set is divided into two levels. Level II codes are commonly referred to as which of the following?
    a. HCPCS
    b. CPT
    c. ICD-10-PCS
    d. ICD-10-CM

13. What is linking the diagnosis and procedure code together called?

   a. Code necessity
   b. Medical necessity
   c. Code linkage
   d. Medical linkage

14. On the CMS-1500 form, in which box are the diagnosis pointers located?

   a. Box 24.A
   b. Box 21.E
   c. Box 24.E
   d. Box 24.D

15. Finish the following sentence: If it's not documented, it _____.

   a. Always happens
   b. Doesn't matter
   c. Can be coded
   d. Never happened

References

Beck, D. E. and D. A. Margolin. 2007 (Spring). Physician Coding and Reimbursement. *Ochsner J* 7(1): 8–15. https://www.ncbi.nlm.nih.gov/pmc/articles/PMC3096340/.

Butler, M. 2018 (June 21). World Health Organization Releases ICD-11. *Journal of AHIMA.* https://journal.ahima.org/2018/06/21/world-health-organization-releases-icd-11/.

Centers for Disease Control and Prevention (CDC). 2015 (November 6). International Classification of Diseases (ICD-10-CM/PCS) Transition–Background. https://www.cdc.gov/nchs/icd/icd10cm_pcs_background.htm.

Centers for Disease Control and Prevention (CDC). 2010 (October 8). Menu of Suggested Provisions for State Tuberculosis Prevention and Control Laws. https://www.cdc.gov/tb/programs/laws/menu/caseid.htm.

Centers for Medicare and Medicaid Services (CMS). 2019a (July 25). HCPCS - General Information. https://www.cms.gov/Medicare/Coding/MedHCPCSGenInfo/index.html?redirect=/medhcpcsgeninfo.

Centers for Medicare and Medicaid Services (CMS). 2019b. CMS 1500. https://www.cms.gov/Medicare/CMS-Forms/CMS-Forms/CMS-Forms-Items/CMS1188854.html.

MedlinePlus. 2019 (November 6). Reportable Diseases. https://medlineplus.gov/ency/article/001929.htm.

World Health Organization (WHO). 2019. ICD-11 for Mortality and Morbidity Statistics. https://icd.who.int/browse11/l-m/en.

World Health Organization (WHO). 2017. History of the Development of the ICD. http://www.who.int/classifications/icd/en/HistoryOfICD.pdf.

World Health Organization (WHO). 2015 (April 14). Report of ICD-11 Revision Review. https://www.who.int/classifications/icd/reportoftheicd11review14april2015.pdf?ua=1.

Resources

Centers for Medicare and Medicaid Services (CMS). 2019 (November 16). Code Sets Overview. https://www.cms.gov/Regulations-and-Guidance/Administrative-Simplification/Code-Sets/index.html.

National Center for Health Statistics (NCHS). 2019. International Classification of Diseases, Tenth Revision, Clinical Modification (ICD-10-CM). https://www.cdc.gov/nchs/icd/icd10cm.htm.

World Health Organization (WHO). 2019. Classifications. http://www.who.int/classifications/icd/en/.

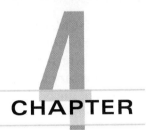

CHAPTER 4

Learning the ICD-10-CM Code Book

Learning Objectives

- Examine the organization, format, notations, and conventions used in the ICD-10-CM code book
- Recognize and utilize general coding guidelines for ICD-10-CM codes

- Examine the structure of ICD-10-CM codes

Key Terms

Accidental intent
Activity
Acute condition
Adverse effect
Assault
Benign neoplasm
Bilateral
Billable code
Carcinoma in situ
Chronic condition
Code first
Combination code
Cross-reference
Definitive diagnosis
Episode of care
Essential modifier
Etiology
Excludes notes
Excludes1
Excludes2
External cause codes
External Causes of Injury Index
First-listed diagnosis

Histologic type
Includes notes
Inclusion terms
Index to Diseases and Injury
Initial encounter
Injury mechanism
Intent
Intentional self-harm
Invalid code
Laterality
Main term
Malignant neoplasm
Manifestation
Metastasis
Morphology
Neoplasm
Neoplasm of uncertain behavior
Nonessential modifier
Not elsewhere classifiable (NEC)
Not otherwise specified (NOS)
Official Guidelines for Coding and Reporting (OGCR)
Patient status

Place of occurrence
Placeholder X
Primary neoplasm
Secondary neoplasm
See also
See condition
Sequela
Sequencing
Seventh character extension
Signs
Specificity
Subsequent encounter
Subterm
Symptoms
Table of Drugs and Chemicals
Table of Neoplasms
Tabular List
Toxic effect
Underdosing
Undetermined intent
Use additional code

Each of the codes sets—ICD-10-CM, CPT, HCPCS, and ICD-10-PCS—have a different intended use, format, and number of characters or digits. They are also published in separate code books, each of which has a different organization, conventions, and guidelines. Therefore, it is necessary to spend some time getting to know the varying code structures, organization of the book, and format and symbols used in each code book, as well as how to find and use the guidelines, and how to use each code book to identify and assign the appropriate codes. This chapter focuses on the many intricacies of the ICD-10-CM code book and code set, which is used for diagnostic coding. Chapter 5 (Learning the CPT and HCPCS Code Books) focuses on learning the procedural coding books. Because ICD-10-PCS coding is mostly used in the inpatient setting, the format of ICD-10-PCS codes and the organization of the PCS code book is discussed in chapter 20 (Inpatient Hospital Services).

ICD-10-CM Organization and Format

The ICD-10-CM code set is used to identify diagnoses and is a publicly available resource. Unlike CPT codes (discussed in detail in chapter 5), which are created, maintained, and copyrighted by the American Medical Association (AMA), ICD-10-CM codes may be compiled and published in a code book by any party. This means that ICD-10-CM code books vary greatly, depending on the publisher. However, even though certain ICD-10-CM code books may have more information such as guidelines, color-coding, or references, the ICD-10-CM codes and code descriptions are all the same, no matter the publisher. This ensures consistency and appropriate code selection across all ICD-10-CM code books. This textbook references the AHIMA *ICD-10-CM Code Book*.

ICD-10-CM codes are some of the longest healthcare codes and require a strict attention to detail, as each character added to the code identifies a specific detail about the patient's healthcare condition. It is important to always code to the highest level of specificity to ensure each and every detail of the patient's condition is reflected in the code.

The ICD-10-CM code book is divided into two major sections: the Index and the Tabular List. Each of these sections is further divided into additional subsections and chapters.

Key to Success

Before getting into specifics of the ICD-10-CM organization and format, if you are using a paper copy of the ICD-10-CM code book, look at the outer edge of the pages of the ICD-10-CM code book. Though it may vary by publisher, the majority of ICD-10-CM code books have a colored outer edge or indented tabs on the side of the page opposite the binding. These colors or tabs identify different sections of the ICD-10-CM book. As you learn how to use the ICD-10-CM code book, these colors or tabs can help you locate and access certain sections in the book. As you learn about the following sections of the code book, flip through these sections and examine their content, layout, and structure.

The Index

The Index to the ICD-10-CM code book is comprised of four different sections. Each of these sections is designed to allow coders to find the main term of the condition, disease, or other reason for a healthcare encounter, and to direct the coder to the code for that condition. For example, a coder seeking the code for pharyngitis (sore throat) can access the Index to find the term *pharyngitis*, which will direct him or her to the code J02.9, Acute pharyngitis, unspecified.

The four individual subsections of the Index each allow the user to look up different types of conditions or reasons for an encounter. These subsections are the Index to Diseases and Injury, the Table of Neoplasms, the Table of Drugs and Chemicals, and the External Cause of Injuries Index.

Key to Success

It is easy to get lost in the hundreds of pages of the ICD-10-CM code book. Because of this, the book commonly lists the condition, location, chapter, or other indicator either on the top corner of the page or on the outer colored edge on each page. Pay attention to these locator terms, as they will be very helpful in guiding you to the correct section of the ICD-10-CM code book.

Index to Diseases and Injury

The Index to Diseases and Injury (often referred to as the Main Index) is the primary index to the ICD-10-CM code book. This is the largest index of the ICD-10-CM code book and allows coders to look up any condition coded with an ICD-10-CM code in alphabetical order, with the exception of the majority of neoplasms, poisonings and adverse effects, and external causes.

When searching for a code using the Main Index, the first step is to find the main term for the condition, disease, or other reason for the encounter. Then check for cross-references, subterms, and nonessential modifiers. Finally, locate the code and verify it in the Tabular List (the alphanumerical listing of all ICD-10-CM codes, discussed as follows). The steps for using the Main Index are discussed in greater detail in the following sections of this chapter and are recapped in figure 4.1.

Find the Main Term

The coder first needs to locate the main term for the condition, disease, or other reason for the encounter. The **main term** is the noun that describes the patient's diagnosis or reason for encounter, such as the term *pharyngitis*. The main terms should be abstracted from the documentation for the encounter. To do this, the coding professional needs to carefully read through the provider's documentation of the encounter, abstract the diagnoses, conditions, or other reasons for the encounter, and then locate the codes for those reasons and assign them on the claim. The rest of the chapters in this textbook will guide the coder through this process until it becomes second nature. Once the main term is located in the Main Index, any cross-references, subterms, or nonessential modifiers must be checked before confirming code selection.

Check Cross-References, Subterms, and Modifiers

Once the main term is located in the Main Index, there may be a cross-reference that informs the coder to "*see* condition." A **cross-reference** instructs the coder to look elsewhere for a code. In this case the "*see* condition" cross reference tells the coder to search for the code by looking up the condition rather than the term he or she initially located. The "*see* condition" cross-reference is very common when looking up diagnoses that are located at specific anatomical sites. For example, Smith is a beginning coder

Figure 4.1. Steps to using the Index to Diseases and Injury (Main Index)

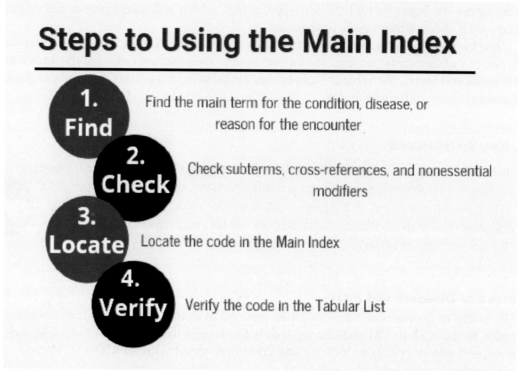

Steps to Using the Main Index

1. Find — Find the main term for the condition, disease, or reason for the encounter

2. Check — Check subterms, cross-references, and nonessential modifiers

3. Locate — Locate the code in the Main Index

4. Verify — Verify the code in the Tabular List

who needs to find the code for knee pain. Using the Index, Smith locates the term *knee* and notes that the term *knee pain* cannot be found; instead, there is a cross-reference that instructs him to "*see* condition." Instead of looking up the word *condition*, Smith must look up the condition of the knee; the knee is in pain, so Smith looks up the term *pain* and discovers that this entry also contains a cross-reference, which instructs the coder to "*see also* painful." The "*see also*" cross-reference instructs the coder to look elsewhere for a code if the precise condition cannot be found in the current index entry. In this case, Smith should *see also* painful if he cannot locate the code for knee pain within the *pain* entry in the Main Index (figures 4.2 and 4.3).

Figure 4.2. ICD-10-CM Main Index example 1

Example: *see* condition

Klumpke (-Déjerine) palsy, paralysis (birth) (newborn) P14.1
Knee —*see* condition
Knock knee (acquired) M21.06-
  congenital Q74.1

Example: *see also*

Pain(s) (*see also* Painful) R52
  abdominal R10.9
    colic R10.83
    generalized R10.84
      with acute abdomen R10.0

Source: Casto 2019, 207, 246.

Key to Success

Cross-references help the coder navigate the Main Index. Sometimes cross-references will have you flipping back and forth through the Main Index searching for a code. This may be frustrating, but don't give up! The more experience you gain from searching for codes, the more you will understand how to navigate through this section to quickly find the code you are looking for.

Figure 4.3. ICD-10-CM Main Index example 1

Example: subterm (essential modifier)

joint M25.50
    ankle M25.57-
    elbow M25.52-
    finger M25.54-
    foot M25.57-
    hand M25.54-
    hip M25.55-
    knee M25.56-
    shoulder M25.51-
    toe M25.57-
    wrist M25.53-

Source: Casto 2019, 247.

After Smith notes the cross-references, he notices there are many subterms under the main term *pain*. **Subterms** are indented under the main term to indicate that they pertain to the main term, and to identify variations of the main term. For example, there are many different types and sites of pain, so the subterms indented beneath the main entry *pain* describe various types or sites of pain. Smith notes that under the main term *pain*, there are quite a few columns of subterms. He searches for the subterm *knee* but notes that he cannot find it. In this case, he must first locate the term *joint*, and then find the specific joint *knee* as a subterm.

Key to Success

Sometimes the subterms are listed in a complex manner. When searching for a condition in which there are numerous subterms in the Main Index, it is a good idea to scan the entire list of subterms to understand how they are listed. When Smith was searching for this term, he had to navigate through multiple subterms, and subterms of subterms. Because of the complexity of ICD-10-CM codes, many publishers include lines down each column of the Index to help coders navigate through the many different subterms. It may also be helpful to use a ruler or straightedge when maneuvering through the Index to keep track of subterms.

Subterms are considered **essential modifiers** because they impact the code that is selected. The location of the pain is an essential modifier that leads the coder to assign a code different than the code for an alternate site of pain. **Nonessential modifiers** are words located in parentheses next to the main term or a subterm in the Index. Nonessential modifiers offer additional information but do not impact code selection. For example, Smith now needs to find the code for pain due to intestinal gas. He now knows to look up the condition—in this case *pain*—and then the type or site of the pain, *intestinal gas pain.* Smith notes that the subterm *intestinal* is not listed in the subterms, but the word *gas* is. Next to the word *gas* is the nonessential modifier *intestinal* in parentheses (see figure 4.4). In this case, the word *intestinal* offers additional information about the gas pain but does not impact the code selection. In other words, it does not change the code that is selected in the way that *knee* did for *knee pain.* Sometimes several nonessential modifiers may be listed next to a main term or subterm in the Index. These just provide more information and help with code selection.

Figure 4.4. ICD-10-CM Main Index example 2

Example: nonessential modifier

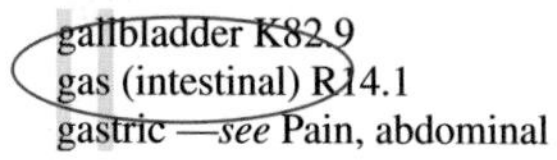

gallbladder K82.9
gas (intestinal) R14.1
gastric —*see* Pain, abdominal

Source: Casto 2019, 247.

Locate and Verify the Code

Once the main term or subterm has been located and any nonessential modifiers and cross-references have been noted, the coder should look to the right of the term to find the ICD-10-CM code. For example, if Smith were looking for the code for knee pain and maneuvered through the index to find the entry *pain, joint, knee,* he would find the code M25.56- to the right of the word *knee* (see figure 4.3). But he is not done yet. Smith now must verify that this is the correct code, especially because the code is listed with a hyphen (-) at the end of it. This means that the code needs an additional digit that must be selected when referencing the Tabular List. If Smith were to assign the code M25.56 without the required sixth character, he would be assigning an invalid code. The additional character that should be assigned to the code M25.56- is found in the Tabular List and, in this case, the code needs one additional digit to identify the laterality of the pain (which knee is in pain—the right or the left). The diagnosis description does not state the laterality, so the correct code is M25.569, Pain in unspecified knee. This information is found within the Tabular List.

The Tabular List is the alphanumerical listing of all ICD-10-CM codes. Not only is it necessary to check the Tabular List to verify the code selected and assign all necessary characters to the code, as in the previous example, but it also contains important information about code selection, sequencing, and guidelines that govern appropriate code selection. The Tabular List and additional characters are discussed in detail in the next section of this chapter.

Key to Success

Default codes are the codes for the unspecified version of a condition and can be easy to overlook. For example, if a coder is looking for the code *pain, unspecified,* then it is not necessary to look any further than the first entry in the Index: Pain(s) (*see also* painful) R52. The code R52 should be assigned for unspecified pain. Default codes are always listed next to the main term in the Main Index and represent the least specified version of that condition.

Complete the exercises in There's a Code for That 4.1, 4.2, and 4.3 to practice identifying the main term, identifying essential and nonessential modifiers, and using the Main Index.

Identify the main term

There's a Code for That

Using the ICD-10-CM-CM code book, identify the main terms for the following diagnostic statements.

1. Knee pain.

   Main term: _____

2. Reactive airway disease.

   Main term: _____

3. Difficulty swallowing.

   Main term: _____

4. Intervertebral disc degeneration.

   Main term: _____

5. Inguinal hernia.

   Main term: _____

Essential versus nonessential modifiers

There's a Code for That

Look up the following terms in the Main Index and identify if the modifier listed is either essential or nonessential (the first one has been completed for you).

	Main term	Modifier	Essential or nonessential
Example	Pachyonychia	congenital	*nonessential*
1.	Strain	back	
2.	Entropion	eyelid	
3.	Cholesterolemia	pure	
4.	Thrush	vaginal	

Using the Main Index

There's a Code for That

Using the Main Index, identify the code for the following diagnostic statements. For this exercise, only locate the code from the Main Index, you do not need to verify the code in the Tabular List.

1. Pneumococcal pneumonia.

   ICD-10-CM code: _____

2. Diaper rash.

   ICD-10-CM code: _____

3. Oropharyngeal dysphagia.

   ICD-10-CM code: _____

(Continued on next page)

4.3

Continued

4. Echolalia.

ICD-10-CM code: _____

5. Muckle-Wells syndrome.

ICD-10-CM code: _____

6. Congenital gastrointestinal tract anomaly.

ICD-10-CM code: _____

In the Index, the Table of Neoplasms follows the Index to Diseases and Injury and is used to locate ICD-10-CM codes for neoplasms, such as benign moles and various cancers.

Table of Neoplasms

Also referred to as the Neoplasm Table, the **Table of Neoplasms** is an index that lists codes for neoplastic conditions such as malignant tumors and diseases, and benign growths. A **neoplasm** is an abnormal growth of tissue and can be fast-growing and invasive, such as malignant cancer, or a benign mass or tumor. The Neoplasm Table is divided first by the anatomic site of the neoplasm, and then the behavior of the neoplasm. There are four different neoplasm behaviors: benign, malignant, carcinoma in situ, or uncertain behavior.

Benign neoplasms are noncancerous growths of tissue, such as a mole or uterine fibroid. They may be problematic and need excision (or removal), but they are not invasive and will not spread to other tissues.

Malignant neoplasms are commonly referred to as cancer. These neoplasms invade surrounding tissues and destroy them and can be fatal. Malignant neoplasms can metastasize—or spread—throughout the body, creating **metastases** (or mets), which are offshoots of the original cancer. Metastases, or metastatic growths, are known as **secondary neoplasms**, or the site of the metastatic growth. The **primary neoplasm** is the where the growth originated. For example, a malignant melanoma of the skin may metastasize to the liver and brain. In this case, the primary neoplasm would be the melanoma, and the secondary neoplasms would be the liver and the brain. Note that even though there are three cancers present (skin, liver, and brain), the metastases are still only referred to as secondary sites (rather than secondary—second and tertiary—third). No matter how many metastases are present, they are still referred to as secondary neoplasms because they are secondary to the primary neoplasm.

Carcinoma in situ (abbreviated as ca in situ) neoplasms are growths of tissue that are potentially cancerous. These growths are not invading other tissues at the time of diagnosis, but may invade other tissues in the future.

Neoplasms of uncertain behavior are neoplasms that have not yet been confirmed as any of the other three types (benign, malignant, or carcinoma in situ). These neoplasms require further evaluation and testing before their behavior can be determined.

It is important to understand the different behaviors of neoplasms because code selection varies depending on the neoplasm behavior. For example, the code for a benign neoplasm of the appendix (D12.1, Benign neoplasm of appendix) differs from the code for a malignant neoplasm of the appendix (C18.1, Malignant neoplasm of appendix). Furthermore, the Table of Neoplasms is divided in such a way as to guide the coder to the correct code based on both the site and behavior of the neoplasm.

The Table of Neoplasms is organized alphabetically by site, and then by the neoplasm behavior. For each site, there are six columns, each of which identify the behavior of the neoplasm. These six columns are: malignant primary, malignant secondary, ca in situ, benign, uncertain behavior, and unspecified behavior (see figure 4.5). A neoplasm of unspecified behavior is one that has not definitively been determined to be either malignant or benign. It is commonly used when a provider is testing the neoplasm to determine its behavior.

Key to Success

As you read through the following sections of text, follow along with your ICD-10-CM code book and note the format, sections, and organization of the following sections of the Index. Take your time and remember to take notes!

To find the code for a neoplasm using the Table of Neoplasms, it is necessary to identify the site of the neoplasm and then the behavior. However, if the coder knows the histologic type of the neoplasm, then it can be located by finding the histologic type of the neoplasm in the Main Index. The **histologic type** of the neoplasm is the specific type of microscopic structure of the neoplastic growth, such as carcinoma, myeloma, or sarcoma. The histology of the neoplasm is also referred to as the **morphology** of the neoplasm, or morphological type of neoplasm. If the morphology of the neoplasm is not known, then it is necessary to refer to the Table of Neoplasms. Often the entry for the morphology or histologic type of the neoplasm in the Main Index refers the coder to the Neoplasm Table.

Figure 4.5. Neoplasm Table

	Malignant Primary	Malignant Secondary	Ca in situ	Benign	Uncertain Behavior	Unspecified Behavior
Neoplasm, neoplastic	C80.1	C79.9	D09.9	D36.9	D48.9	D49.9
A						
abdomen, abdominal	C76.2	C79.8-	D09.8	D36.7	D48.7	D49.89
cavity	C76.2	C79.8-	D09.8	D36.7	D48.7	D49.89
organ	C76.2	C79.8-	D09.8	D36.7	D48.7	D49.89
viscera	C76.2	C79.8-	D09.8	D36.7	D48.7	D49.89
wall—see also Neoplasm, abdomen, wall, skin	C44.509	C79.2	D04.5	D23.5	D48.5	D49.2
connective tissue	C49.4	C79.8-	-	D21.4	D48.1	D49.2
skin	C44.509					
basal cell carcinoma	C44.519	-	-	-	-	-
specified type NEC	C44.599	-	-	-	-	-
squamous cell carcinoma	C44.529	-	-	-	-	-

Source: Casto 2019, 335.

Follow these steps to look up a code in the Neoplasm Table.

1. Identify the morphological type of the neoplasm and look it up in the Main Index. This often leads the coder to the Table of Neoplasms, although this is not always the case. When the morphological type of the neoplasm is an entry in the Main Index, it will lead the coder directly to the code for the neoplasm without having to refer to the Neoplasm Table. If this is the case, then it is still necessary to verify the code in the Tabular List. For example, Marion is looking for the code for right-sided renal cell adenocarcinoma (a cancer of the kidney). She looks up the morphological type of the cancer—*adenocarcinoma*—in the Main Index, then locates the subterm *renal cell*, which leads her to the code C64-. She then verifies this code in the Tabular List and adds the required fourth character, leading her to select the code C64.1, Malignant neoplasm of the right kidney, except renal pelvis. In this example, the Main Index led Marion directly to the code she was searching for. A detailed description of finding codes in the ICD-10-CM code book is discussed later in this chapter.

Key to Success

Note that in figure 4.5 there are some boxes that to do not contain a code but rather a dash (-). This means that there is no possible code for this type of neoplasm. This dash is used throughout the Table of Neoplasms as well as the Table of Drugs and Chemicals to indicate that there is no code option available.

2. When the morphological type of the neoplasm is not known or not specified in the Main Index, the coder must reference the Neoplasm Table and search for the site of the neoplasm. For example, Marion is looking up the code for a malignant neoplasm of the right kidney. Because the morphological type is not specified, she must go directly to the Table of Neoplasms and find the entry for *kidney*. Next to the word *kidney* is a nonessential modifier, *parenchymal*, and there are also a few subterms. Just like the Main Index, the nonessential modifiers in parentheses simply provide more information. The subterms are different—more specific sites—so Marion should scan the subterms to ensure that she has the correct site located.

Key to Success

When locating neoplasms of the skin in the Neoplasm Table, note that the entry for skin neoplasms is very large and it is easy to get lost within this section of the table. It is also important to differentiate between neoplasms of the skin versus neoplasms of deeper tissues or structures. For example, a neoplasm can be in the breast or on the skin of the breast. If the neoplasm is on the skin of the breast, then the coder should reference the entry for *skin*, and then find the subterm for *breast*.

3. Identify the behavior of the neoplasm and select a code. Once the site is found in the Neoplasm Table, identify the behavior of the neoplasm and select the code for the appropriate behavior. For example, Marion is looking for the code for a malignant neoplasm of the right kidney and locates the columns for malignant neoplasms. At this point, Marion has two options—malignant primary or

malignant secondary. Remember that a secondary neoplasm is a growth, or metastasis of the primary neoplasm. Marion's code description does not mention that it is a secondary neoplasm or that it is a metastasis, so she selects the code for the primary neoplasm, C64-.

4. Verify the code in the Tabular List. For example, now that Marion has located code C64-, she must verify the code in the Tabular List and add the fourth character (to represent the laterality of the neoplasm in this case). This leads her to select code C64.1, Malignant neoplasm of right kidney, except renal pelvis. See figure 4.6 for a reminder of the steps to looking up a neoplasm.

Figure 4.6. Steps to looking up a neoplasm

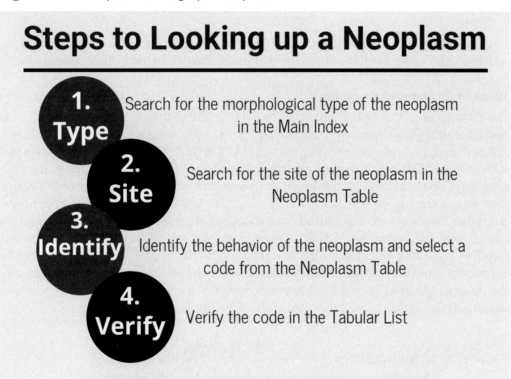

Complete the exercises in There's a Code for That 4.4 to practice using the Table of Neoplasms.

Using the Table of Neoplasms   **4.4**

Using the Table of Neoplasms, identify the codes for the following diagnostic statements. For this exercise, only locate the code from the Index, you do not need to verify the code in the Tabular List.

There's a Code for That

1. Benign neoplasm of the ascending colon.

   ICD-10-CM code: _____

2. Basal cell carcinoma of the skin of the neck.

   ICD-10-CM code: _____

(Continued on next page)

4.4

Continued

3. Primary malignant neoplasm of the vermillion border of the upper lip.

   ICD-10-CM code: _____

4. Secondary malignant neoplasm of the liver.

   ICD-10-CM code: _____

5. Carcinoma in situ of the neck of the pancreas.

   ICD-10-CM code: _____

6. Malignant neoplasm of the bulbourethral gland.

   ICD-10-CM code: _____

The next section of the Index is the Table of Drugs and Chemicals, which allows coders to find codes for toxic effects of chemicals, medicines, and other substances.

Table of Drugs and Chemicals

The third section of the Main Index of the ICD-10-CM code book is the **Table of Drugs and Chemicals** (also referred to as the Table of Drugs), which lists the toxic effects of drugs, chemicals, and other substances (figure 4.7). A **toxic effect** is the result of a toxin—such as a chemical, medicinal, or other substance—on the body. For example, the toxic effect of a chemical may be a burn of the skin. Toxic effect codes are unique because they do not identify the effect of the poisoning, like loss of consciousness or confusion, but rather the substance that caused the toxic effect, the intent of the poisoning, and the encounter. If additional signs, symptoms, or manifestations of the poisoning are present, then they should be coded in addition to the code for the toxic effect code. For example, if a patient came into contact with a toxic substance that caused a burn of the skin, then the coder would need to assign at least two codes: one for the burn of the skin and one to identify the toxin that caused the burn of the skin (from the Table of Drugs).

Figure 4.7. Table of Drugs

Substance	Poisoning, Accidental (unintentional)	Poisoning, Intentional self-harm	Poisoning, Assault	Poisoning, Undetermined	Adverse effect	Underdosing
1-propanol	T51.3X1	T51.3X2	T51.3X3	T51.3X4	—	—
2-propanol	T51.2X1	T51.2X2	T51.2X3	T51.2X4	—	—
2,4-D (dichlorophen-oxyacetic acid)	T60.3X1	T60.3X2	T60.3X3	T60.3X4	—	—
2,4-toluene diisocyanate	T65.0X1	T65.0X2	T65.0X3	T65.0X4	—	—
2,4,5-T (trichloro-phenoxyacetic acid)	T60.1X1	T60.1X2	T60.1X3	T60.1X4	—	—
3,4-methylenedioxy-methamphetamine	T43.641	T43.642	T43.643	T43.644	—	—
14-hydroxydihydro-morphinone	T40.2X1	T40.2X2	T40.2X3	T40.2X4	T40.2X5	T40.2X6

Source: Casto 2019, 357.

Follow these steps to locate and assign a code for a toxic effect.

1. Identify the substance that caused the toxic effect. The Table of Drugs and Chemicals is arranged alphabetically by the name of the substance that caused the toxic effect, so the first step in finding the code for a toxic effect is to identify the substance and find the entry for it in the Table of Drugs. For example, Jamie works in a family practice clinic and she is coding for a patient who had an allergic reaction (rash) to amoxicillin that was prescribed to treat a strep throat infection. This is the first time this patient has been seen for this problem. In this example, the amoxicillin caused the allergic reaction (toxic effect), so Jamie finds the entry for *amoxicillin* in the Table of Drugs. Note that most drugs are listed by their generic names, although this depends on the publisher of the ICD-10-CM code book. There are also subterms and nonessential modifiers for the substances listed in the Table of Drugs, just like the other indices in the ICD-10-CM code book.

2. Identify the intent of the toxic effect. After the substance has been located, the next step is to identify the intent. The **intent** of the toxic effect is the reason why the toxic effect happened. In the ICD-10-CM code book, there are six different intentions that may be identified for a toxic effect code: accidental intent, intentional self-harm, assault, undetermined intent, adverse effect, and underdosing. The code for each intent is located in one of the six corresponding columns. This format is similar to the Table of Neoplasms, with the main term on the left-hand side of the columns and multiple columns that identify different intentions for the toxic effect.

   a. **Accidental intent**. An accidental toxic effect is an unintentional effect of a substance that was either taken inadvertently or in excess. For example, nausea and vomiting are accidental side effects of excessive alcohol consumption. The accidental intent is the default for toxic effects that cannot be identified as intentional, assault, an adverse effect, or underdosing. If the intent is not identified in the documentation, use the code for accidental intent.

   b. **Intentional self-harm**. A toxic effect resulting from intentional self-harm is due to a substance that is taken deliberately as an act of hurting one's self. For example, if a patient consumed an entire bottle of hydrocodone on purpose in an attempted suicide, then this overdose would be intentional self-harm.

   c. **Assault**. A toxic effect that occurs due to assault is one that was purposefully inflicted upon one person by another person, with the intent of hurting the recipient of the substance. For example, if a person spikes someone's drink with Rohypnol (the date-rape drug) to cause a toxic effect, then the intent of this poisoning is assault.

   d. **Undetermined intent**. An undetermined intent of a toxic effect is used only when the intention of the toxic effect cannot be determined to be any of the other types: accidental, intentional, assault, adverse effect, or underdosing. For example, if a patient is found unconscious due to a poisoning caused by a combination of drugs, and the intent of the poisoning cannot be determined to be accidental, intentional self-harm, due to assault, an adverse effect, or an underdose, then the intent "undetermined" should be selected. Use this code option *only* when the documentation states that the intent cannot be determined.

   e. **Adverse effect**. An adverse effect is an unintended effect caused by a substance that is correctly prescribed and administered. Unlike an accidental poisoning, this adverse effect was caused when a patient was supposed to take a substance—and did so correctly—but it still resulted in some sort of unintended consequence. Recall Jamie, who is coding for an allergic rash that was caused by amoxicillin (which was correctly prescribed and correctly administered)—Jamie will select the code the for the "adverse effect" intent of the poisoning, T36.0X5-, Adverse effect of penicillins. The adverse effect code should not be selected when a substance is incorrectly prescribed or administered. For example, if the pharmacy incorrectly filled the prescription or if the patient took too much of the prescribed dose causing a toxic effect, then this would be coded as an accidental poisoning.

   f. **Underdosing.** An underdosing occurs when a patient takes too little of a prescribed substance and suffers an unintended consequence. Even if a patient purposefully underdoses it is not coded as intentional self-harm unless the patient underdosed specifically as an act of self-harm. For example, if a 76-year-old male patient did not take his entire dose of insulin because he either could not afford it or if he simply calculated the dose wrong, then this would be coded with underdosing intent.

3. Verify the code and add the seventh character extension (discussed in detail later in this chapter) for the episode of care. After the intent of the toxic effect has been determined, the next step is correctly identifying a code from the Table of Drugs and Chemicals is to add the seventh character extension to identify the encounter. Note that the seventh characters are *not* listed in the Table of Drugs. The encounter (in this case initial encounter) identifies where the patient is in the timeline of care for their condition. To select the correct encounter, the coder must verify the code in the Tabular List and add the correct seventh character. For example, Jamie is coding that the patient has been seen with this allergic reaction to the amoxicillin prescription for the first time, so she should select the seventh character "A" for initial encounter. Her code is now complete, T36.0X5A, Adverse effect of penicillins, initial encounter. Seventh characters and encounters are discussed in full later in this chapter.

Key to Success

Typically, if a code in the Index does not include the required amount of characters, then it is listed with a hyphen (-) after the code, but this is not the case in the Table of Drugs. Note that none of the codes listed in the Table of Drugs are followed by a hyphen, although each and every one of these codes requires an additional character added to the end of the code. This is done to save space in the Table of Drugs. Be sure to always verify the code in the Tabular, which will remind you to add the seventh character for the episode of care.

4. Check for additional codes and sequencing. After the correct code has been identified, additional codes may be needed to identify the manifestations of the poisoning. The **manifestation** of the poisoning is the sign or symptom that occurred because of the poisoning. These include the signs, symptoms, related conditions, or other manifestations that were caused by exposure to the substance. For example, Jamie found the code for the amoxicillin adverse effect, but she still needs to select a code for the manifestation of the adverse effect—the rash. To do this, she looks up the manifestation in the Main Index, and finds the code R21, Rash and other nonspecific skin eruption. Because Jamie now has two

codes, she must pay attention to the sequencing of the codes. **Sequencing,** or placing the multiple diagnosis codes in the correct order, plays an important part in the coding of toxic effects. Sequencing instructions are listed in the Tabular List section of ICD-10-CM and depend on the intent of the poisoning. Specific sequencing instructions are discussed later in this chapter. See figure 4.8 for a reminder of the steps to using the Table of Drugs and Chemicals.

Figure 4.8. Steps to using the Table of Drugs and Chemicals

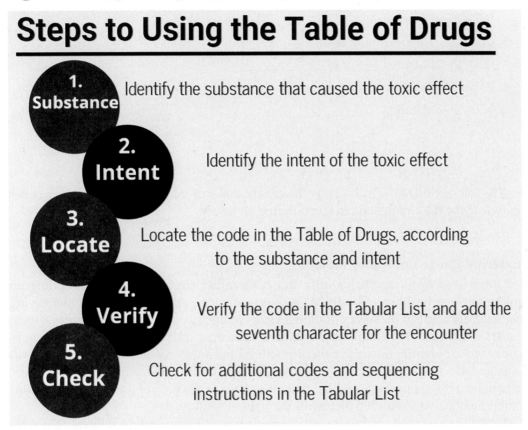

Steps to Using the Table of Drugs

1. Substance Identify the substance that caused the toxic effect

2. Intent Identify the intent of the toxic effect

3. Locate Locate the code in the Table of Drugs, according to the substance and intent

4. Verify Verify the code in the Tabular List, and add the seventh character for the encounter

5. Check Check for additional codes and sequencing instructions in the Tabular List

Complete the exercises in There's a Code for That 4.5 to practice using the Table of Drugs and Chemicals.

Using the Table of Drugs and Chemicals	**4.5**
Using the Table of Drugs and Chemicals, identify the codes for the following diagnostic statements. For this exercise, only locate the code from the Main Index. You do not need to verify the code in the Tabular List or include the seventh character extension. **1.** Accidental poisoning by ammonia gas fumes. ICD-10-CM code: _____	**There's a Code for That**

(Continued on next page)

4.5

Continued

2. Adverse effect of MAO inhibitor.

   ICD-10-CM code: _____

3. Patient was admitted for ingestion of noxious mushrooms as a suicide attempt.

   ICD-10-CM code: _____

4. Patient was admitted to the ICU for acute poisoning by chlorinated insecticide. Patient was applying the insecticide to the outside of his house when the wind blew the substance into his face causing ingestion of the substance.

   ICD-10-CM code: _____

5. Code for ricin poisoning as an assault attempt.

   ICD-10-CM code: _____

6. Poisoning by Hycodan, undetermined intent.

   ICD-10-CM code: _____

The last section of the Index is the External Causes of Injury Index, which lists codes that describe the circumstances surrounding an injury.

External Causes of Injury Index

At times it is necessary to identify the extenuating circumstances surrounding an injury or other healthcare condition. In these instances, one or more codes identifying the external cause of the injury or illness, listed in the **External Causes of Injury Index**, must be included. For example, if a patient suffered a fractured ankle, external cause codes would identify how the patient fractured the ankle: the activity the patient was engaged in and where he or she was when the injury happened, where the patient was when the injury happened, and the patient's status at the time of the injury. These four components give a rounded picture of the patient's injury.

External cause codes provide additional information regarding injuries. They are useful for data analytics purposes such as identifying trends and tracking the volume of injuries caused by certain activities like skateboarding, skydiving, or animal bites. Note, however, that these codes are never used as primary diagnosis codes; they are always sequenced after any codes for actual medical diagnoses (typically the injury). For example, if a patient were bitten by a dog and suffered a wound to the hand, the diagnosis code for the hand wound would be sequenced first, followed by the external cause code for the dog bite, which gives more information about how the injury happened.

Reporting external cause codes varies from state to state. For example, in some states reporting all external causes for all injuries is required, whereas in other states it is not required, and some insurance plans may outright reject external cause codes. External cause codes may be required on claims that deal with motor vehicle accidents or workplace injuries, so they may be necessary in these circumstances even in states that do not require the reporting of external cause codes. For the purposes of this textbook, external cause codes are required whenever known and applicable to describe the extenuating circumstances surrounding an injury.

Key to Success

There are many different types of external cause codes and maneuvering through the Index to External Causes requires thoughtful consideration of exactly what you are searching for. When searching, it is imperative to focus on the type of external cause code—the injury mechanism, place of occurrence, activity, or patient status—and look up each code separately.

Use the following steps to find external cause codes using the External Causes of Injury Index.

1. Identify the extenuating circumstances surrounding the injury. There are four possible codes that may be included to fully describe the external causes of an injury. If each of these circumstances is known, then one code should be assigned for each, for a total of four codes. Once the four components of the external causes have been identified, look up each one in the External Cause Index and find the individual codes for each component. These four components are the injury mechanism, patient activity, place of occurrence, and patient status.

   a. The **injury mechanism** is the way an injury happened. For example, if a patient fell off a ladder and fractured his ankle, the injury mechanism would be the fall from the ladder. This code answers the question: *How did the injury happen?*

   b. The patient's activity should also be identified. The **activity** is what the patient was doing when the injury occurred. For example, if the patient was painting the outside of a building when he fell from the ladder and fractured his ankle, then the activity is painting. This code answers the question: *What was the patient doing when the injury happened?*

   c. The **place of occurrence** is where the patient was when the injury occurred. This should be as detailed as possible to describe the specifics of the location. For example, if the patient was painting the outside of his house, then the code may describe the type of house, such as single-family home or multi-family housing unit. In this example, the place of occurrence would the yard of a single-family house. This code answers the question: *Where was the patient when the injury happened?*

   d. The **patient status** identifies the patient's work context during the accident by identifying if the patient's injury was related to employment, volunteer work, or military status. For example, if the patient was painting the outside of his home during a time when he was not employed and at his leisure, then the patient status would be leisure status. This code helps to answer the question: *Was the patient at work or military duty when the injury happened?*

2. Look up the external causes using the External Cause of Injury Index. This index works very similarly to the Main Index, with cross-references and subterms listed under the main terms. Finding each of the four components can be tricky, however, so it is helpful to know the following tips. For the injury mechanism, it is helpful to search for the main cause or item involved in the injury, such as the term *fall*, and then what the patient fell from: *from, ladder*. When looking up the patient activity, find the word *activity*, and then check the subterms to find the appropriate activity. When looking up the place of occurrence, search for the term *place of occurrence*, and check the subterms for the correct location. Finally, to find

the correct code for the patient status, search for the term *status of external cause* and find the correct patient status in the subterms.

Key to Success

Familiarize yourself with the External Causes of Injury Index by scanning the main terms. This will help when learning how to use the index to find your codes. Start at the beginning of the Index and read through or quickly scan the main terms in each column on each page. Make a note of how the Index is organized so that you can find them easily when you are coding for external causes.

3. Verify the codes in the Tabular List and add the seventh character episode of care when appropriate. Note that the seventh character is not listed in the Index, and unlike the Main Index, the codes that do require a seventh character are not listed with a following hyphen (-). Some External Cause codes may require seventh characters, whereas others may not. Because of this, it is very important to always verify the codes found in the Index by checking the Tabular List. All injury mechanism codes require a seventh character extension to identify the episode of care for the injury. For example, if the patient is still in active treatment for the fractured ankle due to the fall from the ladder, then the episode of care selected for the injury mechanism code would be "A" for initial encounter (discussed in detail later in this chapter). Read through the following example to find the appropriate codes for this patient's injury. Refer to figure 4.9 for a reminder of the steps to using the External Causes of Injury Index and figure 4.10 for an example of how to assign external cause codes.

Figure 4.9. Steps to using the External Causes of Injury Index

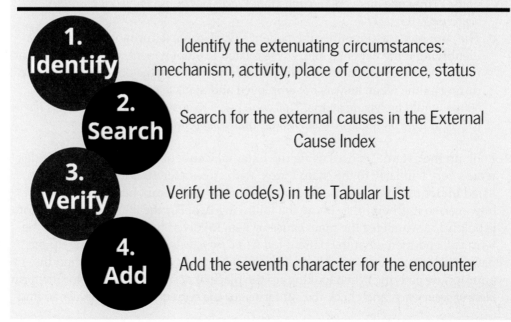

Steps to Using the External Cause Index

1. Identify — Identify the extenuating circumstances: mechanism, activity, place of occurrence, status

2. Search — Search for the external causes in the External Cause Index

3. Verify — Verify the code(s) in the Tabular List

4. Add — Add the seventh character for the encounter

Figure 4.10. External cause codes example

Terrence was in the yard of his single-family home painting the outside of the building during his weekend leisure time, when he fell off his ladder and fractured his left ankle.
Primary injury code: S82.892A, Other fracture of left lower leg, initial encounter
Injury mechanism code: W11.XXXA, Fall on and from ladder, initial encounter
Activity: Y93.H9, Activity, other involving exterior property and land maintenance, building, and construction (*painting outside of building*)
Place of occurrence: Y92.017, Garden or yard in single-family (private) house as the place of occurrence of the external cause
Patient status: Y99.8, Other external cause status (*leisure activity*)

Complete the exercises in There's a Code for That 4.6 to practice using the External Causes of Injury Index.

Using the External Causes of Injury Index

4.6

There's a Code for That

Read the following scenario that describes the external causes of an injury. Using the External Causes of Injury Index, identify the codes for the external causes. For this exercise, only locate the code from the Main Index. You do not need to verify the code in the Tabular List or include the seventh character extension, just list the code found in the Index.

Carter, a 15-year-old high school student, was playing soccer on a public soccer field after school when he was struck by the soccer ball in the face and suffered a broken nose.

1. What is the injury mechanism and for Carter's injury and the ICD-10-CM code for the injury mechanism?

Injury mechanism: _____

ICD-10-CM code: _____

2. What is the place of occurrence and the ICD-10-CM code for the place of occurrence?

Place of occurrence: _____

ICD-10-CM code: _____

3. What was the patient's activity when the injury occurred and the ICD-10-CM code for the activity?

Activity: _____

ICD-10-CM code: _____

4. What is the patient's status and the ICD-10-CM code for the patient's status at the time of injury?

Patient status: _____

ICD-10-CM code: _____

The Tabular List follows the four sections of the Index. This is the largest section of the ICD-10-CM code book and lists all of the actual ICD-10-CM codes and includes instructions and guidelines for the use of selected codes.

Tabular List

The **Tabular List** of the ICD-10-CM code book is the structured list of ICD-10-CM codes, organized alphanumerically and divided into chapters based on body system or condition. The Tabular List includes more than simply a list of ICD-10-CM codes. It employs a specific format to help coders identify valid codes, includes references to guidelines to help with code selection, and employs various symbols, notes, and other conventions to help lead coders to their correct code. The Tabular List is first divided into 21 chapters and each chapter includes a selection of ICD-10-CM codes. Each chapter is formatted similarly and contains the same symbols and other conventions to help coders select the correct code. Finally, there are important guidelines that pertain to using the Tabular List. Depending on the publisher of the ICD-10-CM code book, each chapter may also include the Official Guidelines for Coding and Reporting, which also govern appropriate code selection.

Chapters of the Tabular List

There are 21 chapters in the ICD-10-CM Tabular List. Each chapter is divided based on a specific body system or condition. Several of the individual chapters begin with a new letter of the alphabet, although this is not always the case. Some chapters contain codes from two or more letters of the alphabet, and other chapters contain codes that start with the same letter of the alphabet. Study the list of ICD-10-CM chapters in figure 4.11, paying close attention to the range of codes that are in each chapter.

Figure 4.11. Table of contents of the Tabular List

Table of Contents

1. Certain infectious and parasitic diseases (A00-B99)
2. Neoplasms (C00-D49)
3. Diseases of the blood-forming organs and certain disorders involving the immune mechanism (D50-D89)
4. Endocrine, nutritional and metabolic diseases (E00-E89)
5. Mental, Behavioral and Neurodevelopmental disorders (F01-F99)
6. Diseases of the nervous system (G00-G99)
7. Diseases of the eye and adnexa (H00-H59)
8. Diseases of the ear and mastoid process (H60-H95)
9. Diseases of the circulatory system (I00-I99)
10. Diseases of the respiratory system (J00-J99)
11. Diseases of the digestive system (K00-K95)
12. Diseases of the skin and subcutaneous tissue (L00-L99)
13. Diseases of the musculoskeletal system and connective tissue (M00-M99)
14. Diseases of the genitourinary system (N00-N99)
15. Pregnancy, childbirth and the puerperium (O00-O9A)
16. Certain conditions originating in the perinatal period (P00-P96)
17. Congenital malformations, deformations and chromosomal abnormalities (Q00-Q99)
18. Symptoms, signs and abnormal clinical and laboratory findings, not elsewhere classified (R00-R99)
19. Injury, poisoning and certain other consequences of external causes (S00-T88)
20. External causes of morbidity (V00-Y99)
21. Factors influencing health status and contact with health services (Z00-Z99)

Source: Casto 2019, 472.

Key to Success

It is useful, both as a beginner and as an experienced coding professional, to place tabs at the beginning of each chapter and on codes commonly used in your specialty, to make code location easier. Also, many coding books include a different colored or shaded edge for each chapter that helps to locate codes more quickly.

Key to Success

The letter at the beginning of the codes does not correspond to the type of condition or body area, although it may be helpful to make up letter associations for certain code groups. For example, codes from chapter 15: Pregnancy, childbirth, and the puerperium, all start with the letter *O*. You may choose to associate O codes with *obstetric* conditions.

Formatting and Conventions of the Tabular List

All of the chapters in the Tabular List are formatted similarly so that coders can easily locate and select the appropriate code. Furthermore, the Tabular List also contains a number of conventions that help coders select the correct code and identify if the code chosen is reportable for a certain type of setting, patient, or billing or coding purpose. These include the abbreviations NOS (not otherwise specified) and NEC (not elsewhere classifiable), special highlighting, and symbols on each page to alert the coder to appropriate uses of the codes.

Format of the Tabular List and Specificity

The Tabular List is formatted and organized based on sections, categories, subcategories, and codes. Each chapter is composed of one or more sections, combining conditions that are similar in nature. Sections may include codes from many different categories. All categories are three characters. If a three-character category is not further subdivided, then it is considered a code. As discussed later in the chapter, subcategories can extend codes to four, five, six, or seven characters. Each time a new subcategory is added, it adds more detail to the code (with the exception of placeholders). Three-character categories are listed on the left of the columns, with subcategories and codes indented beneath the category and any additional subcategories.

For a code to be reportable, or valid, it must be extended to the full amount of characters possible. In figure 4.12 it would be incorrect to code E08.0- because there is a more specific code indented beneath it. In this case, the coder should select E08.00, Diabetes mellitus due to underlying condition with hyperosmolarity without nonketotic hyperglycemic-hyperosmolar coma (NKHHC), which is a valid code. There may be as many indentions underneath a category needed to create up to a six-character code.

However, not all individual codes are fully listed in the Tabular List. To save space, the ICD-10-CM code book does not include the seventh character extensions with each code. Instead, the seventh character extension options are listed in a box within the category, and an instructional notation is included in the Tabular List to inform the coder that a seventh character is necessary. This notation differs, depending on the publisher of the ICD-10-CM code book, so it may be a small red dot, check mark, stop sign, or a plus (+) symbol. If the code is not extended to the required number of characters, it is considered an invalid code and cannot be reported on a claim form. A code that has been extended to the full amount of required characters is considered a **billable code**, as it may be reported for billing purposes. Study figure 4.12 to see how this symbol instructs the coder to add more characters to the code.

Figure 4.12. Section, category, subcategory, and code

Diabetes mellitus (E08-E13)

Review coding guideline C.4.a

Category ➡ E08   Diabetes mellitus due to underlying condition

Code first the underlying condition, such as:
  congenital rubella (P35.0)
  Cushing's syndrome (E24.-)
  cystic fibrosis (E84.-)
  malignant neoplasm (C00-C96)
  malnutrition (E40-E46)
  pancreatitis and other diseases of the pancreas (K85-K86.-)

Use additional code to identify control using:
  insulin (Z79.4)
  oral antidiabetic drugs (Z79.84)
  oral hypoglycemic drugs (Z79.84)

Excludes1: drug or chemical induced diabetes mellitus (E09.-)
  gestational diabetes (O24.4-)
  neonatal diabetes mellitus (P70.2)
  postpancreatectomy diabetes mellitus (E13.-)
  postprocedural diabetes mellitus (E13.-)
  secondary diabetes mellitus NEC (E13.-)
  type 1 diabetes mellitus (E10.-)
  type 2 diabetes mellitus (E11.-)

Review coding guideline C.4.a.6.a

Subcategory ➡ + E08.0   Diabetes mellitus due to underlying condition with hyperosmolarity

MCC E08.00   Diabetes mellitus due to underlying condition with hyperosmolarity without nonketotic hyperglycemic-hyperosmolar coma (NKHHC)

⬆

Code   HAC   see Appendix B for HAC conditional logic

Source: Casto 2019, 541.

In figure 4.13, code S04.0 has a plus symbol to the left of it, which indicates that the coder needs to add an additional code, indented below. Code S04.01 also has a plus symbol located to the left of it, so an additional character is needed, and the codes are indented below. The next indented code, S04.011, has a plus symbol as well as the "7th" sign, indicating that an additional character is needed, but there are no more codes indented below. Instead, the coder must refer to the top of the category to find the seventh character extension options, which are usually listed in a box at the beginning of the code category or subcategory. (Note that the formatting of the seventh character options depends on the publisher of the ICD-10 code book. In the AHIMA *ICD-10-CM Code Book*, the seventh character options are located in a gray box). In this case, the coder would have to select one of the seventh character extension options and add it to create a valid code, such as S04.011A, Injury of optic nerve, right eye, initial encounter; S04.011D, Injury of optic nerve, right eye, subsequent encounter; or S04.011S Injury of optic nerve, right eye, sequela. Note that because the codes with the extensions are not listed, it is up to the coder to ensure that the seventh character extensions are added correctly to the necessary codes.

Reporting the code with the most possible characters is referred to as coding to the highest level of specificity. **Specificity** is the amount of detail included within a code description. In other words, the more characters a code has, the more specific it is. Coders must report the code that has the most possible characters.

Figure 4.13. Seventh character additions

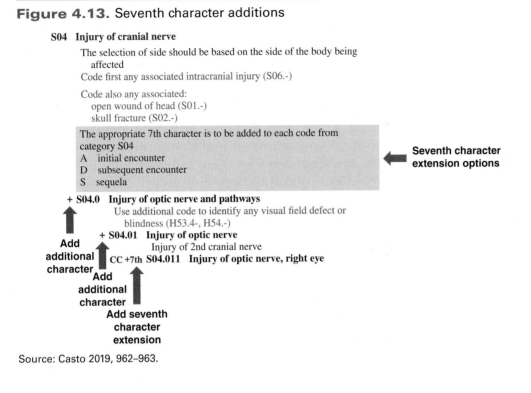

Source: Casto 2019, 962–963.

Key to Success

An easy way to check if the code needs more characters to add specificity is to look for the plus symbol to the left of the code. Remember that this sign also depends on the publisher of the ICD-10 code book. Instead of a plus sign, you might find a small red stop sign, a check mark, or other notation indicating that an additional character is necessary. If the additional character symbol is present, then you must descend to the next level and add another character. If there is no additional character symbol next to the code, then it is a valid code and it may be reported on a claim. Valid codes are also referred to as billable codes, as they are valid for claims and billing purposes.

Abbreviations NOS and NEC

One of the conventions in the Tabular List is the use of two very common and important abbreviations— NOS and NEC. NOS stands for **not otherwise specified**, which means that the healthcare provider's documentation was not specific enough to select a more specific, or detailed, code. For example, if the provider's documentation stated that the condition was *dysphagia, NOS*, then the coder would select the unspecified version of the code for dysphagia, R13.10, Dysphagia, unspecified. The Tabular List may include the abbreviation NOS in the code description to help coders identify unspecified codes.

NEC stands for **not elsewhere classifiable** and indicates that no code exists for a specified condition. In other words, the condition that the coder is searching for does not have a specific code, so the "other" option must be selected. For example, if the provider's documentation specifies that the patient has neurogenic dysphagia, the coder would check the term *dysphagia*, and then look for a code for neurogenic dysphagia specifically. However, no code for neurogenic dysphagia exists. The coder should not select the unspecified version of the condition, because it *was* specified—in this case there is no specific code for it. The coder should select the code to indicate that the condition is not elsewhere classifiable with a specific code, and report code R13.19, Other dysphagia.

When searching for NOS codes in the Tabular List, they may be listed as either NOS or unspecified. NEC codes may be referred to as "other" or "other specified type." Remember: **NOS = Unspecified; NEC = Other**. Note also that both abbreviations may also be found in the ICD-10-CM Index.

Key to Success

Be careful when using unspecified codes. The thousands of specific ICD-10-CM specific codes make it easier to find a code for the exact condition. Therefore, unspecified codes should be reported rarely, as the overuse of unspecified codes can trigger an audit. However, there are many times that unspecified codes are necessary and thus they are still commonly used in the healthcare office. Reporting unspecified diagnoses is discussed further in chapter 8 (Primary Care).

Special Highlighting and Symbols

Many publishers of the ICD-10-CM code book include special highlighting and symbols throughout the Tabular List to help coders identify the proper uses of the codes displayed on the page.

Highlighting is added to help the coder take note of particular guidelines, notations, and special instructions regarding the codes. Highlighting is consistent throughout the code book so that coders can visually pick out the important aspects of the codes and apply that information to help them report the codes correctly. For example, there are instructional guidelines in many codes that have *Includes* and *Excludes* notes (these are discussed later in this chapter). To help coders note these guidelines, they may be highlighted in different colors to help them stand out (see figure 4.14). Note that in the AHIMA *ICD-10-CM Code Book*, the *Includes* note is highlighted in gray, the *Excludes1* note is highlighted in yellow, and the *Excludes2* note is highlighted in green.

There are also symbols or letters that are strategically placed on the pages of the Tabular List. They are commonly placed directly to the right or left of a code and

Figure 4.14. Example of highlighting in the Tabular List

> **K72 Hepatic failure, not elsewhere classified**
> **Includes:** fulminant hepatitis NEC, with hepatic failure
> hepatic encephalopathy NOS
> liver (cell) necrosis with hepatic failure
> malignant hepatitis NEC, with hepatic failure
> yellow liver atrophy or dystrophy
> *Excludes1:* *alcoholic hepatic failure (K70.4)*
> *hepatic failure with toxic liver disease (K71.1-)*
> *icterus of newborn (P55-P59)*
> *postprocedural hepatic failure (K91.82)*
> *Excludes2:* *hepatic failure complicating abortion or ectopic or molar*
> *pregnancy (O00-007, O008.8)*
> *hepatic failure complicating pregnancy, childbirth and the*
> *puerperium (O26.6-)*
> *viral hepatitis with hepatic coma (B15-B19)*

Source: Casto 2019, 734.

provide more information about that code. They function just like footnotes, in that they refer the coder to additional information about that code, located on the bottom edge of the page. Depending on the publisher of the code book, the symbol may be a bullet point, such as a pink dot, or a small letter *M* to indicate that the code is for use on maternal claims only. On the other hand, a green bullet or small letter *N* indicates that the code is for use on newborn records only. Other symbols identify codes for a specific age group, such as pediatric or adult patients, or for a certain gender, either male or female. For example, in figure 4.15, the codes located in this section all have a small pink dot, as well as a small female gender sign next to them. Note that according to the information at the bottom of the page, the pink dot means that this code is applicable for a maternity condition. The gender symbol means that the condition should be used for female patients. Thus, the ICD-10-CM code book indicates that these codes should only be used on maternal records, for female patients.

As a coder, it is important to always pay attention to each and every detail on the page, as it was put there for a reason. Success as a coding professional depends on the ability to pay attention to these small details, understand what they mean, and then use the information to select the most appropriate code. These notes at the bottom of the page provide helpful information and can help coders determine when a code may or may not be appropriate to report.

Figure 4.15. Notations within the Tabular List

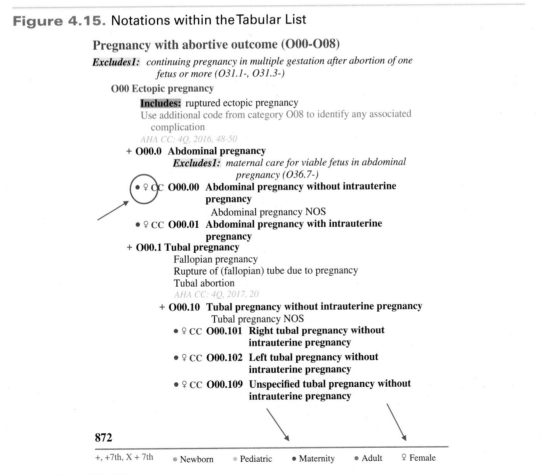

Key to Success

Learning all of the conventions, guidelines, and uses of ICD-10-CM codes can be overwhelming, but don't worry, you don't have to remember everything! In the real world, you should always have access to a code book or other coding resource. As long as you make notes and pay attention to all of the details on the page, you will be a success!

Key to Success

As you learn how to use the Tabular List, make a note of the highlighted terms and symbols in the code book you are using. When you begin using your code book for the first time, note the line of footnotes at the bottom of each page in the Tabular List. These notes help coders recognize what the highlighting means, in addition to other symbols used in the Tabular List. When in doubt, always refer to the bottom of the page to check what the symbol or highlighting means.

Codes and terms may be highlighted throughout the Tabular List to indicate that they may be included within a specific set of codes. This additional highlighting and notation found in the AHIMA *ICD-10-CM Code Book* identifies codes that are manifestation codes (highlighted in pale green, discussed later in this chapter), as well as codes that are unacceptable as a primary diagnosis for an inpatient claim (Unacceptable PDX, highlighted in light blue), HCC codes (highlighted in lavender), codes that are considered a complication or comorbidity (CC) or major complication or comorbidity (MCC), both of which are important in inpatient facility coding, and hospital-acquired conditions (HAC, highlighted in orange). Note that some of these notations may only be important in inpatient facility settings. These are discussed in more depth in chapter 20. See figure 4.16 for an illustration of these notations.

Figure 4.16. Additional notations in the Tabular List

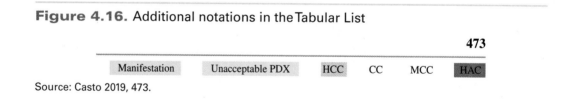

Source: Casto 2019, 473.

Complete the exercises in There's a Code for That 4.7 to test your knowledge of the notations found in the Tabular List.

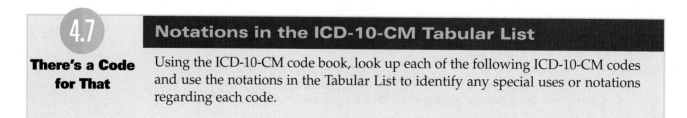

4.7

There's a Code for That

Notations in the ICD-10-CM Tabular List

Using the ICD-10-CM code book, look up each of the following ICD-10-CM codes and use the notations in the Tabular List to identify any special uses or notations regarding each code.

ICD-10-CM Code	Special Use or Notation
1. ____ N42.0, Calculus of prostate	a. Manifestation
2. ____ H93.90, Unspecified disorder of ear, unspecified ear	b. Maternity
3. ____ O32.0, Maternal care for unstable lie	c. Unacceptable PDX
4. ____ T81.19, Other postprocedural shock	d. HCC
5. ____ Z43.0, Encounter for attention to tracheostomy	e. CC
6. ____ N39.0, Urinary tract infection, site not specified	f. Pediatric
7. ____ D63.1, Anemia in chronic kidney disease	g. MCC
8. ____ R10.83, Colic	h. Male
9. ____ R54, Age-related physical debility	i. Adult

Coding conventions—standards and rules that govern how to use the codes in the ICD-10-CM code book—are also found throughout the Tabular List.

Conventions in the Tabular List

In addition to the format, punctuation, and symbols used in the Tabular List, this section also includes conventions for the use of ICD-10-CM codes. Coding conventions are found in the guidelines at the beginning of nearly all ICD-10-CM code books. Some publishers also include chapter-specific guidelines at the beginning of each chapter.

In order to understand guidelines a little better, it is important to discuss the **Official Guidelines for Coding and Reporting (OGCR)**. The OGCR is the set of official guidelines for the use of the ICD-10-CM code set, published by the set of four organizations that make up the Cooperating Parties for ICD-10: AHA, AHIMA, CMS, and NCHS (CMS 2018). So in addition to creating and maintaining the code set, this group also creates the rules that govern how to use it. The OGCR includes general rules that are for use throughout the code set, as well as a large section of chapter-specific guidelines that are applicable to codes specific to certain chapters. Many ICD-10-CM code books include the guidelines in full at the beginning or end of the code book, and others include the full OCGR at the beginning of the code book, as well as the chapter-specific guidelines at the beginning of each chapter. Yet other code books may omit the OCGR completely. The full version of the current year's OGCR can be found on the CMS website, at www.cms.gov.

As the rules on how to use codes, this textbook commonly refers to the OGCR, or guidelines, in the ICD-10-CM code book. When a guideline is especially important for coding purposes, they are included in the text for reference (see figure 4.17).

Conventions are certain guidelines that are applicable to the entire Tabular List, which should be understood before diving into ICD-10-CM coding. Listed as the first section of the OGCR, conventions are general rules for the use of the ICD-10 code book. Some of these conventions have already been discussed in this chapter—such as the abbreviations NEC and NOS, and the use of "other" and "unspecified" codes. Additional important conventions are Includes notes, Excludes notes, "and," "with," "code also," and sequencing instructions, and etiology and manifestation notations.

Figure 4.17. OGCR I.C.1.c. Infections resistant to antibiotics

---

c. Infections resistant to antibiotics

Many bacterial infections are resistant to current antibiotics. It is necessary to identify all infections documented as antibiotic resistant. Assign a code from category Z16, Resistance to antimicrobial drugs, following the infection code only if the infection code does not identify drug resistance.

Source: CMS 2019.

Key to Success

The coding professional needs to know how to locate and use the OGCR, so it is important to understand the configuration of the ICD-10-CM code book you are using and know where to find the OCGR—both the full set and the chapter-specific guidelines. If your book doesn't contain the OGCR, it is a good idea to locate the PDF online and keep it for easy reference.

Includes Notes

Includes notes appear directly underneath a three-character category to further define and give examples of the content that is included in the category. For example, in figure 4.14 the Includes note lists a number of conditions that are included in the category of K72. This means that the conditions listed in the Includes notes may be coded with codes starting with K72.

Inclusion terms are also common throughout the Tabular List. These work similarly to Includes notes, but instead pertain to specific codes rather than a category of codes. Inclusion terms may be synonyms for the condition or a list of various conditions assigned to a specific code. For example, in figure 4.18 the inclusion terms indicate that cholangitic, hematogenic, lymphogenic, and pylephlebitic liver abscesses are all included within the code K75.0, Abscess of liver. Note that the lists of inclusion terms are not exhaustive—so if a term does not appear in the list of inclusion terms, but the condition still fits within the code description, it is still acceptable to assign the code.

Excludes Notes

Excludes notes are the opposite of Includes notes, as they identify conditions that are similar but independent of each other. The ICD-10-CM code set has two types of Excludes notes—Excludes1 and Excludes2. The **Excludes1** note is a pure Excludes note, meaning that the condition listed under the Excludes1 note and the coded condition are mutually exclusive and should never be coded together. For example, a congenital form and an acquired form of a condition cannot be coded together. Looking at figure 4.18, *cholangitis without liver abscess (K83.09)* is listed as an Excludes1 condition, which means that coders should not code K75.0, Abscess of liver, with K83.09, Cholangitis without liver abscess. In this case, the coder would have to select *either* K75.0 *or* K83.09, not both.

Excludes2 notes identify conditions that are "not included here." This means that if the patient had the condition located under the Excludes2 note, then they should code for that condition elsewhere. If the patient has both the condition within the Excludes2 note *as well as* the coded condition, then both of the codes may be reported together, as appropriate. Looking at figure 4.18, *acute or subacute hepatitis NOS (B17.9)* is listed as an Excludes2 note under the K75.0 code. So, if a patient had both an abscess of the liver and unspecified acute or subacute hepatitis, then it would be appropriate for the coder to identify each of the conditions with an individual code: K75.0, Abscess of liver, and B17.9, Acute or subacute hepatitis NOS.

Figure 4.18. Inclusion terms, Excludes1 notes, and Excludes2 notes

```
K75   Other inflammatory liver diseases
        Excludes2:  toxic liver disease (K71.-)
MCC  K75.0  Abscess of liver
              Cholangitic hepatic abscess
              Hematogenic hepatic abscess
              Hepatic abscess NOS
              Lymphogenic hepatic abscess
              Pylephlebitic hepatic abscess
        Excludes1:  amebic liver abscess (A06.4)
                    cholangitis without liver abscess (K83.09)
                    pylephlebitis without liver abscess (K75.1)
        Excludes2:  acute or subacute hepatitis NOS (B17.9)
                    acute or subacute non-viral hepatitis (K72.0)
                    chronic hepatitis NEC (K73.8)
```

Source: Casto 2019, 736.

There is an important exception to Excludes1 notes. Coders may code for both conditions if they are unrelated to each other. The reason for this is that sometimes a diagnosis code is a general code for a condition that can manifest in multiple ways. For example, code F45.8, Other somatoform disorders, includes many different conditions, from teeth grinding to psychogenic dysmenorrhea. Thus, if the initial code is for G47.63, Sleep related teeth grinding—which contains an Excludes1 note for *other somatoform disorders (F45.8)*—then it would be acceptable to code G47.63 *with* F45.8, but only if the condition coded by F45.8 is unrelated to the sleep-related teeth grinding, such as psychogenic dysmenorrhea (teeth grinding and dysmenorrhea are unrelated conditions). Whenever there is confusion regarding whether or not two conditions are related, the coder should query the provider to verify the diagnoses and obtain more information.

And, With, Code Also, *and* Sequencing Instructions

Sequencing, or placing the codes in a particular order, is an important part of ICD-10-CM coding. When sequenced correctly, the diagnosis codes should tell the story of why the patient presented for treatment. Typically, when a patient has more than one healthcare condition, the diagnosis code primarily responsible for the services provided is sequenced before any others. If the patient has two or more diagnoses, each of which requiring the same amount of treatment or management, then either of the diagnoses should be sequenced first. However, there are a few conventions in the Tabular List of the ICD-10-CM code book that instruct coders how to sequence certain conditions, and whether or not to include other codes to identify additional healthcare conditions. These are *and*, *with*, *code also*, and *sequencing instructions*.

When referencing the Tabular List to verify code selection, coders will encounter the term *and*, which should be interpreted to mean *and* or *or*. For example, the code A18.0-, Tuberculosis of bones and joints, can include tuberculosis of the bones, tuberculosis of the joints, or tuberculosis of the bones and joints. This is indicated by the *and* in the code description.

When the term *with* appears in the Tabular, it should be interpreted to mean *associated with* or *due to*. This term presumes a causal relationship between the two conditions linked by the word *with*. For example, K71.1-, Toxic liver disease with hepatic necrosis, codes for hepatic failure (hepatic necrosis) *due to* drugs, as indicated by the word *with*.

The *code also* note informs the coder that two codes may be necessary to fully describe a condition. For example, H35.0-, Background retinopathy and retinal vascular changes, includes the note Code also any associated hypertension (I10). This means that if the patient has a condition classifiable to a code beginning with H35.0-, as well as associated hypertension, then the coder should include a code for *both* conditions. However, this note does not include sequencing instructions regarding which code should be listed first, so the coder must determine the sequencing of the two codes. To determine the code that should be sequenced first, the coder must read through the provider's documentation of the healthcare encounter and identify the primary diagnosis code. Additional instruction on how to assign the primary diagnosis code is provided later in this chapter as well as in chapter 8 of this textbook.

Sequencing instructions are listed in the Tabular List of the ICD-10-CM code book in the same way that *code also* notes are included. They are located beneath a section, category, or subsection, and give coders more information on how to sequence two or more codes. The following are sequencing instructions found in the Tabular List.

- **Code first** instructions list conditions that should be coded before the code identified. For example, there is a *code first* note under J18, Pneumonia, unspecified organism that instructs the coder to Code first associated influenza, if applicable (J09.X1, J10.0-, J11.0-). If the patient had both pneumonia due to unspecified organism and influenza, then the coder would code for each condition with the influenza code first and the pneumonia code second: J11.00, Influenza due to unidentified influenza virus with unspecified type of pneumonia, then J18.9, Pneumonia, unspecified organism.

- **Use additional code** instructions list conditions that should be coded after the identified code. For example, there is a *use additional code* note under D57, Sickle-cell disorders, instructing the coder to Use additional code for any associated fever (R50.81). If the patient had both a sickle cell disorder coded under category D57 and an associated fever, then the fever would be coded in addition to the sickle-cell disorder, ordered as follows: D57.- Sickle-cell disorders, then R50.81, Fever presenting with conditions classified elsewhere.

Etiology and Manifestation

The **etiology** of a disease is the cause of that disease, and the manifestation is the signs and symptoms of the disease (as discussed previously in the chapter). For example, the etiology of streptococcal sore throat is the streptococcal bacteria, whereas the manifestation of the disease is the sore throat and perhaps another symptom like fever. Refer to figure 4.19 for the OGCR related to etiology and manifestation coding.

In ICD-10-CM coding, occasionally the etiology and manifestation of a disease are reported using a **combination code**—one code for both etiology and manifestation. The ICD-10-CM code set contains numerous combination codes, such as diabetes mellitus codes that combine the etiology (diabetes) with the manifestation (retinopathy). So for a patient with diabetes mellitus type 2 with diabetic retinopathy, only code E11.319, Type 2 diabetes mellitus with unspecified diabetic retinopathy without macular edema, would need to be coded to identify both the etiology and the manifestation of the disease.

When the etiology and manifestation are coded separately using two different codes, coders must pay close attention to sequencing guidelines to ensure the correct

Figure 4.19. OGCR I.A.13 Etiology/manifestation convention

---

13. **Etiology/Manifestation Convention ("Code first", "Use additional code" and "In Diseases Classified Elsewhere" Notes)**

    Certain conditions have both an underlying etiology and multiple body system manifestations due to the underlying etiology. For such conditions, the ICD-10-CM has a coding convention that requires the underlying condition be sequenced first, if applicable, followed by the manifestation. Wherever such a combination exists, there is a "use additional code" note at the etiology code, and a "code first" note at the manifestation code. These instructional notes indicate the proper sequencing order of the codes, etiology followed by manifestation.

    In most cases the manifestation codes will have in the code title, "in diseases classified elsewhere." Codes with this title are a component of the etiology/manifestation convention. The code title indicates that it is a manifestation code. "In diseases classified elsewhere" codes are never permitted to be used as first-listed or principal diagnosis codes. They must be used in conjunction with an underlying condition code and they must be listed following the underlying condition. See category F02, Dementia in other diseases classified elsewhere, for an example of this convention.

    There are manifestation codes that do not have "in diseases classified elsewhere" in the title. For such codes, there is a "use additional code" note at the etiology code and a "code first" note at the manifestation code and the rules for sequencing apply.

    In addition to the notes in the Tabular List, these conditions also have a specific Alphabetic Index entry structure. In the Alphabetic Index both conditions are listed together with the etiology code first followed by the manifestation codes in brackets. The code in brackets is always to be sequenced second.

    An example of the etiology/manifestation convention is dementia in Parkinson's disease. In the Alphabetic Index, code G20 is listed first, followed by code F02.80 or F02.81 in brackets. Code G20 represents the underlying etiology, Parkinson's disease, and must be sequenced first, whereas codes F02.80 and F02.81 represent the manifestation of dementia in diseases classified elsewhere, with or without behavioral disturbance.

    "Code first" and "Use additional code" notes are also used as sequencing rules in the classification for certain codes that are not part of an etiology/ manifestation combination.

    See Section I.B. 7. Multiple coding for a single condition.

Source: CMS 2019.

sequencing of the codes. This is common when a condition is caused by an infectious organism. Although some combination codes do exist, it is often necessary to include both the manifestation code and the etiology code for conditions caused by known infectious organisms. For example, category J04, Acute laryngitis and tracheitis requires that the coder Use additional code (B95 to B97) to identify the infectious agent. If the infectious agent is known, then it would be coded after the J04 code, as follows: J04.0, Acute laryngitis, then the code for the infectious agent, B95.0, Streptococcus, group A, as the cause of diseases classified elsewhere.

There are certain codes within the ICD-10-CM code set that can only be used to identify a manifestation of a disease, and in this case *must* be used in combination with the code that identifies the etiology of the condition. Manifestation codes cannot be used alone. The Tabular List of the ICD-10-CM code book typically include some sort of notation to identify manifestation codes, to alert the coder that these codes can only be sequenced after the code for the causative condition (the etiology). In the AHIMA *ICD-10-CM Code Book*, manifestation codes are highlighted in a pale green color (see figure 4.16). For example, codes within the category D63, Anemia in chronic diseases classified elsewhere, are all manifestation codes as they are a manifestation of some sort of underlying cause (the disease classified elsewhere). Note that in the AHIMA *ICD-10-CM Code Book*, all of the codes within category D63 are highlighted green, which indicates that these codes are manifestation codes, and must be sequenced after the code for the underlying etiology. Under each of the manifestation codes, a notation appears to help guide the coder to the code for the underlying condition. For example, code D63.0, Anemia in neoplastic disease, is followed by a notation to Code first neoplasm (C00-D49).

In addition to coding conventions, there are applicable coding guidelines throughout the ICD-10-CM code book that are not chapter specific. That is, they do not apply to only one chapter, but rather to all codes in the book.

OGCR General Coding Guidelines

The ICD-10-CM code book includes general coding guidelines for use with all of the codes in the ICD-10-CM code set. It is important to understand these guidelines, as they govern the way that codes are selected, sequenced, and reported on claims. Note that some guidelines pertain specifically to outpatient (professional) services, and others pertain to the inpatient (facility) setting. Professional outpatient guidelines are discussed here, with inpatient facility guidelines discussed in chapter 20 of this textbook.

Several of these instructions have already been discussed throughout this chapter, but a few remain. Namely, the guidelines on when to code for signs and symptoms versus a definitive diagnosis; sequencing of acute and chronic conditions; laterality; and primary diagnosis. There are additional important guidelines, however, it more useful to discuss these guidelines within the context of actual coding examples. The remaining chapters of this textbook include a discussion of the relevant guidelines when applicable.

Signs and Symptoms versus Definitive Diagnosis

Signs and symptoms are acceptable for reporting purposes only when the definitive diagnosis has not been confirmed by the healthcare provider (see figure 4.20). Signs of a disease or disease process are objective evidence that can be observed or detected by someone other than the individual affected by the condition. For example, a fever would be a sign of a disease process. Symptoms, on the other hand, are subjective evidence of a disease or a disease process experienced by the individual affected by the condition. For example, a headache, lethargy, and nausea would all be symptoms of a disease.

Figure 4.20. OGCR I.B.4, I.B.5, I.B.6

> **4.   Signs and Symptoms**
> Codes that describe symptoms and signs, as opposed to diagnoses, are acceptable for reporting purposes when a related definitive diagnosis has not been established (confirmed) by the provider. Chapter 18 of ICD-10-CM, Symptoms, Signs, and Abnormal Clinical and Laboratory Findings, Not Elsewhere Classified (codes R00.0–R99) contains many, but not all codes for symptoms.
> *See Section I.B.18 Use of Signs/Symptom/Unspecified Codes*
>
> **5.   Conditions that are an Integral Part of a Disease Process**
> Signs and symptoms that are associated routinely with a disease process should not be assigned as additional codes, unless otherwise instructed by the classification.
>
> **6.   Conditions that are not an Integral Part of a Disease Process**
> Additional signs and symptoms that may not be associated routinely with a disease process should be coded when present.

Source: CMS 2019.

Coders should only report signs and symptoms when a definitive diagnosis has not been determined by the healthcare provider. A **definitive diagnosis** is the condition or disease confirmed to be the cause of the signs or symptoms. For example, if a patient presents to the office with the signs and symptoms of fever, headache, lethargy, and nausea, and the doctor determines that the patient has influenza, then influenza is the definitive diagnosis.

When a definitive diagnosis has been identified, it is not acceptable to report the signs and symptoms that are commonly included within the disease process. As these signs and symptoms are integral to a disease process, they are already included within the code description. In the above example, only the influenza diagnosis code would be reported. It is not necessary to report the signs and symptoms of fever, headache, lethargy, and nausea, as these are an integral part of the disease process of influenza.

It is acceptable to code for the signs and symptoms when:

- A definitive diagnosis has not yet been determined. It may take several encounters before a definitive diagnosis is confirmed, and it is common that patients may not return for a definitive diagnosis. In these cases, code for the signs and symptoms.
- Signs and symptoms that are *not* an integral part of a disease process may be reported when present. For example, if the patient also had swelling of the hand and the signs and symptoms of influenza, then the sign of swelling would be reported in addition to the definitive diagnosis of influenza. (CMS 2018)

Acute and Chronic Conditions

Acute conditions have a severe and sudden onset; that is, they occur quickly and are serious in nature. For example, acute bronchitis is typically caused by an infectious organism, producing severe symptoms of coughing that occurs rapidly. **A chronic condition**, on the other hand, is a syndrome or condition that has been in development for a long period of time and is a constant disease state. For example, chronic bronchitis is a constant state of bronchial inflammation that causes a persistent cough. Some conditions may also be referred to as subacute, and others may present with an acute exacerbation of a chronic condition, like a flare-up. These may be referred to as "acute and chronic" or "acute on chronic."

It is important to make the distinction between acute and chronic conditions, as the acuity of the condition impacts the sequencing when a patient present to the office with both the acute and chronic forms of the same condition. Acute conditions are sequenced first. For example, if a patient with chronic bronchitis presents to the healthcare office for treatment of an acute exacerbation, or worsening, of his bronchitis, then it would be appropriate to code for both the acute bronchitis and the chronic bronchitis. In this case, the code for the acute condition would be sequenced before the code for the chronic condition.

Occasionally, there is a combination code that includes both the acute and chronic versions of a condition. If a combination code is available, then it should be used instead of individual codes for the acute and chronic conditions (see figure 4.21).

Laterality

Laterality refers to the side of the body on which a condition appears. The human body has several symmetrical organs. Other than the internal organs, there are two different sides to most of the rest of the human body. ICD-10-CM diagnosis codes capture the side affected by a condition by including the laterality within the code description. Codes exist for right, left, and **bilateral** (affecting both right and left sides) conditions. If the condition does present bilaterally but there is not a bilateral option available, coders should assign the codes for both the right and left sides. When the documentation does not specify the laterality of the condition, it is acceptable to report the code option with unspecified laterality (see figure 4.22).

First-Listed Diagnosis

All diagnosis codes must be supported by documentation from the patient's health record. Once all codes have been identified, it is then necessary to determine the primary reason for the encounter and sequence the codes according to the primary reason for the encounter by using chapter-specific coding guidelines. The **first-listed diagnosis** in outpatient coding is the first diagnosis code listed on a claim when more than one diagnosis code is applicable. It may also be referred to as the primary diagnosis. As previously mentioned, sequencing of diagnosis codes is important, as they tell the story of why the patient presented for treatment in the outpatient setting. Please note that inpatient coding guidelines are different for determining the first-listed condition (called the principal diagnosis in inpatient coding). The guidelines discussed here are for outpatient coding purposes only.

Figure 4.21. OGCR I.B.8, I.B.9

8.   Acute and Chronic Conditions

If the same condition is described as both acute (subacute) and chronic, and separate subentries exist in the Alphabetic Index at the same indentation level, code both and sequence the acute (subacute) code first.

9.   Combination Code

A combination code is a single code used to classify:

- Two diagnoses, or
- A diagnosis with an associated secondary process (manifestation)
- A diagnosis with an associated complication

Combination codes are identified by referring to subterm entries in the Alphabetic Index and by reading the inclusion and exclusion notes in the Tabular List.

Assign only the combination code when that code fully identifies the diagnostic conditions involved or when the Alphabetic Index so directs. Multiple coding should not be used when the classification provides a combination code that clearly identifies all of the elements documented in the diagnosis. When the combination code lacks necessary specificity in describing the manifestation or complication, an additional code should be used as a secondary code.

Source: CMS 2019.

Figure 4.22. OGCR I.B.13

13. Laterality

Some ICD-10-CM codes indicate laterality, specifying whether the condition occurs on the left, right or is bilateral. If no bilateral code is provided and the condition is bilateral, assign separate codes for both the left and right side. If the side is not identified in the medical record, assign the code for the unspecified side.

When a patient has a bilateral condition and each side is treated during separate encounters, assign the "bilateral" code (as the conditions still exists on both sides), including for the encounter to treat the first side. For the second encounter for treatment after one side has previously been treated and the condition no longer exists on that side, assign the appropriate unilateral code for the side where the conditions still exists (e.g., cataract surgery performed on each eye in separate encounters). The bilateral code would not be assigned for the subsequent encounter, as the patient no longer has the condition in the previously-treated site. If the treatment on the first side did not completely resolve the condition, then the bilateral code would still be appropriate.

Source: CMS 2019.

The first-listed diagnosis should be the one chiefly responsible for the healthcare services provided. Any additional coexisting conditions, pertinent patient history or status codes, or diagnoses should be sequenced after the first-listed diagnosis (see figure 4.23). For example, if a patient with diabetes mellitus type 2 presented to the office for treatment of an acute upper respiratory infection, then the first-listed diagnosis would be the one that was primarily responsible for the services provided on that day, with additional conditions sequenced subsequently. In this case: J06.9, Acute upper respiratory infection, unspecified, would be followed by E11.9, Type 2 diabetes mellitus without complications. The patient came in for treatment of the respiratory infection, so the respiratory infection code is sequenced first, followed by the diabetes code. Again, note that this guideline is for the professional outpatient setting, and inpatient facility guidelines may differ (refer to chapter 20).

Sometimes the definitive diagnosis is not known, but the provider has an idea of what it might be. Conditions that are documented as "suspected," "rule out," "probable," or "questionable," should not be coded as they are not confirmed by the healthcare provider. If a condition is "suspected" but not confirmed, then code only for the signs

---

Figure 4.23. OGCR III, III.A

Section III. Reporting Additional Diagnoses

GENERAL RULES FOR OTHER (ADDITIONAL) DIAGNOSES

For reporting purposes the definition for "other diagnoses" is interpreted as additional conditions that affect patient care in terms of requiring:

- clinical evaluation; or
- therapeutic treatment; or
- diagnostic procedures; or
- extended length of hospital stay; or
- increased nursing care and/or
- monitoring

The UHDDS item #11-b defines Other Diagnoses as "all conditions that coexist at the time of admission, that develop subsequently, or that affect the treatment received and/or the length of stay. Diagnoses that relate to an earlier episode which have no bearing on the current hospital stay are to be excluded." UHDDS definitions apply to inpatients in acute-care, short-term, long term care and psychiatric hospital setting. The UHDDS definitions are used by acute-care shortterm hospitals to report inpatient data elements in a standardized manner. These data elements and their definitions can be found in the July 31, 1985, *Federal Register* (Vol. 50, No, 147), pp. 31038–40.

Since that time the application of the UHDDS definitions has been expanded to include all nonoutpatient settings (acute-care, short-term, long-term care and psychiatric hospitals; home health agencies; rehab facilities; nursing homes, etc). The UHDDS definitions also apply to hospice services (all levels of care).

The following guidelines are to be applied in designating "other diagnoses" when neither the Alphabetic Index nor the Tabular List in ICD-10-CM provide direction. The listing of the diagnoses in the patient record is the responsibility of the attending provider.

A. Previous Conditions

If the provider has included a diagnosis in the final diagnostic statement, such as the discharge summary or the face sheet, it should ordinarily be coded. Some providers include in the diagnostic statement resolved conditions or diagnoses and status-post procedures from previous admission that have no bearing on the current stay. Such conditions are not to be reported and are coded only if required by hospital policy.

However, history codes (categories Z80–Z87) may be used as secondary codes if the historical condition or family history has an impact on current care or influences treatment.

Source: CMS 2019.

and symptoms present at the time of the encounter (see figure 4.24). For example, a provider may evaluate a patient with low energy, joint pain, and depression, and suspect that she has hypothyroidism. However, the coder cannot assign the code for hypothyroidism until the provider is certain that it is the patient's definitive diagnosis.

Code all documented conditions that coexist at the time of the encounter and that require or affect patient care, management, or treatment (see figure 4.25). For example, it may be necessary to include a relevant family history code, if that family history has an impact on the current care of the patient. This guideline is especially important in HCC coding (discussed in chapter 2), which requires that coders report all coexisting conditions for risk adjustment purposes. Remember that HCC coding involves identifying and reporting codes that give a full and clear picture of a patient's health. This is more than simply what is required for the payment of a claim, but also includes codes that identify aspects of a patient's health—pertinent personal medical history and status codes, and all other conditions present at the time of the encounter, even if they are not related to the treatment provided that day. Chronic or ongoing diseases may be reported as many times as necessary to report the treatment and care for the ongoing condition.

Figure 4.24. OGCR IV.H

H. Uncertain Diagnosis

Do not code diagnoses documented as "probable", "suspected," "questionable," "rule out," **"compatible with,"** **"consistent with,"** or "working diagnosis" or other similar terms indicating uncertainty. Rather, code the condition(s) to the highest degree of certainty for that encounter/visit, such as symptoms, signs, abnormal test results, or other reason for the visit.

   Please note: This differs from the coding practices used by short-term, acute-care, long-term care and psychiatric hospitals.

Source: CMS 2019.

Figure 4.25. OGCR IV.J

J.   Code All Documented Conditions that Coexist

Code all documented conditions that coexist at the time of the encounter/visit, and require or affect patient care treatment or management. Do not code conditions that were previously treated and no longer exist. However, history codes (categories Z80–Z87) may be used as secondary codes if the historical condition or family history has an impact on current care or influences treatment.

Source: CMS 2019.

ICD-10-CM Code Structure

The structure of ICD-10-CM codes is unique from any other code set. Unlike CPT, HCPCS, or even ICD-10-PCS codes, ICD-10-CM codes are alphanumeric and vary in length, ranging from three to seven characters. Also unique to ICD-10-CM codes is the use of a placeholder X, which keeps the place of a character so that the code can be extended fully to the required amount of characters. And, finally, some ICD-10-CM codes use a character to identify the episode of care, extending the code to the full seven characters.

Code Structure and Format

ICD-10-CM codes range from three to seven characters in length. The length is determined by the requirements for each code and, typically, longer codes (seven characters) contain more detail than shorter codes (three characters), as each additional character adds more detail to the code description. No matter the code length, a decimal point is always placed after the third character in the code, and additional characters are placed after the decimal point. Add as many additional characters as needed in order to code to the full extent, as determined by the ICD-10-CM guidelines (discussed previously in this chapter).

ICD-10-CM codes are alphanumeric, as follows (see figure 4.26):

- The first character is always a letter
- The second character is always a number
- Characters three through seven may be either numbers or letters
- All letters of the alphabet are used with the exception of *U*, which has been reserved for future expansion or updates of the ICD-10-CM code set.

Figure 4.26. ICD-10-CM code structure

ICD-10-CM Code Structure	Examples
• Three to seven characters • First character is always alpha • Second digit is always numeric • Characters three through seven are either alpha or numeric • All letters are utilized (except for *U*)	• R12, Heartburn • J91.0, Malignant pleural effusion • C72.21, Malignant neoplasm of right olfactory nerve • Z3A.20, 20 weeks gestation of pregnancy • H02.821, Cysts of right upper eyelid • S09.21XA, Traumatic rupture of right ear drum, initial encounter

The ICD-10-CM code format is based on a possible length of seven characters total. This does not mean that each code has seven characters. ICD-10-CM codes range from three to seven characters total (see figure 4.27). The first three characters of an ICD-10-CM code are referred to as the category. Codes that start with the same three characters are within the same category. For example, category I11 stands for hypertensive heart disease, so each code that starts with I11 is a type of hypertensive heart disease. In the same manner, I12 stands for hypertensive chronic kidney disease, so each code that begins with I12 is a type of hypertensive chronic kidney disease (see table 4.1).

Figure 4.27. ICD-10-CM code format

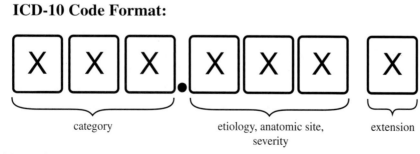

Source: Adapted from DeVault et al. 2014.

The category is followed by a decimal point and a varying number of characters. Note that ICD-10-CM codes range from three to seven codes. This means that there are a number of three-character category codes, such as I10, Essential (primary) hypertension. This code is not further divided as it has no additional characters or details. This is rare, however, as most ICD-10-CM codes do contain additional characters after the decimal point, each of which add further information to the code.

Table 4.1. Categories I10 and I12

I10 Essential (primary) hypertension	I10 Essential (primary) hypertension
I11 Hypertensive heart disease	**I11**.0 *Hypertensive heart disease* with heart failure **I11**.9 *Hypertensive heart disease* without heart failure
I12 Hypertensive chronic kidney disease	**I12**.0 *Hypertensive chronic kidney disease* with stage 5 chronic kidney disease or end-stage renal disease **I12**.9 *Hypertensive chronic kidney disease* with stage 1 through stage 4 chronic kidney disease, or unspecified chronic kidney disease

I13 Hypertensive heart and chronic kidney disease	**I13**.0 *Hypertensive heart and chronic kidney disease* with heart failure and stage 1 through stage 4 chronic kidney disease, or unspecified chronic kidney disease
	I13.1 *Hypertensive heart and chronic kidney disease* without heart failure
	    I13.10 ...... with stage 1 through stage 4 chronic kidney disease, or unspecified chronic kidney disease
	    I13.11 ...... with stage 5 chronic kidney disease, or end-stage renal disease
	I13.2 *Hypertensive heart and chronic kidney disease* with heart failure and with stage 5 chronic kidney disease, or end-stage renal disease

There are four additional characters that may be added to an ICD-10-CM code after the decimal point. Characters four, five, and six each add further detail to the code description, including the etiology (the cause of a disease), anatomic site, and severity of the condition. The meanings of these three characters vary. For example, in table 4.1, the fourth character for category I12 indicates if the hypertensive heart disease presents with or without heart failure. For category I13, the fourth character identifies the stage of chronic kidney disease. For category I13, codes within the subcategory I13.1 each have an additional number that identifies the stage of chronic kidney disease for hypertensive heart and chronic kidney disease without heart failure. Again, these characters have different meanings for each specific code, so it is important to read through each code description and take note of the ways codes change depending on the characters added.

Up to four additional characters may be added after the decimal point, each of which provides more detail to the code. The last possible character—in the seventh location— is referred to as the **seventh character extension**, discussed in detail later in this chapter. This character is always placed in the seventh and last location, and usually represents the **episode of care** for the encounter. The episode of care identifies the patient's place within the care continuum. For example, the episode of care may identify that the patient is still in active treatment status, or is coming in for a subsequent encounter after the active treatment phase has passed.

Seventh Character Extensions and Episode of Care

Each character added to an ICD-10-CM code provides an additional detail, each of which makes the code more specific (see figure 4.28).

Normally, codes that are extended to the seventh character contain a seventh character episode of care identifier. In the majority of cases, the seventh character identifies the episode of care but there are exceptions to this—in rare instances, the seventh character may be used to identify a detail other than the episode of care, such as laterality or fetus in multiple pregnancies. If the seventh character is not added to the code, then it is considered an invalid code and will not be accepted on a claim.

Figure 4.28. ICD-10-CM seven-character code example

S62.512A

Displaced fracture of proximal phalanx of left thumb, initial encounter for closed fracture

S62 – Fracture at wrist and hand level
S62.**5** – fracture of thumb
S62.5**1** – proximal phalanx
S62.51**2** – displaced
S62.512**A** – initial encounter for closed fracture

Character	1	2	3	4	5	6	7
Code	S	6	2	5	1	2	A
Description	Fracture at wrist and hand level			Thumb	Proximal	Displaced	Initial, Closed

CC +7th S62.512 **Displaced fracture of proximal phalanx of left thumb**
　　　　　 HAC 7th character B see Appendix B for HAC conditional logic

A seventh character extension is always placed in the last position (the seventh character) of an ICD-10-CM code and includes more information about the condition or the episode of care for that condition. Although the seventh character most commonly identifies the episode of care, it is also used in obstetrics coding and a few other places in the ICD-10-CM code book. Note that the seventh character extension is not always a letter. In obstetrics coding, the seventh character may be a number, used to identify the fetus in a multiple gestation pregnancy. Seventh character extensions other than the episode of care are discussed when necessary throughout the remainder of this textbook.

For certain conditions, such as fractures, there are up to 16 episodes of care possible. These are discussed in detail in chapter 15 (Orthopedic Services). The three most common episode of care characters found throughout the ICD-10-CM code book are represented by the letters *A*, *D*, and *S*.

- **A- Initial Encounter**. This episode of care is used during the active treatment phase of a condition or when the patient is still receiving treatment for a condition. Note that this does not mean *only* the first time that patient is seen. Episode of care letter *A* may be used multiple times, as long as the patient is still receiving active treatment (for example, if a patient receives wound treatments every day for a complicated wound that requires extensive observation).

- **D- Subsequent encounter**. This episode of care is used when the patient is seen during the healing phase of the encounter and is no longer receiving active treatment for the condition (for example, when a patient presents for cast removal after the healing phase of a fracture is completed).

- **S- Sequela.** A sequela is a condition that is the consequence of a previous disease or injury. Sometimes referred to as a late effect, this letter should be used when a patient is seen for a complication of the condition after the healing phase has been completed. For example, the patient has residual pain in the hip after a hip fracture three years ago.

Review the following examples to see how the encounter affects the episode of care for the patient.

Billy, a five-year-old boy, was playing at a local park feeding the squirrels when he was bit on his left forearm by a squirrel. He presents to the urgent care clinic for cleaning and evaluation of the injury. He is diagnosed with a 1cm puncture wound without foreign body on the left forearm due to the squirrel bite. The urgent care doctor cleaned the wound and placed two stitches, prescribed an oral antibiotic, and ordered the patient to see his PCP the next day.

The diagnosis code assigned by the urgent care doctor would be S51.832-, Puncture wound without foreign body of left forearm. This code is not complete, as it requires a seventh character to identify the episode of care for the visit. In this case, the patient is in the active phase of treatment, so the letter *A* for initial care would be added to the end of the code: S51.832A, Puncture wound without foreign body of left forearm, *initial encounter*.

The next day, Billy presents to his PCP's office for an evaluation of his injury as ordered by the urgent care doctor. His PCP examines the wound and determines that is it healing well at this point, and that Billy should continue to monitor the wound and return to the office in two weeks for removal of his stitches, or sooner if any signs of infection are present.

The diagnosis code assigned by the patient's PCP for this visit would be the same as that assigned by the urgent care doctor: S51.832A, Puncture wound without foreign body of left forearm, *initial encounter*. Notice that even though this is the second time that the patient has been seen for the same wound, he is still in the active phase of treatment. Because of this, the seventh character "A" indicating active care is added to the end of the code.

Three days after Billy was seen by his PCP, his mother brings him into the office because the wound is red, painful, and there is a small amount of pus coming out of the puncture site. After evaluation of the fluid, the doctor determines that the wound is infected, prescribes a different antibiotic, cleans the wound, and replaces the stitches. He then orders the patient to return in two weeks or sooner if necessary.

In this case, the diagnosis code is the same for the wound of the arm: S51.832A, Puncture wound without foreign body of left forearm, *initial encounter*. At this point, the child has been seen three times for the same injury, and each service has been some sort of active care for the patient's injury, so the seventh character "A" for initial encounter is assigned for all three.

Billy presents to the office of his PCP two weeks after the initial injury for removal of stitches and evaluation of the healing status of his wound. His PCP examines the wound, which is well-healed at this point, but is notable for a large scar that has begun to form at the site of the wound. The PCP then removes the two stitches and informs the patient that he no longer has to be seen for this injury.

The diagnosis code for this case would be the same that has been used for the same injury previously, with the exception that the episode of care is different. In this case, the patient is in the healing phase of the injury and is no longer receiving active treatment for the wound. Thus, the seventh character *D*, for subsequent care, replaces the *A* at the end of the code. The code assigned would be as follows: S51.832D, Puncture wound without foreign body of left forearm, *subsequent encounter*.

Three months after the initial injury, Billy's mother returns with him to the office because of a large keloid scar that has formed at the initial injury site. The scar is painful and irritating, and the mother would like to have the PCP evaluate the scar to see if there is anything that they can do. The PCP examines the wound site and diagnoses Billy with a keloid scar due to the initial squirrel bite injury.

For this visit, the PCP assigns a code for the keloid scar that is a sequela of the previous injury, the puncture wound. So two codes are necessary: one to identify the keloid scar and one to identify the previous injury, the puncture wound. The puncture wound diagnosis will be the same as those used previously for the same injury, but since the episode of care is different the seventh character extension will be changed to *S* to recognize that the patient is coming in for a sequela of the injury: S51.832S, Puncture wound without foreign body of left forearm, *sequela*. Refer to table 4.2 for a simplified timeline of these visits.

Table 4.2. Example of episodes of care for an injury

Date	Encounter	Episode of Care
Day 1	Urgent Care for initial injury	A-Initial
Day 2	PCP office for follow-up	A-Initial
Day 5	PCP office for wound infection	A-Initial
Day 22	PCP office for follow-up and suture removal	D-Subsequent
Month 3	PCP office for evaluation of scar	S-Sequela

Key to Success

Rather than thinking of the episode of care letter *A* as the first time a patient is seen, think of it as "Active Care." A = Active Care. The letter *A* should be used for any visit in which the patient is undergoing active care, not necessarily the first time that the patient is seen.

The appropriate episode of care letter should be added to the end of the ICD-10-CM code depending on where the patient presents on their timeline of care. Note that although A, D, and S, are the three most common episode of care identifiers, they are not the only ones. Some fractures have up to 16 different seventh character extensions, each labeled with a letter, which identify the type of fracture, episode of care, and healing status (these are discussed in detail in chapter 15).

Episodes of care extensions are most commonly used with injury codes, such as fractures, burns, and open wounds. They are also used with external cause codes. **External cause codes** identify the circumstances surrounding an injury, poisoning, or adverse event, such as the activity that the patient was engaged in when the injury occurred, where the patient was when the injury took place, and the injury mechanism (how the injury happened). External cause codes are located in the External Causes of Injury Index.

Complete the exercises in There's a Code for That 4.8 and 4.9 to practice identifying seventh character extensions.

4.8

There's a Code for That

Identify the seventh character extension options

Using the Tabular List, identify the possible seventh character extensions for the following codes by locating the seventh character extension options.

1. What are the seventh character extension options for S03.01, Dislocation of jaw, right side?

   Seventh character options: _____

2. What are the seventh character extension options for S12.030, Displaced posterior arch fracture of first cervical vertebra?

   Seventh character options: _____

3. What are the seventh character extension options for H40.221, Chronic angle-closure glaucoma, right eye?

   Seventh character options: _____

4. What are the seventh character extension options for O32.1, Maternal care for breech presentation?

   Seventh character options: _____

4.9

There's a Code for That

Seventh character extensions

Using your understanding of the seventh character extensions *A*, *D*, and *S*, answer the following questions (A-initial, D-subsequent, S-sequela)

1. Melinda was seen for a fracture of her wrist after falling on the sidewalk. This is the first time she has been seen for this injury. What is the episode of care for this encounter?

   Seventh character: _____

2. A patient returned to the orthopedist's office for the removal of a cast on her lower left leg. The fracture was well healed, and the cast was removed. What is the episode of care for this encounter?

   Seventh character: _____

3. Sheila suffered a fracture of her hip five years ago and now presents for treatment of arthritis of her hip due to the fracture. What is the episode of care for this injury?

   Seventh character: _____

> **4.** After initial treatment at the ER, a male patient returned to his primary care
> physician's office for treatment of a wound infection. What is the episode of
> care for this injury?
>
> Seventh character: _____

When assigning seventh character extensions, pay close attention to the guidelines
outlined in the ICD-10-CM code book, as they will specify which extensions to use and
their definitions. Sometimes an ICD-10-CM code is not yet extended to six characters,
but a seventh character is still required. In these cases, a placeholder X must be used to
extend the code to six characters, so that a seventh character may be added.

Placeholder X

In some cases, an ICD-10-CM code requires the use of a seventh character extension
to identify the episode of care, but that code is not yet extended to six characters. For
example, code S02.91-, Unspecified fracture of skull, requires the addition of a seventh
character to identify the episode of care for the visit. However, this code is only five
characters long (see figure 4.29).

This means that the code must be extended to six characters, so that the seventh
character may be added. In this case, it is necessary to insert the placeholder X as the
sixth character, in order to add the seventh character. **Placeholder X** is used to extend
a code to the required number of characters so that a seventh character extension may
be placed. In this example, the letter X is placed in the sixth location, and the correct
episode of care letter (A, D, or S) is placed in the seventh location (see figure 4.30).

The correct code to an unspecified fracture of the skull for an initial encounter
would be S02.91XA, Unspecified fracture of the skull, initial encounter. If the code is

Figure 4.29. Incomplete code example (5 out of 7 characters assigned)

Character	1	2	3	4	5	6	7
Code	S	0	2	9	1		

Figure 4.30. Complete code example (7 out of 7 characters assigned)

Character	1	2	3	4	5	6	7
Code	S	0	2	9	1	X	A

Figure 4.31. Complete code example with three placeholders (characters 4, 5, and 6)

Character	1	2	3	4	5	6	7
Code	W	5	2	X	X	X	A

not extended to seven characters, it is an invalid code. An **invalid code** is not coded to the full extent and may not be used for coding or billing purposes. For example, if an invalid code was sent on a claim for insurance payment purposes, then the insurance company would not pay the claim. It is extremely important to ensure that only valid codes are assigned.

Sometimes, multiple placeholders must be placed to extend a code to the required amount of characters in order to add a seventh character extension. For example, code W52, Crushed, pushed or stepped on by crowd or human stampede, only has three characters. However, a seventh character extension must be added to identify the episode of care for this encounter. In this case, *three* placeholders must be added to extend the code to the correct number of characters, so that the episode of care may be placed in the seventh location (see figure 4.31).

In this example, the correct code for an initial episode of care would be W52.XXXA, Crushed, pushed or stepped on by crowd or human stampede, initial encounter.

The ICD-10-CM code book has conventions and symbols that help coders identify when a seventh character extension is necessary, what the seventh characters are, and when a placeholder is needed. The code book is also carefully organized into a standardized format so coders can locate and assign codes correctly.

Complete the exercises in There's a Code for That 4.10 to practice adding appropriate placeholders.

4.10   Placeholder X

There's a Code for That

Using your understanding of the purpose and function of the placeholder X, answer the following questions.

1. The ICD code for parachutist entangled in object is V97.21-, Parachutist entangled in object, which requires a seventh character to identify the episode of care for this encounter. Which of the following would be the correct way to code for "Parachutist entangled in object, initial encounter"?
   a. V97.21A
   b. V97.XXXA
   c. V97.21XA
   d. V97.21AX

2. Complete the following code for: W54.0-, Bitten by dog, initial encounter

   ICD-10-CM code: _____

3. Complete the following code for: S60.00-, Contusion of unspecified finger without damage to nail, subsequent encounter.

   ICD-10-CM code: _____

4. Complete the following code for: W35.-, Explosion and rupture of boiler, initial encounter.

   ICD-10-CM code: _____

Case Study Diagnoses

PATIENT: Roger Stevenson   **DOB:** 06/23/1931

DATE OF SERVICE: 07/09/20xx

SUBJECTIVE:
Chief Complaint: 88-year-old male here for ER follow-up

History of Present Illness: Patient is here for a hospital follow-up, discharged 3 days ago. He was treated at the hospital for acute stroke. Residual deficit includes paresis of the left hand (patient is right-handed). Current treatment includes baby aspirin. Patient is undergoing physical and occupational therapy. Patient also has type 2 diabetes mellitus, stable on current meds, and hyperlipidemia that has been stable.

Review of Systems:
Constitutional: no fever, no chills, and not feeling poorly.
Eyes: no eye pain, no eyesight problems.
Cardiovascular: no chest pain, patient reports some occasional heart palpitations
Musculoskeletal: lower extremity limb pain, no joint pain or swelling. Weakness of left upper extremity. Weakness of left-hand grip.

Past, Family, Social History:
Current medications reviewed. No known drug allergies (NKDA). Family history of lung cancer (mother). Personal history of hernia repair 10 years ago. Patient is a social drinker and former smoker of cigarettes.

OBJECTIVE:
Physical Examination:
Constitutional: well-developed, vital signs reviewed, no acute distress, healthy weight.
Cardiovascular: heart rate and rhythm were normal, no murmurs heard, apical impulse was normal, no peripheral edema.
Musculoskeletal: normal gait, normal muscle tone. Slight weakness of the left-hand grip. Normal inspection and palpitation of all extremities, full range of motion of the neck, spine and pelvis, and all extremities.
Neurologic: no obvious cranial nerve deficits, no deficits in sensation.
Psychiatric: oriented to person, place, and time. Insight and judgment were intact. Mood and affect were normal. Recent and remote memory was not impaired.

ASSESSMENT and PLAN:

1. Left-sided hemiplegia due to cerebrovascular accident. New onset; improved. Continue with current medication regimen. Refer to neurology and cardiology for follow-up.

2. Diabetes mellitus, type 2, uncomplicated. Well-controlled. Continue with current meds. Discussed potential side effects of medication and goals for monitoring blood sugar.

3. Hyperlipidemia. Uncontrolled for stroke prevention. Discussed course of action and potential side effects of medication. Goal for LDL is < 70.

4. Paroxysmal atrial fibrillation. Rate controlled, no medication other than baby aspirin. Refer to cardiology for further evaluation.

SIGNED: Dr. Terrence Kahn, MD

Use the following steps to select the appropriate diagnosis codes for the case study.

1. Read through the case study in full. As you read, look up any medical terms with which you are unfamiliar. For example, the terms *hyperlipidemia* and *peripheral edema* may not be familiar to you. Use a medical dictionary or medical terminology textbook to define these terms. On your own, look up and define any additional unfamiliar terms.

a. *Hyperlipidemia*:

_____

_____

b. *Peripheral edema*:

_____

_____

2. Review the case study and answer the following question: *Why did the doctor do it?* Search the case study for terms that will identify the healthcare condition. Note the ASSESSMENT section of the documentation, where the provider has listed each of the healthcare conditions observed or addressed during the visit. In the case study, identify the patient's diagnosis (note that there may be multiple diagnoses):

_____

_____

3. Now that you have identified the patient's diagnoses, search the ICD-10-CM code book for the correct code(s) for each condition.

a. Search the Main Index for the name of each condition and search through any applicable subterms and cross-references to locate the appropriate code.

i. _____

_____

ii. _____

_____

iii. _____

_____

iv. _____

_____

b. Verify the codes in the Tabular List. Locate each of the codes identified previously in the Tabular List and refer to any applicable guidelines, notes, and symbols. Does the code selected correctly identify the patient's condition? If yes, list the code here:

i. _____

_____

ii. _____

_____

iii. _____

_____

iv. _____

_____

c. Check the procedure note and ICD-10-CM guidelines and conventions to determine the correct sequencing of the diagnosis codes, if applicable. Correctly sequence the diagnosis codes.

_____

_____

End-of-Chapter Content

Instructions: Indicate whether the following statements are true or false (T or F). For false statements, rewrite the statement on the line below to make the statement true.

1. All ICD-10-CM codes begin with a letter.

_____

_____

2. The first three characters of an ICD-10-CM code are referred to as the subcategory.

_____

_____

3. The maximum amount of characters that an ICD-10-CM code can have is seven.

_____

_____

(Continued on next page)

(Continued)

4. The seventh character of an ICD-10-CM code typically identifies the episode of care.

_____

_____

5. The seventh character A may only be used once for any given injury.

_____

_____

6. The two major divisions of the ICD-10-CM code book are the Index and the Tabular List.

_____

_____

7. Main terms are indented under the subterms to indicate that they pertain to the subterm.

_____

_____

8. Nonessential modifiers impact the code selected from the Main Index.

_____

_____

9. Once the code is located in the Main Index, it is not important to verify the code in the Tabular List.

_____

_____

10. An adverse effect occurs when a substance that is correctly prescribed and administered causes a toxic effect.

_____

_____

Instructions: Choose the best answer.

1. Which of the following is not true regarding ICD-10-CM codes?
   a. The first character may be either a letter or a number
   b. They range from three to seven characters
   c. All letters of the alphabet are used except for the letter *U*
   d. The second character is always a number

2. Which of the following codes would be a valid ICD-10-CM code?
   a. 460.9
   b. Z3A.20.Z
   c. J91.0
   d. P09.X6594

3. What is the purpose of the additional characters after the three-character category code?

   a. They add more detail to the code description
   b. They make the procedure more complicated
   c. They make the ICD-10-CM code more difficult to look up
   d. There are never any characters added to three-character category codes

4. The episode of care extension A, for initial encounter should be used when?

   a. When the patient is receiving follow-up care after an injury has healed
   b. When the patient is pregnant with more than one fetus
   c. When the patient is receiving care for a sequela of an initial condition
   d. When the patient is in the active treatment phase for an injury

5. What is used to extend a code to the required number of characters so that a seventh character extension may be placed at the end of a code?

   a. External cause
   b. Placeholder X
   c. Seventh character extension
   d. A, for initial encounter

6. In which Index would you find the codes for a cancerous tumor?

   a. Main Index
   b. Neoplasm Table
   c. Table of Drugs
   d. External Cause Index

7. In which Index would you find the codes for the mechanism of an injury as well as the place of occurrence for an injury?

   a. Main Index
   b. Neoplasm Table
   c. Table of Drugs
   d. External Cause Index

8. What is the noun that described the patient's diagnosis or reason for encounter?

   a. External cause
   b. Main term
   c. Subterm
   d. Excludes1 note

9. Which cross-reference in the Main Index instructs coders to look elsewhere for a code if the precise condition cannot be found in the current entry?

   a. See also
   b. See condition
   c. Code first
   d. Use additional code

10. Which of the following neoplasm behaviors indicates a cancerous tumor?

    a. Benign
    b. Unspecified
    c. Uncertain behavior
    d. Malignant

11. Which of the following is the structured list of ICD-10-CM codes, organized alphanumerically, and divided into chapters based on body system or condition?

    a. Main Index
    b. Tabular List
    c. Table of Drugs and Chemicals
    d. External Cause of Injury Index

12. A three-digit code is referred to as a:

    a. Category
    b. Subcategory
    c. Section
    d. Subclassification

13. Which note is a pure Excludes note that means two conditions are mutually exclusive of each other?

    a. Excludes1
    b. Excludes2
    c. Includes
    d. Essential modifier

14. Which of the following sequencing instructions tells the coder to place the additional code *after* the current code selected?

    a. Code first
    b. See also
    c. Use additional code
    d. Code also

15. Which of the following is the cause of a disease?

    a. Etiology
    b. Manifestation
    c. Combination code
    d. Underlying infection code

16. In the absence of a definitive diagnosis, what does a coder report?

    a. Suspected conditions
    b. Probable conditions
    c. Integral conditions
    d. Signs and symptoms

17. When a patient has both the acute and chronic versions of the same condition, which is sequenced first?

    a. Acute
    b. Chronic
    c. The combination code
    d. Neither

18. When a condition affects both sides of the body it is:

    a. Lateral
    b. Bilateral
    c. Combination
    d. Acute

19. What is the term for the primary diagnosis listed on outpatient claims?

    a. First-listed diagnosis
    b. Principal diagnosis
    c. Secondary diagnosis
    d. Sequenced diagnosis

References

Casto, A.B., ed. 2019. *ICD-10-CM Code Book*. Chicago: AHIMA.

Centers for Medicare and Medicaid Services (CMS). 2019. ICD-10-CM Official Guidelines for Coding and Reporting FY 2020. https://www.cms.gov/Medicare/Coding/ICD10/Downloads/2020-Coding-Guidelines.pdf.

DeVault, K., A. Barta, and M. Endicott. 2014. *ICD-10-CM Coder Training Manual*. Chicago: AHIMA.

CHAPTER

Learning the CPT and HCPCS Code Books

Learning Objectives

- Understand the structure and purpose of CPT codes
- Examine the organization and format of the CPT code book
- Recognize and utilize the symbols, conventions, and coding guidelines for CPT codes

- Understand the structure and purpose of HCPCS codes
- Examine the organization, format, symbols, and conventions used in the HCPCS code book

Key Terms

Add-on code

Anesthesia section

Category I code

Category II code

Category III code

Eponym

Evaluation and Management
Services section

Indented code

Medicine section

Modifying term

Parenthetical note

Pathology and Laboratory section

Radiology section

Resequenced code

Separate procedure

Special report

Standalone code

Surgery section

Synonym

Table of Drugs

Telemedicine service

Unlisted procedure codes

Diagnostic coding is the first half of coding, and the second half is coding for any procedures performed—reporting the actual services, treatments, and procedures performed by the healthcare provider. There are three code sets that include procedure codes: *International Classification of Diseases, Tenth Revision, Procedure Coding System* (ICD-10-PCS), *Current Procedural Terminology* (CPT), and *Healthcare Common Procedure Coding System* (HCPCS). ICD-10-PCS codes are for procedures performed in the facility inpatient setting. As such, the PCS code book is discussed in chapter 20 (Inpatient Hospital Services) and is not included in this chapter.

As noted in chapter 3 (Basics of Coding), both CPT and HCPCS code sets have been adopted for use by the Centers for Medicare and Medicaid Services (CMS) and are known collectively as HCPCS codes. CPT codes are considered Level I codes, and HCPCS codes are considered Level II codes. Because they are published, created, and maintained by different organizations, it is important to learn the basics of each code book separately, as they differ greatly from one another.

This chapter focuses on the basics of CPT and HCPCS coding, including the structure, purpose, format, and organization and guidelines associated with each code set.

CPT Code Structure and Purpose

CPT codes are five characters in length, beginning with at least four numbers and ending with either a letter or a number. The majority of CPT codes are entirely numeric. Unlike ICD-10-CM codes, CPT codes never change in length. They always remain five characters, no matter how detailed the reported healthcare procedure.

Each CPT code identifies a specific procedure or service performed by the healthcare provider. For example, code 40808, Biopsy, vestibule of mouth, identifies a surgical procedure in which a tissue sample was taken from the inside of the cheek for examination. This code reports the specific surgical procedure performed by the healthcare provider, which will be reported to the insurance company (along with an ICD-10-CM code to identify the medical necessity for the biopsy).

There are unique CPT codes for thousands of different healthcare procedures, ranging from office visits, anesthesia services, and surgeries to radiological services and laboratory procedures. The different types of healthcare services or procedures are divided into three categories and assigned numerical code ranges that are five characters long. Refer to table 5.1 to see the code ranges for different types of procedures.

Table 5.1. CPT code ranges by procedure type

Category Type	Procedure Type	Code Range
Category I	Evaluation and Management	99201–99499
	Anesthesiology	00100–01999, 99100–99140
	Surgery	10021–69990
	Radiology	70010–79999
	Pathology and Laboratory	80047–89398, 0001U–0138U
	Medicine (except Anesthesiology)	90281–99199, 99500–99607
Category II	Supplemental Tracking Measures	0001F–9007F
Category III	New and Emerging Technologies	0042T–0953T

CPT codes are organized with similar procedures grouped together numerically. In other words, similar procedures, or those performed on the same body system, all begin with the same number(s). For example, all evaluation and management (E/M) codes begin with the same two numbers—99—such as 99381, Initial comprehensive preventive medicine evaluation and management of an individual; infant (age younger than 1 year). Similarly, all CPT codes for radiology services, such as 71048, Radiologic examination, chest, 4 or more views, begin with the number 7. As coding professionals learn more about the intricacies of the CPT coding system, these similarities become more apparent. Experienced coders may be so familiar with the CPT code structure that they can simply look at a code and identify the procedure or know on which body system the procedure was performed.

Key to Success

CPT and HCPCS coding are completely different from ICD-10-CM coding. Not only do the codes identify something completely different (a procedure, service, or supply as opposed to a diagnosis), but they are formatted differently as well. At first, these differences may be confusing, but as you work more with all three code sets, recognizing the different code sets and their uses will become second nature.

When assigning CPT codes for services, coders should select the name of the procedure that most accurately describes the service performed, not one that is simply like the code being described. Many times, healthcare procedures vary by only a small detail, such as the time involved in performing the procedure or the approach to a surgical procedure. CPT coding relies heavily on a close reading of the healthcare provider's documentation of the service performed. Any further procedures performed at the same time are reported with additional CPT codes. For example, if a provider performed a biopsy of the vestibule of the mouth and the incision and drainage of a simple pilonidal cyst, then each of these two services would be reported with the appropriate CPT code: 40808, Biopsy, vestibule of mouth, and 10080, Incision and drainage of pilonidal cyst; simple. However, in some instances, multiple procedures are bundled into one code. Bundling is discussed in greater detail in chapter 11 (Surgical Services).

According to CPT guidelines, inclusion of a code in the CPT code set does not indicate the procedure or service will be reimbursed, nor does it indicate endorsement by the American Medical Association (AMA) (AMA 2019). In other words, while a code may exist for a procedure or procedure(s), health insurance coverage is not guaranteed for each code, and reporting a CPT code does not ensure payment for the service.

The CPT Code Book

The AMA publishes the CPT code book on an annual basis and maintains the code set. The two most common versions published by AMA each year are the *CPT Standard Edition*, which is a basic manual that lists the CPT codes, and the *CPT Professional Edition*, an enhanced version of the CPT code book that includes anatomical drawings, extended guidelines, and a three-color format. It is important for first-time coders to have the best code book available; the author of this textbook recommends using the *CPT Professional Edition* while learning to code, as the additional information, guidelines, illustrations, and notes help beginning coders understand the many intricacies of CPT coding.

Like the ICD-10-CM code book, the CPT code book includes a Tabular List of all CPT codes as well as an index and several appendices. CPT codes are divided into three categories, described as follows, with most CPT codes falling within Category I codes (refer to table 5.1). After the Tabular listing of codes (which includes Category I, II, and III codes), are 16 appendices (listed later in this chapter), followed by the Index (also discussed in detail later in this chapter).

Category I codes are the largest set of codes in the CPT code book and are commonly referred to simply as CPT codes. These procedures have been approved by the Food and Drug Administration (FDA), are performed by physicians or other healthcare practitioners throughout the United States at a frequency consistent with their intended clinical use, are consistent with current clinical practice, and have a documented clinical efficacy for treating healthcare conditions (AMA 2019).

Category I CPT Codes

Category I codes are divided into six sections and make up the majority of the CPT code set. These sections group similar procedures together, such as radiology procedures or anesthesia services (see table 5.1). When learning procedural coding, it is important to keep these sections in mind, as the codes in each section are different in nature than those in the other sections. For example, the Pathology and Laboratory section lists codes that report pathology and laboratory services only, even though these services may be performed with procedures from the Radiology, Surgery, or Medicine sections. Ultimately, the sections help coders navigate the code book by grouping similar procedures together. However, codes from different sections of the CPT code book are not exclusive of each other; coders may report procedures from all sections of the CPT code book as necessary.

Guidelines specific to each individual section of the CPT code book are provided at the beginning of each section. These guidelines provide rules on how to use the respective CPT codes and offer additional information and advice about how to code correctly from each section. This textbook refers to CPT guidelines both from the beginning of each of these sections and from within each section of the CPT code book. This chapter also includes a full discussion of common CPT guidelines.

Key to Success

An easy way to see the different sections of the CPT code book is to look at the far edge from the binding, which is either shaded in a different color gray or highlighted in different colors. These varying colors or shades can help you maneuver through the code book to find sections and codes more easily.

Key to Success

As you read about the CPT code book in the following sections, flip through your own copy of the code book and follow along. Familiarize yourself with the location, notations, and format of important components of the CPT code book.

The six sections of Category I CPT codes are Evaluation and Management, Anesthesia, Surgery, Radiology, Pathology and Laboratory, and Medicine.

Evaluation and Management

The first section of Category I codes in the CPT code book is the **Evaluation and Management Services section**, which includes codes 99201 through 99499. E/M codes are perhaps the most important codes in all of professional procedural coding, making up the majority of all codes reported for professional services in both the inpatient and outpatient settings. Also referred to as E&M, E/M codes are used to report any service in which a healthcare professional evaluates and then manages or treats a patient, such as an office sick visit, hospital discharge, routine physical examination, or inpatient critical care visit (among others). E/M codes may be used across all healthcare settings, and as such this section is divided based on the type of E/M service (such as a consultation), place of service (such as in a skilled nursing facility), and patient status (such as new or established patient).

Because of the importance of E/M services, there are a great deal of guidelines governing E/M coding and this textbook will commonly refer to these guidelines as necessary to explain the nuances of E/M coding. Furthermore, because E/M coding is used in all healthcare settings and by all types of qualified healthcare professionals, E/M services will be referenced frequently throughout this text. This textbook introduces E/M coding in chapter 7 (Behavioral Health Services) and includes further detail on E/M code selection in chapter 8 (Primary Care Services).

Key to Success

The first section of the CPT code book, E/M codes, is out of numerical order. E/M codes start with the number 9, which should indicate that they come at the end of the book. However, because E/M codes are common and must be constantly referenced, the CPT code book lists them first so they are easily accessible to coders.

Anesthesia

The **Anesthesia section** lists services that are performed by anesthesiologists, anesthesia assistants, or other healthcare providers to reduce sensation and alleviate pain, usually during surgery or an invasive procedure. Anesthesia services are reported with codes 00100 through 01999.

There are a few different types of anesthesia services, including general anesthesia, moderate sedation, monitored anesthesia care, and regional or local nerve blocks. The anesthesia service codes included in this section are assigned for services used to anesthetize a patient undergoing a surgical procedure, up to and including general anesthesia, such as code 00500, Anesthesia for all procedures on esophagus. Moderate (conscious) sedation and regional and local anesthesia services codes are located in different sections of the CPT code book. For example, moderate sedation codes (99151 through 99157) are located in the Medicine section, and codes for local anesthetic injections, such as 64455, Injection(s), anesthetic agent and/or steroid; plantar common digital nerve(s), are located in their respective surgical subsections. Anesthesia services, including a discussion on general anesthesia coding and coding for moderate sedation anesthesia and local anesthetic injections, are discussed in chapter 12 (Anesthesia and Pain Management Services).

Surgery

The **Surgery section** is the largest of all sections in the CPT code book. It includes codes for all of the invasive procedures that may be performed to treat patients. Surgical procedures are reported with codes 10021 through 69990. The Surgery section is also divided into subsections based on body systems, each of which is further divided based on anatomical regions, organs, or procedure types. These subsections are as follows:

- General (10004–10021)
- Integumentary (10030–19499)
- Musculoskeletal (20100–29999)
- Respiratory (30000–32999)
- Cardiovascular (33016-37799)
- Hemic and Lymphatic (38100–38999)
- Mediastinum and Diaphragm (39000–39599)
- Digestive (40490–49999)
- Urinary (50010–53899)
- Male Genital (54000–55899)
- Reproductive System Procedures (55920)
- Intersex Surgery (55970–55980)
- Female Genital (56405–58999)
- Maternity Care and Delivery (59000–59899)
- Endocrine (60000–60699)
- Nervous (61000–64999)
- Eye and Ocular Adnexa (65091–68899)
- Auditory (69000–69979)
- Operating Microscope (69990)

Healthcare providers from all different specialties may report services from the Surgery section as needed, although most providers specialize in a certain body area or surgery type. For example, a cardiothoracic surgeon specializes in surgeries of the heart, coronary vessels, and organs within the thoracic cavity. Coding for a cardiothoracic surgeon requires an in-depth knowledge of the procedural codes in the cardiovascular system subsection of the CPT code book. The intricacies of these codes are discussed in the context of healthcare specialties throughout the remaining chapters in this textbook.

Radiology

The **Radiology section** lists codes for all of the procedures that use radiant energy to diagnose healthcare conditions, such as x-rays, MRIs, and ultrasounds. This section also includes procedures that use radiant energy to treat healthcare conditions, such as radiation oncology, a special branch of medicine that uses radiation to treat cancerous tumors. Codes in this section range from 70010 to 79999.

Pathology and Laboratory

The **Pathology and Laboratory section** lists codes that represent diagnostic studies on human specimens and tissue samples. Pathology and laboratory codes range from 80047 to 89398 and from 0001U to 0138U. Note that pathology and laboratory codes are for the testing of the sample only; the procurement of the sample, such as biopsy or resection of a tumor, is reported with a different code from the surgery section of the CPT code book. Pathology and laboratory (often abbreviated as path and lab) codes report just the testing of the specimen to determine its pathology. Some path and lab procedures must be performed at specialized testing facilities, whereas others may be done in a regular outpatient clinic setting. As such, this textbook includes pathology and laboratory codes throughout the chapters as necessary, as well as in chapter 14 (Laboratory and Pathology Services).

Medicine

The last section of Category I CPT codes is the **Medicine section**, which includes codes 90281 through 99607. This section is a miscellaneous grouping of all the procedures, treatments, studies, and tests performed on patients that do not belong elsewhere in the book. Some of the procedures are minimally invasive, such as heart catheterizations and vaccination injections, but none are as invasive as the procedures included in the Surgery section. Most of the procedures in this section are noninvasive, such as psychiatry treatments and chiropractic manipulations.

Procedures listed in the Medicine section are performed by an array of different healthcare providers and are commonly performed in the outpatient office setting. This textbook presents these procedures within the context of certain healthcare specialties, along with necessary procedure codes from throughout the rest of the CPT sections.

Key to Success

It is a good idea to place tabs on the outer edges of your code book to help you easily locate the various sections of the CPT book. Even advanced coders utilize tabs to help them quickly locate and assign commonly used codes and important guidelines.

Category II codes are listed in the CPT code book immediately after the Medicine section, which is effectively the end of Category I codes. Category II codes list supplemental tracking codes used for performance measurement. As discussed in chapter 3, performance measurement is the act of tracking a practice or facility's performance against specific measures.

Category II Codes

Category II codes are completely optional; they are not required to be reported on any claim and are not reimbursable, so they are never paid directly. They are intended only to facilitate data collection for performance measurement purposes. Category II codes are supplemental tracking codes that report the performance of a test, evaluation, counseling service, or other procedure that is part of a facility's performance measurement program. For example, code 0545F, Plan for follow-up care for major depressive disorder, documented (MDD ADOL), may be used to report that a practice completed a plan for follow-up care for a patient with major depressive disorder (MDD) documented in the health record. If this MDD follow-up care plan is tracked as part of that practice's performance measures, then a report can be run on how often the follow-up care plans are completed and documented, on which patients, and for which specific diagnoses. Insurance plans may also track and use these codes to measure the practice's performance on specific measures.

Category II codes are five characters in length. The first four characters are numbers, and the last character is always the letter *F*. This format makes the number of characters for Category II codes consistent with the rest of the CPT codes but differentiates them from Category I and Category III codes.

Category III Codes

Category III codes are a set of temporary codes used to report emerging technology, services, procedures, and service paradigms. The use of these codes is integral to the identification and establishment of new healthcare procedures and treatments. Category III codes are five-character codes that begin with four numbers and end with the letter *T*.

Unlike Category I codes, these codes are for technologies and procedures that may not yet have FDA approval or proven clinical efficacy and are not performed frequently throughout the United States. However, this does not mean that the procedures are not clinically effective or that they will never get approval. The purpose of Category III codes is to report emerging services, technologies, and procedures as necessary, and if it is determined that the procedures meet the criteria of a Category I code, then they will be integrated into the Category I code set. In this way, codes for emerging technologies and new procedures can be utilized by physicians across the country for reporting purposes.

Coders should be especially careful when reporting Category III codes, as they are not necessarily covered by insurance. Furthermore, it is important to understand the

Figure 5.1. Decision tree for using unlisted procedures codes

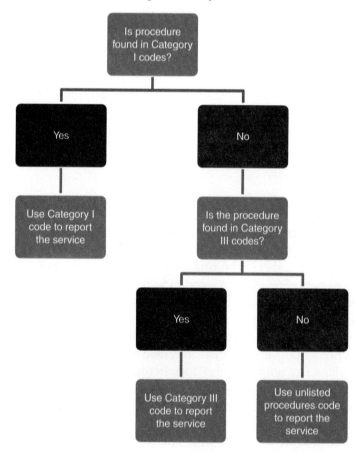

relationship between unlisted procedures and Category III codes. **Unlisted procedures** are useful codes that may be reported when a provider performs a medical procedure that does not have a corresponding CPT code. Unlisted procedures are found in the Category I section of codes in the CPT code book and are not included in the Category III codes. Consider the following example.

A pediatrician commonly sees patients who have fallen in cacti and have multiple small thorns in their extremities. These are small and delicate thorns, and she uses an effective procedure for removing them by placing a piece of sticky tape along the extremity over the thorns and quickly removing the tape, which extracts the thorns.

There is no procedure code in the CPT code set that includes the use of sticky tape to remove foreign bodies from the skin of a patient. Thus, the pediatrician may choose to use an unlisted code to report the service. However, before using an unlisted code, she must first check in the Category III codes section for a code that captures the procedure. If a Category III code exists, then the unlisted procedures code may not be used. Figure 5.1 illustrates this decision-making process.

If it is determined that an unlisted procedure code should be used, then a special report should be sent with the unlisted procedure code to explain the procedure in detail and the rationale for providing the procedure to the patient. Special reports are discussed in more detail in the guidelines section later in this chapter. Review figure 5.2 for a reminder of the three categories of CPT codes and the type of codes included in each category.

Figure 5.2. CPT code categories and sections

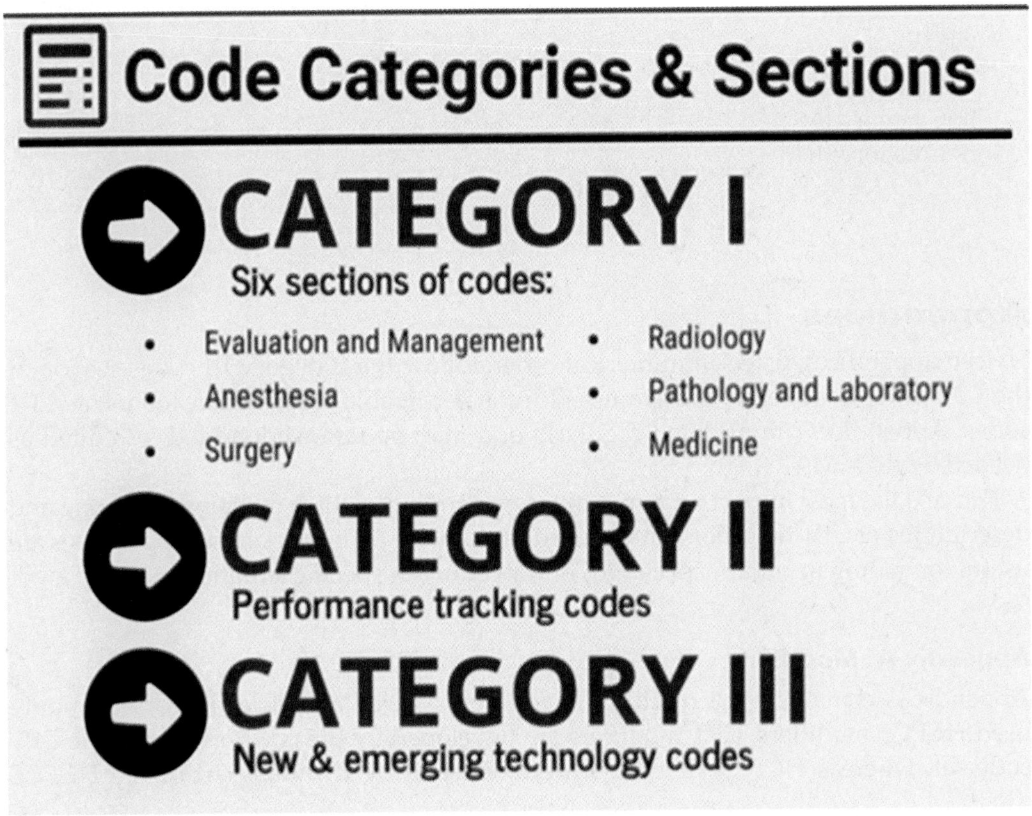

Code Categories & Sections

➡ CATEGORY I
Six sections of codes:

- Evaluation and Management
- Anesthesia
- Surgery
- Radiology
- Pathology and Laboratory
- Medicine

➡ CATEGORY II
Performance tracking codes

➡ CATEGORY III
New & emerging technology codes

Complete the exercises in There's a Code for That 5.1 to test your knowledge of CPT categories.

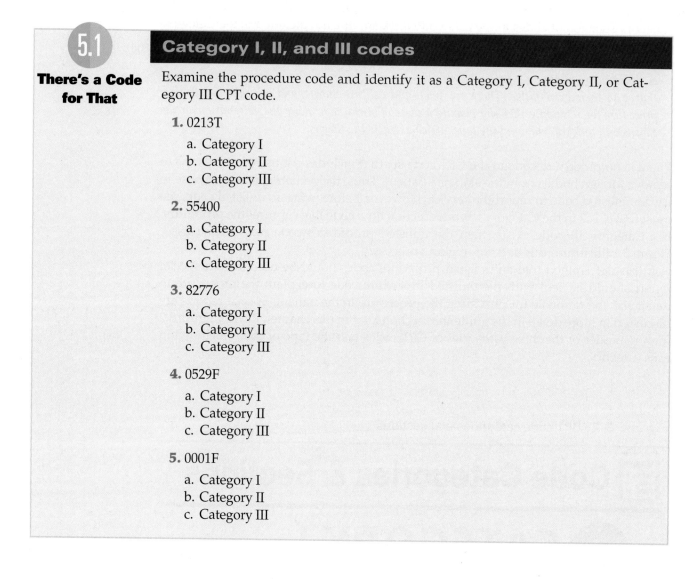

5.1

There's a Code for That

Category I, II, and III codes

Examine the procedure code and identify it as a Category I, Category II, or Category III CPT code.

1. 0213T
   a. Category I
   b. Category II
   c. Category III

2. 55400
   a. Category I
   b. Category II
   c. Category III

3. 82776
   a. Category I
   b. Category II
   c. Category III

4. 0529F
   a. Category I
   b. Category II
   c. Category III

5. 0001F
   a. Category I
   b. Category II
   c. Category III

Appendices

Sixteen appendices, listed in numerical order, follow the Category III codes section of the CPT code book, each containing additional valuable information for using CPT codes. Appendices are updated regularly and may be removed, added, or edited as needed by the AMA.

Perhaps the most important appendix is Appendix A, which contains the listing and descriptions of CPT modifiers (introduced in chapter 3). The remaining appendices are useful for coding in certain specialties or for coding in specific situations.

Appendix A: Modifiers

Appendix A contains a list of all CPT modifiers as well as a selection of commonly used HCPCS modifiers. CPT modifiers are developed by the AMA as part of the CPT code set, whereas HCPCS modifiers are developed by CMS as part of the HCPCS code set. However, HCPCS modifiers may be used to identify certain situations or add further details to a procedure code and are frequently used with CPT codes as well as with HCPCS codes. The list of CPT modifiers in the CPT code book is a complete list, whereas the list of HCPCS modifiers is a shortened list that includes only the HCPCS modifiers most commonly used with CPT codes. The full list of HCPCS modifiers is included in the HCPCS code book, discussed in detail later in this chapter.

As described in chapter 3 (Basics of Coding), modifiers are used to alter the meaning of a code, such as to indicate that a procedure was discontinued after it was begun or that it was an increased procedural service. Modifiers are two characters and are added to the end of a CPT code to provide additional information to the description of the procedure or how it was performed. Sometimes, this added information may impact the way the code is paid, which makes modifiers extremely important to understanding the connection between coding and billing. For example, modifier -22, Increased Procedural Service, should be appended to the code for a procedure that was increased due to some sort of difficulty during the procedure or because of the patient's medical condition. When a service is increased, a higher fee is charged for the procedure in order to include the increased difficulty or extra work that went into performing the service. Appending modifier -22 identifies that the service was increased and explains the increased charge to the insurance company upon receipt of the claim. When a modifier impacts payment, the insurance carrier may request records, a special report, or other justification of the increased charge.

Many CPT modifiers impact payments for specific codes, and the previous example is only one of them. A coder should be aware of all of the different CPT modifiers, as it is his or her responsibility to determine when a specific modifier may or may not be necessary. For example, a coder may read through the provider's documentation of the procedure and notice that the procedure was documented as being "extensive" or taking more than the expected hours to complete due to patient complications. In this instance, the coder must be able to identify that the procedure was increased and append modifier -22 appropriately. When it is difficult to determine whether the procedure did or did not require increased services, it is necessary to query the provider to decide if the procedure should be billed as an increased procedural service or not. As mentioned in chapter 4 (Learning the ICD-10-CM Code Book), querying involves asking the healthcare provider about the specifics of the medical procedure to obtain enough detail about the procedure (or diagnosis) to determine the correct code(s). While appending modifiers may be difficult at first, as coders gain more experience with the codes reported and the specific situations in which the procedure(s) are performed, appending modifiers soon becomes a routine part of coding.

Note that in Appendix A, modifiers are not listed with a preceding hyphen (-). However, it is common in many contexts and publications to include the hyphen to separate the modifier from the end of the CPT code to which it is appended. For example, if code 20200, Biopsy of muscle; superficial, were an increased procedural service, then it may be reported as 20200-22. In the real world, modifiers may or may not have the preceding hyphen, as some insurance payers simply tag the extra digits onto the CPT code (such as 2020022). This requires a certain amount of flexibility when identifying CPT codes and modifiers. Remember that the first five digits are always the CPT code, and the additional two digits are the modifier for the service.

Throughout the rest of this textbook, modifiers (both CPT and HCPCS) and how they may impact reimbursement are discussed, as necessary, in the context of coding procedures in specialty-specific healthcare offices.

There are many different modifiers and it is easy to forget that they are a necessary component of procedural coding. To help remember modifiers and their meanings, it is a good idea to create a set of flash cards with CPT modifiers 22 through 99, as well as the HCPCS modifiers listed in Appendix A, and test yourself. Expert coders can simply read a procedural description and know when a modifier is needed, and which modifier to add to the procedure code.

Appendix B: Summary of Additions, Deletions, and Revisions

Appendix B lists all of the additions, deletions, and revisions made throughout the CPT code set from the previous year's codes. The changes are made either by striking out the text or symbols or by adding new symbols alongside the codes to indicate what has been changed. This appendix is less important for new coders, who may not be familiar with the codes from the previous year. Instead, it is intended for coders who are working in the field and need a quick reference guide to see what has been changed for the new year.

Appendix C: Clinical Examples

Appendix C is made up of a set of clinical examples, which are useful tools for illustrating what the different levels of E/M codes look like across multiple different specialties. Documentation from actual encounters does not need to match the clinical examples. They are provided for informational use only as an aid in E/M code selection.

Appendix D: Summary of CPT Add-On Codes

Appendix D is a list of the add-on codes included in the CPT code set. It is provided only for informational purposes to help coders identify these add-on codes. An add-on code is a CPT code that may not be used alone; instead, it must be added to another CPT code. These are codes that have been specially created to identify additional work, time, body area, or procedures performed in addition to the primary service. For example, code 11200, Removal of skin tags, multiple fibrocutaneous tags, any area; up to and including 15 lesions, is the primary code for the removal of up to 15 skin tags. If the provider removed more than 25 skin tags, the add-on code 11201, Removal of skin tags, multiple fibrocutaneous tags, any area; each additional 10 lesions, or part thereof, would be used to identify the additional amount of skin tags removed by the provider. Add-on codes are identified by a plus symbol in the Tabular List and are discussed in more detail later in this chapter.

Note that the list of add-on codes in Appendix D does not include the code descriptions. Code descriptions are included in the Tabular List.

Appendix E: Summary of Codes Exempt from Modifier -51

Appendix E lists all codes exempt from the use of modifier -51 that are located in the Surgical and Medical sections of codes of the CPT code book. Modifier -51, Multiple Procedures, may not be appended to any of the codes on this list. This is a helpful list, as modifier -51 is one of only two modifiers (along with modifier -63, Procedure Performed on Infants less than 4 kg), that may or may not be appended to specific CPT codes. This list is similar to the list provided in Appendix D and does not include any code descriptions. This is to save space by eliminating the sometimes lengthy code descriptions.

The list in Appendix E is not exhaustive and does not include all codes exempt from usage with modifier -51. This appendix lists only those modifier -51 exempt codes located in the Surgical and Medical sections of the CPT code book. For example, pathology and laboratory codes ranging from 80047 to 89398 are modifier -51 exempt but are not included in Appendix E. Add-on codes are also modifier -51 exempt but are not listed in this section. This again is to save space by eliminating a large number of codes that are by definition exempt from this modifier.

Appendix F: Summary of CPT Codes Exempt from Modifier -63

Appendix F lists all codes that are exempt from modifier -63, Procedure Performed on Infants less than 4 kg. Modifier -63 is typically appended whenever a procedure is performed on any infant that weighs less than 4 kg, except for those procedure codes listed in this appendix. Because certain procedures in the CPT code book are designated as being performed on infants or neonates, the increased complexity of these procedures is already identified without the need for modifier -63. Like the previous two appendices, Appendix F does not include code descriptions; code descriptions are included in the Tabular List.

Appendix J: Electrodiagnostic Medicine Listing of Sensory, Motor, and Mixed Nerves

Appendix J lists nerves that apply to electrodiagnostic services such as nerve conduction tests, electromyography, and neuromuscular junction testing. These procedures are reported with codes 95907 through 95913. Appendix J is included in the CPT code book to enhance the appropriate reporting of these codes. It also includes a table that helps identify the appropriate code and number of units when more than one study is performed, or if more than one area is involved in the study.

Appendix K: Product Pending FDA Approval

Appendix K lists products that are currently pending FDA approval. These codes identify vaccine toxoids and are updated every year. Note, again, that this list does not include any code descriptions; code descriptions are included in the Tabular List.

Appendix L: Vascular Families

Appendix L displays a diagram of the branches of vascular families that may be accessed during a catheterization procedure, assuming that the starting point of catheterization is the aorta. This is a useful diagram to help coders assign codes according to first, second, third, or beyond third order of vascular branch, and is useful in coding catheterizations.

Appendix M: Renumbered CPT Codes–Citations Crosswalk

Appendix M is a listing of crosswalked, deleted, and renumbered codes presented with the associated coding references for the deleted codes. This list helps coders identify previous codes and their replacement codes (like a crosswalk linking the old code to the new code).

This appendix consists of a table with the following columns: Current Code(s), Deleted/Former Code (which was replaced by the current code), Year Code Deleted, and Citations Referencing Former Code—Applicable to Current Code(s). Note that the practice of deleting and renumbering codes is no longer being used for the CPT code set. The codes in Appendix M were deleted between the years 2007 and 2009 and are included in this appendix for reference purposes only (if needed).

Appendix N: Summary of Resequenced CPT Codes

Appendix N is a listing of resequenced codes. As discussed in the following section, some CPT codes are presented out of numerical order. These codes have been resequenced (out of numerical order) so that they are listed with a more appropriate section of codes (such as the same procedure type). Appendix N compiles resequenced codes for easy reference. As CPT codes are updated on an annual basis, they are subject to changes in description of the procedure performed and, as such, may need to be moved to a more appropriate selection of codes. When a code is resequenced, it is listed out of numerical order in the Tabular List with a pound sign next to it (#). Resequenced codes are discussed more in depth later in this chapter.

Like many of the other CPT code book appendices, Appendix N does not include any code descriptions; code descriptions are included in the Tabular List.

Appendix O: Multianalyte Assays with Algorithmic Analyses and Proprietary Laboratory Analyses

Appendix O lists Multianalyte Assays with Algorithmic Analyses (MAAA) administrative codes, some of which are unique to a single clinical laboratory or manufacturer. The list presented in this appendix includes the proprietary name and clinical laboratory or manufacturer, the alphanumeric procedure code, and the code descriptor. Some, but not all, of these codes are also presented in the Category I codes in the CPT code book, and not all MAAA codes are presented in this appendix. This is due to the fact that not all MAAA codes have yet been assigned a Category I CPT code. These tests are listed with a temporary four-digit number followed by the letter *M*, such as 0004M, Scoliosis, DNA analysis of 53 single nucleotide polymorphisms (SNPs), using saliva, prognostic algorithm reported as a risk score, performed or manufactured by ScoliScore™ Transgenomic.

Appendix P: Codes That May Be Used for Synchronous Telemedicine Services

Appendix P, the last appendix in the CPT code book, is a listing of CPT codes that may be used to report a synchronous **telemedicine service**. A telemedicine service is one that links healthcare organizations and patients from diverse geographic locations and transmits text and images for (medical) consultation and treatment; they are also referred to as telehealth services. These procedures must be real-time and involve electronic communication using interactive telecommunications with audio and visual capabilities. They are included in Appendix P for reference. Again, this appendix does not include any code descriptions; code descriptions are included in the Tabular List.

Removed Appendices

As previously mentioned, the CPT code set is updated every year, effective January 1st. These updates reflect changes in clinical and healthcare practice and coding guidelines, and may include new codes, deleted codes, and changed codes. Included in these changes are all of the additional components that constitute CPT coding, including modifiers, code descriptions, and supplementary information and guidance related to the codes. Sometimes this may result in the information in an appendix becoming invalid or obsolete, and in these rare instances, an appendix may be removed entirely from the CPT code book.

Three appendices in the CPT code book have been removed from the current edition. These are Appendix G: Summary of CPT Codes That Include Moderate (Conscious) Sedation, Appendix H: Alphabetical Clinical Topics Listing (AKA—Alphabetical Listing), and Appendix I: Genetic Testing Code Modifiers. Appendices G and H have been removed completely from the CPT code book, whereas the information previously presented in Appendix I is now stored online. Because of the rapid changes to genetic tests, this information is now stored electronically on the AMA website.

Complete the exercises in There's a Code for That 5.2 to test your knowledge of CPT appendices.

CPT Appendices

There's a Code for That   **5.2**

Identify which appendix you would use to locate the following information.

1. CPT modifiers.

   Appendix: _____

2. CPT codes exempt from modifier -63.

   Appendix: _____

3. CPT codes exempt from modifier -51.

   Appendix: _____

4. Clinical examples.

   Appendix: _____

5. Summary of CPT add-on codes.

   Appendix: _____

6. CPT telemedicine codes.

   Appendix: _____

Index

The CPT Index, located directly after the appendices, is the last section of the CPT code book. This Index functions much like the ICD-10-CM Index by listing the main terms of a procedure, then referring the coder to the corresponding CPT code(s). This allows coders to look up the main terms for a procedure to find the correct procedure code. Once the main term is selected, any modifying terms and cross-references are followed until a code can be selected. A more in-depth review of how to locate a CPT code is discussed later in this chapter.

Main Terms

Main terms for a procedure are different than the main terms used to find diagnostic codes. Remember, when coding for healthcare encounters, coders must identify the diagnostic information as well as the procedural information.

To determine the procedure(s) from the documentation, the coder should ask: *What did the doctor do?* The answer to this question should identify the verbs or actions performed by the healthcare provider, such as an examination, a surgical procedure, or other healthcare treatment. To discern the diagnoses from the documentation, the coder should ask: *Why did the doctor do it?* The answer to this question should provide the reasons why the procedure(s) performed by the healthcare provider were medically necessary. Figure 5.3 provides an example of how the procedure(s) and diagnoses are identified from a documentation sample.

Figure 5.3. Identifying procedures and diagnoses

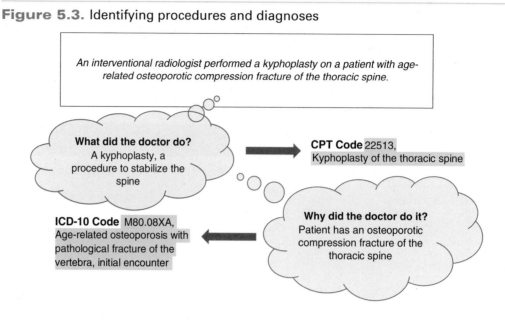

Once a coder has determined the name of the procedure, it is time to search for the main term in the CPT Index. There are four primary classes of main terms:

- *Procedure or service.* This is the action word (verb) for the procedure or service performed (for example, repair, excise, or examine endoscopically).

- *Organ or anatomic site.* This is the organ or anatomic site on which the procedure was performed (for instance, femur, colon, or chest).

- *Condition.* This is the name of the condition that was treated by the procedure (for example, abscess, Lyme disease, or spermatocele).

- *Synonyms, eponyms, and abbreviations.* Synonyms, eponyms, and abbreviations all appear in the CPT Index as main terms. **Synonyms** are words or phrases that have the same meaning as other words or phrases. For example, *removal* and *excision* are synonyms. **Eponyms** are procedures or treatments that are named after a person. These are common in procedural coding, as procedures are commonly named after the healthcare pioneer who invented them. An example of an eponym is *Fredet-Ramstedt procedure*, a specific type of incision into the stomach. Abbreviations are shortened versions of sometimes lengthy procedural names—for instance, EEG is the abbreviation of electroencephalography. Typically, in the CPT Index, abbreviations contain a cross-reference to the full procedural name, rather than listing the CPT codes for the procedure.

Looking at figure 5.3, after asking the question, *what did the doctor do?*, the coder determines that the procedure performed was a kyphoplasty, a procedure to stabilize the spine. This is the term that the coder would look up in the Index before following any modifying terms or cross-references and finally selecting a code to verify in the Tabular List.

Key to Success

If you are having trouble finding a main term in the CPT Index, try to think of as many ways as possible to look up the procedure. For example, if you cannot find the procedure name, search for the body site or anatomic area, the type of condition being treated, and any synonyms, eponyms, or abbreviations that may apply. Sometimes the Index appears to lead you on a wild goose chase, and you may find yourself flipping back and forth throughout it. As you become more familiar with how procedures are listed, this process will become easier.

Modifying Terms and Cross-References

In the Index, once the main term for the procedure has been located, it is necessary to check any modifying terms and cross-references. Modifying terms in the CPT Index are much like subterms in the ICD-10-CM Main Index and function the same way. Modifying terms alter the main term. They are indented below the main term and present different versions of the procedure. For example, the main term *Endoscopy* is modified by the anatomical site of the endoscopy and then divided based on the purpose of the procedure (see figure 5.4). Coders should always review the lists of modifying terms, if available, to ensure correct code selection.

Cross-references direct coders to other main term entries that may need to be referenced. For example, in figure 5.4 the cross-reference "*See* Arthroscopy; Thoracoscopy" informs the coder that if the procedure cannot be found in the list of modifying terms that follow, then he or she should refer to the main terms *Arthroscopy* or *Thoracoscopy*.

Once the term that identifies the procedure has been located, it is necessary to refer to the code on the right-hand side of the column. Sometimes there are multiple codes listed for the procedure referenced in the Index because more than one CPT code may identify the procedure performed. Although they may represent the same procedure, each different code will include a specific detail regarding the procedure, such as the approach to the procedure, the number of elements involved in the procedure, or the exact manner in which the procedure was performed. This is yet another reason why it is important to read code descriptions carefully. When presented with multiple code

Figure 5.4. Endoscopy in the CPT Index

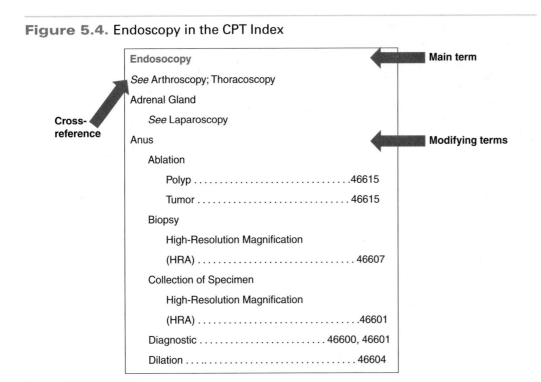

Source: AMA 2019, 957.

options in the Index, search for each one in the Tabular List to ensure that the most appropriate code is selected.

Nonsequential codes are separated with a comma (for example, 43247, 43250, 43251), and if three or more sequential codes apply, then they are separated by a dash (for example, 17106–17108). Sometimes, several nonsequential codes apply, as well as a code range. In these cases, the codes would be separated by both commas and hyphens (for example, 36011, 36012, 36400–36410).

To find a procedure code in the CPT code book, coders must access the Index, locate the main term, refer to any applicable modifying terms and cross-references as necessary, and then locate the code(s) for that procedure. Once the codes are located, it is imperative to verify the codes in the Tabular List (see figure 5.5). The Tabular List of the CPT code book is the listing of Category I, II, and III codes, organized into a special format—sections, subsections, subheading, categories, and codes—for easy code identification and selection.

Figure 5.5. Looking up a CPT code

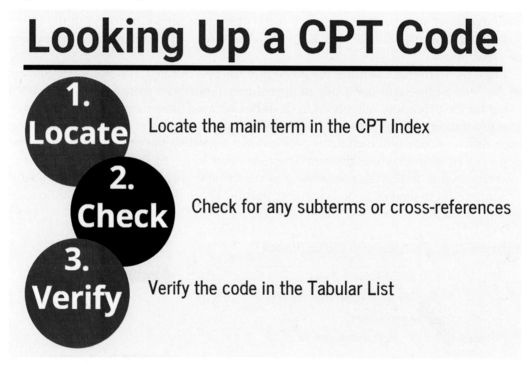

Complete the exercises in There's a Code for That 5.3 to test your knowledge of the CPT Index.

5.3

There's a Code for That

Using the CPT Index

Identify the procedural statement from the following descriptions and then look up the main term in the CPT Index and follow any cross-references and modifying terms. List the code or code ranges given by the CPT Index. The first one is already completed for you. (You do not need to verify the codes in the Tabular for this exercise; simply give the codes listed by the Index).

Example: Surgeon performed an enterotomy for the excision of a lesion.

Procedure name: *Enterotomy, excision, lesion*

Index entry: *44110, 44111*

1. Doctor removed 19 calculi (stones) from the gallbladder of a 35-year-old woman with cholelithiasis.

   Procedure name: _____

   Index entry: _____

2. Salpingectomy with vaginal hysterectomy.

   Procedure name: _____

   Index entry: _____

3. Laparoscopic salpingectomy with vaginal hysterectomy.

   Procedure name: _____

   Index entry: _____

4. Surgeon amputated the gangrenous lower leg of a 75-year-old diabetic woman.

   Procedure name: _____

   Index entry: _____

Format of the Tabular List of CPT Codes

As a reminder, the Tabular List of the CPT code book is divided into three Categories: Category I, Category II, and Category III codes. Category I codes are further divided into six sections: Evaluation and Management, Anesthesia, Surgery, Radiology, Pathology and Laboratory, and Medicine codes (refer to figure 5.2). Although they list different

Figure 5.6. Sections, subsections, subheadings, categories, and codes

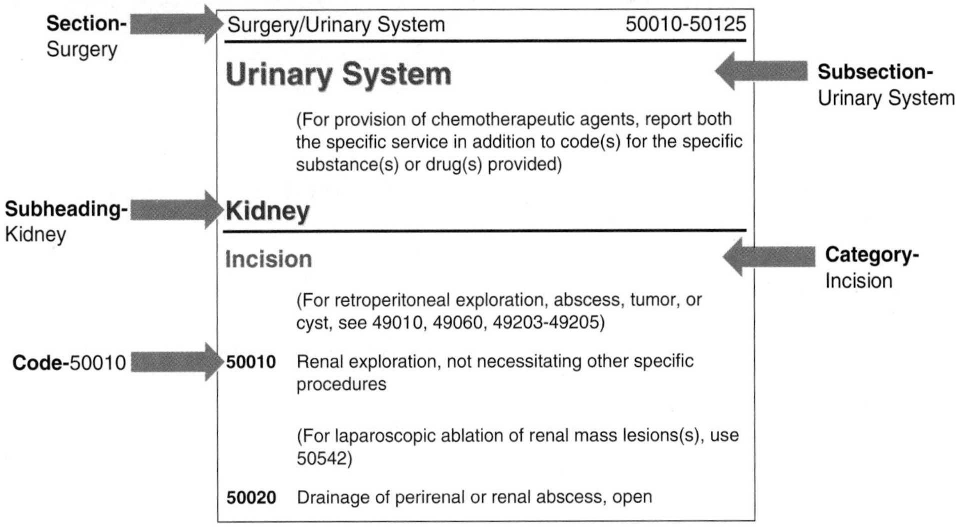

Source: AMA 2019, 361.

types of procedures, the format of each of these six sections is standardized to facilitate understanding and code selection.

Category I sections are each further divided into subsections, subheadings, and finally categories that list the CPT codes and their descriptions (see figure 5.6). Each Category I section begins with a listing of the applicable guidelines for that section, as well as a table of contents. Due to its size, the Surgery section includes a table of contents for each individual subsection.

The subheadings and categories differ among subsections. For example, in the Urinary System example in figure 5.6, the subheadings are the organs within the urinary system: Kidney, Ureter, Bladder, and Urethra. In the Musculoskeletal System subsection, however, there are subheadings that are arranged around the type of procedure—Applications of Casts and Strapping, Endoscopy/Arthroscopy, and so forth. Coders should pay close attention to the subsection, subheading, and category of codes for the procedures for which they are coding, as they can be used to help maneuver through the Tabular List of CPT codes to locate the correct one.

Key to Success

It is a good idea to locate the table of contents for each section as well as the Surgery subsections. When beginning to code from each section, review the table of contents to understand how it is divided as well as the procedures and anatomic sites involved within it. Coders who are familiar enough with the Tabular List may find that they can locate the correct CPT codes without accessing the Index, simply by using the table of contents, subheadings, and categories in each subsection of codes.

Once the code has been identified using the Index, cross-references, and modifying terms, it must be verified in the Tabular List of CPT codes. The Tabular List contains the code descriptions, symbols, conventions, and guidelines to help coders confirm they have selected the right code and ensure they report the code correctly. Complete the exercises in There's a Code for That 5.4 to practice looking up and verifying codes in the CPT code book.

5.4

There's a Code for That

Verifying CPT codes

Read the procedural statement and the CPT code selected and locate the selected CPT code in the Tabular List. Then verify if the CPT code selected is the correct code or not. If it is not the correct code, enter the correct code in the space provided. (The first exercise is done for you).

> Example: Judy selected the code 20606 for an aspiration of an ankle bursa without ultrasound guidance.
> Is this the correct code? *No*
> If not the correct code, enter it here: *20605*

1. Judy selected the code 32561 for the instillation of fibrinolytic agent for the breakup of multiloculated effusion for the third day of fibrinolytic therapy.

Is this the correct code? _____

If not the correct code, enter it here: _____

2. Judy selected the code 61539 for a lobectomy of the temporal lobe with electrocorticography during the surgery.

Is this the correct code? _____

If not the correct code, enter it here: _____

3. Judy selected the code 33724 for the partial repair of the pulmonary vein.

Is this the correct code? _____

If not the correct code, enter it here: _____

4. Judy selected the code 58953 for a bilateral salpingo-oophorectomy with total omentectomy and total abdominal hysterectomy for cancer.

Is this the correct code? _____

If not the correct code, enter it here: _____

CPT Symbols, Conventions, and Guidelines

In the Tabular List of CPT codes, there are many symbols, conventions, and guidelines that help coding professionals navigate the codes and ensure correct code selection. Symbols are placed throughout the Tabular List, as necessary, to identify specific aspects of codes.

Symbols

Symbols are located throughout the Tabular List of the CPT code book as a visual reminder of important details that pertain to certain codes. For example, one symbol identifies codes that are exempt from modifier -51 (as discussed earlier in the chapter). This helps coders to remember that modifier -51 should not be appended to these specific codes.

Symbols are placed on the left-hand side of the code to which they apply. Not all CPT codes have applicable symbols; they only appear when necessary throughout the code listing. In the 2020 CPT code book, there are 10 symbols that apply to CPT codes, each of which identifies a specific aspect of a particular code or codes. These symbols identify add-on codes, new and revised codes and text, modifier -51 exempt codes, codes pending FDA approval, resequenced codes, codes that can be used to report telemedicine services, and duplicate proprietary laboratory analyses (PLA) test codes.

Add-on Codes

Add-on codes are designated by the ✚ symbol. These are procedures commonly carried out in addition to the primary procedure performed. The phrases "each additional" or "(list separately in addition to primary procedure)" are generally found in the description of add-on codes to indicate they should be added onto the code for a primary procedure.

The procedures described by add-on codes include further intra-service work associated with the primary procedure (see figure 5.7). As such, add-on codes *may never be used alone.* They must always be added to a primary procedure code. Furthermore, add-on codes are exempt from modifier -51, Multiple procedures. The full list of add-on codes is included in Appendix D of the CPT code book.

Figure 5.7. Add-on code example

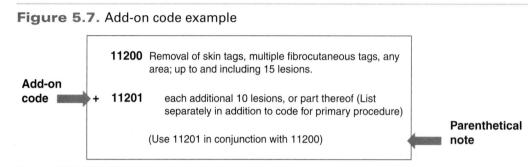

Source: AMA 2019, 83.

In figure 5.7, the add-on code 11201 must be appended to the code for the primary procedure, 11200. The description for code 11200 includes the removal of *up to* 15 lesions, and the add-on code identifies the removal of *each additional* 10 lesions. So, if the procedure was to remove 20 lesions, then the coder should report codes 11200 (for the first 15 lesions) and 11201 (for the additional 5 lesions), which equals 20 total lesions removed. It is permissible to report 11201 for the additional lesions because the code description is for each additional 10 lesions *or part thereof*, which means that the add-on code may be used to report the removal of less than 10 additional lesions.

Note that figure 5.7 also includes a **parenthetical note**—instructions for use of the codes, presented in parentheses throughout the Tabular List. They are intended to prevent errors and help coders report codes appropriately. Parenthetical notes highlight important guidelines, like the addition of a modifier or coding notes indicating when it may be appropriate to report codes together. They are vital in ensuring correct code selection and help coders certify they are reporting CPT codes correctly. For example, the parenthetical note in figure 5.7 states to use 11201 in conjunction with 11200, so if the coder reports 11200 with 11201, he or she knows that is correct.

Key to Success

Parenthetical notes are a very common component of the Tabular List and are easy to overlook. As you are learning coding, it may be helpful to highlight or place a star next to the parenthetical notes throughout the Tabular List to make sure you take them into account when reporting CPT codes.

New and Revised Codes and Text

Each year, the CPT code book is updated to include new and revised codes and guidelines. This includes additions, deletions, and revisions of codes and guidelines. Although these are less important for beginning coders, experienced coders may find that codes used previously have been substantially altered. Therefore, the CPT code book includes three different symbols to identify new and revised codes and code guidelines or text.

New codes added to the CPT code set each year are indicated with a ● (circle) symbol to the left of the code. This symbol is to identify a completely new code that was not included in the code set the previous year.

Revised codes are identified with the ▲ (triangle) symbol. These are codes that have been changed to substantially alter the procedural description. Although the code number itself has not been altered, the description of the procedure for that code has been revised. This may result in having to select a new, more appropriate code than what was used in the previous year.

New and revised text, including CPT guidelines, are identified with the symbols ▶◀ on either side of the text change (two arrows facing each other). One arrow appears to the left of the text when the changes begin, and the other arrow appears to the right of the text after the change ends. Furthermore, in the Professional edition of the CPT code book, the text that includes the changes is listed in green print. In this way, the arrows append the revised or new text, making it easier for coders to identify the specific text in which changes have occurred or that has been newly added. The full list of additions, deletions, and revisions is included in Appendix B of the CPT code book.

Modifier -51 Exempt Codes

Some CPT codes, depending on their use and description, are modifier -51 exempt. These codes are identified with the ⊘ symbol. These codes may not be used with modifier -51 to indicate that they are multiple procedures and have not been designated as add-on codes. For example, code 17004, Destruction (e.g., laser surgery, electrosurgery, cryosurgery, chemosurgery, surgical curettement), premalignant lesions (e.g., actinic keratoses), 15 or more lesions, is listed with the modifier -51 exempt symbol to the left of the code. This means that code 17004 may not be reported with modifier -51. A list of modifier -51 exempt codes is included in Appendix E of the CPT code book.

Codes Pending FDA Approval

Codes that are pending FDA approval are identified with the ⚡ (lightning bolt) symbol. This symbol is used for vaccine codes that have not yet been approved by the FDA but are still included in the CPT code set. For example, code 90666, Influenza virus vaccine (IIV) pandemic formulation, split virus, preservative free, for intramuscular use, is still pending FDA approval but is listed in the Tabular List of the CPT code book with the lightning symbol beside the code. The entire list of codes pending FDA approval is included in Appendix K of the CPT code book.

Resequenced Codes

Resequenced codes are identified with the # (hashtag or pound) symbol. These codes are not placed numerically in the Tabular List and are out of numerical sequence. The symbol is used as a navigational reference to alert coders that the code is found elsewhere. Resequencing allows codes to be placed near codes with related concepts and appropriate families of procedures, regardless of the numerical sequencing.

Because they are out of sequence, these codes may be difficult to locate. For example, physical therapy evaluation services are reported with codes 97161 through 97164. According to the number sequence, these codes should be located after code 97150. However, since these codes have been resequenced, they are listed out of order. In these instances, the CPT book includes a statement to direct the coder where to find these codes. In this case, where code 97161 should be located, the coder will find the following: 97161, Code is out of numerical sequence. See Physical Therapy Evaluation Section. This tells the coder that the code is out of sequence and where he or she can find it. The complete list of resequenced codes is included in Appendix N of the CPT code book.

Telemedicine Codes

The ★ (star) symbol is used to identify codes that may be reported for telemedicine services when they are appended with modifier -95, Synchronous Telemedicine Service Rendered Via a Real-Time Interactive Audio and Video Telecommunications System. The entire list of telemedicine codes is included in Appendix P of the CPT code book.

Duplicate PLA Test Codes

Duplicate proprietary analyses (PLA) codes are identified with the ⊁ symbol. PLA codes identify laboratory procedures that are provided by either a single (sole-source) laboratory or multiple licensed providing laboratories. When one PLA test has an identical CPT description to another PLA test, these codes are identified with the Duplicate PLA Test symbol. For example, codes 0007U and 0020U both have identical descriptions, so both of these codes are appended with the Duplicate PLA Test code symbol. All of the codes identified by this symbol are also located in Appendix O of the CPT code book.

Category I PLA Codes

Codes for Category I proprietary analyses (PLA) are identified with the ↑↓ symbol. A PLA code that has received Category I CPT status is marked with this symbol for easy identification. PLA codes that are not annotated with this symbol have not yet been adopted into the CPT Category I code set.

Conventions and Guidelines

In addition to symbols, there are a few conventions and numerous guidelines found throughout the CPT code book. The conventions are formatting and organizational practices, including the use of standalone and indented codes. Guidelines are found in each section of the CPT code book and differ among the CPT code book sections. However, there are some guidelines that apply to several sections across the CPT code book; these include standalone and indented codes, the time component of codes, unlisted services and special reports, and separate procedures.

Standalone and Indented Codes

To save space in the Tabular List, many codes throughout the CPT code book are indented underneath standalone codes. **Standalone codes** include the full description of the code and do not depend on a parent code to provide more information. **Indented codes** are indented beneath a standalone code and depend on the explanation of the procedure within the standalone (or parent) code to complete the description of the

---

Figure 5.8. Standalone and indented codes

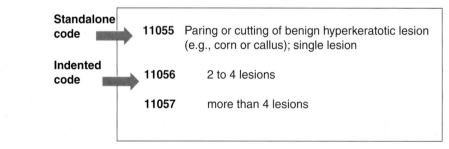

Source: AMA 2019, 80.

indented code. Indented codes begin where the semicolon ends in the standalone code. Coders should replace the portion of the standalone code *after* the semicolon with the description given by the indented code in order to complete the code description. Refer to figure 5.8 for an example of standalone and indented codes.

In figure 5.8, the standalone code is 11055, Paring or cutting of benign hyperkeratotic lesion (eg, corn or callus); single lesion. This means that code 11055 is for the cutting or paring of only *one* single lesion. Code 11056, indented below 11055, is for *2 to 4 lesions*. Because it is indented beneath the code above it, code 11056 pertains to the same procedure, *Paring or cutting of benign hyperkeratotic lesions*, but with a different number of lesions, in this case *2 to 4 lesions*. The full code description for 11056 would thus be interpreted as 11056, Paring or cutting of benign hyperkeratotic lesion (e.g., corn or callus); 2 to 4 lesions. Note that the point of division between the standalone code and the indented code is the semicolon (;) in the standalone code description.

There may be multiple indented codes beneath a single standalone code. As in figure 5.8, there are two indented codes: 11056 and 11057. Each one of these codes pertains to the previous parent standalone code, and they each modify the standalone code in a different way (namely, 11056 is for 2 to 4 lesions, and 11057 is for more than 4 lesions).

Time

Time is an important descriptor in many CPT codes. Some CPT codes are dependent on the amount of time taken for a procedure, from start to finish, and include that amount in the code description. Unless specific guidelines state otherwise, time is the "face-to-face" period that the healthcare professional spends directly with the patient (rather than out of the room or in his or her office working on the patient's health record or treatment). Also, unless specifically indicated in the code description, one unit of time has elapsed once the midpoint has been reached. For example, if the unit of time described in the code is for one hour, then a coder may report that unit once the halfway point has been surpassed (namely, 31 minutes). Similarly, if the unit time were two hours, then the unit could be reported at the 91-minute mark (one full hour for the first 60 minutes, and then the additional hour may be reported after the additional 31-minute mark, so 91 minutes total).

Add-on codes are frequently used with services that require concurrent procedures, or procedures that may be prolonged for a certain amount of time. If add-on codes are present, then the standalone code should be reported first and add-on codes reported according to the number of units necessary to report the full service. See figure 5.9 for an example of a time descriptor in a code, and an add-on time code.

In figure 5.9, the first code, 96360, is for 31 to 60 minutes, and the second code, 96361, is for each additional 60 minutes. Therefore, if the intravenous infusion were performed

Figure 5.9. Coding for time with standalone and add-on codes

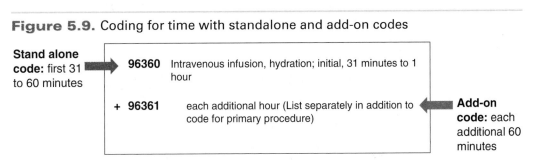

Source: AMA 2019, 731.

for three hours, the appropriate codes would be 96360 (for the first hour) and then 96361 × 2 for the next two hours, equaling three hours total. Notice that the second code would be reported twice to identify two extra hours of the service performed. It is common to report certain procedures more than once. If this is the case, coders can report the services separately (that is, 96360, 96361, 96361), or by changing the number of units (that is, 96360, 96361 × 2).

Unlisted Services and Special Reports

As previously described in this chapter, there may be some services or procedures that are not found in the CPT code set. In these rare instances, a healthcare provider can report the service using an unlisted services procedure code. When an unlisted procedure code is used, the specific service should be described using a special report. A **special report** is included with the reporting of an unlisted procedure or other procedure that is rarely provided, unusual, variable, or new. Special reports should include the following:

- A complete description of the procedure, including the nature of the procedure
- Extent of the procedure performed
- Need for the procedure (that is, the medical necessity for the procedure)
- Amount of time spent on the procedure
- Effort needed to complete the procedure
- Equipment necessary to provide the service

Additional guidelines regarding special reports are found at the beginning of each section or subsection in the Tabular List of the CPT.

Separate Procedures

Some of the procedures or services listed throughout the CPT code book are often carried out as integral components of other procedures or services. These are designated in the Tabular List as a **separate procedure**—a procedure that is commonly part of another, more complex procedure but may be performed independently or be otherwise unrelated to the procedure. Separate procedures codes should not be reported in addition to the code for the primary procedure or service of which it is considered an integral component. For example, code 20100 is designated as a separate procedure: 20100, Exploration of penetrating wound (separate procedure); neck. This means that code 20100 should *not* be reported if is it included as part of a more definitive service, such as repair to major internal structure(s) or blood vessel(s). Consider the following example.

A patient presented to the emergency department with a penetrating stab wound to the upper right thigh. The doctor on call explored the stab wound, including dissection, to determine that it was approximately 1.5 cm deep, noting that there was no damage to any major structures or blood vessels.

In this example, the only procedure performed was the exploration of the wound itself, without a repair done to any major structures or blood vessels. In this case, the doctor would report code 20103, Exploration of penetrating wound (separate procedure); extremity. If the doctor performed a more extensive procedure, then the code reported would be for the more extensive, primary procedure, as in the following example.

A patient presented to the emergency department with a penetrating stab wound to the abdomen. Upon exploration, the doctor on call discovered a small laceration of the liver, which he repaired using a simple suture.

In this example, the doctor did more than simply explore the wound. Upon exploration, it was determined that a more definitive procedure had to be performed (namely, a suture of the liver wound). In this case, a code for the exploration of the wound would not be reported. Rather, the coder would report the code for the definitive procedure: 47350, Management of liver hemorrhage; simple suture of liver wound or injury.

The only time a separate procedure code should be reported is when it is the *only* procedure performed on that body site and is not part of a larger, more definitive procedure. However, a separate procedure may be reported if it was distinct from the other procedures performed at the same encounter. Combine the two previous examples:

A patient presents to the emergency department with a penetrating stab wound to the upper thigh as well as the abdomen. The doctor explores the thigh wound without any additional procedures and then explores the abdomen wound, discovering and repairing a liver wound.

In this example, two codes would be reported; one for the exploration of the upper thigh wound (20103), and another for the repair of the liver (47350). The separate procedure code 20103 should be appended with modifier -59 to identify that it is a distinct procedural service.

Separate procedures have a special relationship with modifier -59. Modifier -59, Distinct procedural service, is used to identify when one procedure is considered separate from another procedure. Because coding is complex and healthcare procedures are performed on all sites of the body, modifier -59 helps to identify when codes that would otherwise be included in other procedures (like separate procedures) are correctly reported in addition to codes for the more definitive procedures. The use of modifier -59 may result in payment for a service that would otherwise be bundled (included) with the payment for another procedure. Because modifier -59 is ambiguous in nature and can lead to coding errors or abuse, it is to be used only as a last resort when no other modifiers better identify the circumstance. Therefore, CMS has developed four different modifiers that can be used in lieu of modifier -59. Check payer guidelines before using the following modifiers, as they may not be accepted by all payers:

- Modifier -XE, Separate encounter, a service that is distinct because it occurred during a separate encounter
- Modifier -XP, Separate practitioner, a service that is distinct because it was performed by a different practitioner
- Modifier -XS, Separate structure, a service that is distinct because it was performed on a separate organ or structure
- Modifier -XU, Unusual non-overlapping service, the use of a service that is distinct because it does not overlap usual components of the main service

In addition to CPT codes, there is one remaining code set to discuss before beginning coding in the outpatient setting. Although not used as frequently as CPT codes, HCPCS codes are an important part of coding that allows coders to report supplies and services provided to patients in the healthcare setting as well as to report services provided to Medicare patients. The last sections of this chapter discuss the structure, purpose, and format of HCPCS codes and the HCPCS code book.

HCPCS Code Structure

HCPCS codes and CPT codes are alike in that they are five-character codes used to report services and procedures provided to patients. However, unlike CPT codes, HCPCS codes begin with a letter rather than a number (for example, K0001, Standard wheelchair). In HCPCS, codes for similar categories of services and supplies are typically grouped together by specific letters (although this is not always the case). For example, HCPCS codes for all ambulance services begin with the letter *A*, and codes for most drugs administered in the healthcare setting begin with the letter *J*. A complete listing of HCPCS code categories is listed later in this chapter.

HCPCS codes are used to report supplies and services to patients in the outpatient setting. However, because the HCPCS Level II code set is created and maintained by CMS, which manages the Medicare health plan, HCPCS codes may be required to report specific services provided to Medicare patients only, such as screenings, annual wellness visits, and vaccinations. The same services provided to non-Medicare patients would be reported with the appropriate CPT codes. Thus, when coding claims for reimbursement purposes, it is important to have the patient's insurance type in mind, as the billing and coding requirements will differ depending on the patient's type of insurance (for a reminder of insurance basics, review chapter 2, Healthcare Billing Basics).

The majority of HCPCS codes are used to report supplies provided to patients in the healthcare setting. Therefore, when coding for healthcare encounters, there is one more question that a coder should ask to ensure that he or she is coding for the encounter completely: *What supply did the doctor provide to the patient?* Note that not all encounters will result in a supply or item being provided to the patient. Because of this, HCPCS supply codes are not necessary for each and every encounter.

The three questions coders should ask themselves are the following:

What did the doctor do? = Procedure code (CPT)
Why did the doctor do it? = Diagnosis code (ICD-10-CM)
What supply did the doctor provide? = Supply code (HCPCS)

Read the following vignette to see how asking these three questions may result in the addition of a HCPCS code.

Rudy is selecting the codes for an encounter for an intrauterine device (IUD) insertion. The patient came in for reproductive management and insertion of an IUD. She is in a monogamous relationship with her husband of five years and has two children. Her second child has just turned six weeks old and she has decided that she would like to get an IUD for contraception. After a brief physical examination and evaluation, the doctor decides that the IUD is appropriate for this patient and inserts the IUD into the patient's uterus. She schedules an appointment in six weeks to ensure appropriate placement of the device.

Rudy is ready to code the encounter and asks herself the first question: What did the doctor do? In this case, the doctor performed a brief E/M service and then inserted the IUD into the patient's uterus. These are her procedure codes, which she will look up in the CPT code book. She then asks herself the second question: Why did the doctor do it? In this case, the doctor performed the IUD insertion for contraceptive management, as requested by the patient. It is important to note that this is not a problem-oriented visit, so the reason for the encounter is not a problem but rather an encounter for reproductive health services. Rudy will search encounter for contraceptive management in the ICD-10-CM code book.

Now that Rudy has her first two questions answered, she must ask the third question: What supply did the doctor provide? In this case, the doctor supplied the patient with the intrauterine device, which she placed in the patient's uterus. Rudy will look up the intrauterine device in the HCPCS code book.

Rudy now has three types of codes to find: the CPT code(s) for the E/M and insertion of the IUD device; the ICD-10-CM code(s) for contraceptive management and insertion of IUD device; and the HCPCS code(s) for the actual intrauterine device.

This third question may be tricky, as it refers not to the equipment or items used to treat the patient but to any nondisposable supplies provided to the patient in the healthcare setting. In this case, the patient was given an IUD, which she will take home with her.

Key to Success

Any disposable supplies provided at the time of service—like gauze, sterile gloves, or lubricating jelly—are not coded with HCPCS codes. These expendable items are paid for by the healthcare office or facility as part of the clinical overhead expense.

As discussed in chapter 3 (Basics of Coding), HCPCS code books differ depending on the book's publisher, so learning HCPCS coding relies on locating the Index and Tabular List. The coder must also follow the same process as CPT coding—locating the main term for the service or supply in the Index, checking subterms and cross-references, and then verifying the code in the Tabular List. These components are discussed in more detail in the last section of this chapter.

The HCPCS Code Book

HCPCS codes are always the same, no matter the publisher. However, the style, format, organization, and content of the HCPCS code book does depend on the publisher, and may vary. Because of this, it is necessary to discuss the sections of the HCPCS manual in general terms, as they may be organized in a different order. The main sections of the HCPCS code book are the Index, the Table of Drugs, list of modifiers, Tabular List of HCPCS Level II codes, and Appendices.

Key to Success

Because HCPCS code books vary, it is a good idea to flip through your book to locate the various sections. Although the HCPCS code book is much smaller than either of the ICD-10-CM or the CPT code books, placing tabs throughout this book for easy reference of important sections and commonly used codes is still recommended.

HCPCS Index

The first section of the HCPCS code book is the Index. This index functions exactly like the indices included in the CPT and ICD-10-CM code books, with a main term listed and available subterms listed beneath the main term. Coders should reference the item, supply, or service they are looking to code in the Index first, which will refer them to a code or range of codes. Coders must then turn to the Tabular List of HCPCS codes to select the appropriate code for the supply provided or the service performed.

Looking up supplies and services in the HCPCS Index is a bit different than using the CPT or ICD-10-CM Index. Rather than searching for the condition or reason for an encounter (as in ICD-10-CM coding), or searching for a service or procedure that was performed on the patient (as in CPT coding), looking for a HCPCS code in the Index usually requires searching for the item that was supplied to the patient. When coding for a supply item, it is necessary to look up the noun or name of the item. For example, for an IUD the coder would look up *intrauterine device* or *intrauterine copper contraceptive.* Use the following when searching for codes in the HCPCS Index:

- Name of the service, test, therapy, or procedure
- Name of the item, prosthetic, orthotic, or equipment supplied
- Name of the drug or medication administered

The entries in the HCPCS code book will differ depending on the publisher of the book. Although CMS publishes an Index to each year's current HCPCS code set, individual publishers are able to rearrange, remove, and add to the Index according to how they believe the information is best presented. Thus, it may be necessary to look up items in a completely different manner than in another book. In one book it may be necessary to search for an augmentative speech generating device under *device, speech generating,* which will lead the coder to E2500, whereas in another book it may be necessary to search for the same device under *Speech generating device,* which leads the coder to the code range E2500 to E2599. Both entries lead to the same area of codes in the Tabular List, even though they were found by searching for different terms.

Key to Success

It is imperative to remain flexible when searching for any term in the Index to a coding book. As the previous example shows, you may have to search for the same supply (or condition in ICD-10-CM coding, or procedure in CPT coding) in different ways. Ultimately, it is the code selection that counts. If you find that you have searched the term in multiple ways and it still leads to the same codes, you can be certain that you have found the right codes.

If a coder is searching for the code for a drug or medicinal substance administered in the healthcare setting—such as an antibiotic shot administered at a doctor's visit—it is necessary to search for the drug in the Table of Drugs (discussed in the next section) rather than in the Index.

Complete the exercises in There's a Code for That 5.5 to practice looking up codes in the HCPCS Index.

5.5 Using the HCPCS Index

There's a Code for That

Identify the HCPCS supply or service from the following descriptions, then look up the main term in the HCPCS Index and follow any cross-references or modifying terms. List the code or code ranges given by the HCPCS Index. The first one is completed for you. (You do not need to verify the codes in the Tabular for this exercise, simply give the codes listed by the Index).

Example: Pathology of blood platelets via pheresis leukocytes reduced and irradiated.
Index entry: *P9037*

1. Body mass index (BMI).

   Index entry: _____

2. Pneumococcal vaccine administration.

   Index entry: _____

3. Dialysis supplies.

   Index entry: _____

4. Monaural hearing aid.

   Index entry: _____

5. Dystrophic nail trimming.

   Index entry: _____

6. Pneumatic ventricular assist device.

   Index entry: _____

Table of Drugs

The Table of Drugs in the HCPCS code book is a reference tool that helps coders find the appropriate HCPCS code for drugs and medications administered in the healthcare setting. It is organized by the name of the drug or medicinal substance, dosage or unit amount given, and method of administration of the drug. The Table of Drugs is discussed in greater detail in chapter 6 (Supplies and Services).

The entries in the Table of Drugs may differ depending on the publisher of the HCPCS code book. Some tables may list drugs by their generic names, whereas others might list drugs by both generic and brand names. When coding for drugs using the Table of Drugs, it may be beneficial to refer to a Physician's Desk Reference (PDR) to help identify specific drugs and the correct routes of administration and unit dosage amounts.

HCPCS Modifiers

HCPCS modifiers are listed in a separate section from HCPCS codes. Modifiers are an important part of coding, so it is important to locate the list of modifiers in the code book table of contents for reference when coding. HCPCS modifiers may be used with either CPT or HCPCS codes, and a small selection of HCPCS modifiers are also found in Appendix A of the CPT code book. These are the most commonly used HCPCS modifiers and are included in the CPT manual for easy reference.

Tabular List of HCPCS Level II Codes

The largest section of the HCPCS code book is the Tabular List of HCPCS Level II codes. HCPCS codes range from A0021 to V5364, and are divided into multiple subsections:

- Transport Services Including Ambulance (A0000–A0999)
- Medical and Surgical Supplies (A4000–A9999)
- Enteral and Parenteral Therapy (B4000–B9999)
- CMS Outpatient Payment System (C1000–C9999)
- Dental Procedures (D0120–D9999)
- Durable Medical Equipment (E0100–E8002)
- Temporary Procedures/Professional Services (G0008–G9987)
- Behavioral Health and/or Substance Abuse Treatment Services (H0001–H2037)
- Drugs Administered in the Medical Setting (J0100–J9999)
- Temporary Codes Established by Different Payers (K0000–K0900), (Q0035–Q9992), (S0012–S9999), (T1000–T5999)
- Orthotics and Prosthetics (L0112–L9900)
- Other Medical Services (M1000–M0301)
- Laboratory Services (P2028–P9615)
- Diagnostic Radiology Services (R0070–R0076)
- Vision and Hearing Services (V2020–V5364)

Coders should familiarize themselves with these sections of their HCPCS code books to help understand the services and supplies coded with this code set.

Each of the major sections includes a heading with a code range. Subheadings are included when necessary, followed by the listing of the HCPCS codes with code descriptions, symbols, and billing notes (see figure 5.10).

Figure 5.10. HCPCS headings, subheadings, and codes

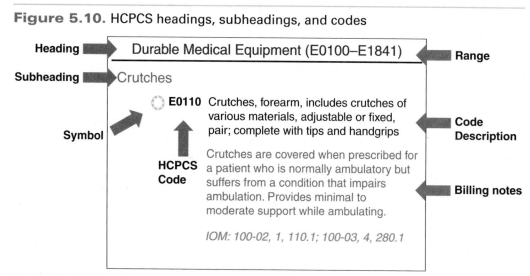

Source: Elsevier 2020, 196.

Not all headings have subheadings, and not all codes have symbols and billing notes. These are added throughout the Tabular List of codes on an as-needed basis. Unlike the CPT code book, the HCPCS code book does not have official guidelines listed before each major section, nor does it have guidelines in the Tabular List. Any special billing considerations, instructions, or advice is listed in the billing notes underneath the code description. Symbols also often refer to billing and coverage guidelines.

HCPCS codes are highly variable when it comes to payment. In other words, some health carriers will pay for certain codes, while others may not. It is important to verify coverage of HCPCS services and supplies before providing them to patients.

Appendices

The last section of the HCPCS code book is the appendices. Typically, HCPCS code books have at least one end-of-book appendix. Sometimes, the Table of Drugs and modifiers are listed in separate appendices, along with lengthy references to Medicare billing guidelines. Other times, the appendicular information at the end of the book includes references to Medicare, billing, or coding guidelines. As always, it is important to be familiar with all sections of the HCPCS code book to be as effective and efficient as possible.

Complete the exercises in There's a Code for That 5.6 to practice looking up and verifying codes in the HCPCS code book.

Verifying HCPCS codes

5.6

There's a Code for That

Read the statement for the HCPCS code selected. Then verify if the HCPCS code selected is the correct code or not. If it is not the correct code, then enter the correct code in the space provided.

1. Judy selected the code E1610 for deionizer water purification system for hemodialysis.

Is this the correct code? _____

If not the correct code, enter it here: _____

2. Judy selected the code L3350 for a heel wedge.

Is this the correct code? _____

If not the correct code, enter it here: _____

3. Judy selected the code V2500 × 2 for two PMMA spherical contact lenses.

Is this the correct code? _____

If not the correct code, enter it here: _____

4. Judy selected the code J3480 for the injection of potassium hydroxide preparation.

Is this the correct code? _____

If not the correct code, enter it here: _____

5. Judy selected the code K0006 for an extra heavy-duty wheelchair.

Is this the correct code? _____

If not the correct code, enter it here: _____

Case Study | Procedures

PATIENT: Cheyenne Savid   **DOB:** 01/04/20xx

DATE OF SERVICE: 01/06/20xx

PROCEDURE: Frenotomy

INDICATIONS: Congenital tongue-tie, problems feeding in newborn

PROCEDURE NOTE:
Risks, benefits, indications, and alternative were discussed, including the risks of infection, bleeding, and pain. Informed consent was obtained from the parents and signed consent form is on file. Before the procedure was performed, a time-out was taken to verify the correct patient, procedure, site, positioning and special equipment.
Baby girl Cheyenne was prepped and draped. A groove director was placed under the tongue to reveal the frenulum. Lingual frenulum was cut with scissors.

ESIMATED BLOOD LOSS: Minimal

COMPLICATIONS: None, patient tolerated the procedure well

SIGNED: Dr. Susan Alameda, DO

Use the following steps to select the appropriate codes for the case study.

1. Read through the case study in full, looking up any medical or procedural terms with which you are unfamiliar. For example, the terms *frenotomy* and *lingual frenulum* may not be familiar to you. Look up these words in a medical dictionary or medical terminology text and provide their definitions as follows. On your own, look up and define any additional unfamiliar terms.

   a. *Frenotomy:*

   _____

   _____

   b. *Lingual frenulum:*

   _____

   _____

Key to Success

As you read through the procedural note and answer the rest of the following questions, make sure to underline, circle, star, and take notes on the case study. This helps to identify key words and phrases and is a helpful tool in understanding complex procedure notes. Use whatever process works best for your understanding!

Take notes!

2. As you read the case study, pay special attention to the actions described by the provider, especially actions that describe the procedure performed. Look for key areas in the documentation, such as the PROCEDURE section, which will identify the name of the procedure performed. Additional information found in the PROCEDURE NOTE is often also helpful, especially for more complicated procedures. This area typically describes the procedure in full, including details that are often important for code selection, such as the approach to the procedure or any additional service performed during the procedure. After you have a good idea of the service performed, answer the question: *What did the doctor do?* Identify the name of the procedure performed in the case study.

_____

_____

Key to Success

Once you have read through the procedural note, make sure you have a good understanding of the procedure itself, how it was performed, and why it was performed. This may require you to research the procedure until you understand exactly how and why it is performed, including multiple variations of the procedure, if necessary. Healthcare coding professionals have the awesome job of getting to learn about a vast array of healthcare conditions and the procedures used to diagnose and treat them. This means that you have your learning cut out for you, but don't despair! The more you learn about healthcare procedures and how they are performed, the better you will ultimately become as a healthcare coding professional.

3. Now that you have the name of the procedure, locate the code for the procedure in the CPT code book.

a. Search the Index for the procedure, examine the options, and list them here.

_____

_____

b. If there are multiple options, identify the most appropriate code option and refer to the code listed in the Tabular section.

_____

_____

c. In the listing of codes, check for any guidelines, important definitions, or parenthetical notes. Does the code selected correctly identify all of the components of the procedure? If yes, then list the code here:

_____

_____

d. Are there any additional procedures that need to be added to identify all of the procedures performed? If yes, follow the previous steps to identify the codes for the additional procedures.

_____

_____

e. Are there any modifiers that need to be added to identify any special circumstance surrounding the procedure(s)? If yes, refer to Appendix A of the CPT code book to assign all appropriate modifiers.

_____

_____

4. Now that the procedure(s) and modifier(s) have been identified, refer to the case study and answer the following question: _Why did the doctor do it?_ To find the reason for the procedure, search for terms that will identify the healthcare condition. Look for key areas in the documentation, such as the INDICATIONS section, which identifies the indications for the procedure (that is, why the procedure was performed, or the patient's diagnosis). From the case study, identify the patient's diagnosis(es).

_____

_____

Key to Success

There are a number of terms used to identify the reason for a procedure, which may be located either at the beginning or the end of a note. Some of these terms include assessment, impression, definitive diagnosis, or indications. Remember that the diagnosis identifies the medical necessity for the procedure performed, so it helps to find the area of the note that identifies why the procedure was performed to correctly identify all of the patient's possible diagnoses.

5. Search the ICD-10-CM code book for the correct code(s) for the case study patient's diagnosis(es). Follow these steps for each of the diagnoses identified.

a. Search the Main Index for the name of each condition, and examine any applicable subterms and cross-references to locate the appropriate code(s).

    i. _____

    ii. _____

b. Verify the code(s) in the Tabular List. Locate the code(s) identified previously in the Tabular Listing of codes and refer to any applicable guidelines, notes, and symbols. Does each code selected correctly identify the patient's condition? If yes, list the code(s) here.

    i. _____

    ii. _____

c. Check the procedure note and ICD-10-CM guidelines and conventions to determine the correct sequencing of the diagnosis codes, if applicable. Correctly sequence the diagnosis codes.

_____

6. Now that the procedure and diagnosis codes have been identified, list them on the CMS-1500 form. Be sure to correctly link the procedure and diagnosis codes. Refer to figure 3.6 for an example.

21. DIAGNOSIS OR NATURE OF ILLNESS OR INJURY Relate A-L to service line below (24E)			ICD Ind.	

A. L_____ B. L_____ C. L_____ D. L_____

E. L_____ F. L_____ G. L_____ H. L_____

I. L_____ J. L_____ K. L_____ L. L_____

24. A.	DATE(S) OF SERVICE						B.	C.	D. PROCEDURES, SERVICES, OR SUPPLIES		E.
	From			To			PLACE OF		(Explain Unusual Circumstances)		DIAGNOSIS
MM	DD	YY	MM	DD	YY		SERVICE	EMG	CPT/HCPCS	MODIFIER	POINTER

End-of-Chapter Content

Instructions: Match the symbols with the appropriate descriptions.

CPT Symbol	Meaning
1. _____ ▶◀	A. Add-on code
2. _____ ✚	B. Modifier -51 exempt
3. _____ ▲	C. Telemedicine code
4. _____ ⁄	D. New code
5. _____ ★	E. New or revised text
6. _____ ●	F. Duplicate PLA test
7. _____ ⊘	G. Resequenced code
8. _____ #	H. FDA approval pending
9. _____ ⊁	I. Revised code
10. _____ ↑↓	J. Category I PLA

Instructions: Choose the best answer.

1. The CPT code answers which of the following questions?

  a. Why did the patient come in?
  b. What did the doctor do?
  c. Why did the doctor do it?
  d. What supply did the doctor provide?

2. The ICD-10-CM answers which of the following questions?

  a. Why did the patient come in?
  b. What did the doctor do?
  c. Why did the doctor do it?
  d. What supply did the doctor provide?

3. The HCPCS code answers which of the following questions?

  a. Why did the patient come in?
  b. What did the doctor do?
  c. Why did the doctor do it?
  d. What supply did the doctor provide?

4. Which of the following types of CPT codes is used for performance measures tracking?

  a. Category I
  b. Category II
  c. Category III
  d. Category IV

(Continued on next page)

(Continued)

5. Which of the following types of CPT codes is composed of all numbers?
   a. Category I
   b. Category II
   c. Category III
   d. Category IV

6. How many sections of Category I codes are there?
   a. 8
   b. 6
   c. 9
   d. 3

7. Which of the following types of CPT codes ends with the letter *T*?
   a. Category I
   b. Category II
   c. Category III
   d. No CPT codes end with the letter *T*

8. If a procedure is not found in either Category I or Category III codes, how do you report the service?
   a. By using a Category II code
   b. By using an unlisted procedures code
   c. By sending a special report
   d. Do not report the service if a code does not exist

9. Which CPT appendix would you use to help identify the branches of a vascular family?
   a. Appendix K
   b. Appendix P
   c. Appendix B
   d. Appendix L

10. Which of the following types of CPT codes is indented beneath a parent code, on which it depends for the full code description?
    a. Standalone code
    b. Indented code
    c. Modifier -51 code
    d. Modifying code

11. What type of codes are used to report supplies provided to patients in the healthcare setting?
    a. CPT
    b. ICD-10
    c. Add-on codes
    d. HCPCS

12. Which of the following would be reported with a HCPCS code?
    a. Chief complaint of cough and runny nose
    b. Kyphoplasty procedure
    c. Fitting of a diaphragm
    d. Diaphragm provided to the patient

13. In which of the following ways would you search for a main term in the HCPCS Index?
    a. Name of the condition
    b. Name of the surgical procedure
    c. Name of the item or equipment supplied
    d. Name of the reason for the encounter

14. Which of the following codes is a HCPCS Level II code?
    a. 0012F
    b. 59050
    c. G0466
    d. 0042T

15. Find the modifiers section in the HCPCS code book. Which of the following is the modifier for Registered Dietitian?
    a. RT
    b. RD
    c. AE
    d. BA

Instructions: Answer the following questions with the appropriate code.

1. Complex repair of the scalp, 10 cm.

   CPT code(s): _____ , _____

2. Debridement of eczematous skin, 20 percent of body surface.

   CPT code(s): _____ , _____

3. Escharotomy, two separate incisions.

   CPT code(s): _____ , _____

4. Appendectomy for ruptured appendix with generalized peritonitis, with intraoperative colonic lavage.

   CPT code(s): _____ , _____

5. Hospital discharge, 30 minutes total.

   CPT code(s): _____

6. Unlisted procedure of the small intestine.

   CPT code(s): _____

7. Unlisted vascular surgical procedure.

   CPT code(s): _____

8. Barium enema colorectal cancer screening.

   HCPCS code(s): _____

9. Insertion of intrauterine device (code for the insertion and the provision of the IUD).

   CPT code(s): _____

   HCPCS code(s): _____

10. Two articulating, spring assisted underarm crutches.

    HCPCS code(s): _____

References

American Medical Association (AMA). 2019. *CPT 2020 Professional Edition*. Chicago: AMA.

Elsevier. 2020. *2020 HCPCS LEVEL II, Professional Edition*. Chicago: AHIMA.

Resources

Centers for Medicare and Medicaid Services (CMS). 2019. 2020 HCPCS Alpha-Numeric Index. https://www.cms.gov/Medicare/Coding/HCPCSReleaseCodeSets/Downloads/2020-HCPCS-Index.pdf.

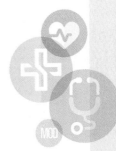

Coding
in the Real World

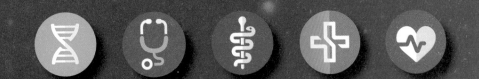

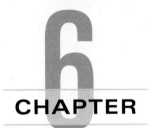

CHAPTER 6

Supplies and Services

Learning Objectives

- Understand the basics of billing and coding; analyze and assign procedural and diagnosis codes to ambulance services
- Understand the basics of billing and coding; analyze and assign procedural and diagnosis codes to durable medical equipment and supplies
- Analyze the HCPCS Table of Drugs and assign HCPCS codes used to report medications given in the healthcare setting

Key Terms

Advanced life support (ALS)
Ambulance modifier
Ambulance supplier
Basic life support (BLS)
Certificate of Medical Necessity (CMN)
Destination
Durable medical equipment (DME)

Durable medical equipment, prosthetics, orthotics, and supplies (DMEPOS)
Emergency transportation
Non-ambulatory
Nonemergency transportation
Origin
Orthotics

Physician's Desk Reference (PDR)
Prosthetics
Route of administration
Services
Supplies
Transportation indicator

In addition to medical and surgical procedures, patients commonly receive a number of miscellaneous supplies and services during healthcare encounters. **Supplies** are items provided to the patient in the healthcare setting, typically designed for long-term or multiple uses. Items that are used to treat the patient or help perform the procedure may also be reported with HCPCS codes. This includes medical equipment for home use (such as a pair of crutches), supplies used in patient care during an admission (such as parenteral nutrition), and medications given to the patient during the encounter (such as an antibiotic injection). **Services** identified by HCPCS codes are miscellaneous services that may be provided to patients in the healthcare setting. Some of these services, such as certain vaccinations, are also identified by CPT codes, whereas other services, such as ambulance transportation services, are identified by codes found in the HCPCS code book only.

Supplies and services are coded using HCPCS Level II codes, as discussed in chapter 5 (Learning the CPT and HCPCS Code Books). While most of these codes are billed by ambulance service or durable medical equipment suppliers, some HCPCS codes (namely those for Medicare-covered services and for drugs or medications administered in the office) are commonly billed in the outpatient setting.

This chapter discusses HCPCS Level II coding within the context of a durable medical equipment office and ambulance supplier, HCPCS codes used for Medicare services in the outpatient setting, and HCPCS codes that are used to bill for drugs and medicinal substances administered in the healthcare setting.

Ambulance and Durable Medical Equipment Services

Durable medical equipment and ambulance suppliers provide a special set of healthcare services. Rather than directly providing services to a patient, such as a surgery or physical examination, durable medical equipment suppliers simply provide supplies that the patient needs in order to maintain or treat his or her health condition. **Ambulance suppliers**, on the other hand, are tasked with transporting a patient with a healthcare need to a provider or facility capable of treating that need. This is usually done in an emergent or urgent situation, and the emergency responders must stabilize and provide a certain level of healthcare services to the patient until he or she can receive care from a healthcare provider. Transportation is also often required in nonemergent situations, when a medically fragile patient is transported from one healthcare appointment or facility to another in order to receive a particular service not offered at the current location, such as a computerized tomography (CT) or magnetic resonance imaging (MRI) scan.

The following sections of this chapter discuss HCPCS and ICD-10-CM coding within the context of an ambulance supplier and durable medical equipment supplier's office. Billing and coding for ambulance services requires a solid understanding of the types and uses of codes, especially HCPCS codes. All ambulance and transportation services are identified by a small selection of HCPCS codes.

Ambulance Coding Basics

There are differences between the various ambulance services identified by HCPCS codes. The first difference is between basic life support and advanced life support services. **Basic life support** (BLS) is a primary level of care used for patients with life-threatening illnesses, injuries, or other severe conditions while they are transported to a facility that can provide them with complete medical care. BLS services focus on adequate blood circulation and a clear airway through the CAB's of life support: Circulation (providing adequate blood supply through chest compressions), Airway (protecting a clear passageway for oxygen), and Breathing (inflating and deflation of the lungs) (American Heart Association 2010). This process is supported by research and ensures the best possibility for survival. **Advanced life support** (ALS) is a higher level of care that includes life-saving protocols to further support airway, breathing, and circulation. ALS services can include manual defibrillation to restart the heart, endotracheal intubation to create an airway, placing a central venous line for venous access, or creating a surgical airway, such as a tracheotomy (opening in the trachea to establish an airway).

The next main difference in ambulance services is between emergency and nonemergency transport. Once the ambulance provider is called, **emergency transportation** responds immediately to the scene of the accident or incident to provide medical assistance and transport to a healthcare facility if necessary. For example, if an ambulance is called to respond to a car accident in which people have been injured, that ambulance arrives as soon as possible to provide healthcare to any injured patients and then transport them to a healthcare facility for further medical care if necessary. On the other hand, **nonemergency transportation** is generally scheduled in advance and used for patient transfers from one facility to another, or to transport **non-ambulatory** patients for healthcare. Non-ambulatory means unable to walk about, so non-ambulatory patients are those who are unable to move around independently, such as a patient confined to a bed. For example, non-ambulatory patients may require transportation for activities of daily living, or transportation to and from healthcare facilities. Patient transfers are commonly performed in a nonemergency setting to transport a patient to a healthcare facility that provides more specialized healthcare.

The last major difference in ambulance services is the type of transportation—air and ground. Transportation is most commonly provided with a ground transportation vehicle, although in certain emergency situations a helicopter may be used to provide faster transport to a healthcare facility. Air ambulance services are provided by either a fixed wing (airplane) or rotary wing (helicopter) vehicle. Ground transportation vehicles vary more and include taxi, wheelchair van, and typical on-ground ambulance carrier. If an HCPCS code does not specify that transportation is provided by either a fixed or rotary wing aircraft (air service), then the code can be used for ground transportation.

There are several additional details needed on ambulance claims, including ambulance origin and destination modifiers, transportation indicators, mileage for both ground and air transportation, and any other services or supplies that were provided to the patient during the transportation service (see figure 6.1).

Ambulance modifiers are required on ambulance claims to identify the origin and destination for each transportation. The **origin** of a transportation service is where the patient was picked up, and the **destination** is where the patient was taken. For example, a patient may be taken from the scene of an accident (origin) to a hospital (destination). Ambulance modifiers are created by combining two letters that are listed in the HCPCS code book before the selection of ambulance codes, before A0021, Ambulance, service, outside state per mile, transport (Medicaid only). These letters are also listed in figure 6.1 for reference. To build a two-letter modifier, the letter that corresponds to the origin is listed first, and the letter that corresponds to the destination is listed last. For example, if the origin were the scene of an accident (S, Scene of accident or acute event), and the destination were a hospital (H, Hospital), then the modifier would be SH, Scene of accident or acute event to Hospital. This modifier would be appended to the end of the HCPCS code, just as in CPT coding. For example, a ground ambulance transport from

Figure 6.1. Ambulance billing details

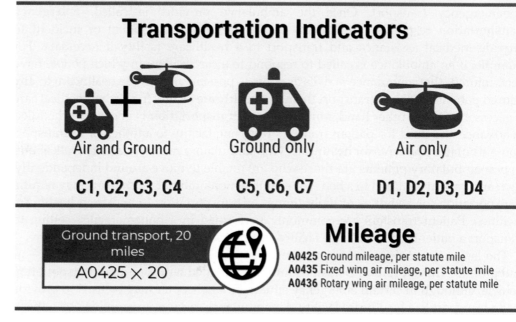

the scene of an accident to a hospital would be coded as such: A0429-SH, Ambulance services, basic life support, emergency transport (BLS-Emergency), Scene of accident or acute event to Hospital.

In addition to the ICD-10 diagnosis and HCPCS ambulance codes, a transportation indicator—a two-character code—is used to identify why the transportation service was medically necessary. These indicators provide more information regarding the circumstances as to why a patient was transported in that particular way. Transportation indicators are not usually listed in the HCPCS manual and may or may not be necessary, depending on the patient's insurance carrier guidelines. The 11 indicators are as follows:

C1 = Transport from low-level facility to higher-level facility
C2 = Transport from one facility to another due to unavailability of service at origin facility
C3 = Response to a major incident or mechanism of injury
C4 = Excessive number of miles driven
C5 = BLS level service provided to an ALS level patient
C6 = ALS level ambulance provided for a BLS level patient
C7 = Intravenous medications required during transport

D1 = Patient condition requires long distance transport
D2 = Traffic patterns necessitating air transport
D3 = Time to get to the patient precludes ground ambulance
D4 = Pick up point not accessible by ground

Transportation indicators C1 through C4 are used for either air or ground transportation. C5 through C7 are used for ground transportation only, and D1 through D4 are used for air transportation only. For example, if a patient was stranded in a desert canyon inaccessible by ground vehicles and suffered a healthcare emergency, then transportation indicator D4, Pick up point not accessible by ground, would be used to identify why rotary wing (helicopter) ambulance transportation was provided.

Transportation indicators are placed in box 19 on the CMS-1500 claim form (see figure 6.2).

Each transportation service provided should be coded with the appropriate HCPCS transportation code, with the number of miles indicated as the number of units for the service. This is done by entering the HCPCS code(s) for the transportation services in box 24.A on the CMS-1500 claim form, with the appropriate number of units identified in box 24.G. For example, if the ambulance service were 20 miles of ground transport, then the HCPCS code A0425 would be entered in box 24.A, with the number of miles identified in box 24.G (see figure 6.3). When multiple units of any HCPCS or CPT code need to be reported on a claim for services, the CPT or HCPCS code is listed, followed by the multiplication symbol (×), and then the number of units. For example, 20 miles of ground transport would be listed as A0425 × 20—A0425 identifies the ground transport and 20 identifies the number of units, in this case miles traveled (refer to figure 6.3).

Additional supplies and services are also coded for ambulance services. HCPCS codes for these supplies include oxygen and oxygen supplies, routine disposable provisions, and esophageal intubation materials.

Figure 6.2. Transportation indicators listed in box 19

Source: CMS 2019a.

Figure 6.3. Entering HCPCS codes on CMS-1500 form

24. A. DATE(S) OF SERVICE						B. PLACE OF SERVICE	C. EMG	D. PROCEDURES, SERVICES, OR SUPPLIES (Explain Unusual Circumstances) CPT/HCPCS | MODIFIER	E. DIAGNOSIS POINTER	F. $ CHARGES	G. DAYS OR UNITS	H. EPSDT Family Plan	I. ID. QUAL.	J. RENDERING PROVIDER ID. #
From MM DD YY			To MM DD YY											
1								A0425			20		NPI	

Source: CMS 2019a.

Key to Success

The selection of HCPCS codes for ambulance services is relatively small, and the more familiar you become with ambulance codes in the A0021 to A0999 range, the easier it will be to ensure that you code all ambulance services correctly.

Diagnosis Coding for Ambulance Services

Emergency personnel on board the ambulance cannot diagnose a patient's condition, but this does not mean they can send a claim for the healthcare services without a diagnosis code. Remember, as discussed in chapter 3 (Basics of Coding), the diagnosis code (ICD-10-CM) on a claim indicates the medical necessity for the service. Therefore, there must be at least one ICD-10-CM code on the claim to prove that the ambulance service was medically necessary.

An emergency responder is not considered a qualified healthcare professional (meaning that they have not received sufficient training to become a physician or mid-level provider). Consequently, an emergency responder cannot determine the patient's diagnosis. He or she must record the signs, symptoms, or complaints of the patient, and code for those only. For example, if an ambulance reports to a home residence where a patient has fallen off a ladder and is complaining of severe arm pain, the code for pain in the arm would be reported on the claim. Once the patient arrives at the hospital, the healthcare providers there will determine the extent of the injury and actual diagnosis (such as a fracture).

The ability to assign a specific diagnosis differs depending on the situation, however. For example, if a patient is being transferred from one healthcare facility to another for an organ transplant or surgery, the ambulance company will have a record of the patient's actual diagnosis, which has been confirmed by a healthcare provider. In this case, the ambulance personnel may report the diagnosis that was given to them by the healthcare provider as medical necessity for the service provided.

When selecting a diagnosis code for an ambulance service, select the correct code according to one of the following three options (figure 6.4):

- Option 1: Select the appropriate code to identify the condition of the patient when they were picked up. These codes identify the patient's signs, symptoms, or other complaint.

- Option 2: Report the diagnosis code that is provided by the treating healthcare provider. This is typically only possible for patient transfers.

- Option 3: Report the ICD-10-CM code for unspecified illness:
  - 69, Illness, unspecified (ICD-10-CM)
  - 99, Ill-defined and unknown cause of mortality (ICD-10-CM)

Figure 6.4. Diagnosis coding for ambulance services

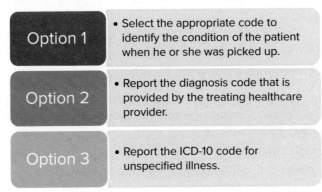

Option 1	• Select the appropriate code to identify the condition of the patient when he or she was picked up.
Option 2	• Report the diagnosis code that is provided by the treating healthcare provider.
Option 3	• Report the ICD-10 code for unspecified illness.

The ambulance service must be fully documented to support all the codes placed on the claim. The presence of detailed documentation for the ambulance service (or lack thereof) determines whether or not the transportation service meets coverage guidelines, which impacts whether the claim is paid by the patient's insurance company. Documentation should always include the details of the trip, including the patient's medical condition and all the services provided to the patient.

Key to Success

In the following sections, selection of codes for the services provided is required. Remember the basics of code selection—examine the documentation to identify the service performed and the patient's diagnosis (when applicable); look up the main term in the Index; verify the code in the Tabular List; check any applicable guidelines, modifiers, and number of units; and assign the code!

Putting It All Together: Coding for Ambulance Services

In order to select the correct code for the service provided, it is important to carefully read the documentation of the service, then access the HCPCS code book Index and find the type of service that was provided. The HCPCS codes for ambulance services range from A0021 to A0999.

Determination of the correct codes for ambulance services relies on the following details:

- Was basic life support (BLS) or advanced life support (ALS) provided during the transport?
- Was the transport emergency or nonemergency?
- What type of transportation was used?
- What was the origin of the transport and what was the destination?
- How many miles were traveled?
- Which transportation indicator is applicable for the service?
- Was there any additional wait time, services, supplies, or personnel utilized during the service?

Study the following examples of appropriate codes for ambulance services. Then complete the exercises in There's a Code for That 6.1 to practice coding for ambulance and transportation services.

Example 6.1. Emergency ambulance service

Patient complaining of severe respiratory distress (shortness of breath) is transported via emergency ALS level 1 ground ambulance from her place of residence to the hospital. Total distance traveled was 8 miles.

HCPCS code: A0427-RH Ambulance service, advanced life support, emergency transport, level 1 (ALS 1-emergency); origin R-Residence; destination H-Hospital
HCPCS code: A0425 × 8 Ground mileage, per statute mile, 8 miles
ICD-10 code: R06.02, Shortness of breath

Example 6.2. Nonemergency ambulance service

A ventilator-dependent geriatric patient is transferred from a skilled nursing facility to home hospice. BLS nonemergency ground transport, 23 miles total. During transfer there was an unexpected death at the nursing facility, and the ambulance had to wait for 90 minutes before the transport could begin.

HCPCS code: A0428-NE Ambulance service, basic life support, nonemergency transport (BLS); origin N-skilled nursing facility; destination E-residential, domiciliary, or custodial facility
HCPCS code: A0425 × 23 Ground mileage, per statute mile, 23 miles
ICD-10 code: Z99.11, Dependence on respirator (ventilator) status

---

6.1

There's a Code for That

Coding for ambulance and transportation services

Enter the correct answer for each of the following practice exercises.

1. Emergency ALS level 2 transport, rotary wing. Code just for the transportation, no mileage, without modifiers.
   HCPCS code: _____

2. Patient was transported from the scene of an accident to the hospital. What modifier would be used?
   HCPCS modifier: _____

3. Patient was picked up at the scene of an accident and transported via helicopter to a transfer pad, where he was then picked up by an on-ground ambulance and transported to a hospital. Helicopter mileage totaled 15 miles. Code only for the hospital transport, including modifier and miles traveled.
   HCPCS code: _____ - _____
   HCPCS code: _____ × _____

4. Patient with severe laceration of the right upper arm was transported from the scene of an accident via helicopter to a hospital. The total distance traveled was 13 miles. Due to heavy traffic conditions, a helicopter was dispatched to pick up the patient rather than an on-ground ambulance.

HCPCS code: _____ - _____

HCPCS code: _____ × _____

Transportation indicator: _____

ICD-10-CM code: _____

5. Nonemergency transport via wheelchair van to patient with quadriplegia and ventilator dependence. Patient was transferred from her residence to a skilled nursing facility, 7 miles total distance traveled.

HCPCS code: _____ - _____

HCPCS code: _____ × _____

ICD-10-CM: _____

ICD-10-CM: _____

Durable Medical Equipment and Supplies

Durable medical equipment (DME) is a category of medical items and supplies used by patients both in and out of the healthcare setting. DME requires the following four characteristics:

- It can withstand repeated use
- It is used to serve a medical purpose
- It is not useful for a person without an illness or injury
- It can also be used in the home setting (outside of the healthcare setting)

For example, a pair of crutches supplied to a 15-year-old with a lower leg fracture are considered durable medical equipment. These crutches are: (1) used on a repetitive basis; (2) serve the purpose of helping the patient to walk; (3) are not useful for a patient without a leg injury or gait abnormality; and (4) are used everywhere that the patient goes, both in and out of the healthcare setting.

One specific type of DME are prosthetics and orthotics. **Prosthetics** are designed to replace all or part of an internal body organ (such as an artificial hip or knee replacement) or to replace an external appendage as an artificial limb (such as a lower leg prosthesis for an amputee). **Orthotics** are instruments that are used on the outside of the body to support, align, or correct deformities, or to improve the movements of joints, the spine, or the limbs (CMS 2019b). The most common types of orthotics are casts, placed on the outside of a body area to immobilize that body area and allow healing of the internal bones.

Durable medical equipment, prosthetics, orthotics, and supplies are often combined using the acronym **DMEPOS**. DMEPOS is a category of DME supplies that includes prosthetics and orthotics. Claims for DMEPOS are paid only if the supply or equipment is considered medically necessary as determined by the healthcare provider and the patient's insurance company. For example, if a patient suffered a minor sprain to his ankle, it may not be necessary to give him a pair of crutches but rather a supportive brace or wrap to immobilize the ankle joint. On the other hand, if a patient suffered a debilitating fracture of the femur, it may be medically necessary to supply the patient with a long leg brace and crutches until the femur bone heals.

Prior authorizations (discussed in chapter 3) may also be necessary before DME supplies are provided to the patient when the patient's health insurance requires determination of medical necessity for the supplied item. For certain DMEPOS items, determination of medical necessity is done by using a **Certificate of Medical Necessity (CMN)** form. A CMN is an official document, completed by the physician and the DME supplier, that details the patient's diagnosis, necessity for the DME supply, and other important patient demographics and information. Usually DMEPOS items that require a CMN are over a certain dollar amount, thus why the additional attestation of medical necessity is required. For example, TRICARE insurance requires a CMN for any DME supply that has a purchase cost of $150 or more (HNFHS 2012). This form serves as proof that the DME supply was medically necessary to treat the patient as required by the patient's health insurance. Figure 6.5 displays a CMN for Positive Airway Pressure (PAP) Devices for Obstructive Sleep Apnea (CMS-10269).

The second page of the CMN contains instructions on how to complete the form. Notice that, according to these directions, some sections should be completed by the physician or physician's office (Sections B and D), whereas the other sections should be completed by the DME supplier (Sections A and C). Any additional health records or documentation of the patient's condition may also need to be sent along with the CMN to ensure the service will be covered. Other items that require a CMN include oxygen, pneumatic compression devices, osteogenesis stimulators, enteral and parenteral nutrition, and seat lift mechanisms, among others.

Once all the billing considerations, such as a CMN or prior authorization, have been addressed, coding for DME is essentially as simple as identifying and reporting the correct HCPCS code(s). Perhaps one of the most problematic parts of coding from the HCPCS code book for beginning coders is locating the correct code in the book itself. Because Index entries vary by publisher and items are listed in various ways, it is sometimes difficult to locate the Index entry for the item being reported. It helps to be as familiar with the HCPCS code book as possible, including knowing where all sections of codes are located and placing tabs throughout the book for easy access.

There are numerous modifiers in the HCPCS code book that may be added to HCPCS codes for DMEPOS to provide more details about the supply or service provided, such as whether the equipment was new or used. HCPCS modifiers can identify the following:

- The type of healthcare provider
- Specifics surrounding anesthesia services
- Body areas, such as specific fingers, eyelids, or coronary arteries
- Laterality (right or left side)
- The number of wounds dressed
- That an advance beneficiary notice (ABN) or waiver of liability was given to the patient
- Specific types of treatments to patients on dialysis or with end-stage renal disease (ESRD)
- Details about the type of equipment provided

Complete the following exercises in There's a Code for That 6.2 to test your knowledge about HCPCS modifiers.

Identifying HCPCS modifiers

6.2

There's a Code for That

In the following exercises, code only for the HCPCS modifier as indicated.

1. Dressing for five wounds.

   HCPCS modifier: _____

2. Left foot, 4th digit.

   HCPCS modifier: _____

3. Right side.

   HCPCS modifier: _____

4. New equipment.

   HCPCS modifier: _____

5. DMEPOS item delivered via mail.

   HCPCS modifier: _____

6. Left main coronary artery.

   HCPCS modifier: _____

7. Administered intravenously.

   HCPCS modifier: _____

8. Upper left eyelid.

   HCPCS modifier: _____

Key to Success

Because HCPCS modifiers are so varied in meaning, it is beneficial to study the list of modifiers and become as familiar with these codes as possible. Read through the HCPCS modifiers section of your HCPCS code book and note the modifier, such as RT, and then the modifier description, such as "Right side." Observe similarities and differences as you review the modifiers and note groups of modifiers that are similar in nature, such as modifiers E1 through E4, which all identify eyelids (E1, Upper left, eyelid; E2, Lower left, eyelid; E3, Upper right, eyelid; E4, Lower right, eyelid).

CPT modifiers are all numeric (they do not contain letters), whereas HCPCS modifiers are all alphanumeric (they contain at least one letter).

MOD

Diagnosis Coding for DME

When a patient requires DME, he or she is generally already under the care of a healthcare practitioner and already has an established diagnosis or condition for

Figure 6.5. Certificate of medical necessity (CMS-10269)

DEPARTMENT OF HEALTH AND HUMAN SERVICES
CENTERS FOR MEDICARE & MEDICAID SERVICES

Form Approved
OMB No. OMB 0938-0679

CERTIFICATE OF MEDICAL NECESSITY   DME 03.03

CMS-10269: POSITIVE AIRWAY PRESSURE (PAP) DEVICES FOR OBSTRUCTIVE SLEEP APNEA

SECTION A: Certification Type/Date: INITIAL ___/___/___ RECERTIFICATION ___/___/___

PATIENT NAME, ADDRESS, TELEPHONE and HICN   SUPPLIER NAME, ADDRESS, TELEPHONE and NSC or NPI #

(___ ___ ___) ___ ___ ___-___ ___ ___ ___   HICN _____   (___ ___ ___) ___ ___ ___-___ ___ ___ ___   NSC or NPI # _____

PLACE OF SERVICE _____	HCPCS CODE	PT DOB ___/___/___; Sex ___ (M/F) ; HT.____(in.) ; WT.____(lbs.)
NAME and ADDRESS of FACILITY if applicable (See Reverse)	_____ _____ _____ _____	PHYSICIAN NAME, ADDRESS (Printed or Typed) PHYSICIAN'S NSC or NPI #: _____ PHYSICIAN'S TELEPHONE #: (___ ___ ___) ___ ___ ___-___ ___ ___ ___

SECTION B: Information in this section may not be completed by the supplier of the items/supplies.

EST. LENGTH OF NEED (# OF MONTHS): _____ 1–99 (99=LIFETIME)   DIAGNOSIS CODES (ICD-9): _____ _____ _____ _____

ANSWERS	ANSWER QUESTIONS 1–7 FOR INITIAL EVALUATION ANSWER QUESTIONS 8–10 FOR FOLLOW-UP EVALUATION (RECERTIFICATION) (Check **Y** for Yes, **N** for No, **D** for Does Not Apply)
☐ Y ☐ N	1. Is the device being ordered for the treatment of obstructive sleep apnea (ICD-9 diagnosis code 327.23)? If YES, continue to Questions 2–5; If NO, Proceed to Section D
___/___/___	2. Enter date of initial face-to-face evaluation
___/___/___	3. Enter date of sleep test (If test spans multiple days, enter date of first day of test)
☐ Y ☐ N	4. Was the patient's sleep test conducted in a facility-based lab?
_____	5. What is the patient's Apnea-Hypopnea Index (AHI) or Respiratory Disturbance Index (RDI)?
☐ Y ☐ N	6. Does the patient have documented evidence of at least one of the following? Excessive daytime sleepiness, impaired cognition, mood disorders, insomnia, hypertension, ischemic heart disease or history of stroke.
☐ Y ☐ N ☐ D	7. If a bilevel device is ordered, has a CPAP device been tried and found ineffective?
___/___/___	8. Enter date of follow-up face-to-face evaluation.
☐ Y ☐ N	9. Is there a report documenting that the patient used PAP ≥ 4 hours per night on at least 70% of nights in a 30 consecutive day period?
☐ Y ☐ N	10. Did the patient demonstrate improvement in symptoms of obstructive sleep apnea with the use of PAP?

NAME OF PERSON ANSWERING SECTION B QUESTIONS, IF OTHER THAN PHYSICIAN (Please Print):

NAME: _____   TITLE: _____   EMPLOYER: _____

SECTION C: Narrative Description of Equipment and Cost

(1) <u>Narrative</u> description of all items, accessories and options ordered; **(2)** Supplier's charge; and **(3)** Medicare Fee Schedule Allowance for <u>each</u> item, accessory, and option. *(See instructions on back)*

SECTION D: Physician Attestation and Signature/Date

I certify that I am the physician identified in Section A of this form. I have received Sections A, B and C of the Certificate of Medical Necessity (including charges for items ordered). Any statement on my letterhead attached hereto, has been reviewed and signed by me. I certify that the medical necessity information in Section B is true, accurate and complete, to the best of my knowledge, and I understand that any falsification, omission, or concealment of material fact in that section may subject me to civil or criminal liability.

PHYSICIAN'S SIGNATURE _____ DATE ___/___/___ (SIGNATURE AND DATE STAMPS ARE NOT ACCEPTABLE)

INSTRUCTIONS FOR COMPLETING THE CERTIFICATE OF MEDICAL NECESSITY
FOR POSITIVE AIRWAY PRESSURE (PAP) DEVICES FOR OBSTRUCTIVE SLEEP APNEA (CMS-10269)

SECTION A: (May be completed by the supplier)

CERTIFICATION TYPE/DATE: If this is an initial certification for this patient, indicate this by placing date (MM/DD/YY) needed initially in the space marked "INITIAL." If this is a revised certification (to be completed when the physician changes the order, based on the patient's changing clinical needs), indicate the initial date needed in the space marked "INITIAL," and also indicate the recertification date in the space marked "REVISED." If this is a recertification, indicate the initial date needed in the space marked "INITIAL," and also indicate the recertification date in the space marked "RECERTIFICATION." Whether submitting a REVISED or a RECERTIFIED CMN, be sure to always furnish the INITIAL date as well as the REVISED or RECERTIFICATION date.

PATIENT INFORMATION: Indicate the patient's name, permanent legal address, telephone number and his/her health insurance claim number (HICN) as it appears on his/her Medicare card and on the claim form.

SUPPLIER INFORMATION: Indicate the name of your company (supplier name), address and telephone number along with the National Provider Identification (NPI) number assigned to you by the National Supplier Clearinghouse (NSC).

PLACE OF SERVICE: Indicate the place in which the item is being used, i.e., patient's home is 12, skilled nursing facility (SNF) is 31, End Stage Renal Disease (ESRD) facility is 65, etc. Refer to the DME MAC supplier manual for a complete list.

FACILITY NAME: If the place of service is a facility, indicate the name and complete address of the facility.

HCPCS CODES: List all HCPCS procedure codes for items ordered that require a CMN. Procedure codes that do not require certification should not be listed on the CMN.

PATIENT DOB, HEIGHT, WEIGHT AND SEX: Indicate patient's date of birth (MM/DD/YY) and sex (male or female); height in inches and weight in pounds, if requested.

PHYSICIAN NAME, ADDRESS: Indicate the physician's name and complete mailing address.

NPI: Accurately indicate the ordering physician's National Provider Identification number (NPI).

PHYSICIAN'S TELEPHONE NO: Indicate the telephone number where the physician can be contacted (preferably where records would be accessible pertaining to this patient) if more information is needed.

SECTION B: (May not be completed by the supplier. While this section may be completed by a non-physician clinician, or a physician employee, it must be reviewed, and the CMN signed (in Section D) by the ordering physician.)

EST. LENGTH OF NEED: Indicate the estimated length of need (the length of time the physician expects the patient to require use of the ordered item) by filling in the appropriate number of months. If the physician expects that the patient will require the item for the duration of his/her life, then enter 99.

DIAGNOSIS CODES: In the first space, list the ICD9 code that represents the primary reason for ordering this item. List any additional ICD9 codes that would further describe the medical need for the item (up to 3 codes).

QUESTION SECTION: This section is used to gather clinical information to determine medical necessity. Answer each question which applies to the items ordered, checking "Y" for yes, "N" for no, or fill in the blank if other information is requested.

NAME OF PERSON ANSWERING SECTION B QUESTIONS: If a clinical professional other than the ordering physician (e.g., home health nurse, physical therapist, dietician) or a physician employee answers the questions of Section B, he/she must print his/her name, give his/her professional title and the name of his/her employer where indicated. If the physician is answering the questions, this space may be left blank.

SECTION C: (To be completed by the supplier)

NARRATIVE DESCRIPTION OF EQUIPMENT & COST: Supplier gives **(1)** a narrative description of the item(s) ordered, as well as all options, accessories, supplies and drugs; **(2)** the supplier's charge for each item, option, accessory, supply and drug; and **(3)** the Medicare fee schedule allowance for each item/option/accessory/supply/drug, if applicable.

SECTION D: (To be completed by the physician)

PHYSICIAN ATTESTATION: The physician's signature certifies **(1)** the CMN which he/she is reviewing includes Sections A, B, C and D; **(2)** the answers in Section B are correct; and **(3)** the self-identifying information in Section A is correct.

PHYSICIAN SIGNATURE AND DATE: After completion and/or review by the physician of Sections A, B and C, the physician must sign and date the CMN in Section D, verifying the Attestation appearing in this Section. The physician's signature also certifies the items ordered are medically necessary for this patient. Signature and date stamps are not acceptable.

Source: CMS 2009.

which the DME supply is necessary. This means that when coding for DME claims, diagnostic coding (ICD-10-CM) relies on the patient's established diagnosis, which should be included on the DME supply request form from the healthcare provider. DME personnel (billers, coders, and administrative staff) are not clinical in nature and are unauthorized to diagnose patients. However, they can and may often be relied upon to abstract healthcare provider notes in order to select an ICD-10 code.

In this sense, medical necessity plays a large part in DME coding. A valid ICD-10-CM diagnosis code is always needed on the claim to indicate medical necessity for the service, and a CMN may also be needed for certain items.

Putting It All Together: Coding for Durable Medical Equipment, Prosthetics, Orthotics, and Supplies

In order to select the correct code for the supply provided, it is important to carefully read the documentation and then access the Index in the HCPCS code book and find the type of supply or equipment provided. Codes for DMEPOS are found throughout the HCPCS code book.

Determination of the correct codes for DMEPOS relies on the following details.

- What type of supply or equipment was provided to the patient?
- What are the details of the supply: amount per unit, size, dosage, frequency, and such?
- Are there any applicable modifiers?

The steps for selecting the correct HCPCS code are similar to those for selecting CPT or ICD-10-CM codes. To find the correct HCPCS code, read through the documentation of the procedure or supply provided, reference the Index to the HCPCS code book, and refer to any subterms or cross-references. Once a code is identified in the Index, that code should be verified in the Tabular section. Refer to chapter 5 for a reminder of the components of the HCPCS code book. Chapter 4 (Learning the ICD-10-CM Code Book) includes a full discussion on identifying and selecting ICD-10-CM codes.

Study the following examples of appropriate codes for DMEPOS. Then complete the exercises in There's a Code for That 6.3 to practice coding for HCPCS supplies and services.

Example 6.3 Patient supply provided

Pediatric patient was supplied with a portable nebulizer machine to be able to provide home breathing treatments for reactive airway disease, new equipment.

HCPCS code: E0570-NU, Nebulizer, with compressor, new equipment
ICD-10-CM code: J45.909, Unspecified asthma, uncomplicated

Example 6.4 Patient supply provided

Patient with pre-diabetes was prescribed a home blood glucose monitor by her PCP. Supplied patient with monitor per physician's orders and educated patient on the proper usage of the equipment.

HCPCS code: E0607, Home blood glucose monitor
ICD-10-CM code: R73.03, Prediabetes

Key to Success

When locating an item in the HCPCS Index, you may find a range of codes listed rather than a single code. In this case, reference each one of the codes within that code range to ensure correct code selection.

Coding for HCPCS supplies and services

6.3

There's a Code for That

Enter the correct answer for each of the following practice exercises.

1. Oxygen mask and two feet of tubing used in the office setting during breathing treatment provided to patient with emphysema.

   HCPCS code: _____

   HCPCS code: _____ × _____

   ICD-10-CM code: _____

2. Wheelchair-bound patient is provided with two replacement arm pads.

   HCPCS code: _____ × _____

3. Rubber colostomy pouch, drainable, with faceplate attached.

   HCPCS code: _____

4. Patient provided with a supply of five occlusive eye patches.

   HCPCS code: _____ × _____

5. Prefabricated wrist sprint.

   HCPCS code: _____

Drugs Administered in the Healthcare Setting

Drugs that are administered in the healthcare setting include injections, chemotherapy drugs, inhaled solutions, and immunosuppressive drugs. They may be administered in a number of different healthcare settings. For example, a patient with a severe bacterial infection presenting to her primary care office may receive an injection of an antibiotic while in the office. On the other hand, a cancer patient presenting for chemotherapy would receive an injection of the chemotherapeutic medicinal substance while in an outpatient cancer treatment center. Unlike over-the-counter or prescription drugs, these drugs are given in the healthcare setting by a healthcare professional, who then monitors the patient to ensure there will be no side effects.

HCPCS Coding for Drugs Administered in the Healthcare Setting

Drugs administered in the healthcare setting are coded using HCPCS codes. Although many of the HCPCS codes for drugs begin with a J (called J-codes), some begin with other letters and are thus found throughout the HCPCS code book. It is important to first search the Table of Drugs to identify the correct substance administered. However, in some instances, the drug is not listed in the Table of Drugs. In these cases, turn to the HCPCS Index and search for the drug by its generic name.

HCPCS codes for drugs administered in the healthcare setting only identify the drug administered and do not include any of the supplies that were used to administer the drug or the procedure code that would be billed for performing the actual administration of the drug. Separate HCPCS codes are used to report additional supplies used to administer the medication, and CPT codes are used to report the procedure performed. Furthermore, ICD-10-CM diagnosis codes are also required to indicate the medical necessity for the drug given. For example, if the patient is receiving a chemotherapy infusion drug for liver cancer, the liver cancer would be identified with an ICD-10-CM code and included on the claim (see figure 6.6).

Figure 6.6. Coding for a chemotherapy infusion

Description	Code type	Description
Medical necessity	ICD-10-CM	C22.8, Malignant neoplasm of liver, primary, unspecified as to type
Procedure	CPT	96401, Chemotherapy administration, subcutaneous or intramuscular; non-hormonal anti-neoplastic
Supply	HCPCS	J1745, Injection, infliximab, excludes biosimilar, 10 mg

Before assigning J-codes, it is important to understand the many routes of administration. The **route of administration** is the way in which the drug is given to the patient. Medications may be administered in numerous ways, and the Table of Drugs takes this into account. There are five routes of injection: intra-arterial (IA), intravenous (IV), intramuscular (IM), intrathecal (IT), and subcutaneous (SC). Other routes of administration include inhaled (INH), oral (ORAL), various (VAR), and other routes (OTH). Coders should select the code for the drug based on the method of administration. Figure 6.7 provides the different routes of administration.

Figure 6.7. Routes of administration

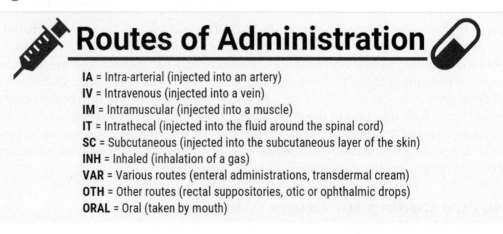

Routes of Administration

IA = Intra-arterial (injected into an artery)
IV = Intravenous (injected into a vein)
IM = Intramuscular (injected into a muscle)
IT = Intrathecal (injected into the fluid around the spinal cord)
SC = Subcutaneous (injected into the subcutaneous layer of the skin)
INH = Inhaled (inhalation of a gas)
VAR = Various routes (enteral administrations, transdermal cream)
OTH = Other routes (rectal suppositories, otic or ophthalmic drops)
ORAL = Oral (taken by mouth)

In the HCPCS manual, the Table of Drugs (introduced in chapter 5) is a list of drugs, their dosages, and the routes of administration, cross-mapped to the corresponding

Table 6.1. Table of Drugs example

Drug Name	Dosage/Unit Per	Route	Code
Nabilone	1 mg	Oral	J8650
Nafcillin			J3490
Naglazyme	1 mg		J1458
Nalbuphine HCL	per 10 mg	IM, IV, SC	J2300
Naloxone HCL	per 1 mg	IM, IV, SC	J2310, J3490
Naltrexone			J3490
Naltrexone, depot form	1 mg	IM	J2315
Nandrobolic L.A.	Up to 50 mg	IM	J2320
Nandrolone decanoate	Up to 50 mg	IM	J2320
Narcan, *see* Naloxone HCL	1 mg	IM, IV, SC	J2310
Naropin	1 mg		J2795

J-code. Although HCPCS code books vary significantly depending on the publisher, the format of the Table of Drugs is similar to table 6.1.

The first column lists the name of the drug by both its generic and brand names. It is helpful to have access to a **Physician's Desk Reference (PDR)**, a compilation of information for prescription drugs to certify that the correct drug is selected for the service.

The second column lists the dosage per one unit of the drug. For example, if the patient received 1 mg of Naloxone, then only one unit was administered. Always pay attention to the dosage or the unit per administration, as this may affect the number of units that are billed for the drug. For example, if the patient were given 2 mgs of Naltrexone, then the coder should select the code for Naltrexone, J2315, Injection, naltrexone, depot form, 1 mg, with the number of units to indicate how much was administered. The correct coding in this case would be J2315 × 2.

The third column identifies the route of administration for the drug in abbreviated form. Many drugs can be given in several different ways, and as such multiple routes of administration may be listed for a single drug. In some cases, codes will differ depending on the route of administration of the drug. Always check for multiple entries of the same drug and verify both the route of administration and the dosage amount.

The last column lists the HCPCS code for the drug administered. Once an HCPCS code has been identified from the Table of Drugs, it is still necessary to verify the code in the Tabular List. For example, once the coder identifies the drug Naloxone HCL, coded in the Table of Drugs to J2310, he or she would then find code J2310 in the Tabular and confirm that the code, dosage, and route of administration is correct (see figure 6.8).

Notice that some of the drugs listed in the Table of Drugs contain a cross-reference to another drug. This cross-reference directs the coder to search for the alternate drug name and then use the code listed for it. For example, in table 6.1, notice that the entry for Narcan refers the coder to *see* Naloxone HCL. The coder may then refer to the entry for Naloxone HCL and code for the drug appropriately. Some drugs are listed multiple times, with different routes of administration. In this case, the code selected should reflect the appropriate route of administration for the drug given.

Figure 6.8. Components of HCPCS drug code descriptions

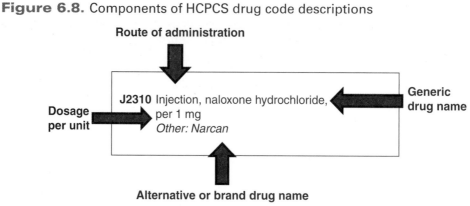

Source: Elsevier 2020, 308.

Putting It All Together: Coding for Drugs Administered in the Healthcare Setting

In order to select the correct code for the drug administered in the healthcare setting, it is important to carefully read the documentation of the service provided, then access the Table of Drugs in the HCPCS manual and locate the drug name. Next, follow all cross-references, locate the correct dosage and route of administration, and find the associated HCPCS code. Be sure to verify the code in the Tabular List before making a final selection; and check the dosage of the drug that was administered to ensure that the correct number of units for the code is selected.

Determination of the correct drug code relies on the following:

- What drug was administered?
- What was the route of administration?
- What was the dosage given?

Study the following examples. Then complete the exercises in There's a Code for That 6.4 to practice coding for drugs administered in the healthcare setting.

Example 6.5 Administration of medication

Patient presented to the ER in severe labor pains, asking for pain relief. This is her first pregnancy and she is dilated 2 cm. Delivery expected in excess of 4 hours. 1 mg of Stadol was administered intravenously.
HCPCS code: J0595, Injection, butorphanol tartrate, 1 mg

Example 6.6 Administration of medication

25-year-old male with gonorrhea received IM injection of Bicillin CR (100,000 units)
HCPCS code: J0558, Injection, penicillin G benzathine and penicillin G procaine, 100,000 units
ICD-10-CM code: A54.9, Gonococcal infection, unspecified

Coding for drugs administered in the healthcare setting

Enter the correct answer for each of the following practice exercises.

1. 20 mg Adalimumab administered subcutaneously.

   HCPCS code: _____

2. A 35-year-old woman with bipolar I disorder was given 0.50 mg of Abilify.

   HCPCS code: _____ × _____

   ICD-10-CM code: _____

   (Tip: Remember to look up the main term *disorder*, and then find the subterm *bipolar*.)

3. A 30-year-old pregnant female with Factor V Leiden deficiency is given 10 mg Lovenox.

   HCPCS code: _____

   ICD-10-CM code: _____

4. A 5-year-old patient presents to the office complaining of acute exacerbation of mild intermittent asthma. He was given 2 mgs of albuterol inhalation solution, concentrated form, via nebulizer machine.

   HCPCS code: _____ × _____

   ICD-10-CM code: _____

Case Study | Procedures and Supplies

PATIENT: Maxine Stewardson   **DOB:** 09/12/1952

DATE OF SERVICE: 01/10/20XX

SUBJECTIVE:
Chief Complaint: 67-year-old female here for right knee pain × 11 months

History of Present Illness: A 67-year-old female presents for intermittent knee pain for the last 11 months. Pain has been at 1/10 but goes as high as 4/10 on some days. She has been taking Tylenol 4 for the pain. She had a right total knee arthroplasty (TKA) approximately 13 months ago. She completed physical therapy, but pain persists.

Review of Systems:
Constitutional: no fever and not feeling tired
Neurological: difficulty walking
Respiratory: no shortness of breath
Cardiovascular: no chest pain
Musculoskeletal: joint pain, joint, swelling, and joint stiffness of the right knee

Past, Family, Social History:
Current medications reviewed. No known drug allergies (NKDA). The patient does not have any blood relatives who had problems with general anesthesia. No previous diagnosis of osteoporosis. The patient has previously been diagnosed with osteopenia. Patient is a current tobacco smoker and does not use recreational drugs.

OBJECTIVE:
Physical Examination:
Constitutional: alert and in no acute distress.
Pulmonary: no respiratory distress.
Musculoskeletal: right knee evaluation reveals well healed scar without concern. There is anterior swelling. There is firmness to the patellar tendon and tenderness to palpation. Patient is able to demonstrate straight raise without extensor lag. Knee extension without weakness. Knee is ligamentously stable in 45- and 90-degree flexion.
Neurologic: sensory exam was normal to light touch and pinprick. Coordination was normal. Deep tendon reflexes were +2 and symmetric.
Psychiatric: the patient was oriented to person, place, and time. Mood and affect were appropriate.

X-RAY RESULTS:
X-RAY KNEE, RIGHT, 4 VIEWS: Findings: Four weight-bearing views of the right knee. Status post right knee arthroplasty. On the lateral view, the patella is more inferior than expected. No evidence of loosening. No fracture or dislocation. Soft tissues are unremarkable.
IMPRESSION: Stable total right knee arthroplasty.

ASSESSMENT and PLAN:

1. Pain of the right knee. Refer to physical therapy. Recommend strengthening program and modalities as indicated for scar tissue. Recommend weight-bearing exercises.

2. Status post right knee joint replacement. X-ray results of the right knee shows TKA without evidence for hardware failure. Without evidence for fracture. Patient provided with pair of metal underarm crutches with pads, tips, and handgrips.

SIGNED: Dr. Murphy Harrison, MD

Use the following steps to select the appropriate codes for the case study.

1. Read through the case study in full. As you read, look up any medical or procedural terms with which you are unfamiliar. For example, the terms *total knee arthroplasty* and *osteopenia* may not be familiar. Use a medical dictionary or medical terminology text to define these terms. On your own, look up and define any additional unfamiliar terms.

   a. *Total knee arthroplasty*:

   _____

   _____

   b. *Osteopenia*:

   _____

   _____

2. Read through the case study and answer the following question: *What did the doctor do?* In this case study, the majority of the documentation identifies the evaluation and management service, otherwise known as an office visit (office visit coding is discussed in the following chapters, so don't worry about this code yet!). However, an additional procedure was performed to evaluate the patient's condition. Review the case study and identify the additional procedure.

_____

_____

3. Locate the code for the procedure in the CPT code book.

   a. Search the Index for the procedure, review the options under the Index entry, and list them here:

_____

_____

   b. If there are multiple options, identify the most appropriate code option and refer to the code listed in the Tabular section.

_____

_____

   c. Locate the code range in the Tabular List of codes and identify the one that most appropriately identifies all components of the procedure performed. Remember to check for any guidelines, important definitions, or parenthetical notes. List the CPT code and description here:

_____

_____

   d. Are there any additional procedures that need to be added to identify all of the procedures performed? If yes, follow the previous steps to identify the codes for the additional procedures.

_____

_____

   e. Are there any modifiers that need to be added to identify any special circumstance surrounding the procedure(s)? If yes, refer to Appendix A of the CPT code book to assign all appropriate modifiers.

_____

_____

4. Now that the procedure(s) and modifier(s) have been identified, re-read the case study and answer the following question: *Why did the doctor do it?* To find the reason for the office visit and x-ray, search for terms that identify the medical condition. Note the ASSESSMENT section of the documentation, where the provider has listed each of the medical conditions he found or addressed during the visit. Identify the case study patient's diagnosis (note that there may be multiple diagnoses).

_____

_____

Key to Success

A number of terms may be used to identify the reason for a procedure, which may be located at either the beginning or the end of a note. Some of these terms include *assessment, impression, definitive diagnosis*, or *indications*. Remember, the diagnosis identifies the medical necessity for the procedure performed, so it helps to find the area of the note that identifies why the procedure was performed to correctly identify all of the patient's possible diagnoses.

5. Now that you have the name of the patient's diagnoses, search the ICD-10-CM code book for the correct codes for these conditions. Follow these steps for each of the diagnoses identified.

   a. Search the Main Index for the name of each condition and search through any applicable subterms and cross-references to locate the appropriate code(s).

      i. _____

      ii. _____

   b. Verify the code(s) in the Tabular List. Locate the code(s) identified previously in the Tabular Listing of codes and refer to any applicable guidelines, notes, and symbols. Does each code selected correctly identify the patient's condition? If yes, list the code(s) here:

      i. _____

      ii. _____

   c. Check the procedure note and ICD-10-CM guidelines and conventions to determine the correct sequencing of the diagnosis codes, if applicable. Correctly sequence the diagnosis codes.

      _____

6. Now that the procedures and diagnoses have been identified, refer to the case study and answer the following question: *What supply did the doctor provide?*

   a. Search through the documentation to determine if the provider supplied the patient with an item that would qualify as a drug administered in the medical setting or a DMEPOS item that would be identified with a HCPCS code. In this case study, what supply item was provided to the patient?

      _____

      _____

   b. Now that you have the name of the item supplied, search the Index of the HCPCS code book for the item and list the code.

      _____

      _____

   c. Locate the code/code range in the Tabular List and find the code that most appropriately identifies the item supplied to the patient.

      _____

      _____

7. List the procedure, diagnosis, and supply codes on the CMS-1500 form. Be sure to identify medical necessity for each service by correctly linking the procedure/supply and diagnosis codes. Refer to figure 3.6 for an example. (Note that the evaluation and management code 9921x has been added for you.)

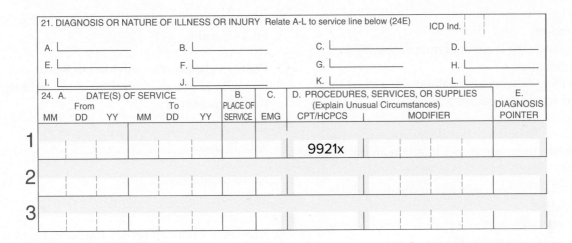

End-of-Chapter Content

Instructions: Match the terms with the appropriate descriptions.

1. _____ Intra-arterial
2. _____ Oral
3. _____ Other routes
4. _____ Various routes
5. _____ Inhaled
6. _____ Intramuscular
7. _____ Intrathecal
8. _____ Intravenous
9. _____ Subcutaneous

A. Rectal suppositories, otic or ophthalmic drops
B. Inhalation of a gas
C. Injected into the fluid around the spinal cord
D. Taken by mouth
E. Injected in to an artery
F. Injected into a muscle
G. Enteral administrations, transdermal cream
H. Injected into the subcutaneous layer of the skin
I. Injected into a vein

Instructions: Choose the best answer.

1. Which of the following types of life support would be used to provide a high level of care with life-saving protocols, such as manual defibrillation?
   a. Basic life support
   b. Advanced life support
   c. Circulation, airway, and breathing support
   d. Level 3 BLS

2. Which of the following types of transportation is scheduled in advance?
   a. Nonemergency
   b. Urgent
   c. Emergency
   d. Ground

(Continued on next page)

(Continued)

3. Why are origin and destination modifiers appended to ambulance services?

  a. To identify why the ambulance service was medically necessary
  b. To identify the route taken by the ambulance company
  c. To justify the amount of mile driven by the ambulance
  d. To identify where the patient was picked up and where the patient was taken

4. Which of the following is the purpose of transportation indicators placed on ambulance claims?

  a. To identify the origin and destination of the transport
  b. To indicate why those particular ambulance services were medically necessary
  c. To support the ICD-10 code selected for the service
  d. To identify the type of injury or illness suffered by the patient

5. Which of the following ways may an emergency technician select a diagnosis for the ambulance services provided to a patient?

  a. Select the last code that was assigned to the patient's chart
  b. Report the code given by a family member
  c. Report the code for unspecified illness
  d. Ask the patient what his or her diagnosis is

Instructions: Answer the following questions with the appropriate code, modifier, or indicator.

1. 1 microgram (MCG) Avonex.

  HCPCS code: _____

2. Ativan, 4 mg.

  HCPCS code: _____ × _____

3. Inhaled Isuprel concentrate, 1 mg.

  HCPCS code: _____

4. 5 mg oral prednisolone.

  HCPCS code: _____

5. 5 micrograms Rebif, administered subcutaneously.

  HCPCS code: _____ × _____

6. Radioelements for brachytherapy, 15 elements.

  HCPCS code: _____ × _____

7. Plaster long-leg cast provided to 8-year-old boy with femur shaft fracture of the right leg (initial encounter).

  HCPCS code: _____
  ICD-10 code: _____

8. Nasal prosthesis.

  HCPCS code: _____

9. ALS level 1 nonemergency transport provided to geriatric patient with terminal brain cancer (malignant neoplasm of brain, unspecified). Picked up from home residence and transferred to custodial facility. Total distance driven was 10 miles.

  HCPCS code: _____ - _____
  HCPCS code: _____ × _____
  ICD-10 code: _____

10. Patient with multiple injuries was transported via rotary wing ambulance from mountain top to hospital. Emergency ALS level 2 support provided during transport, including esophageal intubation and oxygen delivered to patient during transport. 45 miles traveled.

  HCPCS code: _____ - _____
  HCPCS code: _____
  HCPCS code: _____
  HCPCS code: _____ × _____
  Transportation Indicator: _____
  ICD-10 code: _____

References

American Heart Association. 2010. Highlights of the 2010 American Heart Association Guidelines for CPR and ECC. https://www.heart.org/idc/groups/heart -public/@wcm/@ecc/documents/downloadable /ucm_317350.pdf.

Centers for Medicare and Medicaid Services (CMS). 2019a. CMS 1500. https://www.cms.gov/Medicare/CMS-Forms/CMS-Forms/CMS-Forms-Items/CMS1188854.html.

Centers for Medicare and Medicaid Services (CMS). 2019b. Durable Medical Equipment, Prosthetics, Orthotics, and Supplies (DMEPOS) (Rev. 4202, 01-18-19). Chapter 20 in *Medicare Claims Processing Manual.* https://www.cms.gov/Regulations-and-Guidance/Guidance/Manuals/downloads/clm104c20.pdf.

Centers for Medicare and Medicaid Services (CMS). 2009 (December). Certificate of Medical Necessity CMS-10269: Positive Airway Pressure (PAP) Devices for Obstructive Sleep Apnea. https://www.cms.gov/Medicare/CMS-Forms/CMS-Forms/Downloads/cms10269.pdf.

Elsevier. 2020. *2020 HCPCS LEVEL II, Professional Edition.* Chicago: AHIMA.

Health Net Federal Health Services (HNFHS). 2012 (September 12). Does All Durable Medical Equipment Require a Certificate of Medical Necessity? https://www.hnfs.net/content/hnfs/home/tn/prov/provider_news/2012_prov_news_archive/cmn_dme.html.

Resources

Centers for Medicare and Medicaid Services (CMS). 2019. Ambulance (Rev. 4205, 01-18-19). Chapter 15 in *Medicare Claims Processing Manual.* https://www.cms.gov/Regulations-and-Guidance/Guidance/Manuals/downloads/clm104c15.pdf.

Centers for Medicare and Medicaid Services (CMS). 2015. Medical Conditions List and Transportation Indicators. https://www.cms.gov/Medicare/Medicare-Fee-for-Service-Payment/AmbulanceFeeSchedule/Downloads/2015-AFS-Medical-Conditions-Indicators.pdf.

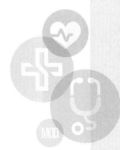

CHAPTER 7

Behavioral Health Services

Learning Objectives

- Understand the basics of billing and coding within the specialty of behavioral health
- Analyze the components of evaluation and management services and interpret evaluation and management coding guidelines for correct code selection

- Examine procedural codes and guidelines for behavioral health services
- Examine diagnosis coding and medical necessity for behavioral health services
- Determine and apply ICD-10-CM, CPT, and HCPCS codes to behavioral health services

Key Terms

Anxiety disorders
Attention-deficit hyperactivity disorder (ADHD)
Behavioral health services
Bipolar disorder
Contributory factors
Coordination of care
Counseling
Depression
Diagnostic and Statistical Manual of Mental Disorders (DSM-5)
Eating disorders
Electroconvulsive therapy (ECT)
Established patient

Examination
History
Inpatient
Interactive complexity
Medical decision-making (MDM)
Mental health
Mental illness
Narcosynthesis for psychiatric purposes
Nature of the presenting problem
New patient
Outpatient
Partial hospitalization
Place of service (POS)

Psychiatrist
Psychologist
Psychotherapy
Remission
Schizophrenia
Screening, Brief Intervention and Referral to Treatment (SBIRT)
SOAP note
Spectrum concept
Substance abuse
Transcranial magnetic stimulation (TMS)

Behavioral health services are treatments and procedures performed by a licensed healthcare professional to address mental illnesses and substance abuse, aiming to promote well-being by preventing or intervening in mental illnesses, substance abuse, and addictive behavior. **Mental health** refers to a person's emotional, psychological, and social well-being. **Mental illness** is a condition that affects a person's thinking, feeling, or mood, and affects a person's ability to perform major life activities and functions each day. **Substance abuse** is the misuse of alcohol or drugs, which impairs a person's ability to meet daily responsibilities at home, work, or school. Behavioral health directly diagnoses, treats, and manages individuals with mental health issues or substance abuse.

Coding for behavioral health requires a basic understanding of evaluation and management (E/M) services provided in the outpatient setting, introduced in chapter 3 (Basics of Coding) and chapter 5 (Learning the CPT and HCPCS Code Books). E/M coding depends on the place of service, level of service, and patient status; and behavioral health coding requires coding accurately for the procedures performed above and beyond the E/M service. It also depends on correctly abstracting diagnostic information to apply diagnosis codes accurately when identifying the medical necessity for the procedures performed.

Behavioral health services are performed in various settings by several different healthcare providers.

Behavioral Health Basics

Behavioral health identifies mental health and substance abuse disorders with diagnostic screenings and tests that help identify specific behavioral disorders and manage treatment of these disorders. Unlike medical services, behavioral health services traditionally have been more restricted in terms of insurance coverage and codes that support medical necessity for the service provided. These services are now commonly covered by most health insurance policies. Approved by Congress in 2008, the Mental Health Parity and Addiction Equity Act (MHPAEA) aimed to expand behavioral health services, including mental health and substance abuse disorder benefits. The Affordable Care Act (ACA), passed in 2010, further expanded these benefits by requiring most insurance plans to cover behavioral health services, including preventive services like depression screenings for adults and behavioral screenings for children.

However, there are still discrepancies with limitations for covered services, types of providers qualified to bill for behavioral health services, the medical necessity to support services, and the actual services performed. Therefore, successful behavioral health coders must always take into consideration the patient's health insurance coverage to ensure that all services performed may be covered by the patient's insurance and are reported properly.

Behavioral health services are performed by a wide variety of providers and because state and insurance requirements vary only certain providers can perform specific services. Additionally, the rates at which the various provider types are reimbursed differ, depending on the provider type—such as psychiatrist, social worker, or clinical psychologist. Behavioral health providers also perform their services in different settings—for example, nursing facilities, assisted living facilities, or via an interactive telemedicine interface—that must be identified on the healthcare claim.

Behavioral Health Providers

Providers who offer behavioral health services differ from those who provide medical services. Although some of them are medical doctors (MDs or DOs), others have specialty credentials that enable them to provide only behavioral health services. Behavioral health providers include

- Psychiatrist
- Clinical Psychologist (CP)
- Clinical Social Worker (CSW)
- Clinical Nurse Specialist (CN)
- Nurse Practitioner (NP)
- Physician Assistant (PA)
- Certified Nurse Midwife (CNM)
- Independently Practicing Psychologist (IPP)

It is important to understand the different types of behavioral health providers because although all of the providers listed are qualified to perform behavioral health services—such as psychotherapy or counseling—their ability to bill and receive payment for their services depends on their degree, license, or credential; the state in which they practice; and the patient's insurance.

For example, a psychiatrist is a medical doctor who is legally authorized to practice in a specific state (or states) and whose behavioral health services are paid at 100 percent by Medicare. This means that Medicare pays the full amount of the allowable charge for a service provided by a psychiatrist. On the other hand, a CSW has a master's or doctoral degree in social work and is legally authorized to perform services in the state in which they work. Medicare pays CSWs 75 percent of the allowable amount for all services. In other words, Medicare pays a CSW only three-quarters of the amount that it would reimburse a psychiatrist. These differences in billing, including state requirements and specific insurance guidelines, vary among states and insurance plans. To learn the specifics of these requirements and guidelines, a coder or biller may have to contact each insurance company individually, as well as the state department of insurance.

Note that mid-level providers (or advanced practitioners), as discussed in chapter 1 (Your Coding Career), include NPs and PAs who also practice in other healthcare specialties. Remember that it is always necessary to check with payer and state regulations to determine any type of billing, coding, or payment differences between provider types.

Because the field of behavioral health is diverse, some behavioral health specialists will further subspecialize within the field. For example, a clinical psychologist may choose to subspecialize in child and adolescent psychiatry, addiction medicine, military and stress-related disorders, or marriage and family therapy.

Key to Success

It is not enough to simply select a code and report it. In addition to reporting the codes correctly, coders must keep the context of the service in mind—including who provided the service, where the service was performed, and which insurance is being billed.

Place of Service

The **place of service (POS)** is the setting of the service, or where the service occurred. Behavioral health services may be performed in several different settings just as healthcare services may be provided in various healthcare settings, depending on the needs of the patient.

There is a special code for each POS in which services occur. A list of POS codes, entitled Place of Service Codes for Professional Claims, can be found at the beginning of the CPT code book. Examples of POS codes are provided in table 7.1.

Because healthcare services are provided in numerous settings, POS codes are important in all healthcare specialties, not just in behavioral health. Therefore, a POS code that corresponds to the setting in which the service occurred must be included on each claim, whether it is a behavioral health or any other healthcare claim for professional services.

POS codes are placed in box 24.B on the CMS-1500 claim form (see figure 7.1). For example, if the service was performed in the office, then POS code 11, for Office, would be placed in box 24.B on the claim form.

Common settings, or places of service, for behavioral health services include the following:

- Outpatient office settings (POS 11)
- Partial hospitalization programs (PHP) (POS 52)
- Community mental health centers (CMHC) (POS 53)
- Inpatient psychiatric facilities (IPF) and hospitals (POS 51)
- Long-term care and nursing facilities (POS 31 and 32)

Table 7.1. Select CPT place of service codes

Place of Service Code(s)	Place of Service Name	Place of Service Description
02	Telehealth	The location where health services and health-related services are provided or received, through a telecommunication system. (Effective January 1, 2017)
03	School	A facility whose primary purpose is education. (Effective January 1, 2003)
07	Tribal 638 Freestanding Facility	A facility or location owned and operated by a federally recognized American Indian or Alaska Native tribe or tribal organization under a 638 agreement, which provides diagnostic, therapeutic (surgical and non-surgical), and rehabilitation services to tribal members who do not require hospitalization. (Effective January 1, 2003)

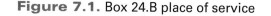

Source: Adapted from CMS 2019a.

Figure 7.1. Box 24.B place of service

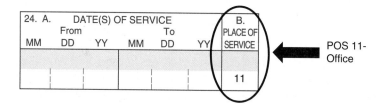

Source: CMS 2019b.

Identifying the POS is one of the many important components of ensuring that the service reported on a healthcare claim is accurate and complete. For example, an inpatient hospital claim must be sent with the appropriate POS code to indicate that the service was completed in an inpatient hospital. Placing the wrong POS code on a claim could result in a misrepresentation of the service performed or a denial of payment for the healthcare claim.

Complete the exercises in There's a Code for That 7.1 to test your knowledge of POS codes.

Identifying the Place of Service

7.1

There's a Code for That

Read the following descriptions of healthcare services. Using the Place-of-Service Codes for Professional Claims section located at the beginning of the CPT code book, identify the appropriate POS code for each of the following scenarios.

1. Patient received an outpatient evaluation of substance abuse in the physician's office.

   POS code:

2. Patient was transported via an air ambulance.

   POS code:

3. Patient presented for a glucose tolerance test at an independent laboratory.

   POS code:

4. Patient received counseling services is a group home.

   POS code:

5. Behavioral health provider commonly performs counseling for patients at the local jail.

   POS code:

After learning the basics of billing for behavioral health services, it is important to study and understand the procedures and procedure codes that are reported for behavioral health services.

Coding for Procedures in Behavioral Health

Most of the procedure codes used by behavioral health providers are evaluation and management (E/M) codes to report the healthcare management of patients, and psychiatry codes to report additional services such as psychotherapy and other treatments.

Key to Success

E/M codes are detailed and contain elements that must be combined to ensure correct code selection. This chapter introduces only the concepts of E/M codes and how to select them. Chapter 8 (Primary Care) further specifies how the levels of each key component are determined. It may be helpful to refer to the basic E/M components in this chapter when reading chapter 8.

E/M Coding in Behavioral Health

E/M codes are used in all healthcare specialties and settings, and by all types of qualified healthcare providers. Thus, they are an extremely important part of all professional outpatient coding, not just behavioral health. Any time a patient receives an *evaluation* by a provider (for instance, a physical examination in conjunction with counseling services), or for *management* of a condition (such as a medication refill request), an E/M code should be reported.

Psychiatrists are medical doctors who specialize in the diagnosis and treatment of mental illnesses. Though they provide psychiatry services, they are also qualified to medically manage behavioral health patients. Many patients needing behavioral health services are given medications to treat their symptoms; others have mental health or substance abuse issues in addition to physical health issues. This requires a level of medical management for some behavioral health patients. Psychiatrists are both qualified and required to perform healthcare E/M services for their patients, as well as any necessary mental health services, such as psychotherapy or group counseling services (discussed later in this chapter).

A **psychologist**, on the other hand, is not a medical doctor but has a terminal degree, such as a PhD, from an educational institution and has been trained in the art of psychology, which is the study of the human mind, emotions, and behavior. Psychologists may provide mental and behavioral health services to patients but are not typically qualified to perform medical procedures and examinations.

This chapter details E/M services by introducing the basic format, function, and components of E/M codes. E/M services are also discussed further in chapter 8. It is important to first present the basic components of E/M codes, and then look at the components comprehensively to determine the correct E/M code.

E/M Coding Basics

E/M codes can be reported for new or established patients, in the inpatient or outpatient setting, and even for telemedicine services. They are used to report the evaluation and management of a patient across all healthcare settings—such as outpatient office visits, inpatient hospital visits, consultations performed in both inpatient and outpatient settings, emergency departments, nursing facilities and rest homes, and home visits. E/M codes are the most commonly used codes in all professional outpatient billing as they are used to report the medical evaluation and management of a patient. Consider the following example.

> *A new patient presents to the office of a psychiatrist in the town where she has just moved. She had been under treatment for depression where she lived previously, and her new psychiatrist performs a medication history, side-effect history, and mental status examination. He then prescribes an antidepressant to the patient.*

In this example, the visit would be reported with an E/M code and only an E/M code since no psychotherapy or any other services were provided.

E/M codes compose the first section of Category I codes in the CPT code book. This section is first organized by the type of service performed. There are also numerous pages of guidelines located before the codes in this section. Some of these guidelines are discussed in the remainder of this chapter, with a more thorough discussion following in chapter 8.

Key to Success

The best way to get an idea of the services reported with E/M codes is to closely look at the table of contents for the E/M section of the CPT code book. Pay close attention to the main headings describing the type of services that may be reported, such as Office or Other Outpatient Services, Hospital Observation Services, and Hospital Inpatient Services. These headings designate the setting in which the service was performed as well as the type of service.

There are three key components of all E/M services: history, examination, and medical decision-making. Each component may be documented at a different level of complexity and may include contributory factors, all of which are combined to report the level of service provided to the patient. Before addressing the three key components, coders must first determine the type of E/M service by defining three factors—type of service, patient status, and place of service.

Three Factors of E/M Codes

To correctly determine the type of E/M service provided, coding professionals must first ask three questions (see figure 7.2).

1. *What is the type of service?* The type of service refers to the kind of E/M encounter given to the patient. For example, was the service an office visit, a consultation, a team conference, or a hospital discharge?

2. *What is the patient status?* There are four different types of patient status—new, established, inpatient, and outpatient. A **new patient** is one who has not received any professional services within the past three years from a healthcare provider or another healthcare provider of the same specialty and subspecialty in the same group practice. An **established patient** is one who has received professional services from the healthcare provider or another healthcare provider of the same specialty and subspecialty in the same group practice within the last three years. An **inpatient** is a patient who has been formally admitted to an inpatient hospital. In behavioral health, it is common that patients are treated in a **partial hospitalization** setting, in which they receive mental health services as an inpatient during the day but are released to go home in the evening. Partial hospitalization services are reported as inpatient services. **Outpatients** are patients seen in the hospital setting who have not been formally admitted, such as those receiving hospital observation services or emergency department services.

3. *What is the place of service?* The POS is where the service was delivered, such as an outpatient office, skilled nursing facility, or hospital setting. Note that the POS also plays a part in determining the patient's status as either inpatient or outpatient. For example, a patient cannot be an *inpatient* in an *office* setting (because patients are not admitted into the office setting). Note also that the POS code reported on the claim must also match the place of service described in the E/M code.

Figure 7.2. Three factors of E/M codes

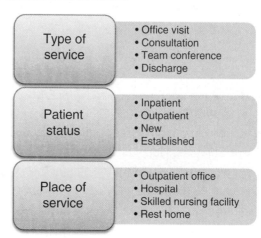

These questions are simply to help understand the basic components of E/M code categories and assist with code selection. The answers to these questions are the components of the E/M service that allow the coder to locate the correct section of E/M service codes to report.

In the following vignette, note how Nidia locates the E/M codes she will use to report an E/M service.

Nidia is learning how to select the codes for the psychiatrist's E/M services. She is coding for a consultation provided to an inpatient with substance abuse in the hospital setting. Before she can determine the level of the service, she must define the three factors of the service, which will allow her to find the correct selection of codes in the E/M section. She asks herself and answers the following questions:

What was the type of service? A consultation
What is the patient status? Inpatient
What is the place of service? Hospital

With this information, she can review the E/M section of the CPT code book to find the codes needed to report this service. Looking at the table of contents in the E/M section, she sees that there is a heading for consultations, with the code ranges next to the types of consultations (see figure 7.3). She knows that she is coding for an inpatient consultation, so she looks at the entry for Inpatient Consultations, New or Established Patient (99251–99255), on page 21 in her book. She then turns to page 21 and finds a range of E/M codes numbered 99251 through 99255.

Figure 7.3. Consultations entry in the E/M table of contents

Source: AMA 2019, 2.

Complete the exercises in There's a Code for That 7.2 to practice finding the correct selection of E/M codes.

7.2

Type of service, patient status, and place of service for E/M codes

There's a Code for That

Read the following evaluation and management statements and determine the type of service, patient status, and place of service. Then use the E/M table of contents to find the correct selection of E/M codes. Note that not all of these components will be available for all E/M services. The first example is done for you.

Psychiatrist performed a consultation on a 35-year-old female inpatient in the hospital setting.

Type of service: consultation

Patient status: inpatient

Place of service: hospital

E/M codes: 99251–99255

POS code: 21

1. Outpatient office visit for a new patient with bipolar disorder.

Type of service: _____

Patient status: _____

Place of service: _____

E/M codes: _____

POS code: _____

2. Subsequent nursing facility care provided to a 78-year-old male admitted to a nursing facility.

Type of service: _____

Patient status: _____

Place of service: _____

E/M codes: _____

POS code: _____

3. Behavior change intervention provided to a new patient (individual) in the office setting.

Type of service: _____

Patient status: _____

Place of service: _____

E/M codes: _____

POS code: _____

4. Initial hospital inpatient service provided to a patient with schizophrenia suffering from panic attack.

Type of service: _____

Patient status: _____

(Continued on next page)

7.2

Continued

Place of service: _____

E/M codes: _____

POS code: _____

5. Emergency department visit provided to a patient in crisis.

Type of service: _____

Patient status: _____

Place of service: _____

E/M codes: _____

POS code: _____

Three Key Components to an E/M Service

There are three key components to an E/M service—history, examination, and medical decision-making—each identifying a specific portion of the service performed by the healthcare provider. Imagine, for example, a typical appointment at the doctor's office: After the patient is roomed by the medical assistant or nurse, the clinical staff will ask a few questions regarding why the patient is in the office on that day and gather baseline vital information about the patient, such as weight and temperature. The healthcare provider will then ask more questions about what is going on with the patient (getting more history) before he or she performs an actual examination of the patient (performing the examination). Finally, the provider determines the patient's diagnosis and plan of treatment (medical decision-making).

The three key components of E/M services are further explained as follows.

- **History** is the subjective information the patient tells the provider at the encounter. There are four elements of the history key component: chief complaint (C/C), history of present illness (HPI), review of systems (ROS), and past, family, social history (PFSH). Keep in mind that this is *subjective* information. The provider typically asks pointed questions to elicit more information from the patient and help determine what to focus on during the physical examination. For example, if the patient says he or she has anxiety (subjective information), then the physician will focus on the portion of the encounter related to the physical symptoms of anxiety (objective information).

- **Examination** is the objective information resulting from a physical examination of the patient. A healthcare provider will perform an examination of specific body areas (BAs) or organ systems (OSs) (discussed in greater detail in chapter 8), depending on the patient's needs. For example, a provider seeing a patient for anxiety may find during the physical examination that the patient has been experiencing heart palpitations. The provider will then perform an examination on the cardiovascular system as well as the neurological and psychiatric systems.

- **Medical decision-making (MDM)** is the portion of the E/M encounter in which the healthcare provider determines the patient's diagnosis and care or treatment plan. The MDM is comprised of the number of possible diagnoses or treatment options, the amount and complexity of data to be reviewed, and the risk of complications or death if the condition were to go untreated. For example, the medical decision-making for a patient with anxiety includes the number of possible diagnoses, such as anxiety, heart palpitations, or any other possible complications; any labs, imaging services, or other healthcare services that should be performed or reviewed; and the risk of complications if the anxiety and heart palpitations are left untreated.

The three key components to an E/M service directly correspond to a common format for health record documentation, called a **SOAP note**. SOAP stands for S, Subjective; O, Objective; A, Assessment; and P, Plan. Commonly used for a problem-oriented visit, this documentation format includes specific sections for the *subjective* information received from the patient, which consists of the chief complaint (C/C), history of present illness (HPI), review of systems (ROS), and past, family, social history (PFSH); the *objective* information (the examination performed by the provider); the *assessment* of the patient's condition (the provider's statement of the clinical impression or diagnosis); and the *plan* (the course of treatment).

For an example of a SOAP note, refer to figure 7.4. Note that this is just a template for the documentation of an E/M encounter and components of this documentation might change. Some healthcare offices have much more complex documentation templates for problem-oriented visits, whereas others might follow a modified version of the template. Either way, it is helpful to compare the components of a SOAP note to the key components of an E/M code.

Figure 7.4. Example of a SOAP note

PATIENT: Date of Birth (DOB):
DATE OF SERVICE (DOS):

SUBJECTIVE:
Chief Complaint:
History of Present Illness:
(Location, Quality, Severity, Duration, Timing, Context, Modifying factors, Associated signs or symptoms)

Review of Systems:
Constitutional
Eyes
Ears, nose, and throat
Cardiovascular
Respiratory
Gastrointestinal
Genitourinary
Musculoskeletal
Integumentary
Neurological
Psychiatric
Endocrine
Hematologic/lymphatic
Allergic/immunologic

Past, Family, Social History:

OBJECTIVE:
Physical Examination:
General appearance

(Continued on next page)

Eyes
Head (including face)
Ears, nose, mouth, and throat (EENT)
Neck
Cardiovascular
Chest (including breasts and axilla)
Respiratory
Abdomen
Gastrointestinal
Genitourinary
Genitalia, groin, buttocks
Back
Musculoskeletal
Extremities
Skin
Neurologic
Psychiatric
Hematologic/lymphatic/immunologic

ASSESSMENT:

PLAN:

SIGNED:

Key to Success

Look carefully at the SOAP note example in figure 7.4 and note that this format has already been used in some of your chapter case studies.

It is helpful to understand how the components of the SOAP note correspond to the elements of an E/M code. As a reminder, the three key components of an E/M code are history, examination, and medical decision-making (MDM). Study figure 7.5 to see how these components can be found in the SOAP note documentation template.

For each of the key components, there are four different levels of work, ranging from low to high levels of work or complexity.

Figure 7.5. SOAP note versus E/M key components

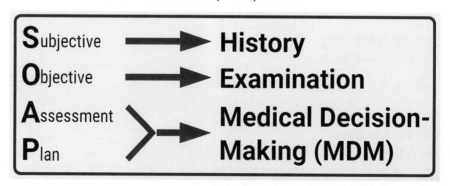

E/M codes are developed this way so that when a provider performs *more* work for a specific E/M service, he or she can bill at a higher level of service and receive more payment for the service. On the other hand, if a provider performs *less* work for a specific service, he or she will bill for a lower level of service and will be paid less for it. In this way, providers can adjust how much they bill for an E/M service according to the amount of work performed for the service. To select the correct E/M code, the coder must determine the level of each of these three key components and then locate the corresponding E/M code. Figure 7.6 illustrates the three key components and how they relate to the levels of service performed.

Figure 7.6. Elements of an E/M code

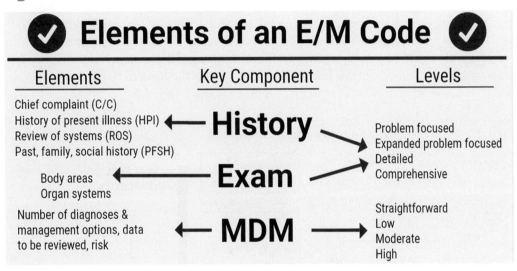

Levels of Key Components

There are four levels of each of the three key components of E/M codes. Each level depends on the amount of work or complexity of the service. For example, if a provider performs a comprehensive examination of all body areas and organ systems on a patient, it is considered a high level of the examination component (comprehensive). On the other hand, if a provider performs only a limited examination of one body area, it would be a low level of the examination component (problem-focused). When selecting the appropriate code for an E/M service, the coder must determine the level of each of the three key components, as follows (see also figures 7.7 through 7.9):

- History. The levels of the history obtained from the patient range from problem focused (lowest level of history), to expanded problem focused (next-highest level), to detailed, and finally comprehensive (highest level of history that can be obtained from the patient). For example, if a provider completed a very low level of history, then the lowest level of this key component would be used to select the level of history for the service: problem focused.

- Examination. The levels of the examination performed by the provider range from problem focused (lowest level of examination), to expanded problem focused, to detailed, and finally comprehensive (highest level of difficulty of the examination component). For example, if a provider completed a very high level of examination (a complete examination of multiple body areas and organ systems), the highest level of this key component would be used to select the level of examination for the service: comprehensive.

- **Medical decision-making (MDM).** The levels of MDM performed by the provider range from straightforward (lowest level of MDM), to low, then moderate, and finally high (highest level of difficulty of MDM). For example, if a patient with a simple problem (such as a small abrasion) was seen by the provider who only needed to perform a very low level of medical decision-making to treat the patient, the lowest level of this key component would be used to select the MDM level for the service: straightforward.

Figures 7.7 through 7.9 illustrate the four levels of difficulty for each of the three key components.

The levels of each key component are based on the amount of work required, information reviewed, or complexity of the data taken into account during each component of the service. For the purposes of this chapter, vignettes, examples, and exercise and review questions will state the level of each key component—for example, *detailed examination* or *low MDM*. Chapter 8 dives deeper into these levels, including how to select the correct level of each key component based on health record documentation. Figure 7.10 illustrates how the levels of the key components impact the level of E/M codes.

Figure 7.7. Levels of the history key component

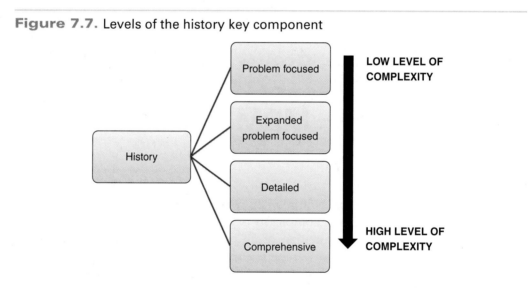

Figure 7.8. Levels of the examination key component

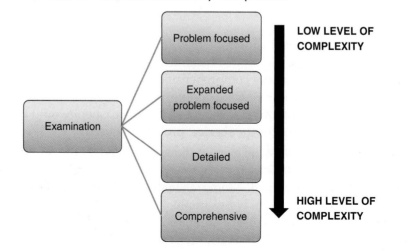

Figure 7.9. Levels of the medical decision-making key component

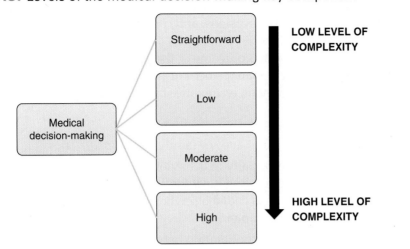

Figure 7.10. Steps to determine the level of E/M code

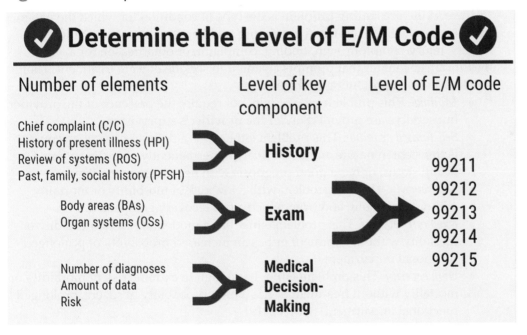

Some E/M services do not depend on the levels of history, exam, and MDM but rather on a contributory factor: counseling, coordination of care, or the nature of the presenting problem.

Contributory Factors

The levels of the three key components are not always necessary for code selection. When the three key components are not applicable to the E/M service (for example, if no standard history or physical examination is performed) and for certain E/M code categories (such as counseling codes), it is necessary to consider the **contributory factors** of counseling, coordination of care, and the nature of the presenting problem, which are used to help determine the level of the E/M service.

- **Counseling** is the discussion between a healthcare provider and a patient or the patient's family. This discussion may include:
  - Diagnostic results, impressions, and/or recommended diagnostic studies
  - Prognosis (the expected outcome of the patient's healthcare diagnosis)
  - Risks and benefits of management or treatment options
  - Follow-up, management, or treatment instructions and compliance advice
  - Risk factor reduction
  - Education of the patient and/or family (AMA 2019)

  It is important to note, especially in behavioral health coding, that the contributory factor of counseling it *not* the same as psychotherapy counseling. Psychotherapy counseling is coded elsewhere in the CPT book and is discussed in the next section of this chapter.

- **Coordination of care** is the cooperation between at least two healthcare practitioners in providing care to a patient. Coordination of care activities might include transfer from one facility to another or may be an agreement on treatment methodologies for a patient between a PCP and a specialist.

- **Nature of the presenting problem** is the type of condition for which the patient is receiving the E/M service. A presenting problem is a disease, condition, illness, injury, symptom, sign, finding, complaint, or other reason for a healthcare encounter that prompts a patient to seek healthcare treatment. There are five levels of presenting problems:
  - *Minimal.* This problem may or may not require the presence of the provider, but services are provided under the provider's supervision.
  - *Self-limited or minor.* This problem either runs a definite prescribed course, is transient in nature and is not likely to permanently alter the patient's health status, or has a good prognosis with healthcare management.
  - *Low severity.* This is a problem with a low risk of morbidity or mortality without treatment, and from which a full recovery is expected.
  - *Moderate severity.* This problem either has a moderate risk of morbidity or mortality without treatment or has an increased probability of prolonged functional impairment.
  - *High severity.* This problem either has a high to extreme risk of morbidity or mortality without treatment or has a high probability of severe, prolonged functional impairment. (AMA 2019)

When counseling or coordination of care is the determining factor of an E/M service, the *time* spent counseling or coordinating care may be used to determine the level of the E/M service. In order to use the *time* component as the determining factor of the E/M service, more than 50 percent of the face-to-face time spent with the patient (in the outpatient setting) or floor/unit time (in a hospital or nursing facility setting) must have been spent on counseling or coordination of care. The amount of time must be clearly documented in the health record and the extent of counseling or coordination of care must be included.

The three key components, contributory factors, and time are all listed in E/M codes, with varying levels. The majority (although not all) of E/M code descriptions are formatted so that coders can clearly select the level of each of these components and select the correct code. It is important to understand the format of these codes to be able to select the appropriate one. Figure 7.11 depicts the anatomy of an E/M code and identifies all these elements in the code description.

Key to Success

Don't worry about remembering all of the intricacies and components of E/M. What is more important as a beginning coding professional is to know where to find the definitions for these components in the guidelines of the CPT code book. Make sure you can locate the E/M guidelines section in the CPT code book. This will ultimately help you make a habit of referring to the guidelines in your code book.

E/M Exceptions for Behavioral Health

Some of the E/M codes used in behavioral health do not fit within the typical format for E/M codes and do not require identification of the levels of any of the key components or contributory factors. These E/M codes are exceptions to the rule. Medical team conferences (99366–99368), smoking and tobacco use/alcohol and/or substance abuse cessation counseling (99406–99409), telephone and online services (99421–99423, 99441–99443), and disability evaluation services (99450) are a few of the other E/M services performed by behavioral health specialists. These codes do not include descriptions of the levels of key components, contributory factors, and patient status, even though they are included within the E/M codes section; they simply describe the service performed

Figure 7.11. Anatomy of an E/M code

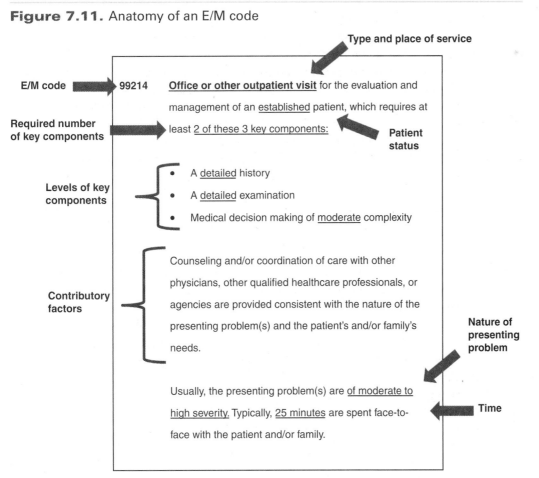

Source: AMA 2019, 13.

(for example, 99406, Smoking and tobacco cessation counseling visit; intermediate, greater than 3 minutes up to 10 minutes).

Selecting the Level of E/M Service

E/M code descriptions are carefully formatted to identify the patient status, type of service, place of service, levels of each of the key components, contributory factors, time, and number of key components that must be met for each specific E/M code. Study figure 7.11 to learn the anatomy of an E/M code.

Each E/M code description identifies of the type and place of service (office or other outpatient visit), the patient status (established), and the required number of key components, as indicated in figure 7.11. The required number of key components and levels that must be met are also identified and listed in the code description (either 2 out of 3, or 3 out of 3 key components). Figure 7.11 illustrates that code 99214 requires 2 out of 3 key components.

Sometimes, the level of *one* key component may exceed the level in the code description, whereas the levels of the other *two* key components are at the levels identified in the code description. For example, a provider might have given a comprehensive (highest level) MDM for an encounter with a detailed history and examination, reported with 99214 (as described in figure 7.11). In this case, the coder must select the code for which all levels as required (either 2 or 3) are *at least* at the level identified in the code description. Two of the levels of the key components must meet or exceed a particular level in order to select that particular code. For instance, because the two lowest levels were detailed the coder cannot select a higher level than detailed. The two common denominators (detailed history and detailed examination) are the basis for code selection. Sometimes, the levels of *two* key components go beyond those identified in the code description. However, if all *three* key components must be met, the coder must select the code in which all three are at least met by the code description.

The next section of the code description contains three bullet points identifying the required level of each key component (history, examination, and MDM). The contributory factors are then listed, followed by the nature of the presenting problem(s) and the time requirement for the code. Remember that time may only be used when more than 50 percent of the time spent face-to-face (in the office or outpatient setting, or on the unit/floor in the inpatient or hospital setting) with the patient is on counseling or coordination of care.

Recall the earlier example of Nidia, who determined that her E/M code was within the 99251 through 99255 range for an inpatient hospital consultation.

*Now that Nidia has found the code range for the service provided, she needs to check the documentation to determine the levels of each of the three key components so she can select the correct code within the 99251 to 99255 code range. Upon looking at the documentation, she determines that the psychiatrist provided a **DETAILED** HISTORY, a **DETAILED** EXAMINATION, and MDM OF **LOW** COMPLEXITY.*

Nidia checks the required key components in each of the code descriptions within the code range 99251 through 99255, and notes that code 99253 also requires a detailed history, detailed examination, and MDM of low complexity. The levels of all three of the key components match, so Nidia knows this is the correct code. She assigns 99253 on the claim.

Complete the exercises in There's a Code for That 7.3 to test your ability to assign codes based on the levels of the three key components.

Selecting the level of E/M services

7.3

There's a Code for That

Read the following E/M statements, determine the level of the E/M service, and assign the E/M code. Remember to check the required number of key components for each service for each category of E/M codes.

1. Office visit for a new patient with an expanded problem-focused history, an expanded problem- focused examination, and straightforward MDM.

   E/M code: _____

2. Office visit for an established patient with depression. Provider performed a comprehensive history, comprehensive examination, and MDM of moderate complexity.

   E/M code: _____

3. Problem-focused history, problem-focused examination, and straightforward MDM for an office visit for an established patient.

   E/M code: _____

4. Initial hospital care provided to a psychiatric patient. Provider performed a comprehensive history and exam, with MDM of moderate complexity.

   E/M code: _____

5. Subsequent hospital care provider to a psychiatric patient. Provider performed an expanded problem-focused history, problem-focused exam, with MDM of low complexity.

   E/M code: _____

6. Outpatient consultation provided to a patient with body dysmorphic disorder. Comprehensive history and detailed examination performed with moderate MDM.

   E/M code: _____

7. Subsequent nursing facility care provided to a 60-year-old woman with paranoid schizophrenia. History was problem focused, examination was expanded problem focused, and MDM was low complexity.

   E/M code: _____

8. Emergency department visit for an 18-year-old female presenting with suicidal ideation and anxiety. Provider performed a detailed history and examination with moderate complexity MDM.

   E/M code: _____

Psychiatry Coding

Most behavioral health codes are found in the Psychiatry subsection of the Medicine section of the CPT code book, in the code range 90785 through 90899. These codes are for diagnostic services, psychotherapy, and other services performed on an individual, family, or group. When using the codes from this section, pay close attention to the service performed, whether or not an E/M service was performed along with the service, who was involved in the service, and the length of time of the service. Codes described in this section include psychotherapy codes, other psychotherapy services or procedures, psychiatric services, and telemedicine services.

Key to Success

As with most of the subsections in the Medicine section, there are a number of guidelines in the Psychiatry section of the CPT code book. When coding from this subsection, be sure to read the guidelines and highlight, underline, make notes, or place a star next to important sections. These guidelines are the rule book for using codes from that section—make sure you utilize them!

Psychotherapy Codes

The most commonly used psychiatry codes for behavioral health providers are psychotherapy codes (90832–90838). **Psychotherapy** is the treatment of mental illness and behavioral disturbance in which the healthcare provider attempts to alleviate the emotional disturbances, reverse or change patterns of behavior, and encourage personality growth and development through discourse with the patient.

Depending on the needs of the patient, psychotherapy sessions can range from 30 to 60 minutes and may or may not be performed with an E/M service (which would be reported with an E/M code). Psychotherapy may be performed on an individual patient, with the patient's family (with or without the patient present), with a multi-family group, or with a non-family group. Special codes exist for psychoanalysis, psychotherapy performed on a patient in crisis, and for psychotherapy performed with interactive complexity. **Interactive complexity** is a psychotherapy service provided to a patient with specific communication factors that complicate delivery of psychiatric procedures. For example, a nonverbal adult might require the use of equipment, other physical devices, an interpreter, or a translator to help overcome communication barriers. This would be reported with the interactive complexity add-on code. For a refresher on add-on codes, see chapter 5.

An important part of coding for psychotherapy services is the use of add-on codes to report all aspects of the service performed. For example, code 90836, Psychotherapy, 45 minutes with patient when performed with an evaluation and management service, is an add-on code that should be reported in addition to the E/M code for the primary procedure. If a provider performed an E/M service on a patient and then provided 45 minutes of psychotherapy, the coder would report one code for each service: the code for the E/M service (such as 99213, Office or other outpatient visit for the evaluation and management of an established patient, which requires two out of three of the following key components: expanded problem-focused history, expanded problem-focused examination, medical decision-making of low complexity), as well as the code for the psychotherapy (90836, Psychotherapy, 45 minutes with patient when performed with an evaluation and management service). If the psychotherapy were also provided with interactive complexity, then the add-on code for interactive complexity would be coded in addition to both the E/M code and the psychotherapy code.

Reporting add-on codes requires close reading, ensuring to account for all components of the patient encounter. In the previous example, the coder should report one code for the healthcare E/M service that was performed and then note that an additional service was performed—the 45 minutes of psychotherapy—and report the appropriate code. Note that under the code description for 90836 is the parenthetical notation: "Use 90836 in conjunction with 99201–99255, 99304–99337, 99341–99350." This tells the coder it is appropriate to report the psychotherapy code with the code for the E/M service.

Key to Success

Add-on codes are often used in addition to other procedure codes to identify certain procedures that are performed together. If the description for the primary procedure does not include the additional services performed, the coder should search for the additional procedures and report any add-on codes, as necessary. As described previously, add-on codes will always include a parenthetical note to identify which service the code may be added to. Pay attention to these notes, as they will help you make sure you are assigning the correct codes! For a refresher on add-on codes, see chapter 5.

Read the following example and notice how Nidia codes for the psychotherapy services performed with interactive complexity on a child.

Lisette, an 8-year-old nonverbal female with autism and bipolar disorder presents for a medication refill and monthly psychotherapy session. She is an established patient. The psychiatrist documents a healthcare evaluation and management encounter with an expanded problem-focused history, expanded problem-focused examination, and medical decision-making of low complexity. She then completes 30 minutes of psychotherapy with the patient using interactive complexity.

Nidia chooses three codes—one for the E/M service, an add-on code for the psychotherapy, and another add-on code for the interactive complexity. She reports the following codes:

- *99213, Office or other outpatient visit for the evaluation and management of an established patient, which requires two out of three of the following key components: expanded problem-focused history, expanded problem-focused examination, medical decision-making of low complexity*
- *90833, Psychotherapy, 30 minutes with patient when performed with an E/M service*
- *90785, Interactive complexity*

Once Nidia has selected her procedure codes, she then must assign the appropriate diagnosis code(s) to identify the medical necessity for the procedures.

When a nonmedical clinician—such as a prescribing psychologist—performs pharmacologic management including prescription and review of medication in addition to psychotherapy services, the add-on code 90863, Pharmacologic management, including prescription and review of medication, when performed with psychotherapy services, should be used. This code was specifically designed for use by psychologists who are licensed to prescribe but cannot bill for an E/M code (because they are not licensed healthcare providers). For example, if a prescribing psychologist performed a 45-minute individual psychotherapy session in addition to pharmacologic management, the coder should report codes 90834, Psychotherapy, 45 minutes with patient, and 90863, Pharmacologic management, including prescription and review of medication, when performed with psychotherapy services.

Other Psychiatric Services or Procedures

In addition to psychotherapy services, a number of treatments and other services can be performed for behavioral health patients. These include

- **Narcosynthesis for psychiatric purposes** (90865), or the administration of sodium amobarbitol (otherwise known as a truth serum), which hinders inhibitions so that a psychiatric interview can be conducted.

- **Transcranial magnetic stimulation (TMS)** treatment (90867-90869) is a noninvasive procedure that utilizes magnetic fields to stimulate areas of the brain, and is used as a treatment for depression that does not respond to medication treatment.

- **Electroconvulsive therapy (ECT)** (90870), involves the application of an electric current to a patient's brain to produce a seizure or series of seizures to alleviate mental illness; primarily depression that is nonresponsive to treatment. If the psychiatrist also administers anesthesia for the service, the anesthesia should be reported separately, in addition to the code for the ECT.

Key to Success

Note that even though the codes described here may not be located in the Psychiatry subsection, they are still used for behavioral health services. It is common to find codes for a certain specialty throughout other sections of the CPT code book.

Codes for these services should be reported in addition to any E/M or psychotherapy services performed at the same session or on the same date of service. Remember that if an E/M service is performed with any additional service, modifier -25 should be appended to the E/M code to distinguish it as a significant, separately identifiable service from the psychiatry service. It is not necessary to append modifier -25 when using an appropriate add-on code. For a refresher on modifiers and their uses, see chapter 5.

Psychiatric Screenings

There are several psychiatric and psychological screenings, tests, and evaluations used to determine the risk of a patient having a mental illness or substance abuse issue, or whether or not the issue is already present. For example, at a six-week postnatal checkup, a mother might receive a postpartum depression screening. Even though this is a mental health screening, it is administered in the primary care setting to determine if the patient needs to be seen by a mental health practitioner. Primary care providers commonly administer mental health screenings to determine if a patient is in need of behavioral health services. After a screening, if it is determined that the patient needs behavioral health services, he or she will be referred to the care of a behavioral health professional. Depending on the insurance billed and the patient's diagnosis, some psychiatric screenings may be covered for primary care providers only, whereas others may be covered for behavioral health providers only.

Ultimately, whether or not the behavioral health provider gives and reports screening services depends on the individual practice. Behavioral health screening services include the following components.

- Psychiatric diagnostic evaluation, with or without medical services (90791 and 90792), which may be provided by a primary care physician.

- Behavior change interventions (99408 and 99409), such as the **Screening, Brief Intervention and Referral to Treatment (SBIRT)**, administered to patients with suspected alcohol or substance abuse. For Medicare patients, coders would use HCPCS codes G0396 and G0397 to report the administration of the same screening; and for Medicaid, coders should report HCPCS codes H0049 and H0050.

- Adaptive Behavior Treatment (97151–97158) services include an array of different psychological, developmental, neurobehavioral, neuropsychological, and emotional and behavioral assessment and treatments. These assessments may be provided by different practitioners, from primary care providers to therapists.

- Health and behavior assessments and interventions (96156–96171) are used to identify the psychological, behavioral, emotional, cognitive, and social factors vital to the prevention, treatment, or management of physical health problems. Behavioral health providers should not report these services if another, more predominant psychiatric service was performed.

Key to Success

Do not forget about the differences in billing requirements for various insurance types. An example of this is in administering drug and alcohol screenings to patients. Commercial insurance requires CPT codes 99406 through 99409, Medicare requires HCPCS codes G0396 and G0397, and Medicaid requires HCPCS codes H0049 and H0050—all for the same services! This is yet one more reason why it is important as a coder to always keep the patient's insurance in mind, as the codes may differ greatly depending on where the claim is sent and the setting in which the services are rendered.

Telemedicine Services

Many of the behavioral health services described in the previous sections may be performed via telemedicine (as noted by the ★ symbol next to the listed codes in the CPT code book). To report a telemedicine service, the coder must report the service with the regular CPT code appended with modifier -95, Synchronous telemedicine service. For example, if a psychiatrist performed 30 minutes of psychotherapy via a telemedicine platform for a nonmobile patient in a rural area, then he or she would report 90832, Psychotherapy, 30 minutes with patient, with modifier -95, Telemedicine service (90832-95).

Modifier -95, Synchronous telemedicine service rendered via a real-time interactive audio and video telecommunications systems must be appended to any service that is performed via a telemedicine platform. When coding for telemedicine services, check for two things: the CPT code must be a telemedicine code (it will have the ★ star symbol next to it in the CPT Tabular List and it will be listed in Appendix P), *and* it must be appended with modifier -95 to identify that the procedure was performed as a telemedicine service.

Complete the exercises in There's a Code for That 7.4 to practice assigning psychiatric procedure codes.

7.4

There's a Code for That

Assigning psychiatric procedure codes

Read the following procedural statements and assign the appropriate psychiatric procedural codes.

1. Psychotherapy for crisis, 30 minutes.

   CPT code: _____

2. Forty-five minutes of individual psychophysiological therapy incorporating feedback training, with supportive psychotherapy.

   CPT code: _____

3. Psychotherapy, 30 minutes, delivered via telemedicine platform.

   CPT code: _____

4. Substance abuse screening assessment and intervention delivered to a Medicare patient, 45 minutes total service time.

   CPT code: _____

5. Sixty minutes psychotherapy performed with interactive complexity.

   CPT code: _____

6. TMS, initial, delivery and management.

   CPT code: _____

Diagnosis Coding for Behavioral Health

Diagnostic coding for behavioral health services is a bit different than diagnostic coding for any other specialty. Rather than utilize the ICD-10-CM code book by itself, behavioral health providers also use the **Diagnostic and Statistical Manual of Mental Disorders**, currently in its 5th edition (DSM-5). Published by the American Psychiatric Association, the DSM-5 is the standard reference for behavioral health practitioners in the United States. For coding purposes, it is used in conjunction with the ICD-10-CM to classify mental illness and substance abuse disorders.

Coders working in the behavioral health field may use a DSM-5 code book to cross reference behavioral health diagnoses with ICD-10-CM codes, although this is not necessary. Although the DSM-5 code book does list associated ICD-10-CM codes along with descriptions of mental disorders, the ICD-10-CM code book is still the standard set of diagnosis codes that should be used for billing and reporting purposes. Ultimately, the DSM-5 is useful for coders because it can help identify the codes that should be used for diagnosed conditions; however, these codes should still be verified using the ICD-10-CM code book. Diagnosis codes for behavioral health and common behavioral health diagnoses are discussed in the following sections.

Diagnosis Codes in Behavioral Health

As in any specialty, ICD-10-CM codes identify the medical necessity for the service performed. Because insurance regulations and guidelines might be stricter regarding behavioral health services, it is important to have a clear understanding of what a patient's insurance plan will accept as medical necessity for specific behavioral health services. For example, transcranial magnetic stimulation (TMS) is typically covered only as a treatment for depression, even though research has shown that it may have a benefit for other mental health conditions such as schizophrenia (Cole et al. 2015). So if a patient were receiving TMS treatment for schizophrenia, this likely would *not* be covered by his or her insurance plan.

The primary diagnosis for behavioral health services should reflect either the reason for the visit or the focus of the treatment. If the patient has multiple diagnoses, then as many diagnoses as necessary should be listed to accurately provide a clinical picture of the patient's mental health status. For example, if a patient is seen for a prescription refill for his attention-deficit hyperactivity disorder, and his co-occurring diagnosis of anxiety is also managed, then two codes would be reported: F90.9, Attention-deficit hyperactivity disorder, unspecified type, and F41.9, Anxiety disorder, unspecified.

It is common for patients with substance abuse disorders to present with co-occurring mental health disorders as well as physical health issues. According to ICD-10-CM coding guidelines, coders should code all documented conditions that coexist at the time of the encounter or visit and require or affect patient care treatment or management. Conditions that previously existed and no longer exist should not be coded. However, patient history codes may be necessary to identify a historical condition that impacts the patient's current care or treatment.

In ICD-10-CM, there is an additional category of codes used to represent psychosocial and environmental problems: codes Z55 to Z65, Persons with potential health hazards related to socioeconomic and psychosocial circumstances. These codes are used to identify additional factors that may have an impact on a patient's mental health or substance abuse issues. For example, if a patient presents with depression due to bipolar disorder, exacerbated by the fact that she was recently separated from her husband of 20 years, then the following codes would be appropriate: F31.31, Bipolar disorder, current episode depressed, mild, and Z63.5, Disruption of family by separation and divorce.

Key to Success

It might be difficult to know what you should code when reading a diagnostic statement. To make sure you have coded all possible diagnoses, a good rule of thumb is to code until you can code no longer. For example, if the diagnostic statement describes relevant patient history codes or social circumstances, check for ICD-10-CM codes to see if there are any codes that correspond to either the history or the social circumstance. This is especially important in HCC coding, which requires that each visit be coded to the full extent.

Most of the diagnosis codes used in behavioral health are found in chapter 5 (Mental, Behavioral and Neurodevelopmental Disorders) of the ICD-10-CM code book. Many of these codes are presented in a **spectrum concept**, including substance abuse, autism, and schizophrenia. This concept identifies that a specific condition may expand from minimal or least-disruptive stage to maximal or most-disruptive stage. For example, the spectrum of substance abuse goes from the earliest stages of the condition (use) to later stages (abuse and dependence). Other mental health disorders are presented in a spectrum, from a minor version of the condition to a more advanced problem.

Codes reported for mental health and substance abuse services often include the following types of specifications.

- Course (for example, in remission or withdrawal)
- Severity (how bad the condition is)
- Frequency (how often it occurs)
- Duration (how long the condition has persisted)
- Descriptive features (clinical features of the condition) (Reichenberg 2014)

Unspecified and other specified (NOS and NEC) versions of behavioral health diagnosis codes are also used; see chapter 4 (Learning the ICD-10-CM Code Book) for a description of NOS and NEC diagnosis codes. Other specified (NEC) codes should be used to identify conditions in which the symptoms of the disorder are present (and documented) but do not fully meet the code description. Unspecified (NOS) codes should be used when the provider has not fully specified the condition and the clinical criteria for the condition have not been fully documented.

The following section discusses common behavioral health conditions that are reported with ICD-10-CM codes.

Common Behavioral Health Diagnoses

Although behavioral health providers can see and treat any mental health disorder, providers commonly specialize in certain disorders. For example, substance abuse requires a specific type of management and course of treatment, so it is common for a provider to treat only substance abuse patients. The following lists some of the more common behavioral health diagnoses.

- **Depression** (F32 to F34) is a mental disorder that affects a person's mood, thoughts, and actions. Symptoms include weight loss or gain, feeling sad or tired, crying for no reason, lack of interest, sleeping too much or too little, thoughts of death and suicide, feeling worthless, and difficulty concentrating. Symptoms must be present every day for at least two weeks to be classified as depression. Codes for depression include many different components and identify the episode (single or recurrent depression), severity (mild, moderate, or severe), and whether or not it presents with psychotic features or if it is in remission. **Remission** is a term that is used to identify that the condition is currently not an issue, such as a temporary recovery. For example, if the depression is in remission, this means that the depression has not recently been an active condition or problem. Furthermore, diagnosis codes for depression identify whether the patient is in full remission or partial remission. Note that codes for depression are HCC codes, so they must be documented in full, as specifically as possible.

- Substance Use and Abuse (F10 to F19) are one of the only behavioral health codes that have applicable official coding guidelines (see figure 7.12). To code accurately for substance abuse or use, the substance must be identified first. There are specific categories available for alcohol, opioids, cannabis, sedatives, hypnotics and anxiolytics, cocaine, other stimulants, hallucinogens, nicotine, inhalants, and other psychoactive substances. It is then necessary to identify the severity of the condition in terms of substance use, abuse, or dependence. According to ICD-10-CM guidelines, only one code should be reported for each substance, according to the following hierarchy (see figure 7.12):

- o If abuse and use are documented for the same substance, code for abuse.
- o If abuse and dependence are documented for the same substance, code for dependence.
- o If use, abuse, and dependence are all documented for the same condition, code for dependence.
- o If use and dependence are documented, code only for dependence.

Codes also identify the course of the substance use—for example, in withdrawal, with intoxication, and in remission. For remission status, the provider needs to document that the patient is in remission in order to be able to report the code for remission status. Note that these are complex codes that require careful reading of the code description. Furthermore, many substance abuse codes are HCC codes, and so special attention must be paid to ensure that they are documented in full and coded to the highest level of specificity.

- **Anxiety disorders** (F40 and F41) are mental disorders that result in constant feelings of worry, fear, and panic when faced with everyday situations. There are many types of anxiety disorders including phobias—that is, fears of specific everyday things like going outside or being in a social environment. Codes for phobias identify the specific fear, and anxiety codes specify the type of anxiety. Note that there is one specific code for a panic attack.

- **Bipolar disorder** (F30 and F31) is a mental disorder that affects a person's mood and behavior by switching from extreme highs (mania) to extreme lows (depression). Symptoms include agitation, restlessness, sleeping less,

Figure 7.12. OGCR I.C.5.b

---

b. **Mental and behavioral disorders due to psychoactive substance use**

1) **In Remission**

Selection of codes for "in remission" for categories F10-F19, Mental and behavioral disorders due to psychoactive substance use (categories F10-F19 with -.11, -.21) requires the provider's clinical judgment. The appropriate codes for "in remission" are assigned only on the basis of provider documentation (as defined in the Official Guidelines for Coding and Reporting), unless otherwise instructed by the classification.

Mild substance use disorders in early or sustained remission are classified to the appropriate codes for substance abuse in remission, and moderate or severe substance use disorders in early or sustained remission are classified to the appropriate codes for substance dependence in remission.

2) **Psychoactive Substance Use, Abuse And Dependence**

When the provider documentation refers to use, abuse and dependence of the same substance (e.g. alcohol, opioid, cannabis, etc.), only one code should be assigned to identify the pattern of use based on the following hierarchy:

- If both use and abuse are documented, assign only the code for abuse
- If both abuse and dependence are documented, assign only the code for dependence
- If use, abuse and dependence are all documented, assign only the code for dependence
- If both use and dependence are documented, assign only the code for dependence.

3) **Psychoactive Substance Use Unspecified**

As with all other unspecified diagnoses, the codes for unspecified psychoactive substance use disorders (F10.9-, F11.9-, F12.9-, F13.9-, F14.9-, F15.9-, F16.9-, F18.9-, F19.9-) should only be assigned based on provider documentation and when they meet the definition of a reportable diagnosis (see Section III, Reporting Additional Diagnoses). These codes are to be used only when the psychoactive substance use is associated with a physical, mental or behavioral disorder, and such a relationship is documented by the provider.

Source: CMS 2019c.

speaking too fast, taking unnecessary risks, laughing uncontrollably, inability to concentrate, and depressed feelings once the manic period is over. Bipolar disorder codes specify the features of the current episode (such as manic or depressed), as well as the severity of the condition, and with or without psychotic features and if it is in remission.

- **Eating disorders** (F50) affect the way a person eats or processes food and nutrition. There are two common types of eating disorders—anorexia nervosa and bulimia. Anorexia symptoms include extreme underweight, constant thoughts about food, weight and body image, refusal to eat, fear of gaining weight, lack of menstruation, and excessive exercise. Bulimia symptoms include too much dieting and exercise, excessive use of laxatives, dehydration, lack of menstruation, poor body image, and going to the bathroom directly after eating.

- **Schizophrenia** (F20 to F29) is a mental disorder that manifests in the symptoms of delusions, hallucinations, paranoia, confused speech, isolation, outbursts of anger, and catatonic behavior that persist for at least one month. When coding for schizophrenia, it is important to note if there is any substance abuse causing the schizophrenia, or if it is related to a brain disease such as epilepsy. These may impact the schizophrenia codes reported.

- **Attention-deficit hyperactivity disorders (ADHD)** (F90) typically occur in school-age children and impact a child's school and social functioning. Symptoms include impulsivity, inattention, difficulty concentrating and following directions, difficulty completing tasks, too much energy, and restlessness. Codes for ADHD differentiate between the type (predominantly inattentive, hyperactive, combined, or other specified type). Note that although this condition is commonly seen in children, these codes can be used for patients of any age.

HCC Coding Corner

Most behavioral health codes are included in hierarchical condition categories (HCC), including depression, substance abuse, bipolar disorder, ADHD, and schizophrenia. Be careful when selecting these codes for HCC reporting purposes! Documentation for behavioral health conditions must be specific enough to support the code selected. This includes specification of the course, severity, frequency, duration, and descriptive features. For example, code F32.9, Major depressive disorder, unspecified, the code for unspecified depression, does not hold any HCC value, whereas all other, more specified types of depression, do hold an HCC value. This illustrates the importance of specific documentation and code description.

Complete the exercises in There's a Code for That 7.5 to practice assigning behavioral health diagnosis codes.

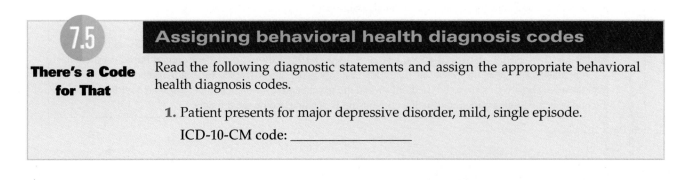

7.5

There's a Code for That

Assigning behavioral health diagnosis codes

Read the following diagnostic statements and assign the appropriate behavioral health diagnosis codes.

1. Patient presents for major depressive disorder, mild, single episode.

   ICD-10-CM code: _____

2. A 10-year-old female with history of childhood abuse presents for treatment of generalized anxiety disorder and moderate recurrent depression.

ICD-10-CM codes: _____ , _____ ,

_____

3. Anorexia nervosa, binge eating/purging type.

ICD-10-CM code: _____

4. Oppositional defiant disorder.

ICD-10-CM code: _____

5. Patient presents for treatment of opioid use. He is opioid dependent, currently in remission.

ICD-10-CM code: _____

6. Patient presents for treatment of chronic post-traumatic stress disorder due to exposure to war while in the military two years ago.

ICD-10-CM code: _____ , _____

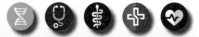

Putting It All Together: Coding for Behavioral Health Services

In order to select the correct code for the behavioral health encounter, it is important to carefully read the documentation and then access each code book to find the procedure or service provided and the corresponding diagnosis or diagnoses to support the medical necessity for the service. Procedural codes for behavioral health services are found in the CPT and HCPCS code books, and diagnosis codes are found in the ICD-10-CM code book.

Determination of the correct codes for behavioral health services relies on the answers to the following questions.

- What service was provided to the patient? Was an E/M service provided in addition to a psychiatric service?
- Are there any applicable modifiers or add-on codes?
- What is the primary condition being treated? This will be the reason for the visit or the focus of the treatment.
- Are there any additional co-occurring mental health or physical health diagnoses?

Study the following vignette demonstrating how to select the appropriate diagnosis and procedure codes. Then complete the exercises in There's a Code for That 7.6 to practice coding for behavioral health.

Now that Nidia is finished with her training, she is responsible for coding the services provided to patients in the behavioral health clinic. She is coding both the procedural and diagnosis codes for the following encounter: A 35-year-old female established patient presented to the office for psychotherapy and medication refill for multiple personality disorder. The physician performed an E/M visit with an expanded problem-focused history and MDM of low complexity, as well as 30 to 45 minutes of psychotherapy with interactive complexity using expressive art therapy.

First, Nidia asks herself: What did the doctor do? The doctor performed an E/M encounter, psychotherapy, and art therapy (interactive complexity). She looks up the procedure codes in the CPT book and finds the following codes.

99213, Office or other outpatient visit for the evaluation and management of an established patient, which requires at least 2 out of 3 of the following: expanded problem-focused history, expanded problem-focused examination, medical decision-making of low complexity

90836, Psychotherapy, 45 minutes when performed with E/M service

90785, Interactive complexity

Now that she has her procedure codes, Nidia asks herself: Why did the doctor do it? The patient presented for treatment of multiple personality disorder. She looks up this condition in the ICD-10-CM code book and finds the following code.

F44.81, Dissociative identity disorder

She then rechecks the documentation to ensure she has coded everything for the encounter and reports the chosen codes on the claim for the service.

7.6   Coding for behavioral health services

There's a Code for That

Read the following documentation from patient encounters and assign the appropriate procedure and diagnosis codes.

1. Patient presents for treatment of recurrent severe depression without psychotic symptoms, which is not responding to combination of medication and psychotherapy treatments. Today she is receiving an initial delivery and management via TMS therapy.

   CPT code: _____

   ICD-10-CM code: _____

2. Narcosynthesis evaluation of a patient with alcohol dependence with alcohol-induced bipolar disorder.

   CPT code: _____

   ICD-10-CM code: _____

3. A 42-year-old new patient is brought into the office by his family for evaluation of alcohol abuse with paranoid delusions. A comprehensive history and examination were performed; MDM was high complexity. Patient was prescribed a neuroleptic and referred to an Alcoholics Anonymous program.

   CPT code: _____

   ICD-10-CM code: _____

4. Initial hospital care provided to a patient with severe psychotic features. A comprehensive history and examination are performed, with high complexity MDM. She was diagnosed with paranoid schizophrenia.

CPT code: _____

ICD-10-CM code: _____

5. Nurse practitioner performed 30 minutes of psychotherapy and pharmacologic management for a patient with moderate bipolar disorder without psychotic features (current episode manic), and generalized social phobia.

CPT codes: _____ , _____

ICD-10-CM codes: _____ , _____

Case Study | Anxiety and Depression Office Visit

PATIENT: Alfred Vincente   **DOB:** 09/18/1983

DATE OF SERVICE: 01/25/20XX

SUBJECTIVE: (Detailed History)
Chief Complaint: Established patient F/U on chronic conditions: anxiety, depression, sleeping disorder

History of Present Illness: Patient presents to clinic today needing medication refills and to follow up on chronic mental health disorders. Patient is an RN who has worked the night shift for many years and has had difficulty returning to the day shift and waking up early in time to get to work. Had been employed by a traveling nurse corp but has recently returned to town to live with elderly parents and take care of his father. Patient is now employed at local psychiatric hospital. Current sleeping medication not always effective. Patient wakes multiple times each night. Gets headaches occasionally. Depression and anxiety are all well-controlled with medication. Needs refills of these.

Review of Systems:
Gastrointestinal: had GI bug a few weeks ago with body aches/pains. Nausea, vomiting, and diarrhea lasted for about 3.5 days, completely resolved now.
Musculoskeletal: body aches/pains with illness about three weeks ago. Completely resolved now.
Integumentary: horizontal ridging in fingernails, worse in first 1 to 3 fingers of each hand, patient concerned.
Psychiatric: anxiety/depression and insomnia controlled on current medication regimen.

Past, Family, Social History:
Current medications reviewed. No known drug allergies (NKDA). Patient drinks recreationally, is not a current tobacco smoker and does not use recreational drugs. Patient is a heterosexual in a monogamous relationship.

OBJECTIVE: (Comprehensive Examination)
Physical Examination:
Constitutional: alert and in no acute distress. Well-nourished and healthy appearing. Thin but appears healthy.
Eyes: pupils were equal in size, round, reactive to light, with normal accommodation. No strabismus was seen.
ENMT: ears and nose were normal in appearance, both tympanic membranes were normal and the nasal mucosa and septum were normal. The oropharynx was normal.
Neck: normal in appearance and supple. The thyroid was not enlarged.
Cardiovascular: heart rate and rhythm were normal and there were no murmurs. No edema seen.
Pulmonary: normal respiratory rhythm and effort, no accessory muscle used noted. Clear bilateral breath sounds.
Abdomen: normal bowel sounds, soft, non-tender and no hepatosplenomegaly.
Musculoskeletal: normal gait and normal movements of all extremities.
Skin: no rash and normal skin turgor.
Neurological: a tremor was seen.
Psychiatric: patient was pleasant, interactive and focused. Oriented to person, place, and time. Affect was normal, insight and judgment were intact, mood was normal, and recent memory was not impaired.
Depression screening: total score 0 (low risk).
Anxiety screening: total score 0 (low risk).

ASSESSMENT and PLAN: (Moderate Complexity MDM)

1. Generalized anxiety disorder. Currently stable and well-controlled with medication. Refill sertraline.

2. Depression, mild, recurrent. Currently stable and well-controlled with medication. Refill gabapentin.

3. Insomnia. Currently uncontrolled. Discontinue Ambien for now and will try hydroxyzine 1 to 2 tablets at bedtime. Reviewed importance of managing and implementing sleep hygiene into self-care.

4. Idiopathic hypersomnia without long sleep time due to night shift schedule. Currently managing but not well-controlled. Refilled phentermine 30 days.

SIGNED: Dr. Susan Alameda, DO

Use the following steps to select the appropriate codes for the case study.

1. Read through the case study in full. As you read, look up any medical or procedural terms with which you are unfamiliar. For example, the terms *hepatosplenomegaly* and *hypersomnia* may not be familiar. Use a medical dictionary or medical terminology text to define these terms. On your own, look up and define any additional unfamiliar terms.

   a. *Hepatosplenomegaly:*

   _____

   _____

b. *Osteopenia*:

_____

_____

2. Review the case study and answer the following question: *What did the doctor do?* In this case study, the documentation is in the SOAP note format. Remember that the components of the SOAP note directly correspond to the key components of an E/M service. Answer the following questions to help you determine the correct E/M code.

a. What is the place of service, type of service, and patient status?

_____

_____

b. Identify the code range for this type of E/M service in the CPT code book and list it.

_____

_____

c. How many key components are necessary to select the level of service for this E/M type?

_____

_____

d. Using the levels of the three key components (as located in the documentation of the visit), identify the correct E/M code for this service.

_____

_____

e. Are there any additional procedures that need to be added to identify all of the procedures performed? If yes, follow the previous steps to identify the codes for the additional procedures.

_____

_____

f. Are there any modifiers that need to be added to identify any special circumstance surrounding the procedure(s)? If yes, refer to Appendix A of the CPT code book to assign all appropriate modifiers.

_____

_____

3. Now that the procedure(s) and modifier(s) have been identified, refer to the case study and answer the following question: *Why did the doctor do it?* To find the reason for the office visit, search for terms that will identify the medical condition. Remember that in the SOAP note format, the diagnoses are included in the Assessment portion of the documentation. This is where the provider lists each of the medical conditions found or addressed during the visit. In this case study, identify the patient's diagnoses.

a. _____

b. _____

c. _____

d. _____

4. Now that you have identified the patient's diagnoses, search the ICD-10-CM code book for the correct codes for these conditions. Follow these steps for each of the diagnoses identified.

   a. Search the Main Index for the name of each condition and search through any applicable subterms and cross-references to locate the appropriate code.

      i. _____

      ii. _____

      iii. _____

      iv. _____

   b. Verify the code(s) in the Tabular List. Locate the code(s) identified previously in the Tabular Listing of codes and refer to any applicable guidelines, notes, and symbols. Does the code selected correctly identify the patient's condition? If yes, list the code(s).

      i. _____

      ii. _____

      iii. _____

      iv. _____

   c. Check the procedure note and ICD-10-CM guidelines and conventions to determine the correct sequencing of the diagnosis codes, if applicable. Correctly sequence the diagnosis codes.

      i. _____

      ii. _____

Key to Success

Pay special attention to Excludes1 and Excludes2 notes. In this case, none of the conditions identified are excluded as per the Excludes1 or Excludes2 notes, but this is not always the case. Remember to always take note of the conditions included in these notes as they will tell you when two conditions may or may not be coded together.

5. Now that the procedure and diagnosis codes have been identified, list them on the following CMS-1500 form. Be sure to identify medical necessity for each service by correctly linking the procedure/supply and diagnosis codes. Please refer to figure 3.6 for an example.

21. DIAGNOSIS OR NATURE OF ILLNESS OR INJURY Relate A-L to service line below (24E)				ICD Ind.	

A. L_____   B. L_____   C. L_____   D. L_____

E. L_____   F. L_____   G. L_____   H. L_____

I. L_____   J. L_____   K. L_____   L. L_____

24. A. DATE(S) OF SERVICE						B. PLACE OF	C.	D. PROCEDURES, SERVICES, OR SUPPLIES (Explain Unusual Circumstances)		E. DIAGNOSIS
From			To			SERVICE	EMG	CPT/HCPCS	MODIFIER	POINTER
MM	DD	YY	MM	DD	YY					
1										
2										
3										

End-of-Chapter Content

Instructions: Indicate whether the following statements are true or false (T or F). For false statements, rewrite the statement on the line below to make the statement true.

1. The behavioral health specialty is comprised of mental health and substance abuse services.

_____

_____

2. A child and adolescent psychiatrist is a subspecialist in the field of behavioral health.

_____

_____

3. The SBIRT is administered to patients with suspected mental illness.

_____

_____

4. Evaluation and management codes are often used in behavioral health coding.

_____

_____

(Continued on next page)

(Continued)

5. A new patient is one who has not been seen by a healthcare provider or another healthcare provider of the same subspecialty in the same group practice within the past two years.

_____

_____

6. The three key components of an E/M service are history, evaluation, and medical decision-making.

_____

_____

7. Contributory factors are the discussion between a healthcare provider and a patient or patient's family.

_____

_____

8. Behavioral health procedural coding is largely comprised of E/M codes and codes in the Psychiatry subsection.

_____

_____

9. The CPT code range 90785 through 90899 includes psychiatry codes used in behavioral health coding.

_____

_____

10. The add-on code for interactive complexity is 90785.

_____

_____

Instructions: Choose the best answer.

1. Which of the following refers to a person's emotional, psychological, and social well-being?
   a. Substance abuse
   b. Mental health
   c. Mental illness
   d. Behavioral health

2. Which of the following is the misuse of alcohol or drugs, which impairs a person's ability to meet daily responsibilities?
   a. Substance abuse
   b. Mental health
   c. Mental illness
   d. Behavioral health

3. What must a behavioral health coder always consider when coding for services?
   a. The age of the patient
   b. The residency status of the patient
   c. The services requested by the patient
   d. The patient's health insurance coverage and limitations

4. What is a request from a provider of services to an insurance company to authorize a service before it is performed?
   a. Referral request
   b. Consultation
   c. Prior authorization
   d. Claim denial

5. What is placed in box 24.B of the CMS-1500 claim form?
   a. Date of service
   b. CPT code(s)
   c. ICD-10 code(s)
   d. Place of service

6. Evaluation and management codes are used to report which of the following?
   a. Healthcare management of a patient
   b. Psychotherapy services
   c. Specialized screenings and diagnostic tests
   d. Electroconvulsive therapy

7. The type of service of an E/M code is which of the following?
   a. The patient's status as new, established, inpatient, or outpatient
   b. The type of evaluation and management encounter that was provided
   c. The setting in which the service was provided
   d. The type of provider that performed the service

8. Which patient type has been formally admitted to an inpatient hospital?
   a. Outpatient
   b. Observation
   c. Inpatient
   d. Initial

9. An established patient is one who has been seen within the last how many years?
   a. Two
   b. Three
   c. Four
   d. One

10. Which of the following is the subjective information the patient tells a provider at the encounter?
    a. History
    b. Examination
    c. Medical decision-making
    d. Evaluation

11. In which portion of an E/M service does the provider make a decision regarding the patient's diagnoses and care or treatment plan?
    a. History
    b. Examination
    c. Medical decision-making
    d. Evaluation

12. How many levels of each of the key components are there?
    a. Four
    b. Three
    c. Two
    d. Six

13. What are counseling, coordination of care, and nature of the presenting problem?
    a. Contributory factors
    b. Time components
    c. Key components
    d. These are not taken into account in E/M coding

14. What is the treatment of a mental illness in which the healthcare provider attempts to alleviate disturbances, reverse or change patterns of behavior, and encourage personality growth and development, through discourse with the patient?
    a. Coordination of care
    b. Evaluation and management service
    c. Psychiatric initial evaluation
    d. Psychotherapy

15. Which of the following is a noninvasive procedure that uses magnetic fields to stimulate areas of the brain?

    a. Mental stimulation
    b. Transcranial magnetic stimulation
    c. Electroconvulsive therapy
    d. Narcosynthesis

16. Which modifier should be reported with telemedicine services?

    a. -51
    b. -25
    c. -95
    d. None

17. When should other specified diagnosis codes be reported?

    a. When identifying conditions in which the symptoms of the disorder are present but do not fully meet the code description
    b. When the provider has not fully specified the condition and the clinical criteria have not been fully documented
    c. When the condition cannot be determined to be one of two variables
    d. When identifying conditions that are not fully specified in the documentation

18. The ICD-10 code book has chapter-specific guidelines on coding which of the following conditions?

    a. Anxiety disorders
    b. Depression
    c. Substance abuse disorders
    d. Attention-deficit hyperactivity disorder

Instructions: Answer the following questions with the appropriate code(s).

1. Psychotherapy provided to a patient in crisis with severe paranoid schizophrenia, 90 minutes total time.

    CPT code(s): _____ , _____

    ICD-10 code(s): _____

2. E/M encounter for established patient in the outpatient office setting, detailed history and examination. Psychotherapy of 45 minutes was also provided to patient with moderate recurrent depression and acute PTSD due to her personal history of childhood neglect.

    CPT code(s): _____ , _____

    ICD-10 code(s): _____ ,

    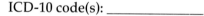 _____ , _____

3. ECT and necessary monitoring performed on 40-year-old female with untreatable depression (severe, recurrent, with psychotic features).

    CPT code(s): _____

    ICD-10 code(s): _____

4. Psychotherapy of 60 minutes provided to a male patient with recurrent depression via a telemedicine platform. His depression has been in remission for three months and is now receiving treatment for agoraphobia and panic attacks.

    CPT code(s): _____

    ICD-10 code(s): _____

5. Family psychotherapy performed without the patient present for a 12-year-old female with chronic PTSD due to the death of her mother approximately one year ago. She also suffers from excoriation disorder and mild intellectual disabilities.

    CPT code(s): _____

    ICD-10 code(s): _____ ,

    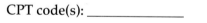 _____ , _____ ,

    _____

References

American Medical Association (AMA). 2019. *CPT 2020 Professional Edition.* Chicago: AMA.

Centers for Medicare and Medicaid Services (CMS). 2019a (November 8). Place of Service Code Set. http://www .cms.gov/Medicare/Coding/place-of-service-codes /Place_of_Service_Code_Set.html.

Centers for Medicare and Medicaid Services (CMS). 2019b. CMS 1500. https://www.cms.gov/Medicare/CMS-Forms/CMS-Forms/CMS-Forms-Items/CMS1188854.

Centers for Medicare and Medicaid Services (CMS). 2019c. ICD-10-CM Official Guidelines for Coding and Reporting FY 2020. https://www.cms.gov/Medicare/Coding/ICD10/Downloads/2020-Coding-Guidelines.pdf.

Cole, J. C., G. Bernacki, A. Helmer, N. Pinninti, and J. P. O'Reardon. 2015 (July–August). Efficacy of transcranial magnetic stimulation (TMS) in the treatment of schizophrenia: A review of the literature to date. *Innovations in Clinical Neuroscience* 12(7-8): 12–19. https://www.ncbi.nlm.nih.gov/pmc/articles/PMC4558786/.

Reichenberg, L.W. 2014. *DSM-5 Essentials: The Savvy Clinician's Guide to the Changes in Criteria.* Hoboken, NJ: Wiley.

Resources

Center for Medicaid and CHIP Services (CMCS). 2014 (July 11). Informational Bulletin: Medication Assisted Treatment for Substance Use Disorders. https://www.medicaid.gov/Federal-Policy-Guidance/downloads/CIB-07-11-2014.pdf.

Centers for Medicare and Medicaid Services (CMS). 2018 (May 22). *MLN Matters*: Medicare Payments for Part B Mental Health Services. https://www.cms.gov/Outreach-and-Education/Medicare-Learning-Network-MLN/MLNMattersArticles/downloads/SE0816.pdf.

Department of Health and Human Services (HHS). 2019. Health Insurance and Mental Health Services. https://www.mentalhealth.gov/get-help/health-insurance.

CHAPTER

Primary Care Services

Learning Objectives

- Understand the basics of billing and coding within the specialty of primary care
- Examine procedural codes and guidelines for primary care services

- Examine diagnosis coding and medical necessity for primary care services
- Determine and apply ICD-10-CM, CPT, and HCPCS codes to primary care services

Key Terms

Annual wellness visit (AWV)

Body area

Care plan oversight (CPO)

Chief complaint (C/C)

Chronic care management (CCM)

Chronic obstructive pulmonary disease (COPD)

CLIA-waived

Congenital condition

Diabetes mellitus

Electrocardiogram (ECG/EKG)

Foreign body

Heart failure

History of present illness (HPI)

Hypercholesterolemia

Hyperlipidemia

Hypertension

Immune globulin

Incision and drainage (I&D)

Initial Preventive Physical Examination (IPPE)

Minor surgical procedure

Organ system

Otitis

Overcoding

Past, family, social history (PFSH)

Perinatal condition

Preventive medicine services

Primary care

Primary care provider (PCP)

Prolonged services

Review of systems (ROS)

Status asthmaticus

Transient hypertension

Transitional Care Management (TCM)

Undercoding

Underdose

Vaccine administration

Vaccine toxoid

Primary care healthcare providers are specialists who provide generalized, day-to-day care to patients. They act as the principal point of care and take responsibility for continuing comprehensive healthcare for patients. These providers also coordinate referrals, diagnostic testing, therapeutic treatments, and coordination of care with other providers from other specialties. There are a handful of specialists that may serve as primary care providers, including family practice, internal medicine, and pediatrics, as well as women's health or obstetrics and gynecology (OB/GYN) practitioners.

Most of the services provided by primary care practitioners are evaluation and management (E/M) services, which is why E/M coding is a major component of primary care coding. Additional services are also performed, such as the administration of vaccines and in-office medical and minor surgical procedures. Patients may be seen in the primary care setting for a vast range of reasons, from signs and symptoms like sore throat and fever to complex health issues such as diabetes mellitus, hypertension, and heart failure.

This chapter discusses the many different services provided within the field of primary care, with a special emphasis on E/M coding that was introduced in chapter 7 (Behavioral Health Services). Additional services provided in the primary care setting are also discussed, including the administration of vaccines, in-office surgical procedures, miscellaneous medical procedures, and in-office laboratory procedures; as well as the top diagnosis codes for this specialty, including routine examinations, signs and symptoms, hypertension, diabetes, and hyperlipidemia/hypercholesterolemia.

Primary Care Basics

There are several types of healthcare specialties that qualify as primary care. Whenever a provider acts as a patient's principal point of contact, coordinates that patient's care with other providers or specialists, and takes primary responsibility for the general healthcare of a patient, he or she is acting as a **primary care provider (PCP)**. For a reminder of the different types of healthcare specialties and the services they provide, refer to chapter 1 (Your Coding Career).

The designation of PCP is important because many health insurance plans require a patient to select a PCP that is contracted and included in the patient's health insurance network. For some plans, the patient must make primary contact with the PCP before they are allowed to see a different provider. For example, if a patient is experiencing a digestive issue, he or she must see the PCP first and obtain a referral to a digestive disease specialist from the PCP before insurance will pay for the visit to the digestive disease specialist. In this way, the insurance company can be sure the patient needs to see the specialist (as determined by the PCP). Furthermore, the PCP can keep track of all the health issues and services provided to the patient.

It is important to note that not all health insurance plans require a referral to see a specialist. Some plans require only that the patient sees an in-network provider. Other plans are much more restrictive and either require prior authorization to see a specialist or may not authorize a visit to the specialist unless certain conditions are met. Because of these varying requirements, coding professionals must understand the relationship between a patient's insurance plan and the services that were requested and received.

Identifying a provider as a patient's PCP is also important in terms of insurance reimbursement, as the payment for health services may be different for a PCP than for a specialist. For example, the copayment amount may differ depending on who the patient sees. A PCP copayment may be $30, whereas a specialist copayment is $50, and an urgent care copayment is $75. There also may be a higher amount of reimbursement, or payment, for PCP services. For example, plan A may pay 90 percent of the allowable amount for PCP charges and send 10 percent to the patient deductible, whereas plan B may pay 75 percent of specialist services and send 25 percent to the patient deductible. Typically, a patient must identify a specific provider as his or her PCP, either over the phone or through the mail; some insurance plans allow patients to choose a PCP via online selection or during registration with the healthcare plan.

One more consideration in terms of coding for primary care services is HCC coding, introduced in chapter 2 (Healthcare Billing Basics). Data from different types of providers is used in HCC coding; however, the base data for this initiative is primary care claims, because PCPs commonly monitor and diagnose patient chronic conditions, such as diabetes or chronic kidney disease, many of which are included in HCC coding.

PCP offices are also more likely to be part risk programs or accountable care organizations (ACOs)—groups of providers collectively accountable for the care they provide patients, that use performance measures to track the quality of the care provided to patients, and that receive payments linked to quality improvement initiatives (refer to chapter 2). ACO performance is evaluated on an annual basis according to specific benchmarks, one of which is the risk score assigned to the beneficiaries for that year. This risk adjustment score is based on the numerous diagnosis codes included in hierarchical condition categories as determined by the diagnosis codes selected for each patient (CMS 2019a). It is important to remember that HCC coding relies on ICD-10-CM diagnosis codes, discussed in a later section in this chapter.

HCC Coding Corner

Remember that in your AHIMA ICD-10-CM code book, HCC codes are identified with lavender highlighting. In the real world, pay special attention to these codes, as they will impact the risk adjustment score for each patient.

Procedural Coding in Primary Care

In primary care, most of the services performed are E/M services because patients often present to a healthcare provider's office for the evaluation of a problem, such as an illness, and the subsequent management of it, perhaps with a medication prescription. Even when patients are not ill, there are office visits for routine examinations or preoperative exams, all of which are also reported with E/M codes. Additional E/M codes include those for special services, such as transitional care management, chronic care management, and care plan oversight services, among many others. Occasionally patients undergo minor surgeries, such as cryosurgery of a wart or the incision and drainage of an abscess, so coders do have to use a few codes from the Surgery section of the CPT code book, in addition to various codes (especially those for vaccinations) from the Medicine section of the CPT code book.

E/M Services

Because the majority of procedures performed by PCPs are E/M services, most of a PCP coder's time is spent assigning E/M codes and checking the provider's documentation to ensure it supports the level of service identified by the E/M code. E/M coding depends on the accurate identification of the numerous components of documentation that together support the levels of each key component and ultimately the E/M code itself.

There are currently two sets of guidelines for the use of E/M codes: 1995 and 1997 documentation guidelines (DGs). In 1995, due to confusion about the interpretation of E/M codes and how to select them, the Centers for Medicare and Medicaid Services (CMS) worked together with the American Medical Association (AMA) to develop a set of E/M documentation guidelines (DGs) to help direct correct code selection. However, these guidelines did not please healthcare specialists, who could not receive credit for an extended examination of a single body system under the 1995 DGs (more on this later in this chapter). In 1997, the DGs were revised to include guidance for specialty providers. But the 1997 DGs were still met with opposition from the physician community. Therefore, CMS mandated that either the 1995 or 1997 DGs may be used to guide E/M code selection, as long as a provider is consistent in which one they use (AAPC 2016). Furthermore, if the healthcare practice is audited, the documentation must clearly show how the specific level of E/M service was chosen based on which DGs (1995 or 1997) were used.

There are multiple elements of each of the three key components: history, examination, and medical decision-making (MDM), first discussed in chapter 7. Remember, the elements of each of the key components are combined, depending on the service documented, to identify the correct level of the key component. This must be done for all three key components, which are then compared to the code descriptions for an E/M service in order to find the correct code (see figure 8.1 or refer to figure 7.10).

Figure 8.1. Determine the level of E/M code

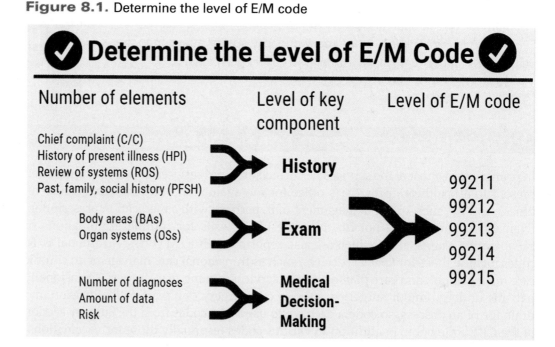

When a healthcare provider performs a complicated service, more elements are included from each of the key components, which raises the level of the E/M service and allows the provider to bill a higher amount. The level of E/M service is comprised of the levels of key components (history, exam, and MDM), so that the higher the levels of key components, the higher the level of E/M service. On the other hand, for a less complicated service less elements from each key component are included, so the level of E/M service is lower and is billed at a lower amount. In this way, doctors can receive a higher amount of payment for more complicated services, and a smaller amount for less complicated services.

It is important to select the appropriate code for the services performed to avoid both undercoding and overcoding. **Undercoding** is the act of coding an E/M service at a level lower than what was performed. For example, if a doctor provided a service that could be billed with a higher level visit, such as a 99214, Office or other outpatient visit for the evaluation and management of an established patient, which requires at least 2 out of 3 of the following key components: *detailed* history, *detailed* examination, medical decision-making of *moderate* complexity, but the coder only bills for a lower level visit, 99213, Office or other outpatient visit for the evaluation and management of an established patient, which requires at least 2 out of 3 of the following key components: *expanded problem-focused* history, *expanded problem-focused* examination, medical decision-making of *low* complexity, the coder is undercoding the visit. The code that should have been reported was for a higher level of service (99214) than what was actually reported (99213). This ultimately means that the doctor is not receiving payment for the service that was actually rendered.

Overcoding, on the other hand, is coding for an E/M service at a level higher than what was performed. For example, coding a level four visit, 99214, Office or other outpatient visit for the evaluation and management of an established patient, which requires at least 2 out of 3 of the following key components: *detailed* history, *detailed* examination, medical decision-making of *moderate* complexity, when only a level three visit, 99213, Office or other outpatient visit for the evaluation and management of an established patient, which requires at least 2 out of 3 of the following key components: *expanded problem-focused* history, *expanded problem-focused* examination, medical decision-making of *low* complexity, was performed would be considered *overcoding.* This is just as dangerous as undercoding, as it can result in a recovery audit performed by an insurance company or another company to uncover overpayments. Overcoding can result in recoupment of overpayments, in addition to more serious allegations such as billing abuse or fraud. See figure 8.2 for an illustration of undercoding versus overcoding.

Coders must understand each of the elements included within each of the key components, so they can combine them correctly and ultimately select the appropriate

Figure 8.2. Undercoding versus overcoding

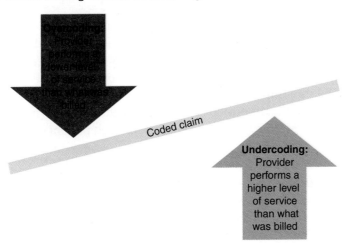

Overcoding: Provider performs a lower level of service than what was billed

Coded claim

Undercoding: Provider performs a higher level of service than what was billed

E/M code. This includes understanding the individual elements involved in the three key components—the elements of history, examination, and medical decision-making. Coding for PCP services also requires a solid understanding of how to code for prolonged services, preventive services, and the modifiers used with E/M codes.

Elements of History

There are four elements of the key component history: chief complaint (C/C), history of present illness (HPI), review of systems (ROS), and past, family, social history (PFSH), as shown in figure 8.3. The level of the history obtained from the patient is based on the levels of each of these four elements. As discussed in chapter 7, there are four levels of history: problem focused, expanded problem focused, detailed, and comprehensive.

Figure 8.3. Elements of history

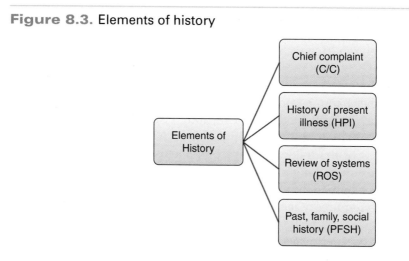

Remember that history is the subjective component of an E/M service. In other words, the history component is just *talking* with the healthcare provider. It is the patient's description of the symptoms, signs, and other complaints, and does not include any components of an actual physical examination. The history component of an E/M code is only an oral account, without any physical examination or determination of the diagnosis or prescription of medications.

Chief Complaint

The **chief complaint (C/C)** is the description of the patient's symptoms, in the patient's own words. This is a concise statement that describes the problem, diagnosis (if known), condition, or other reason for the patient's encounter with the healthcare provider. It should answer the question, *why is the patient in the office today?* For example, a chief complaint could be sore throat and fever or the need for a flu shot. The chief complaint is used to help the healthcare provider understand the reason why the patient seeks treatment. The chief complaint must be recorded for each patient encounter, but it does not impact the level of the history for the encounter.

History of Present Illness

The **history of present illness (HPI)** is a description of the development of the present illness or condition, described chronologically from the first onset of symptoms to the present encounter. The HPI is given by the patient based on questions asked by the healthcare provider. There are eight elements of HPI, each of which explains a different aspect of the current condition.

- *Location*. Where on the body the signs or symptoms are present, such as the throat.
- *Quality*. Characteristics of the signs or symptoms, such as stabbing or aching pain.
- *Severity*. The intensity of the signs or symptoms, often identified on a scale of 1 to 10.
- *Duration*. How long the problem has persisted, such as four days.
- *Timing*. When the signs or symptoms occur, such as every evening or all day long.
- *Context*. The circumstances under which the signs or symptoms occur, such as when walking.
- *Modifying factors*. The circumstances under which the signs or symptoms improve or worsen, such as when taking a deep breath.
- *Associated signs and symptoms*. Any other signs or symptoms related to the chief complaint, such as swelling or itching.

The healthcare provider asks pointed questions crafted around these elements to help narrow the focus of the examination. Depending on the chief complaint, the provider might require information for each of or none of these elements. The level of the HPI is selected based on how many of these elements were covered in the history portion of the E/M service. There are two HPI levels—brief and extended. A brief HPI includes documentation of one to three elements, as described previously. An extended HPI includes documentation of four or more elements, or the status of three chronic conditions (CMS 1995; CMS 1997). Note that according to the 1997 DGs for E/M services, instead of obtaining information on the eight elements of HPI, the provider can document the current status of three or more chronic conditions. This is helpful when a patient presents with multiple chronic conditions, as is often the case in primary care, or for a follow-up or refill of medications. The provider must document the current status of each of the chronic conditions (at least three of them), as stated by the patient.

Read the following example of a patient history and note the eight different elements of HPI.

*A 45-year-old male patient is seen complaining of abdominal pain, nausea with vomiting (three times), diarrhea (five times). He has a constant (**timing**) pain in the abdominal area (**location**), which is stabbing in nature (**quality**). He says that the pain is about a 7 out of 10 (**severity**), and it usually results in nausea and vomiting when he walks around (**context**). Symptoms began yesterday afternoon (**duration**) after eating his lunch. He recalls that the lunch smelled a little "off." He does report that lying on his left side has helped with the pain and nausea a bit (**modifying factor**). He is not experiencing any painful or frequent urination (**associated signs and symptoms**).*

Review of Systems

The **review of systems (ROS)** is a series of questions aimed at obtaining more information regarding signs or symptoms the patient is experiencing. These questions are organized around the following organ systems.

- *Constitutional.* General constitutional signs or symptoms, such as feeling fatigued or weak.
- *Eyes.* Signs or symptoms involving the eyes, such as discharge or visual disturbances.
- *Ears, nose, and throat.* Signs or symptoms involving the ears (such as ringing or pain), the nose (such as rhinorrhea or nose bleeds), and the throat and mouth (such as difficulty swallowing or bleeding gums).
- *Cardiovascular.* Signs or symptoms involving the cardiovascular system, such as chest pain or tightness.
- *Respiratory.* Signs or symptoms involving the respiratory system, such as shortness of breath, cough, or wheezing.
- *Gastrointestinal.* Signs or symptoms involving the gastrointestinal system, such as indigestion or diarrhea.
- *Genitourinary.* Signs or symptoms involving the genitourinary system, such as bedwetting, painful urination, or erectile dysfunction.
- *Musculoskeletal.* Signs or symptoms involving the musculoskeletal system, such as muscle cramps or joint pain or swelling.
- *Integumentary.* Signs or symptoms involving the skin (such as itching or rash) and the breasts (such as breast tenderness or lumps).
- *Neurological.* Signs or symptoms involving the neurologic system, such as dizziness, tingling, confusion, or paralysis.
- *Psychiatric.* Signs or symptoms involving the psychiatric system, such as depression or mood swings.
- *Endocrine.* Signs or symptoms involving the endocrine system, such as elevated blood sugar readings, increases in appetite or thirst, or intolerance to heat or cold.
- *Hematologic/lymphatic.* Signs or symptoms involving the hematologic and lymphatic systems, such as bruising easily and swollen glands.
- *Allergic/immunologic.* Signs or symptoms involving the allergic and immunologic systems, such as allergic reactions to certain foods or medications or frequent sneezing.

Like the answers to the HPI questions, the answers involving a review of systems help the healthcare provider determine the focus of the physical examination. There are three levels of ROS: problem pertinent, extended, and complete. A problem-pertinent ROS is the review of one system. An extended ROS is the review of two to nine systems. A complete ROS is the review of 10 or more systems (CMS 1995; CMS 1997).

Key to Success

Remember, this section of the key component of history—ROS—is still only *talking* with the healthcare provider. It is easy to confuse this section with an examination of each of these body systems, so it is important to keep in mind that this is only a question and answer session between the healthcare provider and patient. The answers to these questions help the provider determine what to observe in the physical examination part of the E/M service.

Past, Family, Social History

The **past, family, social history (PFSH)** is the section of the history component in which the provider asks the patient questions about his or her past healthcare history, family healthcare history, and social habits. These elements may be important in helping the healthcare provider understand the importance of certain signs or symptoms, or may raise further questions or concerns regarding the patient's health.

Past history includes the patient's experiences with childhood diseases, illnesses, operations, hospitalizations, treatments, and medications. Allergies can be accounted for in this section of questioning and in the review of systems, but they can only be accounted for once (either in the ROS or in the PFSH). It is important to keep in mind that these are historical conditions, meaning they are no longer active conditions.

Family history includes relevant family healthcare history, such as history of chronic conditions and malignancies, and other genetic factors like hereditary conditions.

Social history is a review of the patient's current and past social activities. This includes all relevant information regarding high-risk behaviors, such as drinking, smoking, or drug use, as well as environmental factors like the patient's work or home environment.

The amount of questions asked by the provider regarding a patient's PFSH establishes the level of PFSH obtained. There are two possible levels of past, family, social history—pertinent and complete. A pertinent PFSH is the documentation of at least one element from one of the three histories (past, family, and social). A complete PFSH depends on whether the patient is new or established. For new patients, one item from each of the three histories is required; for established patients, one item from two of the three histories is required. Refer to figure 8.4 to see how the elements of history are related to each other (CMS 1995; CMS 1997).

Putting It All Together: Determining the Level of History

The numerous factors of the elements of HPI, ROS, and PFSH are combined to determine the level of history completed for the encounter (see table 8.1). Note that the chief complaint does not factor into these calculations. It is a given that the chief complaint is considered in the documentation for each and every encounter. In table 8.1, the first column lists the level of the key component history, with the next three columns identifying the level of HPI, ROS, and PFSH, respectively, to meet that level of history. For example, a detailed history must have an extended HPI, an extended ROS, and a pertinent PFSH.

According to E/M documentation guidelines, to determine the level of history, three of the three elements must be met or exceeded. The level of each of the elements of the history performed (ROS, HPI, PFSH) must meet or exceed the level performed in order to select that level (CMS 1995; CMS 1997).

For example, if a provider performed an extended HPI, extended ROS, and pertinent PFSH, then the level of history would be detailed (see table 8.2). As another example, if a provider performed a brief HPI, extended ROS, and pertinent PFSH, the level of history performed would be expanded problem focused (see table 8.3). In this case, three out of the three levels must be met or exceeded. Because the level of HPI did not exceed brief, the level of history performed must be selected as expanded problem focused. In other words, the lowest level of *any* element of the HPI is the limiting factor. An HPI higher than the lowest level of any element documented in the HPI cannot be selected.

Figure 8.4. Relationship of the elements of history

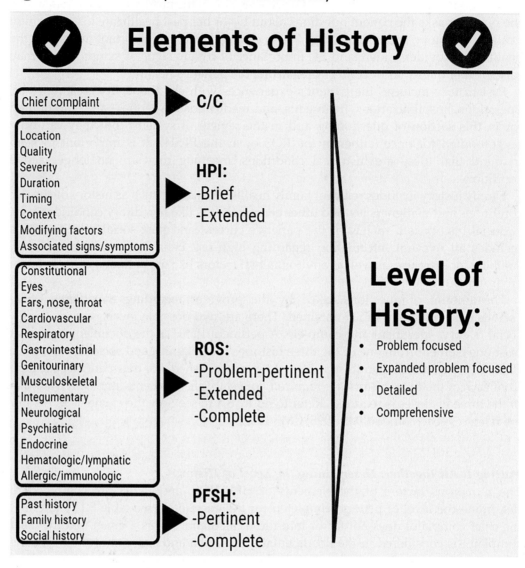

Elements of History

Chief complaint	▶ **C/C**
Location Quality Severity Duration Timing Context Modifying factors Associated signs/symptoms	▶ **HPI:** -Brief -Extended
Constitutional Eyes Ears, nose, throat Cardiovascular Respiratory Gastrointestinal Genitourinary Musculoskeletal Integumentary Neurological Psychiatric Endocrine Hematologic/lymphatic Allergic/immunologic	▶ **ROS:** -Problem-pertinent -Extended -Complete
Past history Family history Social history	▶ **PFSH:** -Pertinent -Complete

Level of History:

- Problem focused
- Expanded problem focused
- Detailed
- Comprehensive

The history is only one of the key components of an E/M service. It is necessary to understand the elements of the remaining two key components—examination and medical decision-making—to determine the level of each and ultimately the level of the E/M service performed. But first complete the exercises in There's a Code for That 8.1 to practice determining the level of history.

Table 8.1. Determining the level of history

Level of History	HPI	ROS	PFSH
Problem focused	Brief	N/A	N/A
Expanded problem focused	Brief	Problem pertinent	N/A
Detailed	Extended	Extended	Pertinent
Comprehensive	Extended	Complete	Complete

Table 8.2. Level of history: Detailed (all levels met)

Level of History	HPI	ROS	PFSH
Problem focused	Brief	N/A	N/A
Expanded problem focused	Brief	Problem pertinent	N/A
Detailed	(Extended)	(Extended)	(Pertinent)
Comprehensive	Extended	Complete	Complete

Table 8.3. Level of history: Expanded problem focused (lowest common denominator)

Level of History	HPI	ROS	PFSH
Problem focused	Brief	N/A	N/A
Expanded problem focused	(Brief)	Problem pertinent	N/A
Detailed	Extended	(Extended)	(Pertinent)
Comprehensive	Extended	Complete	Complete

Determine the level of history

8.1

There's a Code for That

Read the following documentation of the E/M service and determine the level of history for the encounter. You will need to determine the level of each individual element (HPI, ROS, and PFSH), and then determine the level of history provided.

1. Determine the level of HPI from the following encounter: *Established 12-year-old male presents with pain and swelling in his right knee. He plays football at his secondary school and was hit on his knee during a game three days ago by one of the other players. The pain was initially an 8 out of 10, but it quickly subsided to about a 4 out of 10. He now states that it is constantly aching is difficult to walk on, and the pain is worse in the morning. When he lies down and raises his leg with pillows, the pain does subside to a 2 or 3. He does not describe any numbness, tingling, or redness of skin.*

   How many elements of HPI are described in this passage? _____

   What is the level of HPI? _____

2. Determine the level of ROS from the same encounter: *Patient reports feeling generally fine, other than the knee pain. No allergies or immunologic problems, no rash or swelling of any areas other than the right knee, and no bruising. He does report feeling a few muscle cramps in his right thigh, especially at the end of the day after he has been on his feet all day. No tingling in the knee, just constant pain, which goes from a 2 to a 4 out of 10. Pain is generally all over the knee, he cannot tell if it is worse on the front or back, but does seem to be worse on the inner aspect of the knee.*

   How many systems were reviewed in the ROS? _____

   What is the level of ROS? _____

(Continued on next page)

8.1

Continued

3. Determine the level of PFSH from the same encounter. *No known drug allergies, history of arthritis or joint problems, or immunologic problems. No relevant past injuries. No family history of osteoarthritis or joint problems. Patient is active in sports, plays football at school on a daily basis.*

Is this patient new or established? _____

How many elements of the PFSH are documented (how many elements from how many systems)? _____

What is the level of PFSH? _____

4. Using the level of HPI, ROS, and PFSH as determined, what is the level of history for this encounter? _____

Examination

The extent and subject of the examination are determined by the healthcare provider, based on his or her clinical judgment, the patient's history, and the nature of the presenting problem(s). The level of the examination performed is determined by the number of body areas and organ systems observed during the encounter. Remember that the examination is the objective component of an evaluation and management service; it is the physical study of the patient by the healthcare provider. The history is the patient *talking* with the provider, whereas the examination is the provider *doing* the examination.

Body areas are general areas of the body, rather than specific organ systems, that may be examined during an evaluation and management encounter. The CPT code book recognizes the following body areas.

- General appearance
- Head, including the face
- Neck
- Chest, including the breasts and axilla
- Abdomen
- Genitalia, groin, buttocks
- Back
- Each extremity (upper and lower)

Organ systems are the specific groups of organs that may be examined during an evaluation and management encounter. The CPT code book recognizes the following organ systems.

- Eyes
- Ear, nose, mouth, and throat
- Cardiovascular
- Respiratory
- Gastrointestinal
- Genitourinary
- Musculoskeletal
- Skin
- Neurologic

- Psychiatric
- Hematologic/lymphatic/immunologic

The level of the examination performed depends on the number of body areas and organ systems involved in the examination. There are four levels of examination, which range from minimal to more extensive or complete.

- *Problem focused*. This is a limited examination of the affected body area or organ system.
- *Expanded problem focused*. This is a limited examination of the affected body area or organ system and other symptomatic or related organ systems.
- *Detailed*. This is an extended examination of the affected body area or organ system and other symptomatic or related organ systems.
- *Comprehensive*. This is either a general multisystem examination or a complete examination of a single organ system.

The determination of the level of examination is made more complex by the differences in evaluation and management guidelines. Both the 1995 and 1997 DGs require a varying number of elements in order to select a certain level of examination. For example, the 1995 guidelines require documentation of two to seven elements examined to support an expanded problem-focused exam (CMS 1995), whereas 1997 guidelines require six to eleven elements examined (CMS 1997).

The level of the examination depends on the number of body areas or organ systems that were studied (see table 8.4). For example, if one body area was examined, then the level of the exam was problem focused. If eight or more organ systems were examined, then the level of examination was comprehensive. Remember, when determining the level of the evaluation and management code, the coder must use *either* the 1995 *or* the 1997 DGs. The coder may use whichever set of guidelines that are the most beneficial, as long as they are consistent in using the same set of guidelines per each encounter.

Table 8.4. Determining the level of examination

Level of Exam	Exam Components	Number of Body Areas/Organ Systems: 1995 Guidelines	Number of Body Areas/Organ Systems: 1997 Guidelines
Problem focused	Limited exam of affected body area/organ system	1 body area or organ system	1 to 5 body areas or organ systems
Expanded problem focused	Limited exam of affected area and other related/symptomatic organ systems	2 to 7 body areas or organ systems	6 to 11 body areas or organ systems
Detailed	Extended exam of affected area and other related/symptomatic organ systems	Extended exam of 2 to 7 body areas or organ systems	2 areas of examination from 6 organ systems
Comprehensive	General multisystem exam or complete exam of single organ system	8 or more organ systems	2 areas of examination from 9 organ systems

The final key component is medical decision-making; it is the last determination needed before the level of evaluation and management service can be identified. Before reviewing this component, complete the exercise in There's a Code for That 8.2 to practice determining the level of examination.

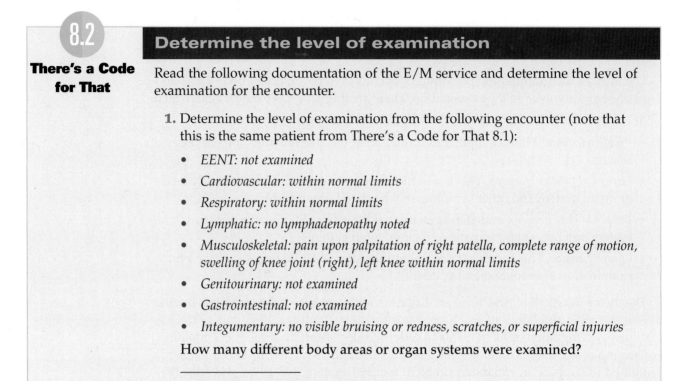

8.2

There's a Code for That

Determine the level of examination

Read the following documentation of the E/M service and determine the level of examination for the encounter.

1. Determine the level of examination from the following encounter (note that this is the same patient from There's a Code for That 8.1):

   - *EENT: not examined*
   - *Cardiovascular: within normal limits*
   - *Respiratory: within normal limits*
   - *Lymphatic: no lymphadenopathy noted*
   - *Musculoskeletal: pain upon palpitation of right patella, complete range of motion, swelling of knee joint (right), left knee within normal limits*
   - *Genitourinary: not examined*
   - *Gastrointestinal: not examined*
   - *Integumentary: no visible bruising or redness, scratches, or superficial injuries*

   How many different body areas or organ systems were examined?

   _____

   What is the level of examination? _____

Medical Decision-Making

The third key component for E/M services is medical decision-making (MDM). As discussed in chapter 7, there are three considerations in determining the level of medical decision-making for an E/M service—number of diagnoses and management options, amount and/or complexity of data to be reviewed, and risk of complications and/or morbidity or mortality (AMA 2017). The levels of work for each of these three elements are identified to determine the level of medical decision-making. If the key component history is *talking*, and the key component examination is *doing*, then the key component medical decision-making is *thinking* (see figure 8.5). The MDM component of an E/M service is the pivotal component in an encounter, and appropriate documentation can guarantee or prevent the accurate selection of the E/M service level. It is important to ensure that the MDM is fully documented.

Figure 8.5. Three key components

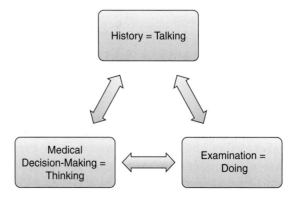

MDM consists of assembling findings from the patient's history and examination, determining a diagnosis (if possible), and weighing the pros and cons of certain treatments, while taking into account the risk of the condition and any additional tests that should be ordered or reviewed. In other words, MDM is the healthcare provider doing what they have been trained to do—use his or her medical expertise to make a decision regarding the patient's condition.

Number of Diagnoses and Management Options
The number of diagnoses and management options is the element of MDM that considers other possible diagnoses or treatment options for the patient, based on the relative difficulty in determining the patient's diagnosis, as well as the status of the problem (such as if it is worsening or stable).

E/M auditing tools are commonly used to help coders determine the exact level of the three key components, including the level of medical decision-making. These audit tools are pre-formatted forms with specific sections for each key component (history, examination, and MDM), and include separate areas to indicate if each element of each key component has been documented or performed (see figure 8.6). These forms usually break down each element into points that can be tallied according to the amount of each element documented in the health record from a specific visit, and then calculated to determine the exact level of each key component.

E/M auditing forms are varied and differ from payer to payer. Some are based on 1995 DGs, whereas others are based on 1997 DGs; and many auditing forms allow the coder to use either 1995 or 1997 DGs. The points system used in the forms may vary from payer to payer, so it is important to check with the insurance payer before using a specific form.

There are four levels of complexity for this element of medical decision-making: minimal, limited, multiple, and extensive. Using a point system aligned with E/M documentation guidelines (either 1995 or 1997, or both), coders can determine which level to choose based on the documentation (see table 8.5). On most audit forms, a minor problem that would likely resolve if the patient had not come in for treatment, may be worth one point. A patient usually has more than one of these minor problems, but only a maximum of two points may be counted no matter the amount of minor problems. Established, stable, or improving conditions would each be worth one point. Established, worsening conditions would be two points. A health problem that is new to the provider, but that does not require any additional workup, is three points (this can only be counted once, even if there is more than one new problem present). A health problem that is new to the provider and requires additional workup would be four points.

The points are added to create a total score for the number of diagnoses and management options, which determines the level of this element, as follows (Novitas 2017).

- Minimal: One point
- Limited: Two points
- Multiple: Three points
- Extensive: Four points

For example, if a patient came saw a provider for a localized rash that did not require any further workup and was already resolving without treatment, this problem would be assigned one point. The level assigned for the number of diagnoses and management options would be *minimal*. On the other hand, if the same patient came in with a severe rash that was worsening by spreading to other areas of the body, and this problem was new to the treating provider who ordered additional workup by testing the patient

Figure 8.6. Example E/M auditing form

History

Refer to data section (table below) in order to quantify. After referring to data, circle the entry farthest to the *RIGHT* in the table, which best describes the HPI, ROS and PFSH. If one column contains three circles, draw a line down that column to the bottom row to identify the type of history. If no column contains three circles, the column containing a circle farthest to the *LEFT*, identifies the type of history.

After completing this table which classifies the history, circle the type of history within the appropriate grid in Section 5.

HISTORY				
HPI: Status of chronic conditions: ☐ 1 condition ☐ 2 conditions ☐ 3 conditions **OR**		☐ Status of 1-2 chronic conditions		☐ Status of 3 chronic conditions
HPI (history of present illness) elements: ☐ Location ☐ Severity ☐ Timing ☐ Modifying factors ☐ Quality ☐ Duration ☐ Context ☐ Associated signs and symptoms		☐ Brief (1-3)		☐ Extended (4 or more)
ROS (review of systems): ☐ Constitutional (wt loss, etc) ☐ Ears,nose, mouth, throat ☐ GI ☐ Integumentary (skin, breast) ☐ Endo ☐ Eyes ☐ Card/vasc ☐ GU ☐ Hem/lymph ☐ Musculo ☐ Neuro ☐ All/immuno ☐ Resp ☐ Psych ☐ All others negative	☐ None	☐ Pertinent to problem (1 system)	☐ Extended (2-9 systems)	☐ *Complete
PFSH (past medical, family, social history) areas: ☐ Past history (the patient's past experiences with illnesses, operation, injuries and treatments) ☐ Family history (a review of medical events in the patient's family, including diseases which may be hereditary or place the patient at risk) ☐ Social history (an age appropriate review of past and current activities)		☐ None	☐ Pertinent (1 history area)	☐ **Complete (2 or 3 history areas)
	PROBLEM FOCUSED	**EXP.PROB. FOCUSED**	**DETAILED**	**COMPRE-HENSIVE**

Examination

Refer to data section (table below) in order to quantify. After referring to data, identify the type of examination. Circle the type of examination within the appropriate grid in Section 5.

Limited to affected body area or organ system (one body area or system related to problem)	**PROBLEM FOCUSED EXAM**
Affected body area or organ system and other symptomatic or related organ system(s) (additional systems up to total of 7)	**EXPANDED PROBLEM FOCUSED EXAM**
Extended exam of affected area(s) and other symptomatic or related organ system(s) (additional systems up to total of 7 or more depth than above)	**DETAILED EXAM**
General multi-system exam (8 or more systems) or complete exam of a single organ system (complete single exam not defined in these instructions)	**COMPREHENSIVE EXAM**

EXAM				
Body areas: ☐ Head, including face ☐ Chest, including breasts and axillae ☐ Abdomen ☐ Neck ☐ Back, including spine ☐ Genitalia, groin, buttocks ☐ Each extremity **Organ systems:** ☐ Constitutional (e.g., vitals, gen app) ☐ Ears,nose, mouth, throat ☐ Resp ☐ Musculo ☐ Psych ☐ GI ☐ Skin ☐ Hem/lymph/imm ☐ Eyes ☐ Cardiovascular ☐ GU ☐ Neuro	☐ 1 body area or system	☐ Up to 7 systems	☐ Up to 7 systems	☐ 8 or more systems
	PROBLEM FOCUSED	**EXP.PROB. FOCUSED**	**DETAILED**	**COMPRE-HENSIVE**

Medical Decision Making

Number of Diagnoses or Treatment Options

Identify each problem or treatment option mentioned in the record. Enter the number in each of the categories in Column B in the table below. (There are maximum number in two categories.)

Number of Diagnoses or Treatment Options

A		B	X	C	=	D
Problem(s) Status		**Number**		**Points**		**Result**
Self-limited or minor (stable, improved or worsening)	Max = 2			1		
Est. problem (to examiner); stable, improved				1		
Est. problem (to examiner); worsening				2		
New problem (to examiner); no additional workup planned	Max = 1			3		
New prob. (to examiner); add. workup planned				4		
				TOTAL		

Multiply the number in columns B & C and put the product in column D. Enter a total for column D.

Bring total to **line A** in Final Result for Complexity (table below)

Amount and/or Complexity of Data Reviewed

For each category of reviewed data identified, circle the number in the points column. Total the points.

Amount and/or Complexity of Data Reviewed

Reviewed Data	Points
Review and/or order of clinical lab tests	1
Review and/or order of tests in the radiology section of CPT	1
Review and/or order of tests in the medicine section of CPT	1
Discussion of test results with performing physician	1
Decision to obtain old records and/or obtain history from someone other than patient	1
Review and summarization of old records and/or obtaining history from someone other than patient and/or discussion of case with another health care provider	2
Independent visualization of image, tracing or specimen itself (not simply review of report)	2
TOTAL	

Bring total to **line C** in Final Result for Complexity (table below)

Use the risk table below as a guide to assign risk factors. It is understood that the table below does not contain all specific instances of medical care; the table is intended to be used as a guide. Circle the most appropriate factor(s) in each category. The overall measure of risk is the highest level circled. Enter the level of risk identified in Final Result for Complexity (table below).

Risk of Complications and/or Morbidity or Mortality

Level of Risk	Presenting Problem(s)	Diagnostic Procedure(s) Ordered	Management Options Selected
Minimal	• One self-limited or minor problem, e.g., cold, insect bite, tinea corporis	• Laboratory tests requiring venipuncture • Chest x-rays • EKG/EEG • Urinalysis • Ultrasound, e.g., echo • KOH prep	• Rest • Gargles • Elastic bandages • Superficial dressings
Low	• Two or more self-limited or minor problems • One stable chronic illness, e.g., well controlled hypertension or non-insulin dependent diabetes, cataract, BPH • Acute uncomplicated illness or injury, e.g., cystitis, allergic rhinitis, simple sprain	• Physiologic tests not under stress, e.g.,pulmonary function tests • Non-cardiovascular imaging studies with contrast, e.g., barium enema • Superficial needle biopsies • Clincal laboratory tests requiring arterial puncture • Skin biopsies	• Over-the-counter drugs • Minor surgery with no identified risk factors • Physical therapy • Occupational therapy • IV fluids without additives
Moderate	• One or more chronic illnesses with mild exacerbation, progression, or side effects of treatment • Two or more stable chronic illnesses • Undiagnosed new problem with uncertain prognosis, e.g., lump in breast • Acute illness with systemic symptoms, e.g., pyelonephritis, pneumonitis, colitis • Acute complicated injury, e.g., head injury with brief loss of consciousness	• Physiologic tests under stress, e.g., cardiac stress test, fetal contraction stress test • Diagnostic endoscopies with no identified risk factors • Deep needle or incisional biopsy • Cardiovascular imaging studies with contrast and no identified risk factors, e.g., arteriogram cardiac cath • Obtain fluid from body cavity, e.g., lumbar puncture, thoracentesis, culdocentesis	• Minor surgery with identified risk factors • Elective major surgery (open, percutaneous or endoscopic) with no identified risk factors • Prescription drug management • Therapeutic nuclear medicine • IV fluids with additives • Closed treatment of fracture or dislocation without manipulation
High	• One or more chronic illnesses with severe exacerbation, progression, or side effects of treatment • Acute or chronic illnesses or injuries that may pose a threat to life or bodily function, e.g., multiple trauma, acute MI, pulmonary embolus, severe respiratory distress, progressive severe rheumatoid arthritis, psychiatric illness with potential threat to self or others, peritonitis, acute renal failure • An abrupt change in neurologic status, e.g., seizure, TIA, weakness or sensory loss	• Cardiovascular imaging studies with contrast with identified risk factors • Cardiac electrophysiological tests • Diagnostic endoscopies with identified risk factors • Discography	• Elective major surgery (open, percutaneous or endoscopic with identified risk factors) • Emergency major surgery (open, percutaneous or endoscopic) • Parenteral controlled substances • Drug therapy requiring intensive monitoring for toxicity • Decision not to resuscitate or to de-escalate care because of poor prognosis

Final Result for Complexity

Draw a line down any column with 2 or 3 circles to identify the type of decision making in that column. Otherwise, draw a line down the column with the 2nd circle from the left. After completing this table, which classifies complexity, circle the type of decision making within the appropriate grid in Section 5.

A	Number diagnoses or treatment options	1 Minimal	2 Limited	3 Multiple	4 Extensive
B	Highest Risk	Minimal	Low	Moderate	High
C	Amount and complexity of data	1 Minimal or low	2 Limited	3 Multiple	4 Extensive
	Type of decision making	STRAIGHT-FORWARD	LOW COMPLEX.	MODERATE COMPLEX.	HIGH COMPLEX.

Source: Novitas Solutions 2017.

MEDICAL DECISION MAKING

for allergies, this would be assigned four points (a new problem with additional workup). The level assigned for the number of diagnoses and management options for this problem would be *extensive*. Refer to table 8.5 and the Number of Diagnoses or Treatment Options within the Medical Decision-making section of the auditing form (figure 8.6) to calculate the previous examples.

Table 8.5. Example of the number of diagnoses and management options

Number of Diagnoses and Management Options	Points
Minor problem (self-resolving)	1 each for a maximum of 2
Established (stable or improving)	1 each
Established (worsening)	2 each
New problem (no additional workup)	3
New problem (with additional workup)	4
Total	

Source: Adapted from Novitas 2017.

The number of diagnoses and management options is only the first part of the calculation to determine the level of medical decision-making for an evaluation and management service. The next component is the amount and/or complexity of data to be reviewed.

Amount and/or Complexity of Data

The amount and/or complexity of data to be reviewed is a measure of the need to order or review tests, or the need to gather and review additional data regarding the patient's condition. The work involved in this element includes planning, scheduling, and performing, as well as reviewing lab tests, radiologic services, and other diagnostic services. It also includes the review of past healthcare history and requesting and reviewing old health records.

There are also four levels of complexity for this element of medical decision-making: minimal or none, limited, moderate, and extensive. A points system aligned with E/M documentation guidelines (either 1995 or 1997, or both), can be used to determine the level of work involved for this element of medical decision-making (see table 8.6). Review of clinical labs, medical tests, and radiological tests would be assigned one point. No matter how many different tests were reviewed, only one point should be assigned for lab or radiologic tests. As many points as necessary may be assigned for tests from the Medicine section of the CPT code book. Examples of how points may be assigned for calculating the amount and/or complexity of data are as follows (Novitas 2017):

- Discussing the results of a test with another healthcare provider = one point.
- Deciding to obtain old records or additional healthcare history from a person other than the patient = one point.
- Reviewing and summarizing data from old records or additional history gathered from a person other than the patient = two points.
- Independent or secondary interpretation of a lab specimen or diagnostic examination results = two points (keep in mind that this is not ordering the test or reviewing another provider's interpretation, but providing a new, independent interpretation of the test results).

Table 8.6. Example of the amount and/or complexity of data

Amount and/or Complexity of Data	Points
Lab ordered or reviewed	1 maximum
Radiologic exam ordered or reviewed	1 maximum
Medicine section test ordered or reviewed	1 each
Discussion of results with performing provider	1
Decision to obtain old records or history	1
Reviewing and summarizing old records, history, or discussion with other health provider	2
Independent interpretation of test results	2
Total	

Source: Adapted from Novitas 2017.

The points are added to create a total score for the amount and/or complexity of data to be reviewed, which determines the level of this element, as follows (Novitas 2017):

- Minimal or none: Zero to one point
- Limited: Two points
- Moderate: Three points
- Extensive: Four points

For example, if a patient came in complaining of a sore throat and the provider chose to perform a strep throat swab in the office (a clinical lab test), then this would be assigned one point (for lab ordered and reviewed). The level for this element would be *minimal*. But if the same patient presented with trouble swallowing and a swallow study was performed (a medicine section test—one point), and the doctor made the decision to order old health records from the patient's previous doctor (one point), as well as discuss the results from a previous swallow study with another healthcare provider (one point), then three total points would be assigned for this element. The level for this element of medical decision-making would be *moderate*. Refer to table 8.6 and the Risk of Complications and/or Morbidity or Mortality table in figure 8.6 for additional factors that may be calculated to identify the level of risk for a patient.

The last component in the calculation of the level of medical decision-making is the risk of complications and/or morbidity or mortality posed by the patient's condition.

Risk of Complications and/or Morbidity or Mortality
The last element that must be considered in medical decision-making is the risk of complications and/or morbidity or mortality from the patient's condition. In other words, how dangerous is the patient's condition? The risk is based on the healthcare provider's determination of the probability that the patient will become seriously ill or diseased, experience complications from the condition, or die. There are a few components considered in this calculation of risk, including the nature of the presenting problem, urgency of the visit, any comorbid (coexisting) conditions, and the need for surgery.

There are four levels of complexity for this element of medical decision-making: minimal, low, moderate, and high. Unlike the other two elements, a points system is not used to determine the level of this element of medical decision-making. According to both 1995 and 1997 DGs, the levels of this element are determined according to the nature of the presenting problem, diagnostic procedures ordered, and management options selected.

- Minimal: One self-limited or minor problem
- Low:
    - Two or more self-limited or minor problems, *or*
    - One stable chronic illness, *or*
    - Acute uncomplicated illness or injury

- Moderate:
    - One or more chronic illnesses with mild exacerbation, progression, or side effects, *or*
    - Two or more chronic stable illnesses, *or*
    - Undiagnosed new problem with uncertain prognosis, *or*
    - Acute illness with systemic symptoms, *or*
    - Acute complicated injury

- High:
    - One or more chronic illnesses with severe exacerbation, progression, or side effects, *or*
    - Acute or chronic illness/injury that poses a threat to life or bodily function, *or*
    - An abrupt change in neurologic status (CMS 1995; CMS 1997)

For example, if a patient presented to the office and the presenting problem was for a referral of allergy medication in a patient with well-controlled allergies, then the level of risk would be low for this patient (one stable chronic illness). On the other hand, if this same patient came in to the office in anaphylactic shock due to an allergic reaction and the provider had to admit the patient to the hospital, then the risk for this patient would be high (acute or chronic illness/injury that poses a threat to life or bodily function). Refer to table 8.6 and the Amount and/or Complexity of Data Reviewed table in the Medical Decision-making section of the auditing form (figure 8.6) to calculate the previous examples.

Once all levels of the three elements of medical decision-making are determined, it is necessary to combine them to determine the level of the medical decision-making for the encounter.

Putting It All Together: Determining the Level of Medical Decision-Making

To determine the level of the medical decision-making for the encounter, it is necessary to identify the number of diagnoses or management options, the amount and/or complexity of data to be reviewed, and the risk of complications and/or morbidity or mortality. There are four levels of MDM: straightforward, low complexity, moderate complexity, and high complexity (see table 8.7). To qualify for a certain level of MDM, **two** out of the **three** levels must be met or exceeded.

For example, if a patient came in for an evaluation and management encounter and the number of diagnoses or treatment options involved was minimal, the data reviewed was limited, and the risk involved was low, then the level of MDM would be *low* because two out of the three levels were met or exceeded (see table 8.8). If, however, the number of diagnoses was extensive, the amount of data to be reviewed was moderate, and the risk involved was low, then the level of MDM for the encounter would be *moderate* (see table 8.9).

Table 8.7. Determine the level of medical decision-making

Level of MDM	Number of Diagnosis or Management Options	Amount and/or Complexity of Data	Risk Involved
Straightforward	Minimal	Minimal or none	Minimal
Low	Limited	Limited	Low
Moderate	Multiple	Moderate	Moderate
High	Extensive	Extensive	High

Table 8.8. Level of MDM: Low (two levels met or exceeded)

Level of MDM	Number of Diagnosis or Management Options	Amount and/or Complexity of Data	Risk Involved
Straightforward	(Minimal)	Minimal or none	Minimal
⇒ **Low**	Limited	(Limited)	(Low)
Moderate	Multiple	Moderate	Moderate
High	Extensive	Extensive	High

Table 8.9. Level of MDM: Moderate (two levels met or exceeded)

Level of MDM	Number of Diagnosis or Management Options	Amount and/or Complexity of Data	Risk Involved
Straightforward	Minimal	Minimal or none	Minimal
Low	Limited	Limited	(Low)
⇒ **Moderate**	Multiple	(Moderate)	Moderate
High	(Extensive)	Extensive	High

For practice determining the level of MDM, complete the exercises in There's a Code for That 8.3 to practice determining the level of medical decision-making.

Determine the level of medical decision-making

8.3

There's a Code for That

Read the following documentation of the E/M service for the patient from There's a Code for That 8.1 and 8.2 and determine the level of MDM for the encounter. You will need to determine both the level of each individual element (HPI, ROS, and PFSH) and then the level of history provided.

1. Calculate the points for the number of diagnoses and management options for this encounter, using the following table: *This is a new problem to the provider today, condition seems stable but will require additional work up to determine diagnosis.*

Number of Diagnoses and Management Options	Points
Minor problem (self-resolving)	1 each for a maximum of 2
Established (stable or improving)	1 each
Established (worsening)	2 each

(Continued on next page)

8.3

Continued

New problem (no additional workup)	3
New problem (with additional workup)	4
Total	

How many points are scored for the number of diagnoses? _____

What is the level of this element of MDM? _____

2. Calculate the points for the amount and/or complexity of data to be reviewed for this encounter, using the following table: *Ordered complete x-ray of right knee, will review radiologist report and follow-up as needed.*

Amount and/or Complexity of Data	Points
Lab ordered or reviewed	1 maximum
Radiologic exam ordered or reviewed	1 maximum
Medicine section test ordered or reviewed	1 each
Discussion of results with performing provider	1
Decision to obtain old records or history	1
Reviewing and summarizing old records, history, or discussion with other health provider	2
Independent interpretation of test results	2
Total	

How many points are scored for the amount and/or complexity of data?

_____

What is the level of this element of MDM? _____

3. Calculate the points for the risk of complications and/or morbidity or mortality for this encounter, using the following table: *Working diagnosis of knee joint pain secondary to injury.*

Level of MDM	Presenting Problem(s)
Minimal	• One self-limited of minor problem
Low	• Two or more self-limited or minor problems • One stable chronic illness • Acute uncomplicated illness or injury
Moderate	• One or more chronic illnesses with mild exacerbation, progression, or side effects • Two or more stable chronic illnesses • Undiagnosed new problem with uncertain prognosis • Acute illness with systemic complications • Acute complicated injury
High	• One or more chronic illnesses with severe exacerbation, progression, or side effects • Acute or chronic illness/injury that poses a threat to life or bodily function • An abrupt change in neurologic status

Source: Adapted from CMS 1995; CMS 1997.

What is the level of this element of MDM? _____

4. Using the level of number of diagnoses, amount and/or complexity of data, and risk, what is the level of MDM for this encounter? _____

_____

Determine the Level of the E/M Service

Once the levels of the three key components have been determined, it is possible to establish the level of the E/M service. As a review from chapter 7, there are three key components to an E/M service—history, examination, and medical decision-making. There are four levels of complexity for each of these key components, as follows.

- History: problem focused, expanded problem focused, detailed, comprehensive
- Examination: problem focused, expanded problem focused, detailed, comprehensive
- Medical decision-making: straightforward, low, moderate, high

Once the levels of each of the three key components are identified, they must be matched to the description of an E/M code, according to how many of the key components are necessary. Look at the description for the following code and notice which of the key components are needed for code selection:

99213, Office or other outpatient visit for the evaluation and management of an established patient, which requires at least 2 of the 3 key components:

- An expanded problem-focused history
- An expanded problem-focused examination
- Medical decision-making of low complexity

This code requires that at least two of the three key components be at or above the level identified in the code description. Some E/M codes require that all three levels of the key components match, such as E/M codes for new patients, initial inpatient or hospital observation care, consultations, and emergency department visits. When this is the case, the levels of all three key components must be at or above the levels identified in the code description.

Use the information from There's a Code for That 8.1, 8.2, and 8.3 to complete the exercises in There's a Code for That 8.4 to practice determining the level of E/M code.

Determine the level of E/M code

8.4

There's a Code for That

Refer to the previous exercises in this chapter and list the following (keep in mind that this is for an established patient office visit):

1. There's a Code for That 8.1

   Level of history: _____

2. There's a Code for That 8.2

   Level of Examination: _____

3. There's a Code for That 8.3

   Level of MDM: _____

4. Using the levels listed previously and your CPT code book, identify the E/M code for this encounter.

   CPT Code: _____

Prolonged Services

In certain circumstances, a healthcare provider may spend an inordinate amount of time with a patient, either face-to-face or without direct patient contact, to manage or treat the patient's condition. These are considered **prolonged services**. These codes are useful for those rare instances when a patient is extremely sick or extra time is required to treat or manage the patient's condition, or to counsel the patient regarding his or her health status. Codes for prolonged services (99354–99416) are used when the healthcare practitioner provides an E/M service that is longer or more difficult than what could be represented by the highest level of E/M code. The prolonged service code is reported in addition to the code for the primary evaluation and management procedure (for example, 99201–99215).

There are three types of prolonged service codes:

- Prolonged services with direct patient contact (99354–99357).
  - Office or other outpatient setting (99354 and 99355)
  - Inpatient or observation setting (99356 and 99357)

- Prolonged services without direct patient contact (99358 and 99359)
- Prolonged clinical staff services with physician or other qualified healthcare professional supervision (99415 and 99416)

All prolonged service codes are time-based codes—the only factor considered during selection of these codes is the extra amount of service time that was provided to the patient. Most prolonged service codes are also add-on codes that must be added to the primary code for the evaluation and management service, such as an outpatient office visit code. For example, code 99354, Prolonged evaluation and management or psychotherapy service(s) (beyond the typical service time of the primary procedure) in the office or outpatient setting requiring direct patient contact beyond the usual service; first hour, identifies one extra hour of direct face-to-face time provided to the patient in the outpatient office setting. Each type of prolonged service has additional add-on codes used to identify additional time *over* the first hour of prolonged service time. For the outpatient office setting, this code is 99355, Prolonged evaluation and management or psychotherapy service(s) (beyond the typical service time of the primary procedure) in the office or outpatient setting requiring direct patient contact beyond the usual service; each additional 30 minutes. Notice that code 99354 counts for the first hour of prolonged services, and code 99355 can be added as many times as necessary for each additional 30 minutes of prolonged service time.

Coding for prolonged services requires a careful calculation of the extra time spent with the patient. Each E/M code identifies a specific amount of time, on which the level of the code should be based (if using time as the determining factor for code selection)—the time spent with the patient that is calculated as part of the initial E/M service. For example, see the description for code 99215 in figure 8.7.

Code 99215 includes 40 minutes of face-to-face time spent with the patient. If the healthcare provider spent 90 minutes in the office face-to-face with the patient, then it would necessitate reporting a prolonged service code because 90 minutes exceeds the 40 minutes reported by code 99215. Note that in order to bill for a prolonged service, the time limit listed in the primary code (like the 40 minutes in code 99215) must be *over* 30 minutes. The prolonged service code should not be reported for anything less than an additional 30 minutes. In the outpatient setting, anything over the first additional 30 minutes, over the 40 minutes identified in the code for the primary procedure, should be reported with a prolonged services code.

Figure 8.7. Code description for 99215

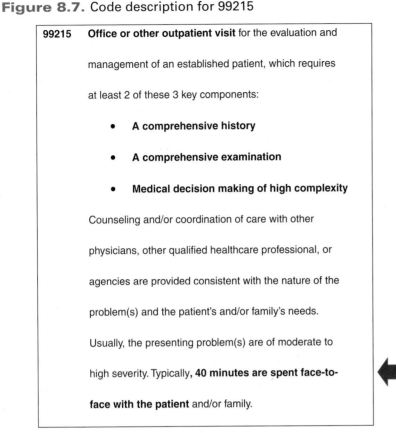

> **99215**   **Office or other outpatient visit** for the evaluation and
>
> management of an established patient, which requires
>
> at least 2 of these 3 key components:
>
> - **A comprehensive history**
>
> - **A comprehensive examination**
>
> - **Medical decision making of high complexity**
>
> Counseling and/or coordination of care with other
>
> physicians, other qualified healthcare professional, or
>
> agencies are provided consistent with the nature of the
>
> problem(s) and the patient's and/or family's needs.
>
> Usually, the presenting problem(s) are of moderate to
>
> high severity. Typically, **40 minutes are spent face-to-**
>
> **face with the patient** and/or family.

◀ Time
(in minutes)

For example, if the patient was treated in the outpatient office setting for 90 minutes, then the codes selected would be as follows: 99215, Office or other outpatient visit for the evaluation and management of an established patient, which requires at least 2 of these 3 key components: comprehensive history, comprehensive examination, and medical decision-making of high complexity, as well as 99354, Prolonged evaluation and management or psychotherapy service(s) (beyond the typical service time of the primary procedure) in the office or outpatient setting requiring direct patient contact beyond the usual service; first hour. 99215 identifies the first 40 minutes, and 99354 identifies the remaining 50 minutes of time. Note that even though only 50 minutes of extra time were spent with the patient, this amount is greater than 30 minutes, so the code can still be reported.

Key to Success

Assigning the correct codes for prolonged services requires careful identification of the total time spent, and then careful selection of the appropriate prolonged services code(s) to account for the correct amount of time. Remember to use your CPT code book as a guide to help you find the correct CPT codes. The CPT Professional Edition includes helpful tables that identify the amount of time spent on the E/M service, as well as how to report the prolonged service codes appropriately.

If the prolonged service is *more* than one hour over the time identified in the primary service, then an add-on code should be reported to identify the additional time. The add-on code should be reported as many times as necessary to identify the full amount of time spent with the patient. For example, if the provider spent 120 minutes (2 hours) in the office face-to-face with the patient, then the codes reported would be as follows: 99215 (Level 5 established patient office visit), 99354 (Prolonged service, first hour), and then 99355, Prolonged evaluation and management or psychotherapy service(s) (beyond the typical service time of the primary procedure) in the office or outpatient setting requiring direct patient contact beyond the usual service; each additional 30 minutes.

Preventive Services

In addition to evaluation and management encounters that involve the three key components of history, examination, and medical decision-making, there is another important type of E/M service common in primary care—preventive medicine services.

Also known as routine general healthcare examinations, routine physicals, checkups, or well-child exams, **preventive medicine services** are comprehensive health evaluations that involve a physical examination and include an age and gender appropriate history, counseling and anticipatory guidance and health risk factor reduction interventions, and the ordering of laboratory and diagnostic procedures. Preventive examinations are usually performed on an annual basis, unless the patient is under the age of three (in which case he or she would receive additional preventive exams throughout the year).

The E/M codes used to report preventive services are significantly more simplistic than outpatient office visit E/M codes. When coding for a preventive service, coders only need to know two things: (1) if the patient was considered new or established and (2) the age of the patient. For example, code 99384, Initial comprehensive preventive medicine evaluation and management of an individual including an age and gender appropriate history, examination, counseling/anticipatory guidance/risk factor reduction interventions, and the ordering of laboratory/diagnostic procedures, new patient; adolescent (age 12 through 17 years) is for a new patient from 12 to 17 years old. This code identifies that the patient is established and the age range of the patient. These are the only two factors used in selecting these codes.

For Medicare beneficiaries, coding for preventive services can be a bit more complicated. Remember that the HCPCS code set contains special codes for Medicare services, and some of these codes identify preventive services. These codes may be used for Medicare beneficiaries instead of the preventive services codes within the CPT code set. Instead of identifying the patient as new or established and the age of the patient, Medicare preventive service codes are selected based on how long the patient has been a Medicare beneficiary and previous services. There are three preventive service codes for Medicare beneficiaries:

- G0402, Initial preventive physical examination; face-to-face visit, services limited to new beneficiary during the first 12 months of Medicare enrollment. This code should be used to report an **Initial Preventive Physical Examination (IPPE)**, provided to a Medicare beneficiary within the first 12 months of enrollment. Also known as the "Welcome to Medicare" visit, this is a once in a lifetime benefit provided to a Medicare recipient, the goal of which is health promotion, disease prevention, and detection. It is only allowed during this first 12-month period, after which the patient may not receive the benefit (CMS 2018a).

- G0438, Annual wellness visit; includes a personalized prevention plan of service (PPS), initial visit. This code should be reported for the first time that a Medicare patient receives an **annual wellness visit (AWV)**, after the first 12 months of enrollment. The AWV is a visit in which a provider should develop and design a personalized prevention plan for the patient's chronic medical conditions and perform various health risk assessments. The initial AWV code may only be reported after the first 12 months of enrollment (ideally a year after the IPPE) (CMS 2018b).

- G0439, Annual wellness visit, includes a personalized prevention plan of service (PPS), subsequent visit. This code is reported for each subsequent AWV provided to a Medicare patient, for as long as necessary.

Key to Success

When it comes to coding for preventive services for Medicare patients, it becomes especially important to understand the exact type of Medicare plan that the patient has, as some Medicare plans may allow additional preventive services in addition to the IPPE and AWV codes listed previously. This is yet one more reason why it is important to understand the very close link between billing and coding.

Coding for preventive services can become more complicated when they are performed on the same day as an additional E/M service. It is common that during a preventive exam, the healthcare provider might encounter an additional problem or abnormality. If the problem or abnormality does not require any additional work, then no additional E/M service codes should be reported. However, if additional work is required to evaluate, treat, or otherwise manage the abnormality, then it may be necessary to include an additional E/M service code.

If a problem or abnormality encountered during a preventive examination is extensive enough to require additional work to perform the key components of a problem-oriented E/M service, then the appropriate office visit code should be reported along with the preventive medicine code. Modifier -25, Significant, separately identifiable service, should be appended to the office visit code to identify that it was a significant, separately identifiable service, provided by the same provider on the same date of service. Refer to chapter 5 (Learning the CPT and HCPCS Code Books) for a reminder of the uses and functions of modifiers.

This scenario is quite common in primary care coding, especially pediatrics, family practice, and internal medicine. Consider the following example.

A one-year-old child presents for a routine preventive examination and vaccinations. While in the office, the parent tells the doctor that the baby has been tugging at her ear lately, has been a bit fussy, and was running a fever the night before. In addition to the comprehensive preventive examination, including the growth and the development of the child and anticipatory guidance, the pediatrician also performs a problem-oriented visit— obtaining a brief history of the present illness; examining the child's ears, eyes, nose and throat; and determining that the child has otitis media (ear infection) and prescribes an antibiotic.

In this scenario, the pediatrician would code for the well-child examination using code 99392, Periodic comprehensive preventive medicine reevaluation and management of an individual including an age and gender appropriate history, examination, counseling/anticipatory guidance/risk factor reduction interventions, and the ordering of laboratory/diagnostic procedures, established patient; early childhood (age 1 through 4 years), as well as 99213, Office or other outpatient visit for the evaluation and management of an established patient, which requires at least 2 of these 3 key components: An expanded problem-focused history; An expanded problem-focused examination; Medical decision-making of low complexity, to report the additional E/M service. The additional E/M code, 99213, would be appended with modifier -25 to indicate that it was a significant, separately identifiable service.

> **MOD**
>
> Modifier -25, Significant, separately identifiable evaluation and management service by the same physician or other qualified healthcare professional on the same day of the procedure or other service, is perhaps one of the most important modifiers in all of procedural coding. Without adding modifier -25, the additional service would be bundled into the primary service (in this case the preventive examination) by the payer. When this happens, the payer only pays for the primary service and does not pay for any of the additional service that was performed. By not effectively using modifier -25, coders may be preventing reimbursement for thousands of dollars to which the healthcare provider is rightfully entitled.

Other than modifier -25, there are a handful of other modifiers that are used with evaluation and management services. They describe different scenarios and provide additional information regarding the primary E/M service.

Modifiers Used with E/M Services

There are several CPT modifiers that are specifically designed for use with E/M services only. They describe modified circumstances, such as modifier -95, Telemedicine service, and can make a significant difference in reimbursement, such as modifier -25, Significant, separately identifiable service. CPT modifiers that may be used with E/M codes include

- Modifier -24, Unrelated E/M service by the same physician or other qualified healthcare professional during a postoperative period. This modifier is used to indicate that an E/M service was performed during a postoperative period for a reason unrelated to the original procedure. This is an important modifier for reimbursement purposes. For example, a 60-year-old male received a pacemaker 20 days ago. Because this is a major procedure, it has a 90-day global period, which means that any routine follow-ups or diagnostic services performed in relation to the pacemaker are bundled into the code for the primary procedure (the code for pacemaker insertion). If the same patient sees the same physician during the postoperative period for a visit unrelated to the pacemaker—such as hypertension—then the coder should append modifier -24 to the E/M code. This will indicate to the payer that the E/M service was *not* related to the pacemaker insertion and it should be paid separately.

- Modifier -25, Significant, separately identifiable evaluation and management service by the same physician or other qualified healthcare professional on the same day of the procedure or other service. As explained previously, this modifier should be appended to an E/M code to identify that it was a separate service from another service performed on the same date. The additional E/M service must be a significant, separately identifiable service from the other service, as substantiated by the documentation in the health record. Modifier -25 should only be appended to an E/M code.

- Modifier -32, Mandated services. This modifier should be appended to a code for a procedure that has been mandated by an official organization, such as a physical examination as required by a third-party payer, government, legislative, or regulatory requirement. Although it can be used with other procedures (when mandated by an official body), it can also be used with E/M service codes.

- Modifier -33, Preventive services. This modifier may not be appended to an E/M code, but it is important to understand in context of preventive services. According to the Affordable Care Act, preventive services must be covered by the patient's health insurance payer at 100 percent, so the patient will not have to pay anything for the service (insurance pays for the entire service because it is a preventive service). This modifier should be appended to a procedure code to identify that it is a preventive service and should be covered at 100 percent by the insurance payer. It should not be used with an E/M code, but rather the code for a preventive procedure, as defined by the US Preventive Services Task Force. For example, a screening colonoscopy may be appended with modifier -33 to identify to the insurance payer that this is a preventive service and should be paid at 100 percent with no patient financial responsibility amount.

- Modifier -57, Decision for surgery. This modifier should be appended on an evaluation and management procedure that resulted in the initial decision to perform a surgery. For example, if a patient comes into the office complaining of intense right lower quadrant abdominal pain, and an immediate need for surgery to remove a burst appendix is determined, then the E/M code for the emergency department service would be appended with modifier -57 to indicate that the E/M service resulted in the decision to perform the surgery.

- Modifier -95, Synchronous telemedicine service rendered via a real-time interactive audio and video communications system. This modifier should be appended to a code to identify that the service was provided through a real-time, interactive communication service. This allows the provider to communicate with the patient who is located at a distant site, and who may not be able to see the provider face to face. The communication between the patient and the provider must be equivalent to substantiate the CPT code selected by the provider, and it must be documented in the health record. If these two conditions are met, then the provider may report the appropriate CPT code for the service, and append modifier -95 to identify that it was performed via a telecommunications system. Remember that only certain CPT codes are eligible for this type of service, and these are identified by the star symbol in the CPT code book. Telemedicine codes are also listed in Appendix P of the CPT code book.

Now, complete the exercises in There's a Code for That 8.5 to practice coding for E/M services.

E/M services

8.5

There's a Code for That

Read the following documentation of the E/M service and code for the encounter.

1. Routine physical examination for newborn infant, never seen in this practice before.

    CPT code: _____

2. Annual wellness exam for 45-year-old female established patient.

    CPT code: _____

(Continued on next page)

8.5

Continued

3. Routine well-child exam of established 2-year-old female. During well check it was found that she had acute serous OM of the right ear. Additional E/M performed with problem-focused history and exam, with MDM of low complexity.

   CPT codes: _____ , _____ - _____

4. A 60-year-old patient seen for a preventive routine physical examination, as mandated by his life insurance policy.

   CPT code: _____ - _____

5. A 15-year-old female was seen in the office and a decision for surgery was made. What modifier would be appended to the E/M service code?

   Modifier: _____

6. Thirty minutes of psychotherapy provided to a patient with agoraphobia via a real-time telecommunications system.

   CPT code: _____ - _____

   ICD-10-CM code: _____

7. Bilateral screening mammography provided to a 55-year-old female patient.

   CPT code: _____ - _____

   ICD-10-CM code: _____

8. Welcome to Medicare visit provided to a 65-year-old male Medicare beneficiary.

   CPT code: _____

Additional E/M Services

Besides office visits and preventive services, as discussed previously, there are a great deal of additional services in the Evaluation and Management section of the CPT code book. Healthcare practitioners may provide some, many, or none of these additional services, but they bear mentioning briefly, as they may be used within the context of primary care. Some of these additional services may include transitional care management (TCM), chronic care management (CCM), and care plan oversight (CPO) services.

Transitional care management (TCM) services, as the name implies, are provided to patients during the transitional period from an inpatient facility to a home setting. These codes cover a month's worth of healthcare services directed toward a patient's care, after they have been discharged from an inpatient facility, such as a hospital follow-up visit. There are only two codes for TCM services that depend on the medical decision-making component (either moderate or high complexity), as well how soon the patient was seen after the discharge (no more than 14 days from the date of discharge). Another important component of these services is the fact that in order to code the service as a TCM (such as a hospital follow-up), the healthcare office must make an interactive contact with the patient within two business days from the date of discharge from the healthcare facility. If this patient contact is not documented in the health record, then the face-to-face visit may not be billed as a TCM service. The two TCM service codes are 99495 and 99496.

Chronic care management (CCM) services are provided to patients with multiple chronic medical conditions, which necessitate the establishment, implementation, revision, or monitoring of a patient care plan. There are two codes for CCM services

(99490 and 99491) that are billed once per month of care and depend on the length of time spent managing the patient's chronic medical conditions during the billing month. Complex chronic care management codes are also available for CCM services that are more complex in nature, such as the need to substantially revise a patient care plan, or services that require more than 60 minutes of clinical staff time per month. Complex CCM services are reported with codes 990487 and 99489.

Care plan oversight (CPO) services are also provided to patients on a monthly basis and are similar in nature to chronic care management services because they involve a month's worth of care provided to a patient. Care plan oversight involves the monthly oversight of the healthcare care plan for a patient in the home health, hospice, or skilled nursing facility settings, and includes healthcare provider time spent coordinating care, completing documentation, reviewing data, and discussions with other healthcare providers. Care plan oversight codes identify the patient healthcare setting and the amount of time per month spent providing care plan oversight services. CPO services are coded with CPT codes 99374 through 99380.

Key to Success

Note that in all of the previous sections, for TCM, CCM, and CPO coding, there are many guidelines and notes in the CPT code book. Make sure to always pay attention to these notes when assigning codes for all services (not just the ones listed here), as they provide invaluable information on what is or is not included in the codes for the services, and how to assign the codes within that section.

Vaccinations

After E/M services, the most common procedures performed by primary care specialists are vaccinations. Often performed alongside an E/M service, especially preventive examinations, vaccinations may be administered on a set schedule, as is the case with infants and children who receive vaccines per a timetable set by the state in which they live. Vaccines also may be given to patients on an annual basis, such as the flu shot, or on an as-needed basis per health recommendations, such as the Tdap (tetanus, diphtheria, and pertussis) vaccine that is recommended for pregnant women and once every 10 years for adults.

It is important to keep in mind that not all injections given in a healthcare office are vaccines. Some are injections of antibiotics or therapeutic substances. These injections are coded differently than vaccinations. **Immune globulins** (codes 90281–90399) are serum globulins extracted from human blood, or recombinant immune globulin products created in a laboratory through genetic modification of human and/or animal proteins. These substances are injected as a post-exposure prophylaxis, meaning that they are given after the patient has been exposed to the disease. For example, the rabies immune globulin (90375, 90376) is given after a patient has been exposed to the rabies virus via an animal bite, scratch, or lick. Although the codes for these injections are listed before the codes for vaccine administrations, vaccine administration codes are not used to report the injection of immune globulins. Rather, the code for the injections of a therapeutic substance should be used (96372, Therapeutic, prophylactic, or diagnostic injection (specify substance or drug); subcutaneous or intramuscular). Pay careful attention to the guidelines before each section of codes to help identify which codes to use.

When coding for vaccines, the coder should understand the two components needed to report a vaccine administration correctly—the administration of the vaccine and the vaccine serum itself. The way the vaccine was administered will also impact the administration codes used. To report a vaccine administration accurately, it is necessary to report two codes, at a minimum. At least one code is required for the administration of the vaccination, and another code is required for the vaccine serum itself (see figure 8.8).

Figure 8.8. Vaccine coding components

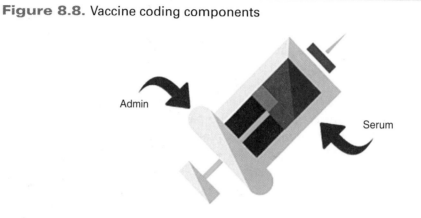

Administration

Vaccine administration is the act of giving the patient the vaccine, such as by injecting the needle into the muscle or spraying the vaccine into the nose or mouth. When coding for the administration of a vaccine, it is important to know the following:

- What was the route of administration: Was it an oral/nasal vaccine, or was it injected?
- The age of the patient: Was the patient under the age of 18 years?
- Was counseling provided to the patient?
- Are there multiple components to the vaccine serum?
- How many vaccines were given and what were they?

There are six different vaccine administration codes, and the coder must know the answers to these questions before he or she can determine which administration codes to report. Vaccine administration codes fall into three categories:

- 90460 and 90461 report administrations that were provided with counseling to pediatric patients.
- 90471 and 90472 report administration of injected vaccines.
- 90473 and 90474 report administration of oral or nasal vaccines.

The most basic vaccine administration codes are 90471, Immunization administration (includes percutaneous, intradermal, subcutaneous, or intramuscular); 1 vaccine, and 90472, Immunization administration (includes percutaneous, intradermal, subcutaneous, or intramuscular injections); each additional vaccine (single or combination vaccine/toxoid). These codes are for the administration of a vaccine via injection (that is, needle), no matter what type of injection is used (for example, intramuscular, intradermal, or subcutaneous). Furthermore, the words "single or combination vaccine/toxoid" are found in parentheses after each code, and indicate that no matter the vaccine serum, if it was given via an injection, then code 90471 should be used to identify the first injection. If a patient received more than one injection, then 90471 is used for the first injection, and the add-on code 90472 is used for each additional injection (see figure 8.9).

Figure 8.9. Example of vaccine injections using 90471 and 90472

A patient received three total vaccines that were administered intradermally.		
90471 (for the first vaccine) 90472 (for the second vaccine) 90472 (for the third vaccine)	OR	90471 (for the first vaccine) 90472 × 2 (for the next two vaccines)

Many third-party payers have specific requirements regarding how they will process vaccine codes. For example, some require the coder to list each individual vaccine administration individually, whereas a different insurance plan may allow coders to report multiple units (illustrated by using the × symbol) and combine administration codes. Still other payers may require the codes to be ordered in a specific manner. What is imperative is that each vaccine serum is reported alongside the appropriate administration codes.

The next vaccine administration codes are 90473, Immunization administration by intranasal or oral route; 1 vaccine, and 90474, Immunization administration by intranasal or oral route; each additional vaccine (single or combination vaccine/toxoid). Again, note that after each code description in parentheses are the words "single or combination vaccine/toxoid," and remember the only thing that matters with these codes is whether the vaccine was delivered orally or intra-nasally. If a patient received more than one oral or nasal vaccine, then the administration of the first vaccine would be reported with 90473 and 90474 would be reported for each additional vaccine (see figure 8.10).

Figure 8.10. Example of vaccine administrations using 90473 and 90474

A patient received two vaccines. One was administered nasally and the other was administered orally.
90473 (for the first vaccine) 90474 (for the second vaccine)

This gets trickier when the vaccines administered are both injected and oral vaccines. It is very common, especially in pediatric patients, that multiple vaccines are given at a single encounter. Often this includes both injected and oral or nasal vaccines and in this case codes 90471 and 90473 (for the first administration) may *never* be used together. One or the other must take precedence. Instead of using both 90471 for the first injected vaccine and 90473 for the first oral/nasal vaccine, either 90471 or 90473 would be used depending on which vaccine was first, and then 90472 and 90474 would be used for the additional vaccines (see figure 8.11).

Figure 8.11. Example of vaccine administrations using a combination of injections and oral/nasal vaccines

A patient received three injected vaccinations, one oral vaccine, and one nasal vaccine.		
90471 (for the first injected vaccine given) 90472 (for the second injected vaccine) 90472 (for the third injected vaccine) 90474 (for the oral vaccine) 90474 (for the nasal vaccine)	OR	90471 (for the first injected vaccine given) 90472 × 2 (for the next two injected vaccines) 90474 × 2 (for the oral and nasal vaccines)

The last two vaccine administration codes necessitate the most attention to detail. These are the only two vaccine administration codes that require counseling by the physician or other qualified healthcare practitioner. They may also only be used with pediatric patients (up to the age of 18). Administration codes 90460, Immunization administration through 18 years of age via any route of administration, with counseling by physician or other qualified healthcare professional; first or only component of each vaccine or toxoid administered, and 90461, Immunization administration through 18 years of age via any route of administration, with counseling by physician or other qualified healthcare professional; each additional vaccine or toxoid component administered, take into account the counseling provided to patients, and were developed in response to the heavy amount of counseling that some healthcare providers must give their patients regarding the safety and efficacy of vaccines. These administration codes were specially developed to capture this extra counseling, for *each component* of *each vaccine* given.

Components are the individual toxoid elements that are present within a vaccine. There are several combination vaccines—such as the MMR vaccine that combines toxoids for measles (M), mumps (M), and rubella (R). This is an example of a three-component vaccine; for the administration of an MMR vaccine, there are three components (measles, mumps, and rubella). 90460 would be used to report the first component, and 90461 (× 2) would be used to report the second and third components (see figure 8.12).

Figure 8.12. Example of component coding using 90460 and 90461

A pediatric patient received the MMR injection with counseling.		
90460 (for the first component)		90460 (for the first component)
90461 (for the second component)	OR	90461 × 2 (for the next two components)
90461 (for the third component)		

If a patient received multiple vaccines, each with several components, then code 90460 (and any additional component administration codes) would be used for each vaccine. For example, if a patient received three vaccines—MMR (three components), DTaP (three components), and flu mist vaccines—then code 90460 would be used *three* times, one for each of the first components. 90461 would be used four times, to report the additional two components for both the MMR and DTaP vaccines (see figure 8.13).

Figure 8.13. Example of component coding using 90460 and 90461 with multiple vaccines

A pediatric patient received an MMR and DTaP injection, and flu mist nasal vaccine with counseling.		
90460 (for the first component of MMR)		90460 (for the first component of MMR)
90461 (for the second component of MMR)		90461 × 2 (for the next two components of MMR)
90461 (for the third component of MMR)		90460 (for the first component of DTaP)
90460 (for the first component of DTaP)	OR	90461 × 2 (for the next two components of DTaP)
90461 (for the second component of DTaP)		90460 (for the one component of flu mist)
90461 (for the third component of DTaP)		
90460 (for the one component of flu mist)		

Key to Success

Note that with administration codes 90460 and 90461, the route of administration does not matter. Codes for vaccine administration provided to a pediatric patient with counseling do not differ depending on whether the vaccine was given orally, nasally, or injected (see figure 8.14).

Figure 8.14. Vaccine administration codes

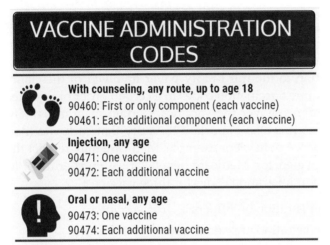

VACCINE ADMINISTRATION CODES

With counseling, any route, up to age 18
90460: First or only component (each vaccine)
90461: Each additional component (each vaccine)

Injection, any age
90471: One vaccine
90472: Each additional vaccine

Oral or nasal, any age
90473: One vaccine
90474: Each additional vaccine

Vaccination coding is not complete without also reporting the serum that was administered. Vaccine serum, or toxoid, codes identify the substance that was injected into the patient.

Vaccine Serums/Toxoids

The **vaccine toxoid** is the actual substance that is injected or given to a patient and that creates an immune response from the patient. There are a number of vaccine toxoid codes, each of which identify the specific substance that was injected into the patient at the encounter. One code should be selected to identify each vaccine administered. When coding vaccine toxoids, it is important to pay attention to the following:

- *The specific toxoid administered.* Codes may describe the formulation of the vaccine, such as 90649, Human papillomavirus vaccine, types 6, 11, 16, 18, quadrivalent (4vHPV) versus 90650, Human papillomavirus vaccine, types 16, 18, bivalent (2vHPV).

- *The age group for the vaccine.* Codes may differ depending on age of the patient, such as 90634, Hepatitis A vaccine pediatric/adolescent dosage, versus 90636, Hepatitis A and hepatitis B vaccine (HepA-HepB), adult dosage, for intramuscular use.

- *The dosing schedule of the vaccine.* Codes sometimes differ, depending on the dosing schedule for which they are formulated, such as 90647, Haemophilus influenzae type b vaccine (Hib), PRP-OMP conjugate, 3 dose schedule, for intramuscular use, versus 90648, Haemophilus influenzae type b vaccine (Hib), PRP-T conjugate, 4 dose schedule, for intramuscular use.

- *The route of administration.* Codes will differ based on the route of administration, such as 90658, Influenza virus vaccine, trivalent, for intramuscular use, versus 90660, Influenza virus vaccine, trivalent, for intranasal use.
- *The components of the vaccine.* As previously discussed, combination vaccines include components for multiple diseases. Pay careful attention to the components included, as there are many similar combinations.

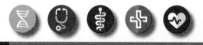

Putting It All Together: Coding for Vaccinations

Procedural coding for vaccines requires *at least* two codes: one for the administration of the vaccine and one for the serum administered. In the real world, it is important to also pay attention to the third-party payer involved in the claim, as the patient's insurance may require vaccination codes in a certain order or reported with additional information in order to cover the vaccines. Certain insurances may also only cover specific vaccines, so it is also important to verify that each vaccine is covered under the patient's insurance policy. For example, Medicare may restrict the number or type of vaccinations covered for Medicare beneficiaries. Furthermore, Medicare requires different vaccine administration codes for three vaccines:

- G0008, Administration of influenza virus vaccine
- G0009, Administration of pneumococcal virus vaccine
- G0010, Administration of hepatitis B vaccine

If a Medicare patient presents for an influenza, pneumococcal, or hepatitis B vaccine, then one of these three vaccine administration codes should be used, rather than the administration codes identified previously (90460–90474). The serum code is still reported with the administration, so if a Medicare patient received an influenza vaccine, then it would be coded as follows: G0008, Administration of influenza virus vaccine, and 90658, Influenza virus vaccine, trivalent (IIV3), split virus, 0.5 mL dosage, for intramuscular use. Complete the exercises in There's a Code for That 8.6 to practice selecting the appropriate vaccine or E/M code.

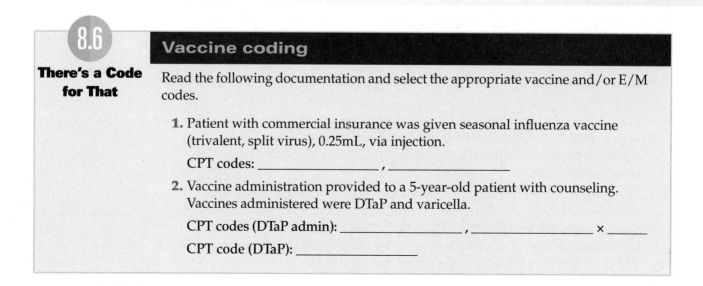

8.6

There's a Code for That

Vaccine coding

Read the following documentation and select the appropriate vaccine and/or E/M codes.

1. Patient with commercial insurance was given seasonal influenza vaccine (trivalent, split virus), 0.25mL, via injection.

   CPT codes: _____ , _____

2. Vaccine administration provided to a 5-year-old patient with counseling. Vaccines administered were DTaP and varicella.

   CPT codes (DTaP admin): _____ , _____ × _____

   CPT code (DTaP): _____

CPT code (varicella admin): _____

CPT code (varicella): _____

3. Patient was given HPV vaccine via IM injection (4vHPV) in the office, patient also received meningococcal conjugate vaccine (MenACWY-TT).

CPT codes (HPV admin and serum): _____ , _____

CPT codes (meningococcal admin and serum): _____ ,

_____

4. Routine physical examination for 18-month-old female with Medicaid. Hepatitis B, IPV, rotavirus (RV5), and influenza (LAIV3) vaccines all given in the office.

CPT code (E/M service): _____

CPT codes (hep B admin and serum): _____ , _____

CPT codes (IPV admin and serum): _____ , _____

CPT codes (rotavirus admin and serum): _____ , _____

CPT codes (influenza admin and serum): _____ , _____

In-Office Procedures

In addition to evaluation and management encounters and vaccinations, primary care providers perform several minor in-office procedures, miscellaneous medical procedures, and certain lab tests. Some of these in-office procedures are specialized in nature—such as avulsion of an ingrown toenail performed by a podiatrist, or removal or insertion of an IUD device performed by a gynecologist. Ultimately, the procedures performed by any provider depend on his or her area of specialty, the needs of the patient, and available resources. It is also important to remember the impact of modifiers on procedures performed at the same time as an evaluation and management service, as these will greatly impact payment for the services provided.

Minor Surgical Procedures

Minor surgical procedures may be found throughout the CPT code book and may be performed across several different healthcare specialties. Unlike major invasive surgeries, **minor surgical procedures** are minimally invasive, in that they only break the skin or mucous membranes and connective tissues. Minor surgical procedures do not require any general anesthesia or respiratory assistance during the procedure. However, they might involve local anesthesia, such as application of a numbing cream to the skin. Some of these in-office medical procedures include

- *Wart cryosurgery.* An integumentary system procedure, cryosurgical removal of warts is a common in-office medical procedure. It involved using a can of medical grade liquid nitrogen to freeze off the nonmalignant lesion and is reported with code 17110, Destruction (e.g., laser surgery, electrosurgery, cryosurgery, chemosurgery, surgical curettement), of benign lesions other than skin tags or cutaneous vascular proliferative lesions; up to 14 lesions.

- *Lysis of penile adhesions.* Common in circumcised male infants, penile adhesions occur when the skin of the glans of the penis adheres to the skin of the shaft of the penis. This must be separated via lysis before it grows together and requires more invasive surgical intervention. It is reported with 54162, Lysis or excision of penile post-circumcision adhesions.

- *Repair of lacerations and suture removal.* Although it is more common for patients to receive sutures in an emergency department or urgent care clinic, some primary care providers may perform simple laceration repairs in-office. Codes for simple repair of the integumentary system (12001–12021), depend on the site of the repair and the total length of the repair. For example, if the doctor sutures three lacerations on the cheek, the lengths of which add up to 3 cm total, then code 12013, Simple repair of superficial wounds of face, ears, eyelids, nose, lips, and/ or mucous membranes; 2.6 cm to 5.0 cm, would be reported. If areas other than the face, ears, eyelids, nose, lips and/or mucous membranes (as listed in this code description) were repaired, then these anatomical sites would be grouped into a different CPT code, as necessary. To code for the simple repair of superficial wounds, both the anatomical sites and the size of the repair are grouped into the same code. Removal of sutures is more common in the primary care office. Most patients who receive sutures in an emergency department or urgent care clinic return to the office of their primary care doctor for removal of the sutures. There is no code that captures the work involved in removing sutures that were placed by another provider. This is because the removal of simple sutures is included in the code for the placement of the sutures; the two procedures are bundled into the same code. Instead, an E/M code that is appropriate to the level of work involved would be reported for the removal of sutures.

- *Biopsy.* Whether or not a primary care specialist performs a biopsy will depend on the needs of the patient and available resources. Typically, more invasive or specialized biopsies, such as the biopsy of a breast lump via fine needle aspiration, are performed by a specialized provider. Simple biopsies, such as the biopsy of a mole or nevus, may be performed by a primary care specialist. This procedure includes the simple shaving, punch, or excision of a portion of the lesion to send to pathology for a biopsy, and would be reported with codes 11102 through 11107, depending on the type of biopsy (tangential, punch, or incisional), and how many biopsies were obtained.

- *Incision and drainage (I&D) of abscess.* **Incision and drainage** is a surgical treatment performed for soft tissue abscesses, for which medical treatment alone is insufficient. In this procedure, the abscess is incised with a sharp blade and drained of material. It is sometimes packed with gauze or other medicinal agents to reduce the infection. Codes for I&D of abscess are 10060, Incision and drainage of abscess (e.g., carbuncle, suppurative hidradenitis, cutaneous or subcutaneous abscess, cyst, furuncle, or paronychia); simple or single, and 10061, Incision and drainage of abscess (e.g., carbuncle, suppurative hidradenitis, cutaneous or subcutaneous abscess, cyst, furuncle, or paronychia): complicated or multiple. When coding for an incision and drainage, it is important to identify the type of cyst or lesion on which the procedure was performed, as there are different codes for the I&D of acne lesions, pilonidal cysts, and for the removal of foreign bodies.

- *Removal of foreign bodies.* A **foreign body** is any unnatural object that is present in the human body. Removal of foreign bodies can be as varied as the removal of a splinter from under the skin, to the removal of a bean stuck in a child's nose or ear. Depending on the site and type of the foreign body, this procedure may be performed in the primary care office or in the hospital setting. For example, the removal of a foreign body from the nose may not be possible in the outpatient setting, if the child is uncooperative or if the foreign body is stuck too far in the nasal cavity to remove with forceps. If this is the case, then the child would be sent to the hospital for general anesthesia or for a more invasive procedure. When coding for foreign body removal, go to the entry for *Removal* in the CPT Index, locate the subterm *Foreign body*, and verify the code selection in the Tabular List.

Medical Procedures

Besides minor surgical procedures, multiple miscellaneous procedures from the Medicine section of the CPT code book are commonly used to report the different procedures and services provided to patients. These procedures range from therapeutic injections, to hearing and visual screening screenings, developmental evaluations, and codes used to report services provided outside normal office hours. The procedures performed will again depend on the type of primary care practitioner, the patients he or she serves, and available resources. They include the following.

- Electrocardiogram (ECG or EKG). ECGs are common procedures that record the heart's electrical activity as a line tracing on paper and can be used to evaluate heart rhythm and function. The code for a routine ECG is 93000, Electrocardiogram, routine ECG with at least 12 leads; with interpretation and report. However, this is not the only ECG code available. Note that the code description read "with interpretation and report." This means that the provider's office both performed the ECG test (which includes placing leads on the patient's chest and performing the procedure), as well as providing a report of the ECG findings. Code 93000 should only be reported if both of these conditions were met. Code 93005, Electrocardiogram, routine ECG with at least 12 leads; tracing only, without interpretation and report should be reported when the office performed the ECG procedure but the healthcare provider did not read and provide a report of the tracing findings. Code 93010, Electrocardiogram, routine ECG with at least 12 leads; interpretation and report only, should be reported when the healthcare provider reviews and provided a report of the ECG tracing, but a different office provides the actual ECG tracing. Keep in mind that there are additional ECG codes within the Cardiography section of the CPT code book. Be sure to read the code descriptions carefully.

Key to Success

The differences in the codes for electrocardiograms describe the technical versus the professional components of the service. The technical component of the service is the performance of the test. The professional component of the service is the healthcare provider's interpretation of the findings of the test. These two components also make up numerous radiology codes as well as some cardiovascular codes, so it is important to keep them in mind as you learn more about the codes in the CPT code book.

- *Therapeutic injections.* Unlike vaccinations, therapeutic injections are given to patients for some sort of therapeutic treatment. For example, a patient may require an injection of an antibiotic in the office to begin antibiotic treatment immediately, or a patient with an intractable migraine may be given a shot of medication to help with the pain immediately. Like vaccine coding, these injections require at least two codes—one for the administration of the injection and one for the substance injected. Code 96372, Therapeutic, prophylactic, or diagnostic injection (specify substance or drug), subcutaneous or intramuscular, should be used to report the intramuscular injection of a therapeutic substance as described previously. The substance injected is reported with the appropriate HCPCS code to identify the medication administered by the injection. These therapeutic substances are reported with the appropriate HCPCS code, found in the Table of Drugs, as discussed in chapter 5.

- *Screenings.* Primary care practitioners, as the first line of care for patients, perform a number of different screenings. These include vision, hearing, psychological, and developmental screenings, among others. These screenings are often performed together with a preventive medicine service to check for any patient abnormalities. If any abnormalities are present, then the primary care practitioner will likely refer the patient to a healthcare specialist, or he or she may order further diagnostic tests. To find the codes for the specific screening service performed, refer to the CPT Index and search under the specific name of the test, or the body area or organ system, and reference the screening performed.

- *Respiratory services.* Respiratory services are common in the primary care office. These include spirometer tests, nebulizer breathing treatments, and pulmonary function tests, and are reported with codes from the Pulmonary subsection, 94002 through 94799.

Laboratory Procedures

The last type of procedures often performed in the primary care setting are in-office laboratory procedures. Whether laboratory procedures are performed in the office and which procedures are performed depend on office specifics. For example, some offices may not perform any laboratory procedures, whereas others might have a **CLIA-waived** status that allows them to perform certain in-office laboratory procedures, such as blood counts and bacterial cultures. CLIA stands for the Clinical Laboratory Improvement Amendments of 1988, which regulates facilities that perform laboratory tests on human specimens. CLIA-waived laboratory tests are simple and have low risk for erroneous results, although they are not error-proof. Some of the laboratory tests that are performed in-office include the following.

- Urinalysis procedures are commonly done to identify a specific substance in the urine, such as glucose, or to indicate if a urinary tract infection is present. They are reported with codes from the Urinalysis subsection of the CPT code book, 81000 through 81099. Usually done with a reactive strip, urine pregnancy tests are administered when a patient may be pregnant and are coded with 81025, Urine pregnancy test, by visual color comparison methods.

- Throat and nasal swabs are performed to obtain a sample of the mucous membrane lining from the back of the throat or nasal passages. Two frequently performed throat swabs are for streptococcus, 87880, Infectious agent antigen detection by immunoassay with direct optical observation; Streptococcus, group A, and mononucleosis, 86308, Heterophile antibodies, screening. Influenza tests are performed via a nasopharyngeal swab and are reported with 87804, Infectious agent antigen detection by immunoassay with direct optical observation; Influenza.

- Blood counts identify the specific amounts of certain cells within a blood sample. For example, a red blood cell count will determine the amount of red blood cells that are present in a blood sample. The code used to report the blood count depends on what type of count it was, such as complete blood count (CBC), white blood cell count (WBC), or red blood cell count (RBC), and other factors that identify the type of hematology procedure performed. They are located in the Hematology and Coagulation subsection of the CPT code book, 85002 through 85999.

It may be necessary to append modifier -QW, CLIA-waived test, at the end of the CLIA-waived laboratory tests performed in your office. This modifier identifies that the procedure was a CLIA-waived test that was performed in your office, rather than sent to a laboratory. This depends on carrier discretion, so some payers might require this and others may not.

Key to Success

Codes for laboratory services might be difficult to locate in the CPT code book. If you are stuck, it is helpful to look up the infectious agent or screening in as many ways as possible and to check all cross-references. Start by searching for the infectious agent by name, or by locating the type of screening, and go from there. It may take some time, but the more familiar you become with laboratory codes, the easier it will be to find what you are looking for.

Modifiers for In-Office Procedures

It is common that an in-office procedure and an evaluation and management procedure are both performed at the same encounter on the same patient. When this happens, it is appropriate to report one code for the evaluation and management service as well as the code for the in-office procedure, as long as the E/M service is a significant, separately identifiable service from the in-office procedure. When this is the case, it is important to remember to append the correct modifiers to the procedure codes as well. Whether or not to add a modifier depends on the insurance payer, as well as the specifics of the encounter. According to CPT guidelines, if an E/M code is billed with any type of additional procedure, modifier -25, Significant, separately identifiable evaluation and management service by the same physician or other qualified healthcare professional on the same day of the procedure or other service, must be appended to the E/M code to identify the E/M service as separately identifiable from the additional procedure. This identifies the E/M as a unique and different service from the other procedure that was performed, so that the insurance payer will pay for each service separately (both the E/M service and the additional procedure). Documentation should clearly identify that an E/M service was performed in addition to the procedure, and that the two services were distinct from each other. Additional important modifiers in the primary care setting include

- Modifier -59, Distinct procedural service. This modifier is used to identify procedures or services, other than E/M services, that are not normally reported together but are appropriate under the circumstances. For example, an E/M service performed with an in-office procedure, such as wart cryosurgery. These two procedures are not commonly reported together, so the cryosurgery code would be appended with modifier -59. Modifier -59 should be used when the documentation supports a different session, different procedure or surgery, different site or organ system, separate excision or incision, separate lesion, or separate injury, not ordinarily encountered on the same day or at the same encounter. Refer to chapter 5 for additional information on modifier -59.

- Modifier -76, Repeat procedure or service by same physician or other qualified healthcare professional. This modifier is useful when a particular procedure must be repeated. For example, if a patient receives a nebulizer breathing treatment in the office to treat asthma with status asthmaticus, and then the provider must administer another nebulizer breathing treatment because the first one was not effective enough, then modifier -76 would be used to indicate the procedure had to be repeated. The procedure code would be billed with two units (depending on how many times the procedure was performed), and appended with modifier -76.

Complete the exercises in There's a Code for That 8.7 to practice selecting the appropriate procedure or E/M codes.

8.7

There's a Code for That

Primary care procedures

Read the following documentation and select the appropriate procedure and/or E/M codes.

1. Newborn seen in the office for suspected urinary tract infection. Doctor performed a detailed history and examination, and moderate complexity medical decision-making for the E/M encounter for this new patient. A straight urinary catheter was inserted to obtain urine sample, and qualitative urinalysis performed.

   CPT code (E/M service): _____ - _____

   CPT code (urinalysis): _____

   CPT code (catheterization): _____

2. Wart cryosurgery performed on three painful warts on 28-year-old female patient.

   CPT code: _____

3. Routine preventive well-child exam performed on established 4-year-old patient. Screening test for visual acuity also performed.

   CPT codes: _____ , _____

Diagnosis Coding in Primary Care

Because primary care specialists are the first point of contact for patients, these providers see healthcare conditions across the entire spectrum of the ICD-10-CM code book. A primary care coder should therefore be familiar with how to select codes from all chapters of the ICD-10-CM code book. Furthermore, because PCPs are often the first healthcare provider that a patient sees when he or she begins to experience problems, they are more likely to see patients with signs, symptoms, and conditions that may not be definitive in nature. For example, a patient with fatigue and thinning hair may need more workup before the provider can diagnose the patient with a specific disease or condition. For the time being, it is necessary to report the patient symptoms, which are typically unspecified in nature. For these reasons, PCPs are more likely to report unspecified (NOS) codes. Therefore, coders should strive to select the most specific code possible, based on the provider's documentation of the patient's healthcare conditions.

Remember, if a provider has documented that a condition is "suspected," "possible," "rule-out," or in any way questions that the patient may not actually have the condition, or if the probable condition is not confirmed, then the diagnosis code for the suspected condition should not be reported. If there is no definitive diagnosis recorded in the patient's health record, then it is necessary to code for the signs and symptoms only. In some instances, the patient may have both a confirmed diagnosis or multiple diagnoses, as well as signs and symptoms for another condition. In this case, it is necessary to code for all documented conditions at the time of treatment.

When coding for primary care services, there are a few chapters in the ICD-10-CM code book with which coders should be more familiar, as well as a few conditions of which they should be especially aware. These are chapter 18 (Symptoms, Signs and Abnormal Clinical and Laboratory Findings, Not Elsewhere Classified); and Z-codes, located in chapter 21 (Factors Influencing Health Status and Contact with Health Services). The end of this section will also discuss some of the top conditions for this specialty, as well as certain conditions that are important in HCC coding.

Signs and Symptoms

Chapter 18 in the ICD-10-CM code book contains codes for signs and symptoms that are reported when a more definitive diagnosis cannot be confirmed. This chapter includes symptoms, signs, abnormal results of clinical or other investigative procedures, and ill-defined conditions regarding which no diagnosis classifiable elsewhere is recorded. According to the OCGR for chapter 18 (see also figure 8.15):

Figure 8.15. OGCR I.C.18.a, I.C.18.b, I.C.18.c

---

18. Chapter 18: Symptoms, Signs, and Abnormal Clinical and Laboratory Findings, Not Elsewhere Classified (R00-R99)

Chapter 18 includes symptoms, signs, abnormal results of clinical or other investigative procedures, and ill-defined conditions regarding which no diagnosis classifiable elsewhere is recorded. Signs and symptoms that point to a specific diagnosis have been assigned to a category in other chapters of the classification.

a. Use of symptom codes

Codes that describe symptoms and signs are acceptable for reporting purposes when a related definitive diagnosis has not been established (confirmed) by the provider.

b. Use of a symptom code with a definitive diagnosis code

Codes for signs and symptoms may be reported in addition to a related definitive diagnosis when the sign or symptom is not routinely associated with that diagnosis, such as the various signs and symptoms associated with complex syndromes. The definitive diagnosis code should be sequenced before the symptom code.

Signs or symptoms that are associated routinely with a disease process should not be assigned as additional codes, unless otherwise instructed by the classification.

c. Combination codes that include symptoms

ICD-10-CM contains a number of combination codes that identify both the definitive diagnosis and common symptoms of that diagnosis. When using one of these combination codes, an additional code should not be assigned for the symptom.

Source: CMS 2019b.

- Codes that describe symptoms and signs are acceptable when a definitive diagnosis has not been established by the provider.
- Codes for signs and symptoms may be reported in addition to a related definitive diagnosis when the sign or symptom is not routinely associated with that diagnosis. The definitive diagnosis should be sequenced before the symptom or sign code.
- Codes for signs and symptoms that are commonly associated with a disease process should not be assigned as additional codes, unless otherwise instructed by ICD-10-CM notations.
- If a combination code exists that includes the definitive diagnosis along with the sign or symptom, it is not necessary to assign an additional code for the symptom.

In short, do not code for signs and symptoms that are routinely associated with a disease process. For example, if the definitive diagnosis is a fractured wrist, then it is not necessary to include a code for wrist pain. On the other hand, if a sign or symptom is not commonly associated with the disease process, it is acceptable to report a sign or symptom code to better describe the condition (for example, a patient experiencing fainting spells in addition to being diagnosed with an ear infection).

Note that not all signs and symptoms are located in chapter 18. Some specific signs and symptoms are located in the chapters for their respective organ system or body area. When searching for diagnosis codes, remember to always search for the main term in the Index, follow all subterms and cross-references, verify the code in the Tabular List, and then follow all necessary ICD-10-CM guidelines. Some of the more common signs and symptoms reported in primary care are

- **Abdominal and pelvic pain (R10).** Abdominal pain codes are specific as to the type and location of the pain. Types include acute abdomen (severe generalized abdominal pain), localized pain, abdominal tenderness, rebound abdominal tenderness, colic, and generalized abdominal pain. The sites for abdominal pain are quite specific, and include left or right upper or lower quadrants, periumbilic, or epigastric sites (see figure 8.16) for an illustration of abdominopelvic regions and quadrants that may be identified by ICD-10-CM codes for abdominal pain. Note that the identifiers "right" and "left" identify the patient's right or left. There are also existing codes for pelvic and perineal pain. Different areas of abdominal pain may be indicative of specific medical conditions, and so the more specific code for the site of the abdominal pain should always be assigned when possible.
- **Fever (R50).** There are five possible fever codes: drug induced, post-procedural, post-vaccination, post-transfusion, or unspecified. If the type of fever is not identified as one of the former types, the NOS code should be selected: R50.9, Fever, unspecified.
- **Chest and throat pain (R07).** Chest pain codes are divided based on the site and type of the chest pain, including pain in throat, chest pain on breathing, precordial pain, pleurodynia, intercostal pain, other specified, or unspecified chest pain. If the chest pain is not identified as one of the former types, then the NOS code should be selected: R07.9, Chest pain, unspecified.
- **Abnormal glucose (R73).** Abnormal glucose codes should be reported when a lab finding has resulted in an atypical reading of the glucose level in the blood.

Figure 8.16. Abdominopelvic regions and quadrants

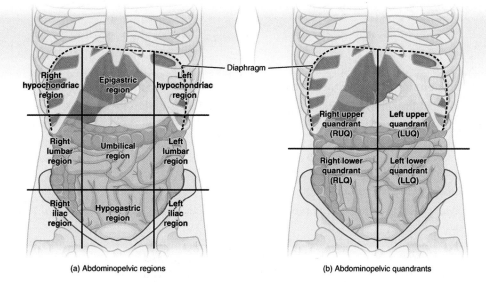

(a) Abdominopelvic regions

(b) Abdominopelvic quandrants

Source: OpenStax 2013.

Codes for abnormal glucose in the signs and symptoms chapter do not include low glucose levels (E16.2, Hypoglycemia), rather only raised or prediabetic levels (hyperglycemia). The codes include impaired fasting glucose, impaired oral glucose tolerance, prediabetes, other specified type of abnormal glucose, or R73.9, hyperglycemia, unspecified.

Z-Codes

Chapter 21 in the ICD-10-CM code book includes numerous codes used in the primary care setting. These codes are different than codes in the other ICD-10-CM chapters, as they do not necessarily identify a medical condition, but rather a reason for an encounter for other health services (for example, a routine preventive or preoperative examination, a vaccination, or for reproductive counseling). Other Z-codes are used to include additional information regarding a patient's health, such as relevant personal or family healthcare history, a past medical event, body mass index, or patient status, such as previous amputation. The official guidelines for the use of codes from this chapter are extensive, so it is important to read and understand these guidelines before selecting codes from it. The following guidelines should be noted (see also figure 8.17):

- Z codes may be used in any healthcare setting, and they may be used as either a first-listed or secondary diagnosis code. Certain Z-codes are designated only as first-listed diagnosis codes. Pay attention to the OGCR when assigning Z-codes, especially as a first-listed diagnosis, because if a Z-code that is not permissible as a first-listed code is sequenced first on a claim, the claim will likely be denied by the patient's insurance.

- Z codes are not procedure codes. They may seem very similar to procedure codes, but do not confuse the two. Z-codes are used to identify the *reason* for a patient encounter. If the encounter is for a preventive examination, then the reason for the encounter is preventive examination (see category Z00, Encounter for general adult medical examination). Keep in mind that both an ICD-10-CM code and a CPT code must be used together to report a healthcare encounter completely.

Figure 8.17. OGCR I.C.21.a, I.C.21.b

Figure 8.17. OGCR I.C.21.a, I.C.21.b

> **21. Chapter 21: Factors Influencing Health Status and Contact with Health Services (Z00-Z99)**
>
> NOTE   The chapter specific guidelines provide additional information about the use of Z codes for specified encounters.
>
> **a. Use of Z codes in any healthcare setting**
>
> Z codes are for use in any healthcare setting. Z codes may be used as either a first-listed (principal diagnosis code in the inpatient setting) or secondary code, depending on the circumstances of the encounter. Certain Z codes may only be used as first-listed or principal diagnosis.
>
> **b. Z Codes indicate a reason for an encounter**
>
> Z codes are not procedure codes. A corresponding procedure code must accompany a Z code to describe any procedure performed.

Source: CMS 2019b.

- There are 16 categories of Z-codes, and not all of them are listed here. It is helpful to read through the OGCR and the description of categories in the chapter to understand the guidelines for each.

Some of the more common Z-codes that are reported in primary care include

- *Persons encountering health services for examinations (Z00 to Z13).* These categories include preventive examinations, such as routine physicals, vision screenings, preoperative examinations, routine gynecological examinations, and screenings for malignant neoplasms and infectious diseases, and screenings for other diseases and disorders. For preventive general examination codes (Z00), it is important to select the appropriate code according to the age of the patient (adult, newborn under 8 days old, newborn 8 to 28 days old, child over 28 days old), and whether or not any abnormal findings were encountered. An abnormal finding includes anything that is considered an additional finding by the healthcare provider. This could range from a problem in growth or development, to an illness or other healthcare condition. Note that when assigning the code for an abnormal finding, this should only be assigned when the abnormal finding is new to the provider. For example, if the provider is seeing a patient for a routine physical and the patient has multiple chronic conditions, but none of them are new or worsening, then the coder should select code Z00.00, Encounter for general adult medical examination without abnormal findings. However, if the same patient with multiple chronic conditions had a new or worsening condition, then coder should select code Z00.01, Encounter for general adult medical examination with abnormal findings, to identify that an abnormal finding was present at that visit. In this case, it may also be necessary to select an additional E/M code to identify any necessary significant, separately identifiable services that were performed on that day in addition to the routine physical examination. See figure 8.18 for the OGCR related to preventive examination services.
- *Patient status codes.* Status codes indicate that a patient is either a carrier of a disease or has the sequelae or residual of a past disease or condition. These codes identify patient status such as the presence of a prosthetic or mechanical device from a past healthcare treatment, the fact that a patient has a healthcare

condition, or a condition that is likely to impact his or her health, acquired absences, and the presence of artificial openings (such as a gastrostomy). See figure 8.19 for the OGCR related to patient status codes.

Figure 8.18. OGCR I.C.21.c.13

---

13) Routine and administrative examinations

The Z codes allow for the description of encounters for routine examinations, such as, a general check-up, or, examinations for administrative purposes, such as, a pre-employment physical. The codes are not to be used if the examination is for diagnosis of a suspected condition or for treatment purposes. In such cases the diagnosis code is used. During a routine exam, should a diagnosis or condition be discovered, it should be coded as an additional code. Pre-existing and chronic conditions and history codes may also be included as additional codes as long as the examination is for administrative purposes and not focused on any particular condition.

Some of the codes for routine health examinations distinguish between "with" and "without" abnormal findings. Code assignment depends on the information that is known at the time the encounter is being coded. For example, if no abnormal findings were found during the examination, but the encounter is being coded before test results are back, it is acceptable to assign the code for "without abnormal findings." When assigning a code for "with abnormal findings," additional code(s) should be assigned to identify the specific abnormal finding(s).

Pre-operative examination and pre-procedural laboratory examination Z codes are for use only in those situations when a patient is being cleared for a procedure or surgery and no treatment is given.

The Z codes/categories for routine and administrative examinations:

Z00	Encounter for general examination without complaint, suspected or reported diagnosis
Z01	Encounter for other special examination without complaint, suspected or reported diagnosis
Z02	Encounter for administrative examination
	Except: Z02.9, Encounter for administrative examinations, unspecified
Z32.0-	Encounter for pregnancy test

Source: CMS 2019b.

HCC Coding Corner

Patient status codes are often important in HCC coding and risk adjustment, as they identify past healthcare conditions and treatments that may still have an impact on the patient's overall health. For example, nearly all codes in category Z94, Transplanted organ and tissue status, qualify as HCC codes. The fact that a patient has a past organ transplant is likely to impact his or her current and future healthcare needs, even though it might not be an issue at the present time.

- *Encounter for inoculation or vaccination.* In strict contrast to the complexity of CPT coding for vaccine administrations, identifying the medical necessity for ICD-10-CM codes is much easier. Code Z23, Encounter for immunization, is to be used to identify the medical necessity for all vaccines or inoculations.

- *Personal and family healthcare history.* There are two types of history codes—personal and family history. Personal history codes explain a patient's past healthcare condition that no longer exists and for which he or she is no longer receiving treatment, but that has the potential for recurrence and therefore may require continued monitoring. For example, an organ transplant or absence of an organ is an important part of personal history that has the potential to impact healthcare needs. Another example of pertinent personal history would

Figure 8.19. OGCR I.C.21.c.3

---

3) Status

Status codes indicate that a patient is either a carrier of a disease or has the sequelae or residual of a past disease or condition. This includes such things as the presence of prosthetic or mechanical devices resulting from past treatment. A status code is informative, because the status may affect the course of treatment and its outcome. A status code is distinct from a history code. The history code indicates that the patient no longer has the condition.

A status code should not be used with a diagnosis code from one of the body system chapters, if the diagnosis code includes the information provided by the status code. For example, code Z94.1, Heart transplant status, should not be used with a code from subcategory T86.2, Complications of heart transplant. The status code does not provide additional information. The complication code indicates that the patient is a heart transplant patient.

For encounters for weaning from a mechanical ventilator, assign a code from subcategory J96.1, Chronic respiratory failure, followed by code Z99.11, Dependence on respirator [ventilator] status.

The status Z codes/categories are:

Z14   Genetic carrier

           Genetic carrier status indicates that a person carries a gene, associated with a particular disease, which may be passed to offspring who may develop that disease. The person does not have the disease and is not at risk of developing the disease.

Z15   Genetic susceptibility to disease

           Genetic susceptibility indicates that a person has a gene that increases the risk of that person developing the disease.

           Codes from category Z15 should not be used as principal or first-listed codes. If the patient has the condition to which he/she is susceptible, and that condition is the reason for the encounter, the code for the current condition should be sequenced first. If the patient is being seen for follow-up after completed treatment for this condition, and the condition no longer exists, a follow-up code should be sequenced first, followed by the appropriate personal history and genetic susceptibility codes. If the purpose of the encounter is genetic counseling associated with procreative management, code Z31.5, Encounter for genetic counseling, should be assigned as the first-listed code, followed by a code from category Z15. Additional codes should be assigned for any applicable family or personal history.

Z16   Resistance to antimicrobial drugs

           This code indicates that a patient has a condition that is resistant to antimicrobial drug treatment. Sequence the infection code first.

Z17   Estrogen receptor status

Z18   Retained foreign body fragments

Z19   Hormone sensitivity malignancy status

Z21   Asymptomatic HIV infection status

           This code indicates that a patient has tested positive for HIV but has manifested no signs or symptoms of the disease.

Z22   Carrier of infectious disease

           Carrier status indicates that a person harbors the specific organisms of a disease without manifest symptoms and is capable of transmitting the infection.

Z28.3   Underimmunization status

Z33.1   Pregnant state, incidental

           This code is a secondary code only for use when the pregnancy is in no way complicating the reason for visit. Otherwise, a code from the obstetric chapter is required.

Z66   Do not resuscitate

           This code may be used when it is documented by the provider that a patient is on do not resuscitate status at any time during the stay.

Z67   Blood type

Z68   Body mass index (BMI)

           BMI codes should only be assigned when **there is an associated, reportable diagnosis (such as obesity).** Do not assign BMI codes during pregnancy.

           See Section I.B.14 for BMI documentation by clinicians other than the patient's provider.

Z74.01	Bed confinement status
Z76.82	Awaiting organ transplant status
Z78	Other specified health status

Code Z78.1, Physical restraint status, may be used when it is documented by the provider that a patient has been put in restraints during the current encounter. Please note that this code should not be reported when it is documented by the provider that a patient is temporarily restrained during a procedure.

Z79	Long-term (current) drug therapy

Codes from this category indicate a patient's continuous use of a prescribed drug (including such things as aspirin therapy) for the long-term treatment of a condition or for prophylactic use. It is not for use for patients who have addictions to drugs. This subcategory is not for use of medications for detoxification or maintenance programs to prevent withdrawal symptoms in patients with drug dependence (e.g., methadone maintenance for opiate dependence). Assign the appropriate code for the drug dependence instead.

Assign a code from Z79 if the patient is receiving a medication for an extended period as a prophylactic measure (such as for the prevention of deep vein thrombosis) or as treatment of a chronic condition (such as arthritis) or a disease requiring a lengthy course of treatment (such as cancer). Do not assign a code from category Z79 for medication being administered for a brief period of time to treat an acute illness or injury (such as a course of antibiotics to treat acute bronchitis).

Z88	Allergy status to drugs, medicaments and biological substances

Except: Z88.9, Allergy status to unspecified drugs, medicaments and biological substances status

Z89	Acquired absence of limb
Z90	Acquired absence of organs, not elsewhere classified
Z91.0-	Allergy status, other than to drugs and biological substances
Z92.82	Status post administration of tPA (rtPA) in a different facility within the last 24 hours prior to admission to a current facility

Assign code Z92.82, Status post administration of tPA (rtPA) in a different facility within the last 24 hours prior to admission to current facility, as a secondary diagnosis when a patient is received by transfer into a facility and documentation indicates they were administered tissue plasminogen activator (tPA) within the last 24 hours prior to admission to the current facility.

This guideline applies even if the patient is still receiving the tPA at the time they are received into the current facility.

The appropriate code for the condition for which the tPA was administered (such as cerebrovascular disease or myocardial infarction) should be assigned first.

Code Z92.82 is only applicable to the receiving facility record and not to the transferring facility record.

Z93	Artificial opening status
Z94	Transplanted organ and tissue status
Z95	Presence of cardiac and vascular implants and grafts
Z96	Presence of other functional implants
Z97	Presence of other devices
Z98	Other postprocedural states

Assign code Z98.85, Transplanted organ removal status, to indicate that a transplanted organ has been previously removed. This code should not be assigned for the encounter in which the transplanted organ is removed. The complication necessitating removal of the transplant organ should be assigned for that encounter.

See section I.C19. for information on the coding of organ transplant complications.

Z99	Dependence on enabling machines and devices, not elsewhere classified

NOTE Categories Z89-Z90 and Z93-Z99 are for use only if there are no complications or malfunctions of the organ or tissue replaced, the amputation site or the equipment on which the patient is dependent.

Source: CMS 2019b.

be a personal history of cancer, which could also impact the patient's current or future healthcare needs. Family history codes are used when a patient has a family member or members who have had a particular disease that poses a risk to the patient—if he or she may also contract the disease, or if the family history impacts the well-being of the patient. History codes are often used together with other ICD-10-CM codes that identify a reason for an encounter. History codes should never be sequenced as the first-listed code. See figure 8.20 for the OGCR related to personal and family history codes.

Figure 8.20. OGCR I.C.21.c.4

---

4) History (of)

There are two types of history Z codes, personal and family. Personal history codes explain a patient's past medical condition that no longer exists and is not receiving any treatment, but that has the potential for recurrence, and therefore may require continued monitoring.

Family history codes are for use when a patient has a family member(s) who has had a particular disease that causes the patient to be at higher risk of also contracting the disease.

Personal history codes may be used in conjunction with follow-up codes and family history codes may be used in conjunction with screening codes to explain the need for a test or procedure. History codes are also acceptable on any medical record regardless of the reason for visit. A history of an illness, even if no longer present, is important information that may alter the type of treatment ordered.

The history Z code categories are:

Z80	Family history of primary malignant neoplasm
Z81	Family history of mental and behavioral disorders
Z82	Family history of certain disabilities and chronic diseases (leading to disablement)
Z83	Family history of other specific disorders
Z84	Family history of other conditions
Z85	Personal history of malignant neoplasm
Z86	Personal history of certain other diseases
Z87	Personal history of other diseases and conditions
Z91.4-	Personal history of psychological trauma, not elsewhere classified
Z91.5	Personal history of self-harm
Z91.81	History of falling
Z91.82	Personal history of military deployment
Z92	Personal history of medical treatment
	Except: Z92.0, Personal history of contraception Except: Z92.82, Status post administration of tPA (rtPA) in a different facility within the last 24 hours prior to admission to a current facility

---

Source: CMS 2019b.

Key to Success

When looking up a history code, go to the entry for *History* in the Index. There are two major divisions under this entry: *family* and *personal*. It is easy to get mixed up between these two sections when searching for a code in the history entry. It is best to draw a line after the family history section, and before the personal history section, to keep these two sections separate.

- **Counseling.** Primary care providers commonly perform different counseling services. As the primary point of contact for healthcare and health services, PCPs must sometimes counsel their patients regarding their health. This counseling includes encounters for contraceptive management (Z30) and counseling for victims of abuse (Z69).
- **Body mass index (BMI).** BMI codes (category Z68) are based on two different scales—adult and pediatric. Pediatric BMI codes identify the weight percentile, either less than 5th percentile, 5th percentile to less than 85th percentile, 85th to 95th percentile, and greater than or equal to 95th percentile for age. Adult BMI codes, on the other hand, identify the specific BMI number, ranging from 19 or less to 70 or greater. Note that BMI codes should never be used as the first-listed diagnosis code, it is only acceptable as a secondary code. Also, according to ICD-10-CM guidelines, BMI codes should only be assigned when there is an associated, reportable diagnosis, such as obesity.

HCC Coding Corner

BMI codes (Z68) are important in HCC coding, but only if they are 40 or over. Codes Z68.41 to Z68.45 are all HCC codes. However, in order to substantiate the diagnosis for HCC coding the additional diagnosis of the patient's obesity must also be included. For example, for a patient with morbid obesity due to excess calories and a BMI of 41, two codes would need to be assigned in order to get full HCC credit for the patient's condition: E66.01, Morbid (severe) obesity due to excess calories, and Z68.41, Body mass index (BMI) 40.0-44.9, adult.

Complete the exercises in There's a Code for That 8.8 to practice assigning primary care diagnoses.

Primary care diagnoses

8.8

There's a Code for That

Read the following documentation and select the appropriate diagnosis code(s).

1. Patient presents with fever, headache, and sore throat. Rapid flu test performed in office is positive for influenza A.

   ICD-10-CM code: _____

2. Patient presents with fever, headache, and sore throat. All labs performed in the office are negative.

   ICD-10-CM codes: _____ , _____ , _____

3. A 40-year-old male presents with lower right quadrant abdominal pain, nausea, and vomiting. STAT CT scan ordered and admitted to hospital.

   ICD-10-CM codes: _____ , _____

4. A 3-day-old female presents for initial routine well-child examination.

   ICD-10-CM code: _____

(Continued on next page)

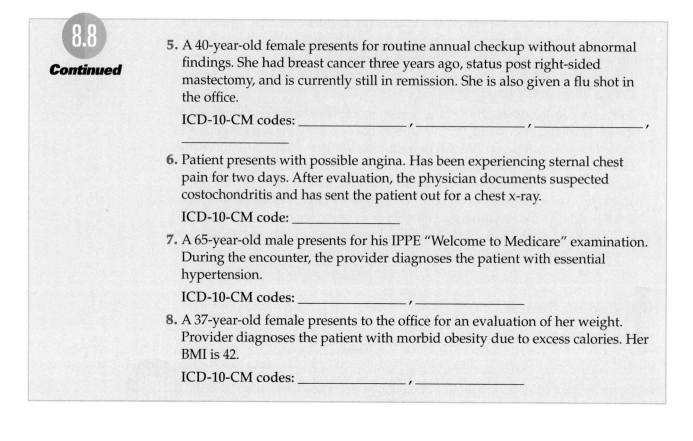

8.8

Continued

5. A 40-year-old female presents for routine annual checkup without abnormal findings. She had breast cancer three years ago, status post right-sided mastectomy, and is currently still in remission. She is also given a flu shot in the office.

ICD-10-CM codes: _____ , _____ , _____ , _____

6. Patient presents with possible angina. Has been experiencing sternal chest pain for two days. After evaluation, the physician documents suspected costochondritis and has sent the patient out for a chest x-ray.

ICD-10-CM code: _____

7. A 65-year-old male presents for his IPPE "Welcome to Medicare" examination. During the encounter, the provider diagnoses the patient with essential hypertension.

ICD-10-CM codes: _____ , _____

8. A 37-year-old female presents to the office for an evaluation of her weight. Provider diagnoses the patient with morbid obesity due to excess calories. Her BMI is 42.

ICD-10-CM codes: _____ , _____

Top Primary Care Conditions

Primary care practitioners see countless conditions ranging from otitis media, to diabetes, to hypertension. The specific conditions seen and treated depend on the specialty of the provider and available resources. For example, a pediatrician is likely to see more ear infections and fewer cases of high blood pressure. An internal medicine doctor is more likely to treat diabetes, hyperlipidemia, and chronic obstructive pulmonary disease.

Available resources also affect the most commonly seen conditions for PCPs. For example, in a rural area the town doctor may see all conditions, as there are few to no specialists who can treat specialized conditions. On the other hand, a PCP in a large city with many specialists close at hand is less likely to treat and manage conditions such as congestive heart failure or neoplastic diseases; instead these patients would be referred to healthcare specialists.

Coders in the primary care setting also need to keep HCC codes in mind, especially if their office belongs to an ACO, as many of these top conditions are included in HCC coding and risk adjustment. Keep an eye out for the (HCC) symbol as you read through this section. This symbol identifies codes that are important in risk adjustment. When coding for these conditions, it is imperative to select codes to the highest level of specificity, based on clear and complete provider documentation.

HCC Coding Corner

Note that many of the conditions discussed in the following section are HCC codes because they are chronic health conditions that will have an impact on the patient's healthcare for the rest of the patient's life. Furthermore, note that the diagnosis documented for many of the following conditions must be as specific as possible, or it may not hold any HCC value. For example, the code for unspecified depression (discussed in chapter 7) is F32.9, Major depressive disorder, single episode, unspecified, and this code does not have an HCC value. On the other hand, the code for moderate depression, F32.1, Major depressive disorder, single episode, moderate, does have an HCC value. The AHIMA version of the ICD-10-CM code book identifies all HCC codes with a lavender highlighting for easy identification.

The following sections discuss the top conditions in primary care coding.

Asthma

Asthma (J45) codes are based on severity—mild, moderate, or severe—and its recurrence, in terms of intermittent or persistent. Each type of asthma is further specified as uncomplicated, with acute exacerbation, or with status asthmaticus. Report the uncomplicated code unless the healthcare provider documents that the patient presents with exacerbation (such as wheezing or shortness of breath), or status asthmaticus. **Status asthmaticus** is an extreme form of asthma exacerbation that does not respond to treatment and can result in hypoxia and ultimately respiratory failure.

Chronic Obstructive Pulmonary Disease

Chronic obstructive pulmonary disease, or COPD, is a lung disease characterized by chronically poor airflow. Symptoms include shortness of breath, chronic cough, and sputum production. Coding for COPD is a bit complicated, as it often presents with additional conditions like chronic or acute bronchitis, emphysema, or another respiratory condition.

To look up COPD in the Index in the ICD-10-CM code book, search first for the term *Disease*, then reference the subterm *pulmonary* or *lung*, then find the subterm *chronic obstructive*. This will lead you to the section of codes in the Index for COPD. Select the code that most closely matches your diagnosis description and verify the code in the Tabular List.

There are three codes for COPD:

- J44.0, COPD with acute lower respiratory infection. Note the guidelines under this code that states to "Code also to identify the infection" such as bronchitis.
- J44.1, COPD with (acute) exacerbation
- J44.9, COPD, unspecified

Coding for COPD gets complicated when a patient presents with COPD and acute lower respiratory infection and acute exacerbation. For example: *A patient with acute bronchitis presents with acute exacerbation of his COPD.* This case would require three codes: one to identify the COPD with acute lower respiratory tract infection (J44.0, COPD with acute lower respiratory infection), one code to identify the COPD as exacerbated (J44.1, COPD with (acute) exacerbation), and one code to identify the acute bronchitis (J20.9, Acute bronchitis, unspecified). This may seem a bit like overcoding, but the two COPD codes are necessary—one to identify the exacerbation and one to identify the additional lower respiratory infection. Figure 8.21 presents the guidelines for COPD coding.

Diabetes

Diabetes mellitus is a common condition in which the body does not control the amount of glucose (sugar) in the blood, and the kidneys excrete large amounts of urine.

Figure 8.21. OGCR I.C.10.a.1

> **10. Chapter 10: Diseases of the Respiratory System (J00-J99)**
>   **a. Chronic Obstructive Pulmonary Disease [COPD] and Asthma**
>   **1) Acute exacerbation of chronic obstructive bronchitis and asthma**
>   The codes in categories J44 and J45 distinguish between uncomplicated cases and those in acute exacerbation. An acute exacerbation is a worsening or a decompensation of a chronic condition. An acute exacerbation is not equivalent to an infection superimposed on a chronic condition, though an exacerbation may be triggered by an infection.

Source: CMS 2019b.

It occurs when the body does not make enough insulin or cannot control the amount of insulin secreted.

Codes for diabetes mellitus are found in chapter 4 (Endocrine, Nutritional, and Metabolic Disease) of the ICD-10-CM code book, in categories E08 through E13. Diabetes codes are complex, and require a close attention to detail, as they identify the type of diabetes and many different complications. Furthermore, additional codes may be required to fully capture all of the patient's conditions. There are five categories of diabetes.

- E08, Diabetes mellitus due to underlying condition. This category should be used when the diabetes is a result of an underlying condition, such as Cushing's syndrome or pancreatitis. When using codes from this category it is important to also identify the underlying condition with an additional code(s), and sequence the diabetes code *after* the code for the underlying condition.

- E09, Drug or chemical induced diabetes mellitus. This category should be used when the diabetes is a result of a drug or chemical. An additional code should be used to identify the toxic effect. If the drug or chemical was not taken or administered correctly, and it resulted in the diabetes, code the toxic effect as a poisoning, and sequence the poisoning code *before* the diabetes code. If the drug or chemical was taken therapeutically and correctly prescribed and administered, code the toxic effect as an adverse effect, and sequence the adverse effect code *after* the diabetes code.

- E10, Type 1 diabetes mellitus. Type I diabetes is also referred to as juvenile or early-onset, and it is insulin-dependent. Patients with type I diabetes must take insulin for the rest of their lives. It usually develops before the age of 40, most cases beginning in early adulthood or during adolescence.

- E11, Type 2 diabetes mellitus. Type 2 diabetes develops later in life and is a result of the body not producing enough insulin for proper function, or when the body creates insulin resistance by not responding to insulin. Type 2 diabetes may be controlled by weight loss, exercise, following a healthy diet, and monitoring blood glucose levels. Some type 2 diabetics must take insulin daily, whereas others may not. Note that according to ICD-10-CM guidelines, if the type of the diabetes is not documented, then the coder should default to type 2 DM.

- E13, Other specified diabetes mellitus. This category should be used for diabetes that does not fit in any other category. This includes diabetes due to genetic defects of beta-cell function, genetic defects in insulin action, post-pancreatectomy diabetes, or postprocedural diabetes.

Once the type of diabetes has been determined, one code should be reported for each complication experienced by the patient. If there are no diabetic complications, report the diabetes code from the correct category without complications (for example, E11.9, Type 2 diabetes mellitus without complications). Except for the uncomplicated codes (one per category), diabetes codes are all combination codes that describe the type of diabetes as well as the complication. Complications that present with diabetes include:

- Hyperosmolarity (with or without coma).
- Ketoacidosis (with or without coma).
- Kidney complications (with nephropathy, chronic kidney disease, or other diabetic kidney complication).
- Ophthalmic complications. Ophthalmic complication codes are very complex. Codes identify the specific type of complication, as well as the laterality of the eye involved. If both eyes are involved, assign the bilateral code. Read these code descriptions carefully to ensure that the code selected correctly identifies all of the specifics of the patient's condition.
- Neurological complications (identify the type of neuropathy or other diabetic neurological complication).
- Circulatory complications (identify if the patient has peripheral angiopathy with or without gangrene, or other specified diabetic circulatory complication).
- Other specified complications. This includes diabetic arthropathy, dermatitis, skin ulcer, foot ulcer, oral disease, hypoglycemia, hyperglycemia, or other specified diabetic complication. Be careful with diabetes with skin ulcer codes, as they require an additional code to identify the site of the ulcer.
- Unspecified complications.

Assign one code for each complication. This may seem like overcoding, but one code must be selected for each complication included in the documentation. If the provider reports that the diabetes is "uncontrolled," "poorly controlled," or "out of control," assign an additional code to identify this complication, as with hyperglycemia (that is, E11.65, Type 2 diabetes mellitus with hyperglycemia).

When assigning codes for diabetes, follow these steps (see also figures 8.22 and 8.23):

1. Determine the type of diabetes (categories E08-E13). If the patient is pregnant, assign a code from category O24, Diabetes mellitus in pregnancy, childbirth, and the puerperium. Note that category O24 includes codes for both pre-existing diabetes in pregnancy and gestational diabetes. Codes for pre-existing diabetes should be used for patients who already had diabetes prior to becoming pregnant. Codes for gestational diabetes should be used for patients who developed diabetes during pregnancy.

2. Select one code for each complication. Assign an additional code for diabetes with hyperglycemia if the condition is identified as uncontrolled. If the patient has many multiple diabetic complications, be sure to assign *one code per complication*.

3. Assign a code for any long-term use of insulin or oral hypoglycemics: Z79.4, Long-term (current) use of insulin, or Z79.84, Long-term (current) use of oral hypoglycemic drugs. Note that neither of these codes should be used with category E10 codes (type 1 diabetes). Because type 1 diabetics must use insulin,

it is implied that they are on long-term use of insulin so it is not necessary to use the code for insulin use. Do not assign either of these codes if insulin is only temporarily given to lower blood sugar. Also note that these codes should be assigned *after* the code(s) for diabetes or diabetic complications.

4. Identify all additional codes and sequence them according to ICD-10-CM guidelines. Additional codes may be required to identify any underlying conditions, toxic effects, stage of chronic kidney disease, the site of a skin ulcer, or other complication or manifestation of the disease. Pay attention to the notes in the Tabular List, as they often indicate how to sequence multiple codes.

Figure 8.22. Diabetes coding

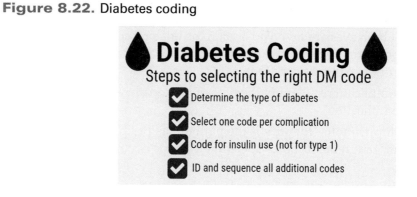

Figure 8.23. OGCR I.C.4.a

---

4. Chapter 4: Endocrine, Nutritional and Metabolic Diseases (E00-E89)

a. Diabetes mellitus

The diabetes mellitus codes are combination codes that include the type of diabetes mellitus, the body system affected, and the complications affecting that body system. As many codes within a particular category as are necessary to describe all of the complications of the disease may be used. They should be sequenced based on the reason for a particular encounter. Assign as many codes from categories E08 – E13 as needed to identify all of the associated conditions that the patient has.

1) Type of diabetes

The age of a patient is not the sole determining factor, though most type 1 diabetics develop the condition before reaching puberty. For this reason type 1 diabetes mellitus is also referred to as juvenile diabetes.

2) Type of diabetes mellitus not documented

If the type of diabetes mellitus is not documented in the medical record the default is E11.-, Type 2 diabetes mellitus.

3) Diabetes mellitus and the use of insulin and oral hypoglycemics

If the documentation in a medical record does not indicate the type of diabetes but does indicate that the patient uses insulin, code E11, Type 2 diabetes mellitus, should be assigned. An additional code should be assigned from category Z79 to identify the long-term (current) use of insulin or oral hypoglycemic drugs. If the patient is treated with both oral medications and insulin, only the code for long-term (current) use of insulin should be assigned. Code Z79.4 should not be assigned if insulin is given temporarily to bring a type 2 patient's blood sugar under control during an encounter.

4) Diabetes mellitus in pregnancy and gestational diabetes

See Section I.C.15. Diabetes mellitus in pregnancy.

See Section I.C.15. Gestational (pregnancy induced) diabetes

5) Complications due to insulin pump malfunction

(a) Underdose of insulin due to insulin pump failure

An underdose of insulin due to an insulin pump failure should be assigned to a code from subcategory T85.6, Mechanical complication of other specified internal and external prosthetic devices, implants and grafts, that specifies the type of pump malfunction, as the principal or first-listed code, followed by code T38.3x6-, Underdosing of insulin and oral hypoglycemic [antidiabetic] drugs. Additional codes for the type of diabetes mellitus and any associated complications due to the underdosing should also be assigned.

(b) Overdose of insulin due to insulin pump failure

The principal or first-listed code for an encounter due to an insulin pump malfunction resulting in an overdose of insulin, should also be T85.6-, Mechanical complication of other specified internal and external prosthetic devices, implants and grafts, followed by code T38.3x1-, Poisoning by insulin and oral hypoglycemic [antidiabetic] drugs, accidental (unintentional).

6) Secondary diabetes mellitus

Codes under categories E08, Diabetes mellitus due to underlying condition, E09, Drug or chemical induced diabetes mellitus, and E13, Other specified diabetes mellitus, identify complications/manifestations associated with secondary diabetes mellitus. Secondary diabetes is always caused by another condition or event (e.g., cystic fibrosis, malignant neoplasm of pancreas, pancreatectomy, adverse effect of drug, or poisoning).

(a) Secondary diabetes mellitus and the use of insulin or *oral* hypoglycemic drugs

For patients with secondary diabetes mellitus who routinely use insulin or oral hypoglycemic drugs, an additional code from category Z79 should be assigned to identify the long-term (current) use of insulin or oral hypoglycemic drugs. If the patient is treated with both oral medications and insulin, only the code for long-term (current) use of insulin should be assigned. Code Z79.4 should not be assigned if insulin is given temporarily to bring a secondary diabetic patient's blood sugar under control during an encounter.

(b) Assigning and sequencing secondary diabetes codes and its causes

The sequencing of the secondary diabetes codes in relationship to codes for the cause of the diabetes is based on the Tabular List instructions for categories E08, E09 and E13.

(i) Secondary diabetes mellitus due to pancreatectomy

For postpancreatectomy diabetes mellitus (lack of insulin due to the surgical removal of all or part of the pancreas), assign code E89.1, Postprocedural hypoinsulinemia. Assign a code from category E13 and a code from subcategory Z90.41-, Acquired absence of pancreas, as additional codes.

(ii) Secondary diabetes due to drugs

Secondary diabetes may be caused by an adverse effect of correctly administered medications, poisoning or sequela of poisoning.

See section I.C.19.e for coding of adverse effects and poisoning, and section I.C.20 for external cause code reporting.

Source: CMS 2019b.

Heart Failure

Heart failure, also called congestive heart failure or CHF, is a condition in which the heart cannot pump enough blood to meet the body's needs. Heart failure can only affect one or the other side of the heart, and it can be acute, chronic, or acute on chronic. Codes for heart failure (I50) will depend on the site of the failure and its acuity. Heart failure and hypertension are closely related, and many guidelines exist for hypertensive heart failure, discussed as follows.

Hyperlipidemia/Hypercholesterolemia

Hyperlipidemia is a condition in which there are high levels of lipids, or fats, in the blood. **Hypercholesterolemia** is a condition in which there are high levels of cholesterol in the blood. Codes for both conditions are included in the same category: E78, Disorders of lipoprotein metabolism and other lipidemias.

Hypertension

Hypertension, or high blood pressure, is a common health condition. Because of its systemic effects on the body, hypertension can result in heart disease and heart failure, as well as chronic kidney disease. When coding for hypertension, pay special attention to additional heart or kidney conditions, and follow all guidelines in the ICD-10-CM code book to ensure the selection of all necessary codes. There are five categories of hypertension, as follows.

- I10, Essential (primary) hypertension. This is high blood pressure without any related heart disease or chronic kidney disease, which is not a result of an underlying condition.

- I11, Hypertensive heart disease. This category of hypertension should be used when heart disease is a result of hypertension, or if the provider documents "hypertensive heart disease." If the provider documents a different cause of the heart disease, use one code for the heart disease and code I10, Essential (primary) hypertension. Codes differ depending on if the patient presents with or without heart failure. If the patient has heart failure, use an additional code to identify the heart failure (I50, Heart failure).

- I12, Hypertensive chronic kidney disease. This category should be used when a patient has both hypertension and chronic kidney disease (CKD). However, if the provider documents a cause other than hypertension, use code I10, Essential (primary) hypertension, along with the code identifying the CKD. Codes differ based on the stage of chronic kidney disease, either stage 5 CKD or end-stage renal disease (ESRD), or stage 1 through 4 or unspecified CKD. Either way, an additional code to identify the stage of CKD should be included, sequenced after the code for the hypertension as follows:
  - N18.1, Chronic kidney disease, stage 1
  - N18.2, Chronic kidney disease, stage 2 (mild)
  - N18.3, Chronic kidney disease, stage (moderate)
  - N18.4, Chronic kidney disease, stage (severe)
  - N18.5, Chronic kidney disease, stage
  - N18.6, End-stage renal disease (ESRD)

- I13, Hypertensive heart and chronic kidney disease. This category is to be used when the patient has both hypertensive heart disease as well as hypertensive chronic kidney disease. As in the previous categories, codes differ based on the stage of CKD as well as whether the heart disease presents with or without heart failure. Assign an additional code to identify the stage of CKD, as well as to identify the heart failure (if present).

- I15, Secondary hypertension. Secondary hypertension is due to an underlying condition. Assign one code for the hypertension and one code for the underlying disease. Sequencing of the two codes will depend on which condition is the primary reason for the encounter.

There are additional types of hypertension codes, such as category I16, Hypertensive crisis, which is an acute severe increase in blood pressure, and codes include I16.0, Hypertensive urgency, I16.1, Hypertensive emergency, and I16.9, Hypertensive crisis, unspecified. Additional codes exist for hypertension within certain organs, such as pulmonary hypertension, hypertension in the vessels of the eye and the brain, and hypertension complicating pregnancy, childbirth, and the puerperium. Hypertensive crisis can occur with underlying hypertension. If this is the case, then follow the ICD-10-CM guidelines to "Code also any identified hypertensive disease (I10–I15)."

Also called "white coat syndrome," **transient hypertension** is a temporary elevated high blood pressure reading, without the diagnosis of hypertension. It is assigned code R03.0, Elevated blood pressure reading without diagnosis of hypertension, and should be used until a diagnosis of hypertension is established. See figure 8.24 for the OGCR pertaining to hypertension.

Figure 8.24. OGCR I.C.9

---

9. Chapter 9: Diseases of the Circulatory System (I00-I99)

a. Hypertension

The classification presumes a causal relationship between hypertension and heart involvement and between hypertension and kidney involvement, as the two conditions are linked by the term "with" in the Alphabetic Index. These conditions should be coded as related even in the absence of provider documentation explicitly linking them, unless the documentation clearly states the conditions are unrelated.

For hypertension and conditions not specifically linked by relational terms such as "with," "associated with" or "due to" in the classification, provider documentation must link the conditions in order to code them as related.

1) Hypertension with Heart Disease

Hypertension with heart conditions classified to I50.- or I51.4-I51.7, I51.89, I51.9, are assigned to, a code from category I11, Hypertensive heart disease. Use an additional code(s) from category I50, Heart failure, to identify the type(s) of heart failure in those patients with heart failure.

The same heart conditions (I50.-, I51.4-I51.7, I51.89, I51.9) with hypertension are coded separately if the provider has documented they are unrelated to the hypertension. Sequence according to the circumstances of the admission/encounter.

2) Hypertensive Chronic Kidney Disease

Assign codes from category I12, Hypertensive chronic kidney disease, when both hypertension and a condition classifiable to category N18, Chronic kidney disease (CKD), are present. CKD should not be coded as hypertensive if the provider indicates the CKD is not related to the hypertension.

The appropriate code from category N18 should be used as a secondary code with a code from category I12 to identify the stage of chronic kidney disease.

See Section I.C.14. Chronic kidney disease.

If a patient has hypertensive chronic kidney disease and acute renal failure, an additional code for the acute renal failure is required.

3) Hypertensive Heart and Chronic Kidney Disease

Assign codes from combination category I13, Hypertensive heart and chronic kidney disease, when there is hypertension with both heart and kidney involvement. If heart failure is present, assign an additional code from category I50 to identify the type of heart failure.

The appropriate code from category N18, Chronic kidney disease, should be used as a secondary code with a code from category I13 to identify the stage of chronic kidney disease.

See Section I.C.14. Chronic kidney disease.

The codes in category I13, Hypertensive heart and chronic kidney disease, are combination codes that include hypertension, heart disease and chronic kidney disease. The Includes note at I13 specifies that the conditions included at I11 and I12 are included together in I13. If a patient has hypertension, heart disease and chronic kidney disease then a code from I13 should be used, not individual codes for hypertension, heart disease and chronic kidney disease, or codes from I11 or I12.

For patients with both acute renal failure and chronic kidney disease an additional code for acute renal failure is required.

(Continued on next page)

Figure 8.24. *(Continued)*

4) Hypertensive Cerebrovascular Disease

For hypertensive cerebrovascular disease, first assign the appropriate code from categories I60-I69, followed by the appropriate hypertension code.

5) Hypertensive Retinopathy

Subcategory H35.0, Background retinopathy and retinal vascular changes, should be used with a code from category I10 – I15, Hypertensive disease to include the systemic hypertension. The sequencing is based on the reason for the encounter.

6) Hypertension, Secondary

Secondary hypertension is due to an underlying condition. Two codes are required: one to identify the underlying etiology and one from category I15 to identify the hypertension. Sequencing of codes is determined by the reason for admission/encounter.

7) Hypertension, Transient

Assign code R03.0, Elevated blood pressure reading without diagnosis of hypertension, unless patient has an established diagnosis of hypertension. Assign code O13.-, Gestational [pregnancy-induced] hypertension without significant proteinuria, or O14.-, Pre-eclampsia, for transient hypertension of pregnancy.

8) Hypertension, Controlled

This diagnostic statement usually refers to an existing state of hypertension under control by therapy. Assign the appropriate code from categories I10-I15, Hypertensive diseases.

9) Hypertension, Uncontrolled

Uncontrolled hypertension may refer to untreated hypertension or hypertension not responding to current therapeutic regimen. In either case, assign the appropriate code from categories I10-I15, Hypertensive diseases.

10) Hypertensive Crisis

Assign a code from category I16, Hypertensive crisis, for documented hypertensive urgency, hypertensive emergency or unspecified hypertensive crisis. Code also any identified hypertensive disease (I10-I15). The sequencing is based on the reason for the encounter.

11) Pulmonary Hypertension

Pulmonary hypertension is classified to category I27, Other pulmonary heart diseases. For secondary pulmonary hypertension (I27.1, I27.2-), code also any associated conditions or adverse effects of drugs or toxins. The sequencing is based on the reason for the encounter, except for adverse effects of drugs (See Section I.C.19.e).

Source: CMS 2019b.

Infectious Diseases

As primary care practitioners are often the first line of healthcare, they see many different types of infectious diseases. These may range from localized antibiotic resistant infections and urinary tract infections to respiratory conditions, such as the common cold, bronchitis, or pneumonia. Many times, if there is no definitive diagnosis, it is necessary to code for the signs and symptoms of the disease, such as fever or sore throat.

Otitis

Otitis, otherwise known as an ear infection, can occur in the outer ear canal as *otitis externa* (H60, Otitis externa), or in the middle ear, *otitis media* (H65, Nonsuppurative otitis media, H66, Suppurative and unspecified otitis media, H67, Otitis media in diseases classified elsewhere). It is a common condition in pediatric patients. Codes for otitis depend on the type of ear infection and the laterality (either right, left, or bilateral). When coding for otitis, it is important to also code for any known exposure to or use of tobacco or tobacco products, as this results in the selection of an additional code. This includes environmental exposure to tobacco, such as second-hand smoke. Some otitis media codes are combination codes that include associated ruptured tympanic membrane (ear drum), whereas others are not. If an associated ruptured tympanic membrane is present, and it is not included in the code description, then assign an additional code to identify the rupture. Always pay attention to the guidelines and notes in the Tabular List, as they will often indicate when an additional code, such as rupture of tympanic membrane, is necessary.

Pediatric Conditions

Pediatricians see patients under 18 years old, including newborns, and may need to select codes for congenital or perinatal conditions. A **congenital condition** is one that was present at or before birth, and a **perinatal condition** is one that occurs at or during childbirth and may occur up to 6 weeks post-delivery. Perinatal conditions are found in chapter 16 (Certain Conditions Originating in the Perinatal Period) of the ICD-10-CM code book. These codes are generally assigned during the birth or delivery record for the newborn and resolve before the patient is discharged. For example, a preterm infant born at 36 weeks' gestation with meconium aspiration would have the following code assigned: P07.39, Preterm newborn, gestational age 36 completed weeks, and P24.00, Meconium aspiration without respiratory symptoms. These codes may be assigned as long as necessary if the condition persists, throughout the lifetime of the patient. See figure 8.25 for the OGCR for perinatal conditions.

Underdosing

Unlike an overdose, in which a patient takes too much of a certain substance, or an adverse effect, when a patient takes something correctly prescribed but suffers some sort of problem due to the substance taken, an **underdose** occurs when a patient does not take the properly prescribed amount of a medication. When a patient presents to the PCP's office and is suffering an ill-effect because he or she is not taking medication as prescribed, it should be coded as an underdose.

When coding for an underdose, the primary code should identify the problem being experienced by the patient as a result of the underdose, followed by the underdose code. For example, if a type 2 diabetic patient is suffering from high blood sugar episodes because she keeps forgetting to take her medication regularly (and hence underdosing), then the codes would be as follows: E11.65, Type 2 diabetes mellitus with hyperglycemia, and then T38.3X6A, Underdosing of insulin and oral hypoglycemic [antidiabetic] drugs, initial encounter. The additional code Z91.130, Patient's unintentional underdosing of medication regimen due to age-related debility, would also be assigned to identify the patient's noncompliance with her medication regimen (in this case unintentional because she keeps forgetting). Remember that underdosing codes are located in the Table of Drugs, as discussed in Chapter 4. To correctly select an underdose code, identify the substance in the Table of Drugs and select the appropriate code from the "Underdosing" column. See figure 8.26 for the OGCR related to underdosing.

As previously mentioned, primary care practitioners see patients with diagnoses from across the spectrum of available ICD-10-CM codes. When coding for primary care services, it is important to pay attention to the many different signs and symptoms, and when they should be reported rather than, or in addition to, a definitive diagnosis. HCC coding also requires that documentation be complete, clear, and as specific as possible so coders can report all appropriate codes necessary for risk adjustment coding.

Figure 8.25. OGCR I.C.16.a.1–I.C.16.g

---

16. Chapter 16: Certain Conditions Originating in the Perinatal Period (P00-P96)

For coding and reporting purposes the perinatal period is defined as before birth through the 28th day following birth. The following guidelines are provided for reporting purposes

a. General Perinatal Rules

1) Use of Chapter 16 Codes

Codes in this chapter are <u>never</u> for use on the maternal record. Codes from Chapter 15, the obstetric chapter, are never permitted on the newborn record. Chapter 16 codes may be used throughout the life of the patient if the condition is still present.

2) Principal Diagnosis for Birth Record

When coding the birth episode in a newborn record, assign a code from category Z38, Liveborn infants according to place of birth and type of delivery, as the principal diagnosis. A code from category Z38 is assigned only once, to a newborn at the time of birth. If a newborn is transferred to another institution, a code from category Z38 should not be used at the receiving hospital.

A code from category Z38 is used only on the newborn record, not on the mother's record.

3) Use of Codes from other Chapters with Codes from Chapter 16

Codes from other chapters may be used with codes from chapter 16 if the codes from the other chapters provide more specific detail. Codes for signs and symptoms may be assigned when a definitive diagnosis has not been established. If the reason for the encounter is a perinatal condition, the code from chapter 16 should be sequenced first.

4) Use of Chapter 16 Codes after the Perinatal Period

Should a condition originate in the perinatal period, and continue throughout the life of the patient, the perinatal code should continue to be used regardless of the patient's age.

5) Birth process or community acquired conditions

If a newborn has a condition that may be either due to the birth process or community acquired and the documentation does not indicate which it is, the default is due to the birth process and the code from Chapter 16 should be used. If the condition is community-acquired, a code from Chapter 16 should not be assigned.

6) Code all clinically significant conditions

All clinically significant conditions noted on routine newborn examination should be coded. A condition is clinically significant if it requires:

- clinical evaluation; or
- therapeutic treatment; or
- diagnostic procedures; or
- extended length of hospital stay; or
- increased nursing care and/or monitoring; or
- has implications for future health care needs

Note: The perinatal guidelines listed above are the same as the general coding guidelines for "additional diagnoses", except for the final point regarding implications for future health care needs. Codes should be assigned for conditions that have been specified by the provider as having implications for future health care needs.

b. Observation and Evaluation of Newborns for Suspected Conditions not Found

1) Use of Z05 codes

Assign a code from category Z05, Observation and evaluation of newborns and infants for suspected conditions ruled out, to identify those instances when a healthy newborn is evaluated for a suspected condition that is determined after study not to be present. Do not use a code from category Z05 when the patient has identified signs or symptoms of a suspected problem; in such cases code the sign or symptom.

2) Z05 on Other than the Birth Record

A code from category Z05 may also be assigned as a principal or first-listed code for readmissions or encounters when the code from category Z38 code no longer applies. Codes from category Z05 are fur use only for healthy newborns and infants for which no condition after study is found to be present.

3) Z05 on a birth record

A code from category Z05 is to be used as a secondary code after the code from category Z38, Liveborn infants according to place of birth and type of delivery.

c. Coding Additional Perinatal Diagnoses

1) Assigning codes for conditions that require treatment

Assign codes for conditions that require treatment or further investigation, prolong the length of stay, or require resource utilization.

2) Codes for conditions specified as having implications for future health care needs

Assign codes for conditions that have been specified by the provider as having implications for future health care needs.

Note: This guideline should not be used for adult patients.

d. Prematurity and Fetal Growth Retardation

Providers utilize different criteria in determining prematurity. A code for prematurity should not be assigned unless it is documented. Assignment of codes in categories P05, Disorders of newborn related to slow fetal growth and fetal malnutrition, and P07, Disorders of newborn related to short gestation and low birth weight, not elsewhere classified, should be based on the recorded birth weight and estimated gestational age.

When both birth weight and gestational age are available, two codes from category P07 should be assigned, with the code for birth weight sequenced before the code for gestational age.

e. Low birth weight and immaturity status

Codes from category P07, Disorders of newborn related to short gestation and low birth weight, not elsewhere classified, are for use for a child or adult who was premature or had a low birth weight as a newborn and this is affecting the patient's current health status.

See Section I.C.21. Factors influencing health status and contact with health services, Status.

f. Bacterial Sepsis of Newborn

Category P36, Bacterial sepsis of newborn, includes congenital sepsis. If a perinate is documented as having sepsis without documentation of congenital or community acquired, the default is congenital and a code from category P36 should be assigned. If the P36 code includes the causal organism, an additional code from category B95, Streptococcus, Staphylococcus, and Enterococcus as the cause of diseases classified elsewhere, or B96, Other bacterial agents as the cause of diseases classified elsewhere, should not be assigned. If the P36 code does not include the causal organism, assign an additional code from category B96. If applicable, use additional codes to identify severe sepsis (R65.2-) and any associated acute organ dysfunction.

g. Stillbirth

Code P95, Stillbirth, is only for use in institutions that maintain separate records for stillbirths. No other code should be used with P95. Code P95 should not be used on the mother's record.

Source: CMS 2019b.

Figure 8.26. OGCR I.C.19.e.5.c.

(c) Underdosing

Underdosing refers to taking less of a medication than is prescribed by a provider or a manufacturer's instruction. Discontinuing the use of a prescribed medication on the patient's own initiative (not directed by the patient's provider) is also classified as an underdosing. For underdosing, assign the code from categories T36-T50 (fifth or sixth character "6").

Codes for underdosing should never be assigned as principal or first-listed codes. If a patient has a relapse or exacerbation of the medical condition for which the drug is prescribed because of the reduction in dose, then the medical condition itself should be coded.

Noncompliance (Z91.12-, Z91.13- and Z91.14-) or complication of care (Y63.6-Y63.9) codes are to be used with an underdosing code to indicate intent, if known.

Source: CMS 2019b.

When assigning an underdosing code, at least two codes are required—one for the negative effect of the underdosing, and one to identify the underdosing itself. To find the underdosing code, it is necessary to go to the Table of Drugs in the ICD-10-CM code book and refer to the drug that the patient was supposed to be taking. The sixth column in the Table of Drugs lists the underdosing codes. It is still necessary to verify the code in the Tabular List and identify the episode of care for the encounter. For a refresher on using the Table of Drugs and assigning encounters for services, refer to chapter 4. Complete the exercises in There's a Code for That 8.9 to practice assigning top primary care diagnosis codes.

8.9

There's a Code for That

Coding for top primary care diagnoses

Read the following documentation and select the appropriate diagnosis code(s).

1. Diabetes, unspecified.

   ICD-10-CM code: _____

2. Patient presents with type 2 diabetes mellitus with mild bilateral nonproliferative diabetic retinopathy without macular edema, and diabetic cataract in the right eye. She is on long-term use of oral hypoglycemic drugs.

   ICD-10-CM codes: _____ , _____ , _____

3. Diabetes secondary to Cushing's disease. Patient seen today for treatment of her Cushing's.

   ICD-10-CM codes: _____ , _____

4. Patient presents for follow-up on her recently diagnosed type 2 diabetes. Her healthcare conditions are also significant for essential hypertension, hyperlipidemia, and obesity due to excess calories. Her current BMI is 34.

   ICD-10-CM codes: _____ , _____ , _____ , _____ , _____

5. A 10-year-old male with juvenile diabetes presents for management of his condition. He is currently well-controlled with his current insulin regimen.

   ICD-10-CM code: _____

6. Hypertensive heart disease with acute systolic heart failure.

ICD-10-CM codes: _____ , _____

7. Patient is seen for management of his hypertensive CKD (stage 3). He also has DM2 with peripheral neuropathy and CHF (congestive heart failure), which is not related to the hypertension.

ICD-10-CM codes: _____ , _____ ,

_____ , _____

8. COPD and acute bronchitis.

ICD-10-CM codes: _____ , _____

9. Pediatric patient presents with moderate persistent asthma with acute exacerbation. He is exposed to secondary smoke in the home.

ICD-10-CM codes: _____ , _____

10. A 7-year-old male presents to the office of his pediatrician for evaluation of his moderate persistent asthma.

ICD-10-CM codes: _____

11. A 60-year-old patient presents to the PCP for follow-up on his chronic conditions: hypertension, DM2, COPD, and hypercholesterolemia.

ICD-10-CM codes: _____ , _____ ,

_____ , _____

12. A 3-day-old female seen by her pediatrician for neonatal jaundice.

ICD-10-CM codes: _____

Putting It All Together: Coding for Primary Care Services

To select the correct codes for a primary care encounter, it is important to carefully read the documentation, then access each code book to find the procedure or service provided as well as the corresponding diagnosis or diagnoses to support the medical necessity for the service. Procedural codes for PCP services are found in the CPT and HCPCS code books, and diagnosis codes are found in the ICD-10-CM code book.

Determination of the correct codes relies on the answers to the following questions.

- What services were provided to the patient?
  - Was an E/M service provided?
  - Were any in-office medical procedures provided?
  - Were any in-office surgical procedures performed?
  - Were any in-office labs completed?
- Are there any applicable modifiers or add-on codes?
- What is the primary condition being treated? The primary reason for the encounter should be the first-listed diagnosis.
- Are there any additional signs, symptoms, conditions, or Z-codes that should be reported? Follow all ICD-10-CM guidelines.

Study the following vignette and note how to select the appropriate diagnosis and procedure codes. Then complete the exercises in There's a Code for That 8.10 to practice coding for primary care services.

One year ago, Audrey graduated from a health information management program. She learned the basics of evaluation and management coding and is preparing to take her coding certification exam in six months. Currently, she is working as a coding professional in a large primary care group practice and has learned a lot about primary care in general. Audrey is getting better at selecting the correct level of E/M code, even though the process is still a bit confusing for her. She is currently working on the following encounter.

History: *A 67-year-old female presents for medication follow-up. She is currently taking 10 mg gabapentin every four hours to control symptoms of peripheral neuropathy. She is not taking any other medications and is not allergic to any medications. Her neuropathy began seven years ago, when she noticed tingling and stabbing pains in her fingers and toes. Some days she notes that her entire arms begin to tingle and feel achy all over. She reports that she must take her prescribed dosage every four hours as directed or her symptoms reappear. Today, she has a slight burn on her right hand, which happened as she was baking a cake. She reports that her hands are difficult to control at times.*

Exam: *Patient looks well, awake and well-oriented to surroundings. Eye, cardio, respiratory, and gastro all within normal limits. Skin is notably dry in patches. Complete range of motion of both arms and legs, neuro exam of toes reveals slight pain to the touch and lack of response to stimuli in three of the left toes. Hand grip strength is generally strong, but lower on the right hand than the left.*

MDM: *Based on patient's reports, peripheral neuropathy seems to be controllable with current dosage of gabapentin. Continue meds as prescribed and follow up in six months.*

First, Audrey asks herself: What did the doctor do? The doctor performed an E/M encounter. There were no additional medical or surgical procedures or lab tests. She now begins to audit the E/M encounter to determine the correct code. The first component that she audits is the history component, and Audrey scores it as follows:

A 67-year-old female presents for medication follow-up (chief complaint)*. She is currently taking 10 mg gabapentin every four hours to control symptoms of peripheral neuropathy* (PFSH: past medical–current medications)*. She is not taking any other medications, and is not allergic to any medications* (PFSH–past medical– no allergies)*. Her neuropathy began seven years ago* (HPI: duration)*, when she noticed tingling and stabbing* (HPI: quality) *pains in her fingers and toes* (HPI: location)*. Some days she notes that her entire arms begin to tingle and feel achy all over* (ROS: neurologic)*. She reports that she must take her prescribed dosage every four hours as directed or her symptoms reappear* (HPI: modifying factors)*. Today, she has a first degree burn on her right hand, which happened as she was baking a cake* (HPI: context)*. She reports that her hands are difficult to control at times* (ROS: neurologic)*.*

Audrey has scored the following for the history component for this encounter:

- *HPI-5 elements, level of HPI is* extended
- *ROS-1 element, level of ROS is* problem pertinent
- *PFSH-2 from past medical, level of* pertinent

Level of History	HPI	ROS	PFSH
Problem focused	Brief	N/A	N/A
Expanded problem focused	Brief	Problem pertinent	N/A
Detailed	Extended	Extended	Pertinent
Comprehensive	Extended	Complete	Complete

She determines that the level of history *for the encounter is* detailed.

Now, Audrey scores the examination component of the encounter, as follows:

> *Patient looks well, awake and well-oriented to surroundings* (general appearance). *Eye, cardio, respiratory, and gastro exams all within normal limits* (eye, cardiovascular, and gastrointestinal organ systems). *Skin is notably dry in patches* (integumentary organ system). *Complete range of motion of both arms and legs, neuro exam of toes reveals slight pain to the touch and lack of response to stimuli in three of the left toes* (neurological organ system). *Hand grip strength is generally strong, but lower on the right hand than the left* (neurological organ system).

Audrey has scored the following for this component:

- *Limited exam of affected area and other related/symptomatic organ systems*

Level of Exam	Exam Components	Number of Body Areas/ Organ Systems: 1995 guidelines	Number of Body Areas/Organ Systems: 1997 guidelines
Problem focused	Limited exam of affected body area/organ system	1 body area or organ system	1 to 5 body areas or organ systems
Expanded problem focused	Limited exam of affected area and other related/ symptomatic organ systems	2 to 7 body areas or organ systems	6 to 11 body areas or organ systems
Detailed	Extended exam of affected area and other related/ symptomatic organ systems	Extended exam of 2 to 7 body areas or organ systems	2 areas of examination from 6 organ systems
Comprehensive	General multisystem exam or complete exam of single organ system	8 or more organ systems	2 areas of examination from 9 organ systems

She determines that the level of examination *for the encounter is* expanded problem focused.

Now Audrey scores the final component of the encounter, medical decision-making:

Based on patient's reports, peripheral neuropathy seems to be controllable with current dosage of gabapentin. Continue meds as prescribed and follow up in six months.

- *Number of diagnoses: Established problem—stable (peripheral neuropathy, controllable, continue meds as prescribed), 1 point. Level is minimal.*
- *Amount of data to be reviewed: None. Level is none (minimal).*
- *Risk of complications, morbidity, or mortality: One stable chronic condition. Level is minimal.*

Audrey has scored the following for this component:

Level of MDM	Number of Diagnosis and Management Options	Amount and/or Complexity of Data	Risk Involved
Straightforward	Minimal	Minimal or none	Minimal
Low	Limited	Limited	Low
Moderate	Multiple	Moderate	Moderate
High	Extensive	Extensive	High

She determines that the level of MDM for the encounter is straightforward.

Now that Audrey has all three levels of the key components, she determines the type of service, place of service, and patient's status in order to find the correct section of codes in the E/M section of the CPT code book. This is an outpatient office visit for an established patient, so Audrey goes to codes 99211 through 99215 in the CPT code book, and selects the code that matches the following (remember that for established patients, only two out of the three levels of the key components are required to match):

- *Detailed history*
- *Expanded problem-focused examination*
- *Straightforward medical decision-making*

Audrey's code is: 99213, Office or other outpatient visit for the evaluation and management of an established patient, which requires at least 2 out of 3 of the following: expanded problem-focused history, expanded problem-focused examination, medical decision-making of low complexity.

Now that she has her procedure code, Audrey asks herself: Why did the doctor do it? The patient presented for a follow-up on her established diagnosis of peripheral neuropathy. She also has a first degree burn on her right hand. She looks up these conditions in the ICD-10-CM code book and finds the following codes:

Neuropathy, peripheral (Audrey uses the default code as there are no more specifics on the type of neuropathy): G62.9, Polyneuropathy, unspecified.
Burn, hand, right, first degree, initial encounter: T23.101A, Burn of first degree of right hand, unspecified site, initial encounter.

She then rechecks the documentation to ensure she has coded everything for the encounter and reports the chosen codes on the claim for the service.

Coding for primary care services

8.10

**There's a Code
for That**

Read the following documentation from patient encounters and assign the appropriate procedure and diagnosis codes.

1. An 18-month-old established female presents with acute suppurative OM of the right ear with rupture of tympanic membrane. Physician performed a E/M service with detailed history, expanded problem-focused exam, and MDM of low complexity. During the exam, a large accumulation of impacted cerumen was noted in the left ear, which was removed with instrumentation by the physician.

   CPT codes: _____ - _____ , _____

   ICD-10-CM codes: _____ , _____

2. A 72-year-old female presents for treatment of treatment-resistant urinary tract infection. She came in two days ago and urine culture was taken, which tested positive for MRSA. Provider performed a problem-focused history and examination, with moderate complexity medical decision-making.

   CPT codes: _____

   ICD-10-CM codes: _____ , _____

3. A 45-year-old female presents to the office of her internist with anemia in CKD, stage 3. Internist performs a detailed history, detailed examination, and MDM of moderate complexity. CBC (automated and automated differential WBC count) performed in office indicates that anemia is improving.

   CPT codes: _____ , _____

   ICD-10-CM codes: _____ , _____

4. A 67-year-old established male patient is seen in the clinic with DM2 and mild nonproliferative diabetic retinopathy with macular edema, as well as a diabetic cataract on his right eye. His DM is controlled daily with insulin. Physician performed a detailed history and with comprehensive examination and medical decision-making of high complexity. Due to worsening of visual problem, physician also performed a bilateral visual acuity screen and referred the patient to an ophthalmologist.

   CPT codes: _____ , _____

   ICD-10-CM codes: _____ , _____ , _____

5. A 45-year-old male presents for routine physical examination. Patient is a healthy middle-aged male, no abnormal findings. Flu shot (IIV3) also administered in the office.

   CPT codes: _____ , _____ , _____ ,

   ICD-10-CM codes: _____ , _____

PATIENT: Korben Brother

DATE OF SERVICE: 12/01/20XX

Outpatient office visit, established patient.

SUBJECTIVE:
Chief Complaint: Follow-up on chronic conditions: DM2, COPD, hypertension, heart failure, and hyperlipidemia

History of Present Illness: Patient states that he has been doing well with his COPD control since his last visit. He has not had to use his rescue inhaler recently. Last time he used the inhaler was 2 weeks ago. Chronic diastolic heart failure diagnosed 3 years ago, as a result of his hypertension. Hyperlipidemia status—the patient's last LDL was 87 mg/dL at last preventive examination. He has adjusted his diet and is hoping to see a drop in labs today. He is compliant with his medication regimen. Denies medication side effects. Hypertension has been controlled lately as per blood pressures taken at home. Diabetes is controlled per patient since his last visit. Diabetic complications include hypertension, hyperlipidemia and coronary artery disease. Checks his blood sugars sporadically.

Review of Systems:
Constitutional: feels good recently.
Pulmonary: no dyspnea on exertion, no reduced exercise tolerance, no cough, not coughing up increased sputum, no wheezing.
Cardiovascular: denies lower extremity edema, denies fatigue, denies orthopnea, and denies paroxysmal nocturnal dyspnea.
Neurological: no neuropathy noted, no numbness to the feet.
Gastrointestinal: no vomiting, not peptic ulcers.
Integumentary: no skin ulcers, dry skin on extremities and feet.
Endocrine: diabetes has been controlled since last visit, no urinary frequency.

Past, Family, Social History:
Current medications reviewed. Patient does not smoke. Patient admits to exercise noncompliance. Allergic to penicillins, sulfa drugs. No known food allergies. Negative relevant surgical history.

OBJECTIVE:
Physical Examination:
Constitutional: well-nourished, healthy appearing, alert, oriented and in no acute distress.
EENT: The sclera and conjunctive were normal and pupils were equal in size, round, reactive to light, with normal accommodation.
Neck: the neck was supple, normal in appearance, and no neck mass was observed.
Pulmonary: no respiratory distress, normal respiratory rhythm and effort, clear bilateral breath sounds heard on auscultation.
Cardiovascular: heart rate and rhythm were normal, no gallops heard, no murmurs heard, carotid pulses normal with no bruits, pedal pulses were full and no edema seen.
Musculoskeletal: normal gait, no clubbing of the fingernails, no joint swelling seen, and the muscle tone was normal.

Diabetic foot exam: right and left foot appear normal. The toes of the right and left feet appear normal. The vascular exam shows normal capillary refill of the right toes. Posterior tibialis: right 2+. Dorsalis pedis: right 2+. Sensory exam of the right foot shows normal tactile sensation with monofilament testing. The vascular exam shows normal capillary refill of the left toes. Posterior tibialis: 2+. Dorsalis pedis: left 2+. The sensory exam on the left foot shows normal tactile sensation with monofilament testing. The vascular exam shows normal capillary refill of the left toes. No assistive device required for ambulation and normal gait.

Skin: normal skin color and pigmentation, no rash and no skin lesions.

Neurological: cranial nerves 2–12 were intact, the sensory exam was normal to light touch and pinprick and the motor exam was normal.

Psychiatric: oriented to person, place, and time, insight and judgment were intact, the affect was normal and the mood was normal.

ASSESSMENT and PLAN:

1. Hypertensive heart disease with chronic diastolic heart failure. Stable. Reassess at next visit.

2. COPD. Stable. Monitor.

3. Diabetic hyperlipidemia. Diabetes is not well controlled due to noncompliance with exercise regimen. He will resume a regular exercise regimen and will reassess in 4 months.

4. Diabetic hypertension. Stable. No medicine changes. Monitor.

5. Healthcare maintenance: Tdap shot given in office today via IM injection.

SIGNED: Dr. Susan Alameda, DO

Use the following steps to select the appropriate codes for the case study.

1. Read the case study in full. As you read, look up any medical or procedural terms with which you are unfamiliar and use a medical dictionary or medical terminology text to define the unfamiliar terms.

2. Review the case study and answer the following question: *What did the doctor do?* In this case study, the documentation is in the SOAP note format. Remember that the components of the SOAP note directly correspond to the key components of an E/M service. Answer the following questions to help you determine the correct E/M code.

   a. What is the place of service, type of service, and patient status?

   _____

   _____

   b. Identify the code range for this type of E/M service in the CPT code book and list it.

   _____

   _____

   c. How many key components are necessary to select the level of service for this E/M type?

   _____

   _____

d. Carefully read through the documentation and determine the levels of the three key components of the E/M service.

   i. History:

   _____

   _____

   ii. Examination:

   _____

   _____

   iii. Medical Decision-Making:

   _____

   _____

e. Using the levels of the three key components (as located in the documentation of the visit), identify the correct E/M code for this service.

   _____

   _____

3. Are there any additional procedures that need to be added to identify all of the procedures performed? Use the CPT code book to identify all additional necessary procedure codes.

   _____

   _____

   a. Are there any modifiers that need to be added to identify any special circumstance surrounding the procedure(s)? If yes, refer to Appendix A of the CPT code book to assign all appropriate modifiers.

   _____

   _____

4. Now that the procedure(s) and modifier(s) have been identified, refer to the case study and answer the following question: *Why did the doctor do it?* To find the reason for the office visit, search for terms that will identify the medical condition. Remember that in the SOAP note format, the diagnoses are included in the Assessment portion of the documentation. This is where the provider has listed each of the medical conditions found or addressed during the visit. In this case study, identify the patient's diagnoses.

   a. _____

   b. _____

   c. _____

   d. _____

   e. _____

5. Now that you have identified the patient's diagnoses, search the ICD-10-CM code book for the correct codes for these conditions. Follow these steps for each of the diagnoses identified.

a. Search the Main Index for the name of each condition and search through any applicable subterms and cross-references to locate the appropriate code.

i. _____

ii. _____

iii. _____

iv. _____

v. _____

b. Verify the code(s) in the Tabular List. Locate the code(s) identified previously in the Tabular Listing of codes and refer to any applicable guidelines, notes, and symbols. Does the code selected correctly identify the patient's condition? If yes, list the code(s).

i. _____

ii. _____

iii. _____

iv. _____

v. _____

c. Check the procedure note and ICD-10-CM guidelines and conventions to determine the correct sequencing of the diagnosis codes, if applicable. Correctly sequence the diagnosis codes.

_____

6. Now that the procedure and diagnosis codes have been identified, list them on the CMS-1500 form. Be sure to identify medical necessity for each service by correctly linking the procedure/supply and diagnosis codes. Please refer to figure 3.6 for an example.

21. DIAGNOSIS OR NATURE OF ILLNESS OR INJURY Relate A-L to service line below (24E)			ICD Ind.	
A. L_____	B. L_____	C. L_____	D. L_____	
E. L_____	F. L_____	G. L_____	H. L_____	
I. L_____	J. L_____	K. L_____	L. L_____	

24. A. DATE(S) OF SERVICE						B. PLACE OF SERVICE	C. EMG	D. PROCEDURES, SERVICES, OR SUPPLIES (Explain Unusual Circumstances) CPT/HCPCS	MODIFIER	E. DIAGNOSIS POINTER
From MM	DD	YY	To MM	DD	YY					
1										
2										
3										

End-of-Chapter Content

Instructions: Indicate whether the following statements are true or false (T or F). For false statements, rewrite the statement on the line below to make the statement true.

1. Primary care practitioners specialize in the care of neoplasms.

   _____

   _____

2. A women's health practitioner may be considered a primary care practitioner.

   _____

   _____

3. PCP stands for primary care patient.

   _____

   _____

4. HCC coding is not important for accountable care organizations.

   _____

   _____

5. Most of the procedures performed by primary care providers are E/M encounters.

   _____

   _____

6. HPI stands for history of the patient's illness.

   _____

   _____

7. There are four different elements that make up the key component of history.

   _____

   _____

8. The key components of history and examination are both made up of the same elements.

_____

_____

9. Modifier -25 may not be appended to evaluation and management services.

_____

_____

10. Biopsy is an example of a minor surgical procedure that would be performed in the office.

_____

_____

Instructions: Choose the best answer.

1. In some health insurance plans, patients are required to select which of the following?

a. A patient care coordinator
b. A primary care provider
c. Designated procedure codes
d. Mental health services

2. Which of the following is the best description of an ACO?

a. A group of patients who engage in risk management reduction
b. A billing and coding group that specializes in auditing claims
c. A group of healthcare providers that collectively utilizes performance measures
d. A group of insurance companies that engages in risk adjustment education

3. Which of the following types of CPT is most commonly billed in primary care coding?

a. Evaluation and management codes
b. Vaccination codes
c. In-office surgical procedure codes
d. Medicine codes

4. The elements of the key component history are: chief complaint; history of present illness; past, family, social history; and which of the following?

a. Body areas
b. Organ systems
c. Risk
d. Review of systems

5. What is the act of coding an E/M service at a level lower than what was performed?

a. Undercoding
b. Overcoding
c. Fraud
d. Abuse

6. Which of the following describes an organ system?

a. A specific organ system that may be examined during an E/M encounter
b. A general area of the body that may be examined during an E/M encounter
c. A specific area of the body that is reviewed in the review of systems
d. A general organ system that is reviewed in the review of systems

7. In E/M coding, which key component asks the question: How dangerous or risky is the patient's healthcare condition?

a. History
b. Examination
c. Medical decision-making
d. None of the above

8. In coding for vaccines, the two codes that must be reported are the administration and which of the following?

a. Administration
b. Serum
c. Immune globulin
d. Therapeutic substance

9. Which of the following best describes an encounter that includes a comprehensive health evaluation and anticipatory guidance?

   a. Evaluation and management encounters
   b. Preventive services
   c. Chronic care management
   d. Vaccination administration

10. When two E/M services are performed on the same day, which modifier is necessary to report?

    a. Modifier -32
    b. Modifier -95
    c. Modifier -24
    d. Modifier -25

11. Which of the following vaccine administration codes would be used for an injection provided to a pediatric patient with counseling?

    a. 90471
    b. 90473
    c. 97632
    d. 90460

12. Which of the following vaccine administration codes would be used for a nasal administration of a flu vaccine?

    a. 90471
    b. 90473
    c. 97632
    d. 90460

13. Offices may perform laboratory procedures in the office if they are which of the following?

    a. Provider approved
    b. Sent to the patient deductible
    c. Pre-authorized by the insurance plan
    d. CLIA-waived

14. Which of the following modifiers should be appended to a procedure that was repeated on the same date of service?

    a. Modifier -59
    b. Modifier -QW
    c. Modifier -76
    d. Modifier -XU

15. In ICD-10-CM coding, Z-codes are used to report which of the following reasons for encounter?

    a. Signs and symptoms
    b. Preventive examinations
    c. Patient history
    d. Patient status

16. For hypertension with CKD, one code should be selected for the hypertension, and another code for the:

    a. Heart failure
    b. Diabetes
    c. Stage of CKD
    d. End-stage renal disease

Instructions: Answer the following questions with the appropriate code(s).

1. A 56-year-old female with DM2 presents with recently diagnosed mild open-angle bilateral glaucoma and right eye cataract. Her diabetes is poorly controlled with daily insulin use. (Remember to use an additional code for hyperglycemia because the DM is identified as poorly controlled). Provider performed a detailed history, comprehensive examination, and high complexity MDM. Referred to endocrinologist.

   CPT code(s): _____

   ICD-10-CM code(s): _____ ,

   _____ , _____ , _____ ,

   _____ , _____

2. A 56-year-old new male patient is seen for stage 4 CKD with congestive heart failure due to hypertension. Provider performed a detailed history and exam with MDM of moderate complexity.

   CPT code(s): _____

   ICD-10-CM code(s): _____ ,

   _____ , _____

3. A 21-year-old female is seen with severe persistent asthma with acute exacerbation. Pulse oximetry taken in the office revealed oxygen level of 88 percent. Pressurized nebulizer breathing treatment immediately administered using albuterol sulfate inhalation solution. Post-neb oxygen level was a steady 95 percent. Provider performed a problem-focused history, detailed examination, and high complexity MDM.

CPT code(s): _____ , _____ ,

_____

ICD-10-CM code(s): _____

4. A 65-year-old male Medicare patient presents for his IPPE "Welcome to Medicare" visit and routine EKG as part of his IPPE benefit. During the encounter, the provider diagnoses the patient with psoriasis. He is also evaluated for his type 2 diabetic polyneuropathy and diabetic cataract, both of which are well-controlled.

HCPCS codes: _____ , _____

ICD-10-CM codes: _____

References

American Academy of Professional Coders (AAPC). 2016. *Study Guide: CEMC Evaluation and Management.* Salt Lake City, UT: AAPC.

American Medical Association (AMA). 2019. *CPT 2020 Professional Edition.* Chicago: AMA.

Centers for Medicare and Medicaid Services (CMS). 2019a (December). Shared Savings Program: For Providers. https://www.cms.gov/Medicare/Medicare-Fee-for-Service-Payment/sharedsavingsprogram/for-providers.

Centers for Medicare and Medicaid Services (CMS). 2019b. ICD-10-CM Official Guidelines for Coding and Reporting FY 2020. https://www.cms.gov/Medicare/Coding/ICD10/Downloads/2020-Coding-Guidelines.pdf.

Centers for Medicare and Medicaid Services (CMS). 2018a (August). Initial Preventative Physical Examination. https://www.cms.gov/Outreach-and-Education/Medicare-Learning-Network-MLN/MLNProducts/Downloads/MPS_QRI_IPPE001a.pdf.

Centers for Medicare and Medicaid Services (CMS). 2018b (August). Annual Wellness Visit. https://www.cms.gov/Outreach-and-Education/Medicare-Learning-Network-MLN/MLNProducts/Downloads/AWV_Chart_ICN905706.pdf.

Centers for Medicare and Medicaid Services (CMS). 1997. 1997 Documentation Guidelines for Evaluation and Management Services. https://www.cms.gov/Outreach-and-Education/Medicare-Learning-Network-MLN/MLNEdWebGuide/Downloads/97Docguidelines.pdf.

Centers for Medicare and Medicaid Services (CMS). 1995. 1995 Documentation Guidelines for Evaluation and Management Services. https://www.cms.gov/Outreach-and-Education/Medicare-Learning-Network-MLN/MLNEdWebGuide/Downloads/95Docguidelines.pdf.

Novitas Solutions. 2017. E/M Documentation Auditor's Instructions. https://www.novitas-solutions.com/webcenter/content/conn/UCM_Repository/uuid/dDocName:00004966.

OpenStax. 2013. Regions and Quadrants of the Peritoneal Cavity. Digital Image. https://cnx.org/contents/F-TuqKAF@3/Anatomical-Terminology#fig-ch01_06_05.

Resources

American Health Information Management Association (AHIMA). 2019. *ICD-10-CM Code Book: 2020.* Chicago: AHIMA.

Beck, D. and D. Margolin. 2007. Physician Coding and Reimbursement. https://www.ncbi.nlm.nih.gov/pmc/articles/PMC3096340/.

Centers for Disease Control and Prevention (CDC). 2018. Waived Tests. https://wwwn.cdc.gov/clia/resources/waivedtests/.

Menahem, S., A. Nazarenko, and P. Shvartzman. 2014 (March 25). Minor surgical procedures and musculoskeletal injections by primary care physicians—an Israeli experience. *Israel Journal Health Policy Research* 3:12. https://www.ncbi.nlm.nih.gov/pmc/articles/PMC3987677/.

Practice Management Institute (PMI). 2012. *E/M Coding Workshop.* San Antonio: Assistex, Inc.

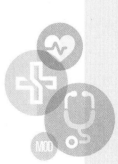

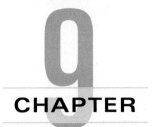

CHAPTER

Eye and Vision Services

Learning Objectives

- Understand the basics of billing and coding within the specialties of optometry and ophthalmology
- Examine procedural codes and guidelines for eye and vision services
- Examine diagnosis coding and medical necessity for eye and vision services
- Identify and apply ICD-10-CM, CPT, and HCPCS codes to optometry and ophthalmology cases

Key Terms

Acquired condition
Comprehensive ophthalmological services
Cortical cataract
Enucleation
Evisceration
Exenteration
Extracapsular cataract extraction (ECCE)
Glaucoma
Goniolens
Intermediate ophthalmological services

Intracapsular cataract extraction (ICCE)
Intraocular pressure
Keratoplasty
Lifestyle impairments
Macular degeneration
Nuclear cataract
Ocular adnexa
Ophthalmologist
Ophthalmology
Optometrist
Optometry

Paired organs
Phacoemulsification
Pseudophakia
Refraction
Refractive surgery
Retinal detachment
Slit lamp
Strabismus
Subcapsular cataract
Trabeculectomy
Vision insurance

Eye and vision services are performed by two different yet interrelated healthcare specialists—optometrists and ophthalmologists. **Optometrists** examine the eyes for visual defects, such as myopia (nearsightedness), and prescribe lenses to correct the defect (either glasses or contact lenses). **Ophthalmologists** specialize in pathology and diseases of the eyeball and perform surgeries to correct eye problems.

Often, to determine visual acuity, optometrists see patients with defects in vision and perform vision screenings and **refractions**. A refraction is a test performed to determine if a patient has any abnormalities with his or her vision; it is used to identify the appropriate prescription for eyeglasses or contact lenses. However, optometrists sometimes see patients with medical problems of the eye, such as a corneal ulcer, and provide medical treatment. Therefore, optometrists sometimes see patients with vision diagnoses, and other times they see patients with medical diagnoses. This results in complications when billing and coding for eye services, as some healthcare insurance plans will pay for vision procedures, while others will only pay for medical procedures.

This chapter discusses the basics of coding for optometry and ophthalmology services, for both visual and medical conditions. This includes the differences between the two specialties, in addition to the different procedures and diagnoses used in coding for eye and vision services. Eye services also employ a special set of ophthalmology evaluation and management (E/M) codes that may be used as an alternative to medical E/M codes—making eye and vision services an interesting offshoot from general coding.

Optometry and Ophthalmology Basics

There are two major divisions within eye and vision services—optometry and ophthalmology—each of which provides a specific type of service. An optometrist is a specialist in **optometry**; practitioners in this field perform examinations of the ophthalmological system, in addition to providing medical treatment and management of eye conditions. For example, an optometrist would perform an evaluation and management of a patient's ophthalmological system as well as a refraction to determine any visual defects. Then the optometrist would provide a prescription for corrective lenses to correct any visual defect.

On the other hand, an ophthalmologist is a specialist in **ophthalmology**. Practitioners in this field specialize in the anatomy, physiology, and pathology of diseases of the eyeball; they also perform medical and surgical procedures on the eye. For example, an ophthalmologist would be the healthcare provider to repair a retinal detachment or perform an intraoperative lens procedure.

It is important to understand the distinction between the two types of providers to understand which codes are reported in each of these specialties. Billing and coding for eye and vision services is also particularly unique because of the difference between vision insurance and healthcare insurance, as identified by the diagnosis code submitted to identify the medical necessity for the service (see figure 9.1).

Billing and Coding Basics

The difference between optometrists and ophthalmologists is more than just a side note. Because the two specialties are inherently different, there are major differences in billing and coding for their respective services. The first important thing to note is the difference between insurance plans. Depending on the type of service and the patient's diagnosis, it is necessary to send the claim for services to either a *vision* insurance plan or a *healthcare* insurance plan. Furthermore, documentation requirements to support medical necessity for eye and vision services are more extensive and a simple statement of patient diagnosis may not be enough to support certain services.

Figure 9.1. Optometry versus ophthalmology

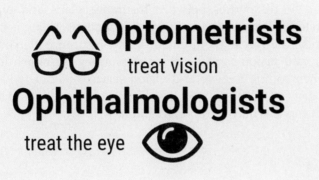

Type of Patient Insurance

Like behavioral health services, certain vision services are not covered under healthcare insurance. Rather, these services are paid under a separate vision insurance policy. **Vision insurance** is similar to health insurance, but it only covers services related to visual acuity assessments, refractions, and corrective lenses. Services covered by vision insurance typically include

- Routine (ophthalmological) wellness examinations
- Contact lens fitting
- Hardware, such as frames and lenses

Vision insurance plans vary widely. For example, some plans cover contact lens fitting, while others may not. Many also place limits on the frequency of services, such as one wellness examination per year. There are also limits on the amount of payment for services—such as insurance will pay $150 for a pair of glasses (spectacles) with lenses, but any amount over the $150 the patient would have to pay out of pocket.

Healthcare insurance covers services that are necessary due to a *medical* diagnosis. Even though services are performed on the eye, they are covered by healthcare insurance if the patient has a medical condition that affects the eye, such as diabetes mellitus. Services covered by healthcare insurance for eye procedures include:

- Office visits
- Diagnostic tests
- Surgical procedures
- Office procedures due to a medical diagnosis

Unlike vision insurance, healthcare insurance has few limitations on the number or frequency of visits. Instead of once per year, patients may receive medical eye services as often as medically necessary. Because it does not cover vision services, healthcare insurance does not pay for lenses, frames, or contact lenses. In short: Vision insurance pays for eyesight care, and medical insurance pays for eye care.

Vision and healthcare insurance are not always separate. It is possible to have a plan with combined coverage, so a patient may have one plan that covers both medical and vision procedures. Other insurance plans—such as Medicaid and Medicare—include coverage for certain vision services through the healthcare plan. For example, most Medicaid plans permit one eye screening per year and allow a certain amount of coverage for lenses (eyesight care) in addition to covering injuries or medical conditions of the eyes, like corneal lacerations or glaucoma (eye care).

When coding, the differences between insurance plans and types of insurance cannot be understated. Because the majority of outpatient coding is used for payment, it is helpful to know the special requirements of the insurance plan being billed. Codes reported for eye and vision services differ, depending on which insurance plain is being billed. When coding for eye and vision services, either for an optometrist or an ophthalmologist, it is necessary to first identify the patient's insurance plan and determine which services may be reported and how.

Key to Success

The rest of this chapter discusses the numerous codes used for different insurance plans and services. Do not get preoccupied with these billing differences as you are learning ICD-10-CM and CPT coding. It is more important to focus on learning how to code accurately by correctly reporting the procedure performed and the condition treated. Differences in billing will become more significant when you are a more experienced coder.

Healthcare versus Vision Diagnoses

It is important to differentiate between vision diagnoses and medical diagnoses of the eye. When coding for vision services (billed through vision insurance), use only vision diagnosis codes from the ICD-10-CM code book for conditions that affect eyesight and require corrective lenses, such as codes for amblyopia or presbyopia. When coding for medical eye services (billed through healthcare insurance) the necessary ICD-10-CM diagnosis code can be used to identify the condition affecting the eyes, such as foreign body on the eye or diabetic retinopathy, both of which are medical problems impacting the eyes.

Specific diagnostic coding information for common conditions is discussed later in this chapter. First, it is important to briefly discuss instances in which more than a simple diagnosis code is needed.

Medical Necessity for Eye Services

Before discussing the specific diagnosis codes used in eye and vision services, medical necessity for eye procedures should be addressed, as the requirements to support medical necessity for some procedures are more extensive than simply stating the diagnosis code.

Medical necessity to support procedures that treat such conditions as cataracts, capsular opacification, and blepharoptosis, must identify lifestyle impairments suffered by the patient due to the condition. **Lifestyle impairments** are descriptions of how the patient's eye condition has negatively impacted his or her lifestyle, including

- How decreased vision affects daily living activities
- Eyelids that rest on the eyelashes
- Restriction of peripheral vision
- Continued complaints of glare, or lack of distance or near vision
- Patient must raise eyelashes to see better

These functional impairments and ones like them must be documented before the surgery to correct the condition. If additional surgeries are needed, then the new lifestyle impairments must be sufficient to support the medical necessity for the new service. To ensure that the patient's diagnosis qualifies as a lifestyle impairment, and that the service provided will be considered medically necessary, it may be necessary to contact the patient's insurance payer to confirm that the service will be covered. Some insurance policies may require a prior authorization for certain services before they may be provided.

As a coder in an optometry or ophthalmology practice, coding may entail more than simply selecting and reporting a code. Certain services may need to be reported with health records, or with pre-certification or preauthorization documents that support the need for the procedure.

Anatomy and Physiology of the Eye and Ocular Adnexa

The eye and ocular adnexa are some of the most complex structures in the human body. To ensure correct code selection, it is necessary to be familiar with the anatomy and physiology of the eye. The Eye and Ocular Adnexa section in the CPT code book is organized anatomically, starting with the eye and then moving to the adnexa and accessory structures. Review figure 9.2 and identify the following:

- Eyeball
- Anterior segment (consists of the cornea, anterior chamber, anterior sclera, iris, ciliary body, and lens).
- Posterior segment (consists of the vitreous, retina, choroid, and posterior sclera)

Ocular adnexa are the accessory structures of the eye, including the extraocular muscles, eyelids, lacrimal system, orbit, and optic nerve and pathways. Surgical procedures on these structures are also found in the Eye and Ocular Adnexa subsection of the CPT code book (with the exception of the optic nerve and pathways, found in the Nervous System subsection). Review figures 9.2 through 9.4 and identify the following:

- Extraorbital muscles
- Eyelids
- Conjunctiva
- Lacrimal System

Figure 9.2. Anatomy of the eye

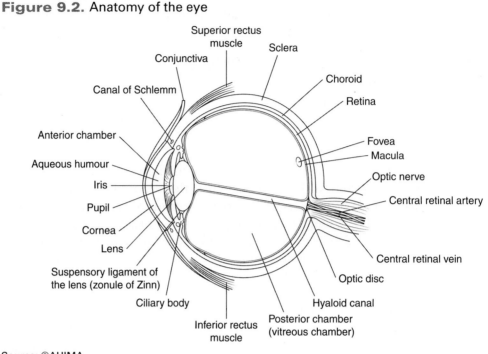

Source: ©AHIMA.

Figure 9.3. Extrinsic eye muscles

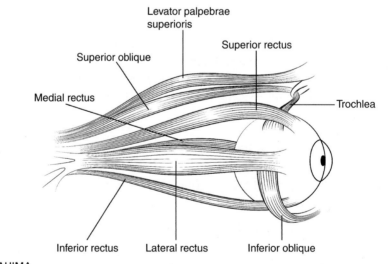

Source: ©AHIMA.

Key to Success

The medical terms for eye and ocular structures may be unfamiliar to most coders, especially those new to the field. As you read this chapter (and other chapters with distinct terminology), be sure to use a high-quality medical dictionary. Learning the terminology now will ensure that you have what it takes to complete a certification exam or begin working as a coder in this field.

Figure 9.4. Lacrimal apparatus

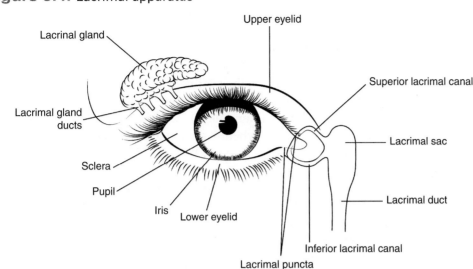

Source: ©AHIMA.

Procedural Coding in Optometry and Ophthalmology

Procedural coding for optometry and ophthalmology services is based on a unique set of procedure codes. Although eye service providers may bill E/M codes, there are several other sections in the CPT code book that are specifically devoted to the eye. The majority of eye and vision service codes are located in three different areas of the CPT code book: the E/M section, the Eye and Ocular Adnexa subsection in the Surgery section, and the Ophthalmology subsection of the Medicine section. Additional codes from the Radiology section (ultrasounds of the eye and orbital contents) and Category III (new and emerging eye technology) codes may also be used for eye and vision services.

Key to Success

The specialty of eye and vision services will determine which codes you use most often. For example, optometry coding relies more on evaluation and management of eye conditions and healthcare services, so coding for an optometrist will require spending most of your time in the E/M and Medicine sections of the CPT code book. On the other hand, ophthalmology coding relies heavily on the surgical procedure performed by the ophthalmologist, so coding within this specialty may require you to spend more time in the Surgery section of the CPT code book. Whatever the specialty in which you work, it is necessary to remain flexible and code for the service that was performed rather than coding only from one section of the book.

Coding for eye and vision services is perhaps best understood by dividing the two specialties—optometry coding and ophthalmology coding. However, it is first necessary to discuss the E/M codes that may be used by either specialty, including when to use ophthalmology E/M codes rather than medical E/M codes, and vice-versa. Finally, this section discusses the handful of modifiers that are often used in optometry and ophthalmology services.

Ophthalmology E/M Services

Coding for eye and vision encounters varies from medical services because there is a special selection of E/M codes used only for ophthalmological services. Eye specialists can use E/M codes (Office or Other Outpatient Services, 99201–99215), from the E/M section of the CPT code book or ophthalmological service E/M codes (Ophthalmology, 92002–92499) from the Medicine section of the CPT code book.

There are four ophthalmological service E/M codes that are divided depending on patient status (new or established) and level of the service (intermediate or comprehensive). These codes are used when a provider performs an evaluation of the ophthalmological system, including history, general observation, external and ophthalmoscopic examinations, gross visual field, and sensorimotor examination. These are integrated services and medical decision-making cannot be separated from the examining techniques used. Unlike medical E/M codes, ophthalmological services do not include a history related to all aspects of the patient's health, such as a review of all body areas or organ systems, nor do they include a physical examination or more than just the ophthalmological system. They focus only on the eye and accessory structures. The four ophthalmology E/M codes are as follows.

- 92002, Ophthalmological services: medical examination and evaluation with initiation of diagnostic and treatment program; *intermediate, new patient*
- 92004, Ophthalmological services: medical examination and evaluation with initiation of diagnostic and treatment program; *comprehensive, new patient*
- 92012, Ophthalmological services: medical examination and evaluation with initiation or continuation of diagnostic and treatment program; *intermediate, established patient*
- 92014, Ophthalmological services: medical examination and evaluation with initiation of diagnostic and treatment program; *comprehensive, established patient*

There are two levels of complexity for ophthalmological services—intermediate and comprehensive (see table 9.1). **Intermediate ophthalmological services** include an evaluation of a new or existing condition complicated with a new diagnosis. **Comprehensive ophthalmological services** include a general evaluation of the complete ophthalmological system. An ophthalmologist may also decide to use a medical E/M code (discussed as follows), instead of one of the four ophthalmology E/M codes. Note also that these ophthalmological services codes (92002–92014) are to be used in conjunction with codes to report any other services performed on the same date.

Table 9.1. Ophthalmological services E/M codes

Ophthalmologic Services	Intermediate	Comprehensive
New	92002	92004
Established	92012	92014

Notice that the last two digits in the ophthalmological services codes are the same as if they were medical E/M codes. A low-level intermediate E/M encounter for a new patient is coded with 99202, Office or other outpatient visit for the evaluation and management of a new patient, which requires these three key components: an expanded problem-focused history; an expanded problem-focused examination; straightforward medical decision-making; and the low-level ophthalmologic services encounter for a new patient is coded with 92002, Ophthalmological services: medical examination and evaluation initiation of diagnostic and treatment program; intermediate, new patient. Correspondingly, the higher-level E/M code is 99214, Office or other outpatient visit for the evaluation and management of an established patient, which requires at least 2 of these 3 key components: a detailed history; a detailed examination; medical decision-making of moderate complexity; and the comprehensive level ophthalmological services codes is 92014, Ophthalmological services: medical examination and evaluation of diagnostic and treatment program; comprehensive, established patient. However, ophthalmological services should not be coded when the provider performs an evaluation of the patient's ophthalmological system for a medical diagnosis.

E/M codes (99201–99215) may be used in lieu of the ophthalmological services codes when the provider performs an encounter for a medical diagnosis that involves more than the patient's ophthalmological system. For example, if an optometrist performs a routine visual examination of a patient with diabetic retinopathy, she would use an E/M code (99201–99215) rather than an ophthalmological services code (92002–92014).

Both sets of E/M codes are used by either optometrists or ophthalmologists, depending on the circumstances of the encounter. Figure 9.5 shows examples of each type of encounter.

Figure 9.5. E/M and ophthalmological services examples

Case #1: Evaluation and Management Code	Case #2: Ophthalmological Services Code
A 68-year-old new patient presented to the office of an ophthalmologist for an eye checkup. He states that his glasses might be "slightly off." After further questioning, he states that his vision has been slightly blurry for the past three months, at all distances. Ophthalmologist performed a comprehensive history, comprehensive eye examination with refraction and diagnosed the patient with a senile nuclear cataract and glaucoma suspect (moderate complexity MDM). Additional testing in the office included pachymetry and retinal photos. Will follow up in one week for intraocular pressure and optical coherence tomography.	A 68-year-old established patient presents to the ophthalmology office for his follow-up from one week ago. Ophthalmologist performed an intermediate examination and diagnosed the patient with primary open-angle glaucoma. Optical coherence tomography and extended visual field examination was performed in the office. Prescribed Xalatan and will follow up in two weeks.
Procedure codes:	**Procedure codes:**
99204, Level 4 E/M encounter, new patient 92015, Determination of refractive state 76514, Ophthalmic ultrasound, diagnostic; corneal pachymetry, unilateral or bilateral (determination of corneal thickness) 92250, Fundus photography with interpretation and report	92012, Ophthalmological services; intermediate, established patient 92133, Scanning computerized ophthalmic diagnostic imaging, posterior segment, with interpretation and report; optic nerve 92083, Visual field examination, with interpretation and report; extended examination
Diagnosis codes:	**Diagnosis codes:**
H25.10, Age-related nuclear cataract, unspecified eye H40.009, Preglaucoma, unspecified, unspecified eye	H40.1190, Primary open-angle glaucoma, unspecified eye, stage unspecified
Justification of code use:	**Justification of code use:**
In this case, the patient came in for just a checkup, but the provider completed a comprehensive history, examination, and moderate MDM, and found two significant medical problems: cataracts and glaucoma suspect.	In this case, the patient came in for an evaluation of an existing condition complicated by a new diagnostic problem, with initiation of diagnostic and treatment program.

Besides E/M services, there are several additional procedures performed on the eyes and accessory structures. It is helpful to discuss these services separately, depending on if they are optometry or ophthalmology services, as well as briefly cover some of the modifiers used in coding optometry and ophthalmology procedures.

Optometry Procedures

Optometry services are focused on the health and wellness of the eye and the ability to see. Optometry procedures are surgically noninvasive and do not include surgical treatments of the eyes. These procedures consist mostly of eye examinations, the provision of glasses and corrective lenses, screenings and diagnostic tests for eye conditions, and miscellaneous ophthalmological services.

Eye Exams and Refractions

Eye examinations are coded with either medical E/M codes or with ophthalmological services E/M codes, as described in the previous section. It is important to note that eye examination codes do not include refraction. A refraction test is a component of a typical eye examination performed by an optometrist for a corrective lens prescription and may be coded separately from the eye examination itself using code 92015, Determination of refractive state.

After a refraction is performed, it may be determined that the patient needs glasses or corrective lenses. However, using this refraction code depends on the patient's insurance policy. If the patient has Medicaid, there are two HCPCS codes that include the refraction in addition to the eye examination: S0620, Routine ophthalmological examination *including refraction*, new patient, and S0621, Routine ophthalmological examination *including refraction*, established patient. Notice that in the example presented in figure 9.6, the encounter description is the same, yet the procedure codes billed differ based on the patient's insurance coverage.

Figure 9.6. Examples of refraction coding

Case #1: Commercial Insurance	Case #2: Medicaid
Intermediate eye examination performed on 10-year-old established female patient, including refraction.	*Intermediate eye examination performed on 10-year-old established female patient, including refraction.*
Procedure codes:	**Procedure code:**
92012, Ophthalmological services; intermediate, established patient 92015, Determination of refractive state	S0621, Routine ophthalmological examination including refraction, established patient

Glasses and Corrective Lenses

Many optometry offices also provide glasses and corrective lenses to their patients, which are coded using the appropriate HCPCS or CPT code.

HCPCS codes for vision services (V2020–V2799) are used to bill various supplies such as corrective lenses. The act of refracting the patient's vision or performing any actual procedures on the patient's vision are reported with CPT codes and are discussed as follows. These HCPCS codes are used to report the corrective lenses or other vision products that are supplied to the patient. They include

- Frames
- Spectacle lenses (single vision, bifocal, trifocal, and variable asphericity)

- Contact lenses
- Low vision aids
- Prosthetic eyes
- Intraocular lenses
- Miscellaneous vision services

As previously mentioned, CPT codes are used to report the procedures specific to fitting contact lenses, either for correcting a patient's vision or for managing a health condition. They include the following:

- 92071, Fitting of contact lens for treatment of ocular surface disease. This code is used when a contact lens is prescribed to provide dressing to the eye. For example, a contact lens may be fitted over a corneal abrasion to act as a bandage and allow healing.
- 92072, Fitting of contact lens for management of keratoconus, initial fitting. Keratoconus is a condition in which the cornea of the eye protrudes in a cone shape. Contact lenses for keratoconus help to reshape the cornea and restore vision.
- Contact lens services. These services include the prescription and fitting of contact lenses and the instructions and training of the wearer. Incidental revision of the lens during the trial period is also included in these services (for example, fitting a different set of lenses within the trial period if the initial pair were uncomfortable or did not fit well). These services are coded with 92310 through 92317, and depend on the type of lens, the condition being treated, and the individual that is completing the fitting component of the contact lens service. In addition to the contact lens fitting, the appropriate HCPCS V-code (as listed previously) should also be used to identify the lenses supplied to the patient.

For example, when a patient goes into the office for the fitting of contact lenses, the actual fitting and prescription of the lens is reported with the appropriate CPT code. The lens itself is reported with the appropriate HCPCS code.

Screenings and Miscellaneous Eye Services

Similar to medical specialties, optometrists perform a number of different screenings used to either test for a specific condition (such as glaucoma), or to test for visual acuity. There are also several different ophthalmological services performed by optometrists.

- G0117 and G0118, Glaucoma screening for high risk patient, is used for Medicare patients who meet the criteria for a glaucoma screening.
- 92020, Gonioscopy (separate procedure), is an examination of the front part of the eye (the anterior chamber), between the cornea and the iris. This examination is used to determine a buildup of pressure, which could indicate glaucoma.
- 92100, Serial tonometry (separate procedure) with multiple measurements of intraocular pressure over an extended time period with interpretation and report, same day (eg, diurnal curve or medical treatment of acute elevation of intraocular pressure) is yet another way to screen for glaucoma. This consists of multiple measurements of intraocular pressure over an extended period of time on the same day. Note that a tonometry measurement is included in an ophthalmological examination, and this procedure is designated as a separate procedure. It should be reported only if it is the sole procedure performed on the date of service.

- 76514, Ophthalmic ultrasound, diagnostic; corneal pachymetry, unilateral or bilateral (determination of corneal thickness) is performed for various reasons, including screening for keratoconus and glaucoma.

Additional codes for miscellaneous ophthalmological services, visual acuity assessments, and ophthalmoscopy codes are also listed throughout the Ophthalmology subsection of the CPT code book. Minor surgical procedures are also performed by optometrists. Keep in mind that these procedures are not invasive surgeries, like those performed by ophthalmologists.

Figure 9.7. Slit lamp examination of the eye

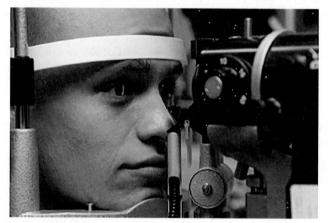

Source: US Air Force, Seltmann 2012.

Minor Surgical Procedures

Minor surgical procedures performed by optometrists are minimally invasive, and usually are done to treat a minor or uncomplicated problem. They include the following:

- 65205–65222, Removal of foreign body, external eye. These codes report the removal of a foreign body from the external eye, including the cornea or conjunctiva. Foreign bodies that are deeper than the external eye may require patient anesthesia and a more complex removal. These codes depend on the depth of the foreign body, the area from which the foreign body was removed, and whether or not a slit lamp was used. A **slit lamp** is a high-intensity light that can be focused into a thin sheet to shine into the eye. Slit lamps are commonly used during eye examinations to find abnormalities in the anterior of the eye (see figure 9.7).

- 65435, Removal of corneal epithelium; with or without chemocauterization (abrasion, curettage). Also called corneal epithelial debridement, this procedure treats irregularities of the epithelium (skin) of the cornea.

- 67820, Correction of trichiasis; epilation, by forceps only. Trichiasis in a condition in which the eyelashes are ingrown or misdirected and must be manually removed using forceps and a biomicroscope.

- 68761, Closure of the lacrimal punctum; by plug, each. In this procedure, the provider inserts a small plug into the lacrimal punctum, which reduces drainage from the eye. It is often performed as a treatment for dry eye syndrome.

Complete the exercises in There's a Code for That 9.1 to practice coding optometry procedures.

Optometry procedures

9.1

Read the following documentation of the optometry service and code for the encounter.

There's a Code for That

1. Comprehensive ophthalmological examination with refraction performed on an established patient with senile nuclear sclerosis and hypermetropia.

   CPT codes: _____ , _____

2. Optometrist performed a comprehensive ophthalmological examination on a new patient with open angle glaucoma and type 1 diabetes mellitus. Additional procedures included a bilateral corneal pachymetry, scanning computerized ophthalmic diagnostic imaging (SCODI) of the anterior segment, and extended bilateral visual field examination using Humphrey visual field analyzer.

   CPT codes: _____ , _____ , _____ ,
   _____

3. Routine ophthalmological examination with refraction performed on an established Medicaid patient. Optometrist furnished patient with spectacle frames with lenses. Lens #1 (right): single vision, plano to 1.75. Lens #2 (left): single vision, plano to 1.90. Both with anti-reflective coating. (Hint: Since this is a Medicaid patient, use the appropriate HCPCS code for the service. Supplies are also coded with HCPCS codes. Modifiers should identify the right and left sides).

   HCPCS codes: _____ , _____ , _____ ,
   _____ , _____ , _____ , _____

4. Patient with pain in the left eye was found upon examination (new patient, level 3 encounter) to have a foreign body in the cornea. Optometrist removed FB from the cornea with slit lamp assistance. Hint: Upon examination, the provider made the decision to perform the FB removal surgery.

   CPT codes: _____ , _____ , _____

Ophthalmology Procedures

Ophthalmologists may perform both medical and ophthalmological E/M services, but their specialty is focused on surgical interventions to treat eye conditions. Procedures consist of several specialized eye surgeries, but the most common are refractive surgeries, trabeculectomies, cataract surgeries, orbital surgeries, and strabismus surgery.

Key to Success

At the beginning of the Eye and Ocular Adnexa subsection in the Surgery section of the CPT code book, note the statement placed before the listing of CPT codes: *Do not report code 69990 in addition to codes 65091–68850.* Codes 65091 through 68850 are all Eye and Ocular Adnexa surgery codes. Code 69990, Operating microscope, should be reported when a surgical microscope is employed during microsurgery. However, the use of a surgical microscope is integral to ophthalmological procedures, and so it may not be reported separately when coding from this subsection of the CPT code book.

Refractive Surgeries

Refractive surgeries are performed to reshape the cornea of the eye and improve eyesight. They may be either elective or functional. Elective refractive surgery would be done solely to improve idiopathic myopia, hyperopia, and astigmatism, and would be elected by the patient so they would no longer have to wear glasses or corrective lenses. Functional refractive surgery would be done to correct a defect in vision due to a medical diagnosis, such as a traumatic injury. The surgery is performed by using a laser to re-shape the cornea and only takes a few minutes.

There are a number of different codes for refractive surgeries, which differ depending on the reason for the surgery and the type of surgery performed.

- Laser-assisted refractive surgeries are procedures in which a laser is used to incise the eye and reshape the cornea. The two most common are
    - S0800, Laser in situ keratomileusis (LASIK). Although it is not covered by Medicare, a handful of commercial insurance payers may pay for LASIK surgery to correct vision conditions.
    - S0810, Photorefractive keratectomy (PRK), is the second most common refractive laser surgery (after LASIK).
- If astigmatism is a result of ocular trauma or has been surgically induced, refractive surgery may be performed to reshape the cornea and restore vision. These procedures are coded with 65772, Corneal relaxing incision for correction of surgically induced astigmatism, and 65775, Corneal wedge resection for correction of surgically induced astigmatism.
- If none of the previous codes are applicable because of differences in the manner in which the procedure was performed, it would be appropriate to use 66999, Unlisted procedure, anterior segment of the eye, for either LASIK or PRK.

Trabeculectomy

A **trabeculectomy** is performed as a treatment for glaucoma, by lowering the **intraocular pressure** (the pressure inside the eyeball). The ophthalmologist uses a laser to open a drainage canal in the eye to allow for the outflow of aqueous humor by removing a part of the trabecular meshwork of the eye. The resulting outflow of aqueous humor drains into a bleb on the upper portion of the eye, covered by the eyelid. By draining the pressure of the aqueous humor, a trabeculectomy may slow the damage caused by glaucoma but cannot restore any vision lost from glaucoma (see figure 9.8). Procedure codes for trabeculectomies include the following:

- 66170, Fistularization of sclera for glaucoma; trabeculectomy ab externo in absence of previous surgery, and 66172, Fistularization of sclera for glaucoma; trabeculectomy ab externo with scarring from previous ocular surgery or trauma (includes injection of antifibrotic agents). These codes are the basic trabeculectomy codes for the treatment of glaucoma.
- 65850, Trabeculotomy ab externo, and 65855, Trabeculoplasty by laser surgery are performed for congenital glaucoma. These procedures are less invasive than trabeculectomies and are less likely to cause cataracts.
- 65820, Goniotomy. Also performed as a treatment for congenital glaucoma, this procedure uses a device called a **goniolens** (an ophthalmic endoscope) to see the anterior chamber of the eye and make an incision into the trabecular meshwork, reducing intraocular pressure. Note that if the goniolens is used, the add-on code 66990, Use of ophthalmic endoscope, should also be reported.

Figure 9.8. Trabeculectomy

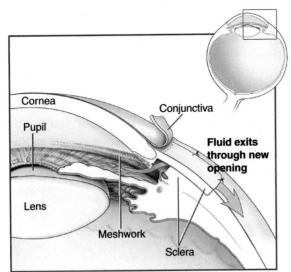

Cornea

Pupil

Conjunctiva

Fluid exits through new opening

Lens

Meshwork

Sclera

Source: NEI 2006.

Key to Success

Be careful when reading and selecting surgical procedure codes, as differences in procedure names are usually only a few letters. For example, a trabecul*ectomy* is a completely different procedure than a trabecul*otomy*. Reading either of these terms too quickly makes it easy to miss the small differences in spelling and may ultimately result in selecting the wrong code.

Cataract Surgery

Cataracts are a common cause of vision loss and affect, to some degree, over half of all adults over the age of 65 (Johns Hopkins University 2017). A cataract occurs when the lens, which lies behind the iris and pupil of the eye, becomes clouded, impeding vision.

There are three main types of cataracts.

- **Nuclear cataracts** form in the nucleus of the lens and are often associated with aging. They may also be referred to as senile cataracts.
- **Subcapsular cataracts** form at the back of the lens and are more common in individuals with diabetes mellitus or patients on high doses of steroids.
- **Cortical cataracts** begin on the peripheral edges of the lens and work their way inward toward the center. (AAO 2017)

Cataract surgery consists of replacing the clouded lens with an artificial lens to restore vision. It is a commonly performed surgery that takes about 30 minutes to complete. **Phacoemulsification** is a technique used during extracapsular cataract excision that uses ultrasound vibrations to break up the cloudy lens and extract it through a small hollow tube. There are two types of cataract extractions (note that all of these procedures include the placement of the intraocular lens prosthesis):

- **Extracapsular cataract extraction (ECCE).** In this procedure the lens is either broken up via phacoemulsification or it is surgically removed in one piece, leaving the lens capsule intact. ECCEs are reported with the following codes:

- 66982, Extracapsular cataract removal with insertion of intraocular lens prosthesis (1-stage procedure), manual or mechanical technique (eg, irrigation and aspiration or phacoemulsification), complex, requiring devices or techniques not generally used in routine cataract surgery (eg, iris expansion device, suture support for intraocular lens, or primary posterior capsulorrhexis) or performed on patients in the amblyogenic developmental stage
  - 66984, Extracapsular cataract removal with insertion of intraocular lens prosthesis (1 stage procedure), manual or mechanical technique (eg, irrigation and aspiration or phacoemulsification); without endoscopic cyclophotocoagulation.
- **Intracapsular cataract extraction (ICCE)**. This procedure removes both the lens and the lens capsule and is performed only in rare cases. ICCE is reported with code 66983, Intracapsular cataract extraction with insertion of intraocular lens prosthesis (1 stage procedure).

Orbital Surgery

Orbital surgeries are performed to treat defects resulting in acquired absence of the eye, eye tumors, or for removal of the eye for medical reasons.

Codes for the removal of ocular contents are based on the extent of the removal:

- **Evisceration** of the ocular contents is the removal of the contents of the globe of the eye, while leaving the remaining structures intact. This procedure is coded with
  - 65091, Evisceration of ocular contents; *without implant*, or
  - 65093, Evisceration of ocular contents, *with implant*.
- **Enucleation** is removing the eyeball while leaving the orbital structures intact, including the extraocular muscles. Codes for enucleation are divided depending on whether an implant was placed after the removal of the eye, and whether the extraocular muscles were attached to the implant (if placed). They are
  - 65101, Enucleation of eye, *without implant*,
  - 65103, Enucleation of eye; *with implant, muscles not attached to implant*, and
  - 65105, Enucleation of eye; *with implant, muscles attached to implant*.
- **Exenteration** of the orbit includes the removal of the eye and ocular adnexa. These codes are based on the extent of the removal. They are
  - 65110, Exenteration of orbit (does not include skin graft), removal of orbital contents; only,
  - 65112, Exenteration of orbit (does not include skin graft), removal of orbital contents; with therapeutic removal of bone, and
  - 65114, Exenteration of orbit (does not include skin graft), removal of orbital contents; with muscle or myocutaneous flap.

Strabismus Surgery

Strabismus is a misalignment of the eye muscles that can be surgically corrected by repositioning and strengthening the muscles of the eye. Codes for strabismus surgery (67311–67340) are based on the type or muscle (horizontal, vertical, or superior oblique), and the number of extraocular muscles involved in the procedure.

Keratoplasty

Keratoplasty is a corneal transplant, a procedure that replaces the cornea with a donor cornea graft. Code assignment for keratoplasty procedures is based on the thickness of the corneal graft and includes

- Partial thickness grafting, 65710, Keratoplasty (corneal transplant); anterior lamellar,
- Full thickness grafting, 65730, Keratoplasty (corneal transplant); penetrating (except in aphakia or pseudophakia), 65750, Keratoplasty (corneal transplant); penetrating (in aphakia), and 65755, Keratoplasty (corneal transplant); penetrating (in pseudophakia), and
- Grafting of the endothelium through a scleral tunnel, 65756, Keratoplasty (corneal transplant); endothelial.

Modifiers Used in Eye and Vision Services

There are a handful of important modifiers that a coder may need to append to eye and vision service codes. They identify the laterality of the procedure (either right or left), as well as the specific eyelid being worked on (when applicable). Additional modifiers may identify specific stages of the operative period, or the decision for surgery. Note that these additional modifiers may be used for any surgical procedure, not just surgical procedures on the eye or ocular adnexa.

- Modifier -LT, Left side and modifier -RT, Right side. Theses modifiers are used with paired organs to identify the side of the body on which the procedure was performed. For example, if the patient had strabismus surgery on the right eye, the modifier -RT should be appended to the strabismus surgery code. These modifiers should be used for any paired organ, such as limbs or ears, not just for eye procedures.
- Eyelid modifiers are used to identify the specific eyelid on which the procedure is being performed. It is not necessary to also use the -RT or -LT modifiers with these, as the laterality is already built into the modifier.
    - Modifier -E1, Upper left, eyelid
    - Modifier -E2, Lower left, eyelid
    - Modifier -E3, Upper right, eyelid
    - Modifier -E4, Lower right, eyelid
- Modifier -54, Surgical care only. This modifier is used when the surgeon performed only the surgery on the patient and did not provide either the pre- or postoperative care. For example, if the ophthalmologist performed an extracapsular cataract extraction (ECCE) and then transferred the care of the patient to an optometrist, he would bill the code for the ECCE (66984) with modifier -54 to indicate that he performed only the surgery on the patient: 66984-54, Extracapsular cataract removal with insertion of intraocular lens prosthesis (1 stage procedure), manual or mechanical technique (eg, irrigation and aspiration or phacoemulsification); without endoscopic cyclophotocoagulation, *surgical care only*. The payment for the surgery will be reduced accordingly.

If you are not sure whether or not to include the laterality or eyelid modifiers, append the modifiers to the appropriate procedure codes, just in case. It is better to have a modifier and not need it than to need a modifier and not have it. Usually, if an informational modifier is reported and the insurance plan does not require the modifier, they will simply ignore it. However, if the insurance *does* require the modifier and it was not reported, they may deny the charge.

- Modifier -55, Postoperative management only. This modifier should be appended when one healthcare provider performed the surgical procedure and a different healthcare provider performed the postoperative care. It should be appended to the code for the primary procedure, when reported by the provider who only managed the postoperative care. For example, an optometrist postoperatively manages a patient that just received an ECCE. He would report the code for the ECCE with modifier -55: 66984-55, Extracapsular cataract removal with insertion or intraocular lens prosthesis, manual or mechanical technique (eg, irrigation and aspiration or phacoemulsification); without endoscopic cyclophotocoagulation, *postoperative management only*. Even though the optometrist did not perform the cataract removal, it is coded as if he did, but with modifier -55 appended to identify that it was the postoperative care only. Modifier -55 will result in a minimal payment for the service, according to the work that was performed; for example, about 20 percent of the regular payment amount.

- Modifier -57, Decision for surgery. This modifier is important in coding, as it can indicate that a decision for surgery was made during an E/M encounter. For example, if it were determined during the encounter that a patient with glaucoma needed surgical intervention to treat the condition, then modifier -57 would be appended to the E/M code.

- Modifier -58, Staged or related procedure or service by the same physician or other qualified healthcare professional during the postoperative period. This modifier should be used when a procedure is performed in stages, and it should be appended to the second or subsequent code for the additional stage of surgery. For example, a surgeon performed a blepharoplasty (plastic repair of the eyelid), which was reported with code 67971, Reconstruction of eyelid, full thickness by transfer of transconjunctival flap from opposing eyelid; *up to two-thirds of eyelid, 1 stage or first stage*. It was determined that this surgical repair was not sufficient, the patient returned to the operating room on a different day after the initial surgery, and a second stage of the repair was done. The second stage repair should be reported as 67975, Reconstruction of eyelid, full thickness by transfer of transconjunctival flap from opposing eyelid; *second stage*, appended with modifier -58, as such: 67975-58.

Complete the exercises in There's a Code for That 9.2 to practice coding ophthalmology procedures.

9.2   Ophthalmology procedures

There's a Code for That

Read the following documentation of the ophthalmology service and code for the encounter.

1. Photocoagulation of localized retinal lesion of the right eye.

   CPT code: _____

2. Laser-assisted in situ keratomileusis.

   HCPCS code: _____

3. Goniotomy performed on 2-year-old female with congenital glaucoma with ophthalmological endoscopic assistance.

   CPT code: _____ , _____

4. ECCE with insertion of IOL prosthesis.

   CPT code: _____

5. Excision of two chalazion on right upper eyelid.

   CPT code: _____

Diagnostic Coding in Optometry and Ophthalmology

Diagnostic codes used in optometry and ophthalmology include a vast range of conditions affecting the eye and ocular adnexa as well as comorbid conditions, as discussed in chapter 2 (Healthcare Billing Basics), like hypertension or diabetes mellitus, which may complicate or even cause eye diseases. Diagnosis codes used in eye and vision services can be separated into two main types: screenings, or examinations, and eye conditions.

Key to Success

Diagnosis codes should be selected carefully, taking into account the patient's insurance—whether it is vision or healthcare insurance. Remember that healthcare insurance will not pay for an examination or treatment of a vision condition or general eye wellness examination. Rather, healthcare insurance will only pay for eye services performed for an actual medical diagnosis.

Eye Screenings and Examinations

Routine wellness examinations are performed on the ophthalmological system by optometrists and ophthalmologists, just as they are performed on the entire physical body by primary care practitioners. Optometrists perform annual wellness examinations to check for disease processes and to care for the vision of patients with vision needs. If, after examination, an optometrist discovers indicators for a disease, he or she will determine if there is a need for a further diagnostic test for the suspected condition. The diagnosis codes used to identify the medical necessity for these services depend on the type of service performed and whether any abnormalities or disease conditions were encountered.

- Z01.00, Encounter for examination of eyes and vision, without abnormal findings, and Z01.01, Encounter for examination of eyes and vision, with abnormal findings, should be used when a patient presents for a routine eye wellness examination. If no abnormal findings are encountered, code Z01.00 should be reported. Similar to coding for preventive physical examinations, if any abnormal findings are encountered, then code Z01.01 should be reported, with secondary codes to identify the abnormality. This includes any abnormal condition, even a vision problem. For example, if a patient is seen for a routine eye check and it is discovered that he or she has irregular astigmatism of the right eye, then the coder should report Z01.01, Encounter for examination of eyes and vision, with abnormal findings, along with H52.211, Irregular astigmatism, right eye.

- Z13.5, Encounter for screening of eye and ear disorders, should be reported when a patient presents for a diagnostic test for an eye condition and there was no diagnosis confirmed as a result of the test. For example, if a patient comes in for a diagnostic screening for macular degeneration and the diagnosis of macular degeneration is confirmed at that visit, only the code for macular degeneration should be reported. On the other hand, if the diagnosis of macular degeneration was *not* confirmed, then the code for the diagnostic screening (Z13.5) should be reported. If specific signs and symptoms that prompted the test are present, the coder should report the codes for the signs and symptoms. The screening code should be reported only if the diagnostic test was ordered without any signs, symptoms, illness, or injury recorded.

- Z96.1, Presence of intraocular lens, should be reported for any patient who has an intraocular lens prosthesis (pseudophakia).

Diagnostic Eye Coding

Besides eye screenings and examinations, optometrists and ophthalmologists commonly see a number of different medical diagnoses of the eye. There are specific guidelines when it comes to coding for eye conditions, including laterality, diabetic complications, and congenital conditions.

Laterality and Eyelids

Because the eyes are paired organs, which are symmetrically placed on the body, many of the diagnosis codes for eye conditions specify the laterality of the condition. Remember that in CPT coding, specific modifiers (-LT, Left side; -RT, Right side; and -50, Bilateral procedure) identify the laterality of the procedure. Laterality also exists in ICD-10-CM coding for eye conditions. However, in ICD-10-CM coding, laterality is identified by selecting the correct diagnosis code for the laterality documented rather than adding a modifier to identify the laterality, as in CPT coding. It is important to be particularly careful when coding for eye conditions and the procedures performed on them, to ensure that the laterality identified in the ICD-10-CM code matches the laterality identified by the CPT modifier (if applicable). If the laterality specified in the CPT procedure does not match the laterality specified in the ICD-10-CM diagnosis code, or vice-versa, then insurance may deny the claim.

The laterality of the eye conditions may be specified as right, left, or bilateral. If there is no laterality specified in the documentation, then the unspecified laterality code should be reported. For conditions affecting the eyelids, diagnosis codes may specify the exact eyelid affected by the condition. They include the right upper, right lower, left upper, and left lower eyelids. As with the laterality, if the specific eyelid is not documented, the code for the unspecified eyelid should be selected. For example, the codes for stye (H00.01-, Hordeolum externum) identify both the eyelid involved (upper or lower) as well as the laterality of the condition (right or left). A stye on the upper right eyelid would be coded as H00.011, Hordeolum externum right upper eyelid. However, if the provider's documentation did not specify which side (laterality) or eyelid on which the stye was located, then the unspecified version of the code would be reported (H00.019, Hordeolum externum unspecified eye, unspecified eyelid). Many eye conditions require detailed documentation to ensure that the correct laterality and eyelid are identified in the code.

Key to Success

When selecting diagnosis codes for eye conditions, be sure that the laterality (or eyelid) of the diagnosis code matches the laterality (or eyelid) identified by the CPT modifier. For example, if the procedure code modifier is -RT for a right-sided procedure, then the diagnosis code should identify that the condition affected the right eye. If the laterality or the eyelids do not match, then it may cause problems with claim processing.

Diabetic Eye Complications

Chronic high blood sugar, like that which happens with diabetes mellitus, can have negative effects on the eyes, and it is common for eye conditions to develop as a result of diabetes. When this happens, it is necessary to code for both the eye condition and the diabetes, by type. The following diabetes codes are combination codes that identify both the type of diabetes and the ophthalmological complication. Notice that they all end with the character "3" to identify the diabetic complication as "ophthalmic":

- E08.3-, Diabetes mellitus due to underlying condition with ophthalmic complications
- E09.3-, Drug or chemical-induced diabetes mellitus with ophthalmic complications
- E10.3-, Type 1 diabetes mellitus with ophthalmic complications
- E11.3-, Type 2 diabetes mellitus with ophthalmic complications
- E12.3-, Other specified diabetes mellitus with ophthalmic complications

If no combination code exists that identifies both the diabetes and the complication, then it is necessary to code for the two conditions separately.

Use the following steps to look up diabetes with ophthalmic complications and code for them correctly. Remember that one code should be used to identify each diabetic complication, so if the patient has multiple ophthalmic conditions, then one code should be reported to identify each individual complication.

1. Identify the type of diabetes: diabetes due to underlying condition, drug or chemical-induced diabetes, type 1, type 2, or other specified diabetes.
2. Identify each ophthalmic complication: diabetic retinopathy, diabetic cataract, diabetic macular edema, or other diabetic ophthalmic complication. Diabetic retinopathy codes are very specific and identify the type of retinopathy (proliferative or nonproliferative), the severity (mild, moderate, or severe), and whether it presents with or without macular edema.
3. If no combination code exists that identifies both the diabetes and the complication, then select the code for *other diabetic complication,* such as E11.39, Type 2 diabetes mellitus with other diabetic ophthalmic complication, and add an additional ICD-10-CM code to identify the specific complication.
4. Assign one code per diabetic complication, which may include multiple ophthalmic complications as well as other non-ophthalmic diabetic complications.

Congenital versus Acquired Conditions

A congenital condition is one that was present at or before birth. An **acquired condition**, on the other hand, is one that develops over the course of a person's life. Congenital conditions affect every part of the human body, not just the eyes, so the difference between congenital and acquired conditions should be kept in mind for coding for conditions throughout the ICD-10-CM code book.

Congenital conditions are all coded from chapter 17 (Congenital Malformations, Deformations, and Chromosomal Abnormalities) of the ICD-10-CM code book. Acquired conditions of the eyes are coded from chapter 7 (Diseases of the Eye and Adnexa) of the ICD-10-CM code book. If a condition is stated as *congenital*, then it should be coded from chapter 17. To look up a congenital anomaly in the ICD-10-CM code book, search for the condition in the Main Index and then select the congenital version of the condition. For example, when searching for congenital aphakia (absence of the lens of the eye), look up the term *aphakia* in the ICD-10-CM Main Index, and then reference the subterm *congenital*, which leads you to code Q12.3. Verify the code in the Tabular List: Q12.3, Congenital aphakia.

Eye Conditions

Coding for eye conditions usually requires knowledge of the laterality of the condition, as well as specifics of the severity of the condition. Generally speaking, coders should report one code for each eye condition, per eye, unless the condition presents bilaterally and a bilateral code exists. Top diagnoses for eye conditions include glaucoma, injuries, cataracts, macular degeneration, vision problems, and retinal detachments, all of which can be found in the Main Index of the ICD-10-CM code book and verified in the Tabular List.

Glaucoma

Glaucoma (H40–H42) is a buildup of intraocular pressure that causes damage to the eye's optic nerve over time and may eventually lead to irreversible vision loss. Treatments for glaucoma include medication and surgical intervention (trabeculectomy, as previously discussed). There are many types of glaucoma, which may be caused by injury to the eye, inflammatory conditions, severe eye infections, or a blockage of blood vessels in the eye. They are as follows:

- Open-angle glaucoma, also called wide-angle glaucoma, in which the trabecular meshwork of the eye does not properly allow for the outflow of aqueous humor
- Angle-closure glaucoma, also called chronic angle-closure or narrow-angle glaucoma, in which drainage of aqueous humor from the eye due to the angle between the iris and cornea being too narrow
- Congenital glaucoma (Q15.0, Congenital glaucoma), when a child is born with glaucoma due to a congenital defect in the eye's drainage structure
- Secondary glaucomas, which occur as a result of another condition or circumstance, and include glaucomas secondary to trauma, inflammation, other eye disorders, drug use, or underlying medical condition, such as poorly controlled diabetes or hypertension.

ICD-10-CM codes for glaucoma are perhaps the most specific eye condition codes, many of which require seven characters, so a coder must be careful with code selection and pay attention to the Official Guidelines for Coding and Reporting (OGCR) for this condition. As many codes as possible should be assigned to identify the type of glaucoma, the affected eye, and the stage of the glaucoma. When a patient has bilateral glaucoma and both eyes are documented as having the same type and stage of glaucoma, then the bilateral code option should be selected. If the glaucoma is bilateral but the stage or type is different, then one glaucoma code for each eye should be assigned rather than the bilateral code option. If the stage of the glaucoma cannot be determined, the code option for *indeterminate* stage is used. This is different from *unspecified* stage, which should be used when the documentation does not specify the stage of glaucoma. Refer to figure 9.9 for the OGCR related to coding for glaucoma.

Figure 9.9. OGCR I.C.7.a

---

7. **Chapter 7: Diseases of the Eye and Adnexa (H00-H59)**

   a. **Glaucoma**

      1) **Assigning Glaucoma Codes**

      Assign as many codes from category H40, Glaucoma, as needed to identify the type of glaucoma, the affected eye, and the glaucoma stage.

      2) **Bilateral glaucoma with same type and stage**

      When a patient has bilateral glaucoma and both eyes are documented as being the same type and stage, and there is a code for bilateral glaucoma, report only the code for the type of glaucoma, bilateral, with the seventh character for the stage.

      When a patient has bilateral glaucoma and both eyes are documented as being the same type and stage, and the classification does not provide a code for bilateral glaucoma (i.e. subcategories H40.10, H40.11 and H40.20) report only one code for the type of glaucoma with the appropriate seventh character for the stage.

      3) **Bilateral glaucoma stage with different types or stages**

      When a patient has bilateral glaucoma and each eye is documented as having a different type or stage, and the classification distinguishes laterality, assign the appropriate code for each eye rather than the code for bilateral glaucoma.

      When a patient has bilateral glaucoma and each eye is documented as having a different type, and the classification does not distinguish laterality (i.e. subcategories H40.10, H40.11 and H40.20), assign one code for each type of glaucoma with the appropriate seventh character for the stage.

      When a patient has bilateral glaucoma and each eye is documented as having the same type, but different stage, and the classification does not distinguish laterality (i.e. subcategories H40.10, H40.11 and H40.20), assign a code for the type of glaucoma for each eye with the seventh character for the specific glaucoma stage documented for each eye.

      4) **Patient admitted with glaucoma and stage evolves during the admission**

      If a patient is admitted with glaucoma and the stage progresses during the admission, assign the code for highest stage documented.

      5) **Indeterminate stage glaucoma**

      Assignment of the seventh character "4" for "indeterminate stage" should be based on the clinical documentation. The seventh character "4" is used for glaucomas whose stage cannot be clinically determined. This seventh character should not be confused with the seventh character "0", unspecified, which should be assigned when there is no documentation regarding the stage of the glaucoma.

Source: CMS 2019.

Key to Success

Be careful when selecting codes for glaucoma, as many of them require a seventh character extension to identify the stage of the condition. If the glaucoma is due to an underlying condition, underlying eye disorder, or an adverse effect, additional codes are needed to identify the causative conditions. Pay attention to the notes in the Tabular List, as they will indicate when an additional code may be necessary.

Eye Injuries

Eye injuries are coded from chapter 19 (Injury, Poisoning, and Certain Other Consequences of External Causes) of the ICD-10-CM code book, from category S05, Injury of eye and orbit. Remember that all injury codes require a seventh character extension to identify the encounter (A-initial, D-subsequent, S-Sequela). To code for an injury of the eye, check the documentation for the specific type of eye injury (contusion, laceration, penetrating wound) and the laterality of the condition. Bilateral eye injury codes do not exist, so if there are both right- and left-sided injuries, assign one code per ocular injury.

Cataracts

Diagnosis codes for cataracts (H25, H26, H28) specify the type and laterality of the condition. Types include age-related (also called senile), infantile or juvenile, traumatic (resulting from a traumatic injury), complicated (by neovascularization, other eye disorder, or glaucoma), drug-induced, or secondary cataract. If the same cataract presents bilaterally, assign the bilateral code option. If the condition presents bilaterally but the type of cataract is different, assign one code for each side. Additional codes may be needed to identify the underlying disease or eye condition, or the causative substance in drug-induced cataracts. As usual, pay attention to the notes in the Tabular List, as they will indicate when an additional code may be necessary.

Macular Degeneration

Macular degeneration (H35.3-) is a deterioration of the central portion of the retina, called the macula. In its early stages macular degeneration does not affect eyesight, but as the disease progresses patients may experience blurry or wavy vision, and in its most severe stages it can lead to complete loss of the central area of vision. Be diligent when reporting codes for macular degeneration, as some require seven characters while others require only six. Codes for nonexudative (or dry) and exudative (or wet) age-related macular degeneration (AMD) require seven characters. The seventh character identifies the stage of the AMD.

Vision Impairments

Because optometrists treat vision and refractive disorders, there are several commonly coded diagnoses for vision impairments (H52 and H53). These include myopia (nearsightedness), astigmatism, presbyopia (farsightedness), and other visual disturbances such as scotomas (blind spots) and color blindness.

Retinal Detachment

A retinal detachment (H33) occurs when the retina, a layer of tissue at the back of the eye, detaches from the eye tissues. It causes irreversible and immediate vision impairment and requires urgent treatment. Diagnosis codes for retinal detachments identify the laterality of the condition as well as the type of tear: retinal break, single break, multiple breaks, giant retinal tear, retinal dialysis, or total retinal detachment.

Coding for eye and vision diagnoses requires an eye for detail, as many codes require identification of the laterality and severity of the condition; and most ICD-10-CM codes are six to seven characters long, making these codes some of the more complex diagnosis codes in ICD-10-CM coding.

Complete the exercises in There's a Code for That 9.3 to practice assigning optometry and ophthalmology diagnosis codes.

Diagnostic coding for optometry and ophthalmology

9.3

There's a Code for That

Read the following documentation and assign the appropriate diagnosis code(s) for the encounter.

1. Patient presents for a routine eye exam with no abnormal findings.

   ICD-10-CM code: _____

2. Patient presents for a routine eye examination. During the exam, it is noted that the patient has developed regular astigmatism of the right eye since the last visit. Spectacle glasses were provided as well as lenses with anti-reflective coating.

   ICD-10-CM codes: _____ , _____

3. Patient is a known diabetic (type 2), diagnosed with proliferative diabetic retinopathy with macular edema of the right eye and proliferative diabetic retinopathy without macular edema of the left eye.

   ICD-10-CM codes: _____ , _____

4. Congenital cataract in a 1-year-old female patient.

   ICD-10-CM code: _____

5. Patient has primary open-angle glaucoma of the right and left eyes, mild stage.

   ICD-10-CM code: _____

6. A 28-year-old male hockey player presents for evaluation of his partially resolved cataract of the left eye, which is a late effect of blunt force trauma to the eye from a hockey stick. (Hint: Remember that a late effect is a sequela of a previous injury).

   ICD-10-CM codes: _____ , _____

7. Age-related macular degeneration.

   ICD-10-CM code: _____

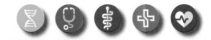

Putting It All Together: Coding for Eye and Vision Services

To select the correct codes for an eye and vision service encounter, a coder must carefully read the documentation, then access each code book to find the procedure or service provided and the corresponding diagnosis or diagnoses to support the medical necessity for the service. Procedural codes for optometry and ophthalmology services are found in the CPT and HCPCS code books, and diagnosis codes are found in the ICD-10-CM code book.

Determination of accurate codes relies on the answers to the following questions.

- What services were provided to the patient?
  - Was an E/M service provided? Was it a E/M service or an ophthalmological E/M service?
  - Were any additional procedures performed?
  - Was a surgery performed?
- Are there any applicable modifiers or add-on codes?
- Is there a definitive diagnosis for the encounter? If yes, this should be the first-listed diagnosis code. If no, then use the appropriate eye screening code. If signs or symptoms are present, code for the signs and symptoms.
- Are there any additional signs, symptoms, conditions, or Z-codes for screenings, examinations, or patient history that should be reported?

The following vignette demonstrates how to select the appropriate diagnosis and procedure codes for an ophthalmological service. After studying the vignette, complete the exercises in There's a Code for That 9.4 to practice diagnostic and procedural coding for eye and vision services.

Terrence is coding an encounter for a 42-year-old female that was seen yesterday at her optometrist's office. The woman has been suffering from bilateral dry-eye syndrome for many years and has elected for punctal occlusion. After a level 4 medical examination with a detailed history and examination and moderate MDM of this established patient, the optometrist closed the left and right lacrimal punctum via plug occlusion.

First, Terrence asks himself: What did the doctor do? The doctor performed a level 4 medical examination for an established patient, and then inserted four plugs into the patient's lacrimal ducts (right upper, right lower, left upper, and left lower lacrimal ducts). He assigns code 99214 for the E/M service, and determines that the code for the lacrimal occlusion is 68761. Because the doctor plugged all four of the lacrimal ducts, he assigns the code four times with the appropriate modifier to identify the location of the procedure:

99214, Office or other outpatient visit for the evaluation and management of an established patient, which requires at least 2 of these 3 key components: a detailed history, a detailed examination, medical decision-making of moderate complexity

68761-E1, Closure of the lacrimal punctum; by plug, each (upper left eyelid)

68761-E2, Closure of the lacrimal punctum; by plug, each (lower left eyelid)

68761-E3, Closure of the lacrimal punctum; by plug, each (upper right eyelid)

68761-E4, Closure of the lacrimal punctum; by plug, each (lower right eyelid)

Now that he has his procedure codes, Terrence asks himself: Why did the doctor do it? In this case, the patient has bilateral dry-eye syndrome. He looks up the condition in the ICD-10-CM code book and finds the following code:

H04.123, Dry eye syndrome of bilateral lacrimal glands

He then rechecks the documentation to make sure he has coded everything for the encounter, and reports the chosen codes on the claim for the service.

Diagnostic and procedural coding for eye and vision services

Read the following documentation and assign the appropriate CPT, HCPCS, and ICD-10-CM code(s) for the encounter.

1. Extended ophthalmoscopy with retinal drawing, with interpretation and report. Patient has been experiencing visual discomfort and visual halos, and has vitreous floaters of the left eye.

   CPT codes: _____

   ICD-10-CM codes: _____ , _____ , _____

2. Ophthalmologist performed a strabismus surgery of the left eye on two horizontal muscles (medial rectus muscle), and one vertical muscle (superior rectus muscle), employing posterior fixation technique, without muscle recession. Patient is a 22-year-old female with monocular esotropia of the left eye.

   CPT codes: _____ - _____ , _____ - _____ ,
   _____ - _____

   ICD-10-CM codes: _____

3. Repair of retinal detachment via photocoagulation on a 62-year-old with retinal detachment with single break of the right eye.

   CPT codes: _____ - _____

   ICD-10-CM codes: _____

Case Study | Eye and Vision Services—Blepharoplasty

PATIENT: Myriam Ahmed

DATE OF SERVICE: 08/29/20XX

PREOPERATIVE DIAGNOSIS: Bilateral upper lid dermatochalasis inhibiting upward visual field.

POSTOPERATIVE DIAGNOSIS: Bilateral upper lid dermatochalasis inhibiting upward visual field.

PROCEDURE: Bilateral upper lid blepharoplasty.

ANESTHESIA: Local injection of 1% Xylocaine with epinephrine mixed with 0.5% Marcaine in a 1:1 ratio.

PROCEDURE IN DETAIL: The patient was brought to the operating room where she was anesthetized as described. After marking the eyelid skin with a marking pen, attention was first directed to the right eye. An incision was made along the marked lines and a skin/muscle flap was excised and removed from the field. The orbital septum was opened and orbital fat was excised in a graded fashion using a clamp and cautery technique. Hemostasis was accomplished throughout by means of bipolar cautery. The left eye was operated on in an identical fashion. The wounds were then closed with running 6-0 nylon suture. The wounds were dressed. The patient went to the recovery room in stable condition to be instructed in postoperative care.

SIGNED: Dr. Georgia Singh, MD

Use the following steps to select the appropriate codes for the case study encounter.

1. Read the case study in full. As you read, look up any medical or procedural terms with which you are unfamiliar and use a medical dictionary or medical terminology text to define the unfamiliar terms.

2. Review the case study and answer the question: *What did the doctor do?* Identify the name of the procedure performed.

_____

_____

Key to Success

Once you have read through the procedural note, make sure you have a good understanding of the procedure itself, how it was performed, and why it was performed. This may mean you have to research the procedure until you understand exactly how and why it is performed, including multiple variations of the procedure, if necessary.

3. Locate the code in the CPT code book for the procedure identified.
   a. Search the Index for the procedure and search through the options.

   _____

   _____

   b. If there are multiple options, identify the most appropriate code option and refer to the code listed in the Tabular section.

   _____

   _____

   c. In the listing of codes, check for any guidelines, important definitions, or parenthetical notes. Select the code that correctly identifies all of the components of the procedure.

   _____

   _____

d. Are there any additional procedures that need to be added to identify all of the procedures performed? If yes, follow the previous steps to identify the codes for the additional procedures.

_____

_____

e. Are there any modifiers that need to be added to identify any special circumstance surrounding the procedure(s)? If yes, refer to Appendix A of the CPT code book to assign all appropriate modifiers.

_____

_____

4. Now that the procedure(s) and modifier(s) have been identified, refer to the case study and answer the following question: *Why did the doctor do it?* In the case study, identify the patient's diagnosis (note that there may be multiple diagnoses).

_____

_____

5. Now that you have identified the patient's diagnoses, search the ICD-10-CM code book for the correct code for this condition.

a. Search the Main Index for the name of the condition and search through any applicable subterms and cross-references to locate the appropriate code.

_____

b. Verify the codes in the Tabular List. In the Tabular Listing of codes, locate the code identified and refer to any applicable guidelines, notes, and symbols. Does the code selected correctly identify the patient's condition? If yes, list the code.

i. _____

ii. _____

c. Check the procedure note and ICD-10-CM guidelines and conventions to determine the correct sequencing of the diagnosis codes, if applicable. Correctly sequence the diagnosis codes.

_____

6. Now that the procedure and diagnosis codes have been identified, list them on the following CMS-1500 form. Be sure to correctly link the procedure and diagnosis codes. Refer to figure 3.6 for an example.

21. DIAGNOSIS OR NATURE OF ILLNESS OR INJURY Relate A-L to service line below (24E)			ICD Ind.	
A. _____	B. _____	C. _____	D. _____	
E. _____	F. _____	G. _____	H. _____	
I. _____	J. _____	K. _____	L. _____	

24. A. DATE(S) OF SERVICE		B. PLACE OF SERVICE	C. EMG	D. PROCEDURES, SERVICES, OR SUPPLIES (Explain Unusual Circumstances) CPT/HCPCS MODIFIER	E. DIAGNOSIS POINTER
From MM DD YY	To MM DD YY				

HCC

End-of-Chapter Content

Instructions: Indicate whether the following statements are true or false (T or F). For false statements, rewrite the statement on the line below to make the statement true.

1. Optometrists treat vision and ophthalmologists surgically treat eye conditions.

_____

_____

2. Vision insurance pays for your eyes, and healthcare insurance pays for your glasses.

_____

_____

3. There are five ophthalmological E/M encounter codes.

_____

_____

4. Optometrists and ophthalmologists may code for encounters with either E/M codes or ophthalmological E/M codes.

_____

_____

5. Ophthalmology procedures are typically noninvasive.

_____

_____

6. A trabeculectomy is a procedure to treat cataracts.

_____

_____

7. Eyelid modifiers should be used on diagnosis codes to identify the laterality of the eyelid.

_____

_____

8. Congenital eye conditions are present at birth.

_____

_____

Instructions: Choose the best answer.

1. Which of the following types of insurance would pay for an optometrist to perform a routine eye examination?

a. Healthcare insurance
b. Vision insurance
c. Dental insurance
d. Insurance will not pay for this service

2. Which of the following is a good example of a lifestyle impairment that would prove medical necessity for an ophthalmological service?

a. Inability to get a job due to poor life management skills
b. Patient must lose weight to function better
c. Restriction of peripheral vision
d. The statement of the diagnosis

3. Which of the following is included as a component of the ocular adnexa?

a. Cornea
b. Anterior chamber
c. Vitreous
d. Conjunctiva

4. If an optometrist performed an examination of the ophthalmological system for presbyopia, which of the following E/M codes might she report?

a. 99213
b. 92002
c. 99214
d. 92015

5. Which of the following would be an appropriate code for the fitting of a contact lens for a corneal abrasion injury?

a. 92071
b. 92310
c. 92072
d. 92311

6. LASIK is one type of which type of surgery?

a. Phacoemulsification
b. Cataract surgery
c. Refractive surgery
d. Goniotomy

7. If a patient has two types of glaucoma, one in each eye, how should it be reported?

a. With one code to identify both of the conditions
b. With a bilateral code
c. With one code for each condition to identify them individually
d. With two codes for the same type of glaucoma, with a right and left modifier

8. Which of the following conditions is a buildup of intraocular pressure?

a. Cataracts
b. Macular degeneration
c. Retinal detachment
d. Glaucoma

Instructions: Answer the following questions with the appropriate code(s).

1. A 30-year-old female patient presented to the office with a central corneal ulcer of the right eye. Level 4 E/M performed for this new patient, with fitting of contact lens. Gas permeable scleral contact lens provided to the patient in office.

CPT code(s): _____

ICD-10-CM code(s): _____

2. Evisceration of left eye with implant due to malignant neoplasm of left eye.

CPT code(s): _____

ICD-10-CM code(s): _____

3. A 67-year-old male presents for routine eye examination, intermediate ophthalmological E/M encounter performed with no new treatment plan established. Patient's history is relevant for cataract surgery two years ago, and he has an intraocular lens in the left eye. He also has presbyopia and irregular astigmatism.

CPT code(s): _____

ICD-10-CM code(s): _____

References

American Academy of Ophthalmology (AAO). 2017 (October 4). Cataract. http://eyewiki.org/Cataract.

Centers for Medicare and Medicaid Services (CMS). 2019. ICD-10-CM Official Guidelines for Coding and Reporting FY 2020. https://www.cms.gov/Medicare/Coding/ICD10/Downloads/2020-Coding-Guidelines.pdf.

John's Hopkins University. n.d. Cataracts FAQ. http://www.hopkinsmedicine.org/wilmer/conditions/cataracts_faq.html.

National Eye Institute (NEI). 2006 (June). Conventional Surgery to Treat Glaucoma. Digital Image. Wikimedia Commons. https://commons.wikimedia.org/wiki/File:Conventional_surgery_to_treat_glaucoma_EDA11.JPG.

US Air Force, D. Seltmann. 2012 (April). Luke AFB Eye Exam. Digital Image. Wikimedia Commons. https://commons.wikimedia.org/wiki/Category:Slit_lamp#/media/File:Luke_AFB_eye_exam.jpg.

American Medical Association (AMA). 2013. *Advanced Anatomy and Physiology for ICD-10-CM/PCS*. Salt Lake City, UT: Contexo Media.

Asbell, R.L. 2004 (February 1). Coding for corneal surgery requires distinction between cosmetic and functional. *Ocular Surgery News U.S. Edition*. http://www.healio.com/ophthalmology/news/print/ocular-surgery-news/%7B17138fd4-b050-4108-a2b5-5639286885ac%7D/coding-for-corneal-surgery-requires-distinction-between-cosmetic-and-functional.

Blue Cross Blue Shield of Rhode Island. 2013 (September 5). Payment Policy | Ophthalmology Examinations and Refractions: Correct Coding and Benefits Adjudication. https://www.bcbsri.com/sites/default/files/polices/Opthalmology_Examinations.pdf.

Cibis, G.W. 2017 (March 13). Primary Congenital Glaucoma Treatment & Management. https://emedicine.medscape.com/article/1206081-treatment#d9.

Centers for Medicare and Medicaid Services (CMS). 2018 (April). Medicare Vision Services. https://www.cms.gov/Outreach-and-Education/Medicare-Learning-Network-MLN/MLNProducts/downloads/VisionServices_FactSheet_ICN907165.pdf.

The Coding Institute (TCI). 2017 (February). Use Expert Examples to Avoid These Common Eye Coding Errors. *Ophthalmology and Optometry Coding Alert* 20(2): 9–16. https://codinginstitute-upload.s3.amazonaws.com/product_images/afc0ba_opc.jpg.

Vijaya, L., P. Manish, G. Ronnie, and B. Shantha. 2011 (January). Management of Complications in Glaucoma Surgery. *Indian Journal of Ophthalmology* 59(Suppl1): S131–S140. https://www.ncbi.nlm.nih.gov/pmc/articles/PMC3038515/.

Resources

American Academy of Ophthalmology (AAO). 2017 (October 30). Enucleation. http://eyewiki.org/Enucleation.

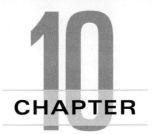

CHAPTER

Urgent Care and Emergency Department Services

Learning Objectives

- Understand the basics of billing and coding in urgent care and emergency department services
- Examine procedural codes and guidelines for urgent care and emergency department services
- Examine diagnosis coding and medical necessity for urgent care and emergency department services
- Determine and apply ICD-10-CM, CPT, and HCPCS codes to urgent care and emergency department services

Key Terms

Appendicitis

Burn codes

Cardiopulmonary resuscitation (CPR)

Closed procedure

Corrosion

Dislocation reduction

Emergency services

Emergent

Endotracheal intubation

Foreign body (FB)

Hemothorax

Incision and drainage (I&D)

Lumbar puncture

Lund-Browder classification

Moderate (conscious) sedation

Motor vehicle accident (MVA)

Myocardial infarction

Nasal packing

Open procedure

Oximetry

Penetrating wound

Pleural effusion

Pneumothorax

Professional component

Rule of nines

Sepsis

Septic shock

Systemic inflammatory response syndrome (SIRS)

Technical component

Thoracostomy

Tracheostomy

Tracheotomy

Urgent care

Urgent care and emergency department (ED) services are provided on an as-needed basis to patients with urgent and **emergent** (life-threatening) healthcare issues. Although they sound similar, urgent care and emergency department services should not be confused, as they each provide a different level of service to patients, depending on their healthcare needs.

This chapter discusses the basics of coding for both urgent care and emergency department services, which include a wide range of procedure and diagnosis codes. It also discusses the differences between the two healthcare settings—including services provided, evaluation and management (E/M) codes used, and the types of healthcare providers who practice in each setting. Coding for urgent care and emergency department services requires the ability to differentiate between signs and symptoms versus a definitive diagnosis, the ability to effectively utilize many portions of both the CPT and ICD-10-CM code books, and an understanding of the difference between urgent and emergent services and conditions.

Urgent Care and Emergency Department Basics

Coding for urgent care and emergency department (ED) services requires a solid understanding of both the CPT and ICD-10-CM code books as well as how to read, interpret, and apply the coding guidelines while keeping in mind the billing and coding differences between the two settings. It also entails an understanding of how the billing details of the facility may impact coding for services performed in each setting, respectively. Although both types of facilities treat patients who have immediate healthcare needs, the level of urgency differs between the two settings. Furthermore, because of the differences in the available resources and urgency of the healthcare services, pricing structure and reimbursement also differ greatly.

Please note that some EDs may report ICD-10-PCS codes, depending on how the facility is organized. This chapter discusses ICD-10-CM, CPT, and HCPCS codes in the setting of the ED or urgent care clinic only. ICD-10-PCS coding is discussed in chapter 20 (Inpatient Hospital Services).

Urgent Care Services

Urgent care services are provided to patients who need healthcare for non–life-threatening situations, illnesses, or injuries. Most urgent care practices are open after-hours and on weekends and have on-site x-ray and laboratory access.

Urgent care services are provided to patients who need services urgently but are not in danger of losing life or limb, such as when a patient's regular doctor is not available and he or she cannot wait for an appointment. For example, a pediatric patient rapidly develops a fever and rash on a Friday evening, but the child's regular doctor's office is closed for the weekend. The parent of the child can take him or her to an urgent care clinic for an examination, any necessary lab tests, and a medication prescription.

Urgent care clinics take patients on a walk-in basis, without scheduling an appointment beforehand. Though the patient has the benefit seeing a healthcare provider without an appointment, it also means that patients are generally seen on a first-come, first-seen basis and may need to wait a long time. Urgent care centers are typically non–hospital-based and open seven days a week for usually 13 or more hours each day, so healthcare services are almost always available.

Because urgent care clinics are not primary care practices and provide care to patients only on an as-needed basis, claims for urgent care services must be submitted with a specific place-of-service (POS) code; refer to chapter 7 (Behavioral Health Services) for a refresher on place of service codes. Urgent care centers are designated as outpatient offices but are not considered primary care offices, as their purpose is to treat outpatients seeking immediate healthcare. When billing for services provided at an urgent care clinic, it is necessary to use POS code 20, Urgent Care Facility, on the CMS-1500 form when sending claims to third-party payers. According to the CPT code book, POS code 20 should be used for any "location, distinct from a hospital emergency room, an office, or a clinic, whose purpose is to diagnose and treat illness or injury for unscheduled, ambulatory patients seeking immediate medical attention" (AMA 2019). The POS code is listed in box 24.B of the CMS-1500 claim form (see figure 10.1).

Figure 10.1. CMS-1500 box 24.B: Place-of-service code 20, Urgent Care Facility

24. A. DATE(S) OF SERVICE						B. PLACE OF SERVICE	C. EMG
From			To				
MM	DD	YY	MM	DD	YY		
						20	

Source: CMS 2019a.

Because the basic structure of the clinic is an outpatient facility that provides healthcare encounters at a level of care lower than an emergency room (for instance, operations and complex medical procedures are not possible at urgent care centers), it is necessary to use outpatient office E/M codes when billing for urgent care encounters. Coders should report codes 99201 through 99215 (Office or Other Outpatient Services) for E/M encounters provided to patients in the urgent care setting.

Emergency Department Services

Emergency services are provided to patients in a life-threatening situation, when loss of life or limb is imminent. These patients are in immediate need of an x-ray, surgical procedure, or interventional procedure for trauma or other life-threatening situations. An example of an emergency is a patient with a severe laceration of the arm from a chainsaw injury who is at risk of losing either his life or his limb (see figure 10.2).

Figure 10.2. Urgent versus emergent

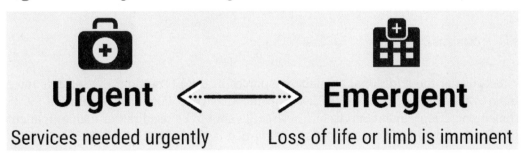

Emergency services are provided in a designated ED or emergency room (ER), which is a hospital-based facility open 24 hours a day. Like urgent care clinics, patients do not need an appointment to be seen in an ED; however, patients in the ED are not seen on a first-come, first-seen basis. ED services are allocated so that patients with the most severe injuries or illnesses are seen before patients with less severe or life-threatening situations. For example, if a patient with a high fever signs into the ED before the patient with the arm laceration, the ED will take the arm laceration patient for treatment before the patient with the fever. This arm injury is more life-threatening than the fever. This may result in patients waiting much longer for treatment at an ED than they would at an urgent care clinic, depending on the reason for the visit.

Billing and coding for ED services requires an understanding of the different POS and E/M codes used to bill for services performed there. There is also a separate box on the CMS-1500 form to identify emergent services.

Key to Success

Emergent patients may present to the urgent care, and urgent patients may present to the ED. Both care settings may see the same patients, and it is very common for urgent care centers to recommend that very sick or complicated patients go to the ED or call an ambulance for transport to the ED. Neither setting will turn away patients, which may result in a nonemergent patient presenting to the ED to wait a long time before receiving services, depending on the acuity of the other patients at the ED.

Place of Service and Fees for Emergency Department Services

The ED is a designated portion of a hospital that is open to patients 24 hours a day and used to diagnose and treat illnesses, injuries, and other life-threatening conditions. As a designated space apart from the hospital, the ED has its own POS code. When billing for services that were performed in the ED, it is necessary to use POS code 23, Emergency Room-Hospital, as the place of service. POS code 23 should be used for "a portion of a hospital where emergency diagnosis and treatment of illness or injury is provided" (AMA 2019). The POS code is listed in box 24.B of the CMS-1500 claim form (see figure 10.3).

Figure 10.3. CMS-1500 box 24.B: Place-of-service code 23, Emergency Room-Hospital

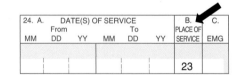

Source: CMS 2019a.

Because of the additional available resources in the ED setting, ED services have their own section of E/M codes listed in the CPT code book: 99281 through 99288 (Emergency Department Services). These codes should be used rather than outpatient E/M codes when E/M encounters are performed in the ED setting.

Key to Success

When coding for services, the POS code must match the type of service performed. For example, if you report an ED E/M code but the POS code does not indicate that the place of service was the ED, then the insurance company will not pay for the claim. POS codes are easy to overlook, but they are a fundamental component of coding for services.

Box 24.C, Emergency

On the CMS-1500 claim form, there is an additional area that must be completed when coding for emergency services. Box 24.C, Emergency, should be filled out with a "Y" to identify that the service was provided on an emergent basis (see figure 10.4). If the service is not an emergency, the box can be left blank.

This is an important designation to make, as emergency services are usually excluded from prior authorization requirements for medical procedures. For example, if a patient emergently presented to the ER with a severe head injury and a computerized tomography (CT) scan was performed to rule out a subdural hematoma, this service would be indicated as an emergency in box 24.C of the CMS-1500 claim form. On the other hand, if a patient came into the outpatient office with a severe headache and the doctor wanted to order a CT scan, then a prior authorization or quality review would likely be needed before the service would be authorized by the insurance, because the headache is not an emergency. This is yet another example of the close connection between the intricacies of healthcare coding and billing for reimbursement.

Figure 10.4. CMS-1500 box 24.C: Emergency

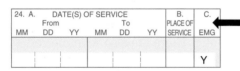

Source: CMS 2019a.

Various procedures, including E/M services, labs, some surgeries, radiological procedures, and medical procedures are performed in the urgent care and ED settings, and coders will utilize all areas of the CPT and HCPCS code books to code these encounters. ICD-10-CM coding is just as varied; patient conditions in the urgent care and ED settings range from anxiety attacks to severe traumatic injuries.

Procedural Coding for Urgent Care and ED Services

Urgent care services are provided to patients who need care right away. Emergency services are provided to patients in a life-threatening situation. Because the line between urgent and life-threatening situations is sometimes difficult to discern, urgent care clinics and EDs provide some of the same services.

However, there are some important differences. First, the E/M codes used in either setting are completely different. Urgent care clinics use codes 99201 through 99215 to report E/M services, whereas EDs use E/M codes 99281 through 99288 for the same purpose. Urgent care services are also less invasive than those provided in the ED, as surgical procedures performed in the urgent care setting are typically minor. Both urgent care clinics and EDs perform medical evaluations and services, x-rays, and labs, but EDs perform more surgically complex procedures that require a specialized level of medical training. EDs must also keep more resources on-hand, such as a sterile operating room, advanced imaging equipment, and the ability to perform more complex laboratory tests.

Procedures Performed in the Urgent Care Setting

Procedures performed in the urgent care setting range from simple E/M encounters to more complex healthcare encounters that may involve laboratory tests, x-rays, or other imaging procedures. Additional medical procedures, such as breathing treatments or injections, may also be performed in the urgent care setting. Urgent care clinic resources are more limited than ED resources, and staff are not trained to treat all emergency situations. Therefore, an urgent care clinic will sometimes call for an ambulance to transport a patient to the hospital.

The E/M codes used in the urgent care setting range from 99201 to 99215; they are the same as those used in outpatient facility billing and the primary care settings, as discussed in chapter 8 (Primary Care Services). As a reminder, codes 99201 through 99205 are for new patients, and codes 99211 through 99215 are for established patients. Urgent care centers may see new or established patients, so it is important to remember how to differentiate the two. Refer to chapter 7 for the basics on how to determine if a patient is new or established. These guidelines are also located in the E/M guidelines section of the CPT code book.

For a review of the key components of E/M codes and how to select the level of E/M code based on the provider documentation, refer to chapter 7 and chapter 8 of this text.

Besides healthcare E/M services, urgent care clinics perform countless procedures, all aimed at diagnosis and initial treatment of medical conditions. These procedures are either diagnostic or therapeutic. There are also revenue codes that identify the urgent care encounter as a special service and can pay an extra amount for the service.

Diagnostic Procedures

Diagnostic procedures performed in the urgent care setting include lab tests and blood analysis, x-rays, oximetry, and electrocardiograms (ECGs). These tests are designed to evaluate the severity of the patient's condition or to determine the patient's definitive diagnosis.

Laboratory Tests

Laboratory tests are designed to determine patient diagnosis, mostly for infectious diseases such as strep throat, influenza, bacterial and fungal infections, and sexually transmitted infections (gonorrhea, chlamydia, herpes). Common blood tests performed are complete blood counts (CBC), lipid panels, basic metabolic panels (BMET) and comprehensive metabolic panels (CMP), hepatic function panels, thyroid stimulation hormone tests, and tests for heterophile antibodies. Note that this is not a comprehensive list of all lab tests performed at urgent care centers. Laboratory procedures are coded from the Laboratory and Pathology section of the CPT code book. To look up a laboratory procedure, it helps to first look under the entry *Pathology and Laboratory* in the Index, and then find the subterm(s) for the substance being tested for, such as angiotensin converting enzymes (ACE). Another way to look up a lab procedure is to search for the type of lab test performed, such as *Blood Cell Count*, and then find the subterm(s) for the type of blood count performed. All laboratory procedure codes are located in the Pathology and Laboratory section of the CPT code book and start with the number 8. Laboratory services are discussed in greater detail in chapter 14 (Laboratory and Pathology Services) of this textbook.

X-rays and Imaging Procedures

X-rays and imaging procedures are found in the Radiology section of the CPT code book. When coding for x-rays, go to *X-ray* in the Index and search for the subterm that identifies the body area imaged. For example, a patient coming into the urgent care clinic with a wrist injury would likely receive an x-ray of the wrist to rule out a fracture. To look up this x-ray, go to *X-ray* in the Index and find the subterm *wrist*. This leads you to code range 73100 through 73110. Next, go to that range of codes in the Radiology section of the CPT code book, where there are two codes available for wrist x-ray. (Note that code 73115, Radiological examination, wrist, arthrography, radiological supervision and interpretation, is an arthrography code, which uses contrast material into the joint to diagnosis joint problems.)

- 73100, Radiologic examination, wrist; *2 views*
- 73110, Radiologic examination, wrist; *complete, minimum of 3 views*

In this example, the two codes for x-ray of the wrist differ based on the number of views. The number of views refers to the number of images taken at different angles during the x-ray. For example, the x-ray technician may take two views—one anterior-view x-ray of the wrist and one lateral-view x-ray of the wrist. Each view creates an image from a different angle and may help to diagnose a fracture or other condition.

CPT codes for most x-rays differ based on the number of views taken during the x-ray. If the x-ray code is described as *complete*, then it will identify the minimum number of views required for a complete x-ray. Anything over that number of views is included in the code. For example, if the x-ray tech took four views of the wrist, the appropriate code selection for the procedure would be 73110, Radiologic examination, wrist; *complete, minimum of 3 views*.

Oximetry

Oximetry is a noninvasive test that measures a patient's oxygen saturation level. A sensor is placed over a portion of the body with thin skin with vascular structures underneath, such as the fingertip or earlobe or, in the case of infants, a foot. Oximetry is performed to determine if the patient is in any type of respiratory distress by measuring whether the level of oxygen in the blood is decreased. Normal pulse oximetry levels are between 95 and 100 percent, and anything under 90 to 92 percent is considered low (Hackethal 2017). A patient who has a low blood oxygen level may be started on oxygen, a breathing treatment, or additional interventions, depending on how low the oxygen reading is. The CPT codes for oximetry differ, depending on the number of readings taken. Note that there is no code for the delivery of oxygen.

- 94760, Noninvasive ear or pulse oximetry for oxygen saturation; *single determination*
- 94761, Noninvasive ear or pulse oximetry for oxygen saturation; *multiple determinations (eg, during exercise)*
- 94762, Noninvasive ear or pulse oximetry for oxygen saturation; *by continuous overnight monitoring (separate procedure)*

Electrocardiogram

As discussed in chapter 8 , an electrocardiogram (ECG or EKG) measures the electrical impulses of the heart and can be used to identify arrhythmias and other heart issues. Codes for ECGs range from 93000 to 93042 and differ depending on the type of ECG taken and the work involved in the test. The most common codes are the following:

- 93000, Electrocardiogram, routine ECG with at least 12 leads; *with interpretation and report*
- 93005, Electrocardiogram, routine ECG with at least 12 leads; *tracing only, without interpretation and report*
- 93010, Electrocardiogram, routine ECG with at least 12 leads; *interpretation and report only*

Note that the codes differ based on interpretation and report, and tracing. There are two components to an ECG: the work involved in taking the test (which includes placing the leads and performing the test), and the interpretation of test results and written report of the findings. Tracing is the work involved in taking the test, also called the **technical component** of the test. The interpretation and report make up the **professional components** of the test, which consist of the healthcare provider interpreting the results from the test, determining a diagnosis or next steps in treatment or diagnosis, and providing a written report of his or her findings. Because most urgent care centers own the testing equipment, perform the test (technical component), and employ the healthcare provider who reads and interprets the report (professional component), urgent care centers typically bill for codes that include both components (93000, Electrocardiogram, routine ECG with at least 12 leads; with interpretation and report). If the facility performs only one portion of the service (technical or professional), then they would bill *only* for the service performed. For example, if the provider on staff is not qualified or trained to read the ECG, then he or she may bill only for 93005, Electrocardiogram, routine ECG with at least 12 leads; tracing only, without interpretation and report.

Therapeutic Procedures

Therapeutic procedures are performed to treat either a confirmed diagnosis or a patient's signs or symptoms in the urgent care clinic. Most of the time, treatments are minimal or initial enough to ensure the patient is not in any immediate medical danger. The patient is then referred to his or her primary care physician or healthcare specialist for follow-up and definitive treatment. In some cases, the patient may be advised to go to the hospital via ambulance. Therapeutic procedures include injections, vaccinations, breathing treatments, injury treatments, and wound repair.

Injections

Injections are given to treat medical conditions therapeutically with a medicinal substance. Injections should not be confused with vaccinations and are *not* coded, with vaccination administration codes. Rather, code 96372, Therapeutic, prophylactic, or diagnostic injection (specify substance or drug); subcutaneous or intramuscular, is used to identify the administration of the medicinal substance, with a separate HCPCS code identifying the substance injected. For example, if a patient with a severe bacterial infection presents to the urgent care clinic, the healthcare provider may choose to inject an antibiotic in the office rather than wait for a prescription to be filled and oral antibiotics taken. This encounter would be coded with CPT code 96372 for the injection procedure and an HCPCS code for the antibacterial substance injected into the patient (such as J0696, Injection, ceftriaxone sodium, per 250 mg). Note that the medicinal substance injected is a *supply* provided to the patient, and as such these codes are located in the HCPCS code book. Search the Table of Drugs for the substance and pay attention to the route of injection and amount per unit. For a refresher on coding from the Table of Drugs, refer to chapter 6 (Supplies and Services).

Vaccinations

Vaccinations are also given in the urgent care setting, such as the seasonal flu vaccine or a tetanus vaccine administered to a patient with an injury from a rusty nail. Refer to chapter 8 for the basics of vaccine coding. The only difference between coding for vaccines in the urgent care setting rather than the primary care setting would be the change of the POS code to identify the place of service when the vaccination was administered.

Breathing Treatments

Breathing treatments are given to patients in respiratory distress or if they have a low blood oxygen level due to an asthma exacerbation, respiratory infection, or other respiratory condition like pneumonia or chronic obstructive pulmonary disease (COPD). Breathing treatments use pressurized air mixed with a steroid solution that is inhaled by the patient. This procedure helps open airway passages to allow the patient to breathe more easily. To find the codes for breathing treatments, search in the Index under the term *Inhalation Treatment*, and select the subterm for the type of breathing treatment administered.

Treatment for Injuries

Injury treatments provided in the urgent care setting depend on the type of injury suffered by the patient. Urgent care centers are not trained nor equipped to operate on patients, perform casting procedures, or repair complex injuries (these would be performed in the emergency department or hospital setting). Furthermore, urgent care centers do not have healthcare providers who are trained in all medical procedures, such as setting fractures or reducing dislocations. Because of these limitations, most of the injury treatments performed are aimed at stabilizing the injury and reducing pain or discomfort so the patient may receive more definitive treatment from his or her PCP, a specialty provider, or in the inpatient hospital. For example, an injury treatment for a fracture would include the application of a temporary splint to immobilize the fracture until the patient could be seen by an orthopedist (bone doctor). Any splint, brace, or other immobilizing device would be reported with the appropriate HCPCS codes to identify the device, and the application or provision of the device would be included in the E/M code for the visit. An immobilizing device, otherwise known as an *orthotic device* or *orthosis*, is an externally applied device designed for a particular body area to protect and support injuries, reduce pain, and assist in the healing process; orthotic devices are discussed in chapter 6. To look up orthotic devices in the HCPCS code book, search under the term *Orthotic additions*, or search by the body area (wrist, ankle, hand).

If more than one injury is treated, the procedure that required the most work is reported first, with less work-intensive procedures listed thereafter. This should also correspond with the injury diagnosis codes, as they should also be listed before the codes for less severe injuries (this is discussed in greater depth in the diagnosis coding section of this chapter).

Wound Repair

Wound repair codes (12001–13160) are found in the Integumentary section of the CPT code book. Complex, penetrating, or otherwise life-threatening wounds are seen in the emergency setting. Wounds such as lacerations, cuts, abrasions, and superficial injuries are treated in urgent care; and wound repair consists primarily of repairs of the skin such as suturing, stapling, or cleaning and bandaging wounds on the skin. Would repair codes are divided into three types—simple, intermediate, and complex repairs, and code selection depends on the site and size of the wound. If the wound is repaired using adhesive strips as the only repair material, then the wound repair is included in the E/M code and not coded separately.

- Simple wound closure codes (12001–12021) are used when the wound is superficial or involves subcutaneous tissues but does not involve any deeper structures. This type of repair requires only one layer of closure.

- Intermediate wound repair codes (12031–12057) are used for wounds that require layered closure of one or more of the deeper layers of subcutaneous tissue and superficial fascia, in addition to closure of the skin (see figure 10.5). Closure of wounds that are heavy in particulate matter or otherwise require extensive cleaning are also categorized as intermediate.

- Complex wound repair codes (13100–13160) are used for wounds that require more than layered closure, such as scar revision, debridement due to traumatic lacerations or avulsions, extensive undermining, stents, or retention sutures. Because of the complex nature of this type of repair, it is less commonly performed at urgent care centers than the two former types of wound repair.

Figure 10.5. Intermediate wound repair (layered skin closure)

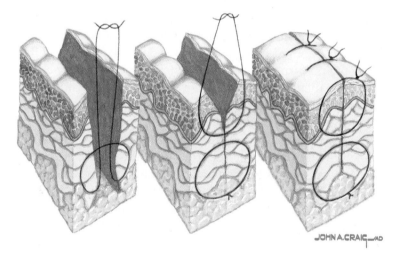

JOHN A. CRAIG

When coding wound repair, pay attention to three important components of wound repair codes:

- *The site of the wound repair.* Each wound repair code identifies a group of anatomical regions, all of which may be included in the same repair code. For example, code 13120, Repair, complex, *scalp, arms, and/or legs*; 1.1 cm to 2.5 cm, groups repairs of the skin on scalp, arms, or legs.

- *The size (in centimeters) of the repair.* Each wound repair code identifies the total size of the repair, for that specific anatomical site. For example, code 13120, Repair, complex, scalp, arms, and/or legs; *1.1 cm to 2.5 cm*, identifies a total repair of 1.1 to 2.5 centimeters total for those specific body areas. Note that 1 inch equals 2.54 centimeters.

- *The complexity of the repair*. Each repair code identifies the complexity of the repair procedure, in terms of simple, intermediate, or complex. For example, code 13120, Repair, *complex*, scalp, arms, and/or legs; 1.1 cm to 2.5 cm, identifies a complex repair of the skin on the specified anatomical sites.

Combine the lengths of the wounds of like complexity from each group of body sites. For example, if there is a 1.0 cm simple repair of the right cheek, a 0.5 cm simple repair of the left cheek, and a 0.75 cm repair of the forehead, the repairs would be added together—because they are the same complexity (simple) and the same body site (face)—to total a simple repair of the face of 2.25 cm. The code selected in this example would be 12011, Simple repair of superficial wounds of face, ears, eyelids, nose, lips and/or mucous membranes; 2.5 cm or less. The coder should add the lengths of wound of the same complexity and body area as defined by the CPT codes (see figure 10.6).

Figure 10.6. Wound repair

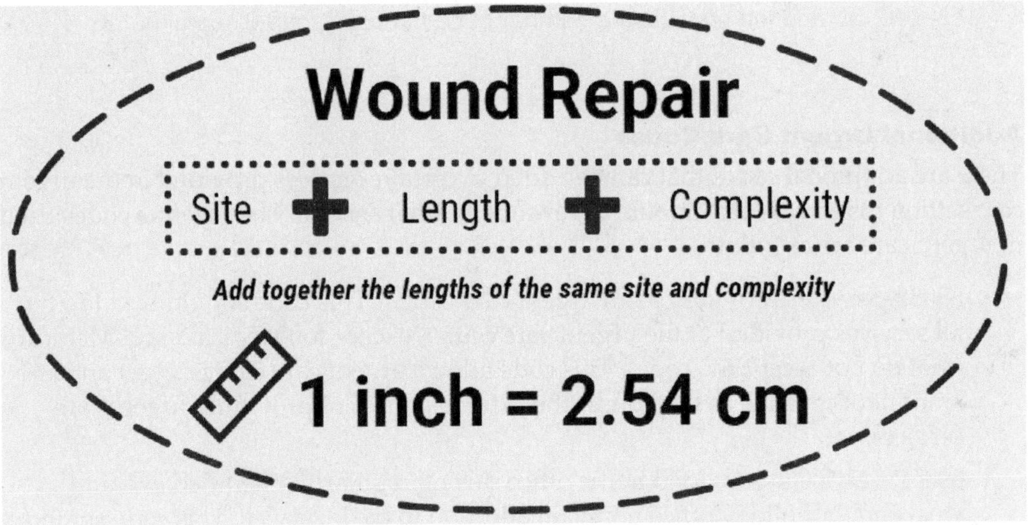

Wound Repair

Site **+** Length **+** Complexity

Add together the lengths of the same site and complexity

1 inch = 2.54 cm

Wounds of different complexities or body area should be coded separately. For example, if the wound repair was a 1.0 cm *simple* repair of the right cheek and a 0.75 cm *intermediate* repair of the left cheek, then the two codes selected would be 12011, Simple repair of superficial wounds of face, ears, eyelids, nose, lips and/or mucous membranes; 2.5 cm or less, and 12051, Repair, intermediate, wounds of face, ears, eyelids, nose, lips and/or mucous membranes; 2.5 cm or less.

Just as in coding for injury treatments, sequence the more complex wound repair code first, followed by the less complex wound repair code(s).

According to CPT guidelines, when more than one classification of wound is repaired (in terms of anatomical site, size, and complexity), the most complicated repair should be listed first, followed by the less complicated repairs. Additional repair codes should be appended with modifier -59, Distinct procedural service, to identify that the repair procedures were distinct from each other. If any nerves, blood vessels, or tendons were repaired as part of a complex repair service, then these procedures should be coded separately and appended with modifier -59 to indicate that these procedures were distinct from the primary service.

MOD

Key to Success

Remember to read through CPT guidelines before each category of codes, as they spell out specific coding scenarios and when to use specific modifiers. For example, before the category of codes for wound repair, there are a great deal of guidelines, which detail exactly how to select and use the codes, in addition to when modifier -59 may be appropriate to append.

Key to Success

All wound repair codes are reported in centimeters. The conversion factor from inches to centimeters is 1 inch to 2.54 centimeters. Therefore, if the documentation reads 1 inch, this should be converted to 2.54 centimeters. To perform the conversion, multiply the number of inches by 2.54, and the result is the number of centimeters. For example, if the wound repair was 1.5 inches, then multiply the number of inches (1.5) by 2.54, and the result is the number of centimeters, or 3.81 centimeters.

Additional Urgent Care Codes

There are additional codes that can be added to certain services provided in the urgent care setting to increase the amount of revenue for that service. The revenue codes used in urgent care are as follows.

- S9088, Services provided in an urgent care center. This code should be added to all services provided at the urgent care center, except for Medicaid and Medicare (that do not accept the code). This code allows urgent care clinics to get an extra amount of revenue to help offset the extra expenses of providing urgent care services.

- 99051, Service(s) provided in the office during regularly scheduled evening, weekend, or holiday office hours, in addition to basic service. This code should be used only for services that are provided during evening hours (typically after 5 p.m.), on the weekend (Saturday or Sunday), or on a holiday regularly scheduled by the urgent care clinic. This code should be added to the basic service provided, but only for those services that occur at the off-times as indicated by the code description. Like the previous code, it is designed to obtain additional revenue to offset costs by regularly staying open during off-hours.

- S9083, Global fee urgent care centers, should be used only when there is a specific agreement between the urgent care center and the insurance company. To see if this fee is necessary, the healthcare practice would have to verify by calling the insurance company to see if it is required. This is a global fee. If using this code, the urgent care does not charge for any specific services provided during the patient encounter; rather, they are reimbursed a set fee for the global urgent care charge.

The procedures performed in the urgent care setting are less invasive, less costly, and less severe in nature. Procedures performed in the ED setting are by nature more invasive, more costly, and more dangerous due to the life-threatening nature of the patient's medical condition.

Complete the exercises in There's a Code for That 10.1 to practice assigning procedure codes for urgent care services.

Read the following documentation and select the appropriate procedure and/or E/M codes.

1. An 8-year-old female new patient seen after having sustained a wrist injury from a fall on the playground at school. She appears in acute distress. Complete x-ray of the wrist confirms Colles' fracture of the left wrist. Wrist was immobilized using compression bandages and referral was given for patient to see ortho next week. Expended problem-focused history and examination, with moderate medical decision-making (MDM).

   CPT code (E/M service): _____

   CPT code (x-ray): _____

   CPT code (revenue code): _____

2. A 12-year-old established Medicaid patient seen for fever and sore throat during evening hours. Mother reports that the entire family has been sick for the last week, and now her daughter has reported feeling ill. Streptococcal (group A) swab performed in the office is negative. CBC (automated with automated WBC count) shows low WBC count. Prescribed amoxicillin and follow up with PCP if not improved in a week. Detailed history and examination with moderate complexity MDM.

   CPT code (E/M service): _____

   CPT code (labs): _____ , _____

   CPT code (revenue code): _____

3. Patient seen for multiple wound repairs after having walked through a plate glass window. Following wounds were repaired: simple repair of 7 cm laceration on right upper thigh, 3 cm laceration of right hip, and 2 cm on abdomen. Intermediate double layer repair done on a 3 cm laceration of the right forearm, 2 cm laceration on right shoulder, and 2.75 cm laceration on forehead. (Remember, when sequencing codes for injuries, sequence the repair for the worst injury first, followed by the least complex repairs.)

   CPT codes: _____ , _____-_____ ,

   _____-_____

   CPT code (revenue code): _____

4. A 25-year-old sexually active established male patient presents during weekend hours, suspecting that he has a UTI. Gonorrhea immunoassay tests positive. Azithromycin prescribed. Detailed history performed with moderate complexity MDM.

   CPT codes: _____ , _____

   CPT code (revenue codes): _____ , _____

Procedures Performed in the ED Setting

Procedures performed in the ED setting are by nature more complex and riskier, due to the life-threatening medical conditions of the patients. However, some patients who present to the ED for treatment are not experiencing true life- or limb-threatening situations. These patients will still be treated, but their services will be more similar to those performed in an urgent care setting. Note that one difference between urgent care and ED procedures is in the treatment of fractures. Where an urgent care center may provide a temporary cast and refer the patient to an orthopedist for definitive treatment, an ED may provide the definitive treatment for the fracture. Fracture diagnosis and treatment is discussed in detail in two later chapters in this text: chapter 13 (Radiology and Imaging Services) and chapter 15 (Orthopedic Services).

E/M encounters in the ED setting are assigned to a special code range of E/M services: emergency department services (99281–99288). Additional procedures performed in the ED include life-saving surgical procedures and other less invasive procedures.

E/M Encounters in the Emergency Department

Emergency department E/M encounters are coded from the Emergency Department Services section of the CPT code book, with codes 99281 through 99288. While there are many similarities between these codes and outpatient office E/M codes, there are a couple of notable differences.

First, all of the key components of the E/M service are the same—history, examination, and medical decision-making; the levels and elements of each key component; and the nature of the presenting problem included in the code description. However, the component of time is *not* a consideration in E/M coding for ED encounters. Because of the variable intensity of the nature of ED services, and because most providers see many patients at multiple times throughout their services, it is difficult to determine the total time spent on any ED service, so it is not included in the code descriptions.

Key to Success

Time is a factor in many E/M codes, including outpatient office and inpatient E/M services. However, time is *not* a component of code selection for E/M services rendered in the ED setting. Coders should not use time as a deciding factor for the level of service provided in the ED and instead rely on the complexity of the service performed.

There is also no differentiation between new or established patients in the ED setting, as there is no additional classification of codes for new patients versus established patients. When coding for E/M services in the ED, coders should rely on the documentation of the level of history, examination, and medical decision-making while considering the nature of the presenting problem. Note that these E/M codes require all three key components to match the level described in the code description in order to select the code.

Surgical Procedures

Surgical procedures performed in the ED are performed to treat the patient's illness or injury (such as the reduction of a dislocated shoulder or incision and drainage of an abscess), to help diagnose the patient (for example, a lumbar puncture), or to help stabilize the patient before he or she is taken to the operating room or is admitted to the hospital for another procedure (such as endotracheal intubation, or chest tube placement). An inherent component of many of these procedures is conscious sedation, administered by the ED provider to help reduce the sensation of pain during the procedure. Additional procedures performed in the ED setting include foreign body removals and penetrating wound explorations.

Emergency Intubation and Tracheostomy

An emergency intubation is performed to open the airway to prevent asphyxiation. There are two types of intubations—endotracheal and tracheostomy.

An **endotracheal intubation** (also called intubation) is performed to maintain an open airway, or to allow the administration of certain drugs, such as anesthesia. On critically ill patients, an emergent intubation is performed to help ventilate the lungs and prevent asphyxiation and airway obstruction. The procedure is performed by carefully inserting a laryngoscope through the mouth and into the larynx to help view the procedure, and the endotracheal tube is placed directly in the trachea. The laryngoscope is then removed, and the endotracheal tube is left in place (see figure 10.7).

To code for an emergency endotracheal intubation, report code 31500, Intubation, endotracheal, emergency procedure.

Figure 10.7. Endotracheal intubation

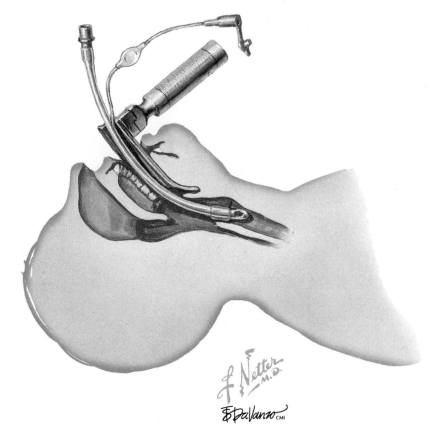

An emergency tracheostomy is performed for the same reasons as an emergency endotracheal intubation—to open the airway to prevent asphyxiation or to allow ventilation of the lungs. However, this procedure is performed when the mouth or upper airway is compromised due to either trauma or obstruction of the upper airway. In this procedure, a **tracheotomy** is performed, which cuts through the trachea to allow for the insertion of a tracheostomy tube, or trach tube (Ahmadinejad 2011). The trach tube is then left in place to allow for ventilation (see figure 10.8). The **tracheostomy** is the connection that is established by the insertion of the tube.

Figure 10.8. Tracheostomy

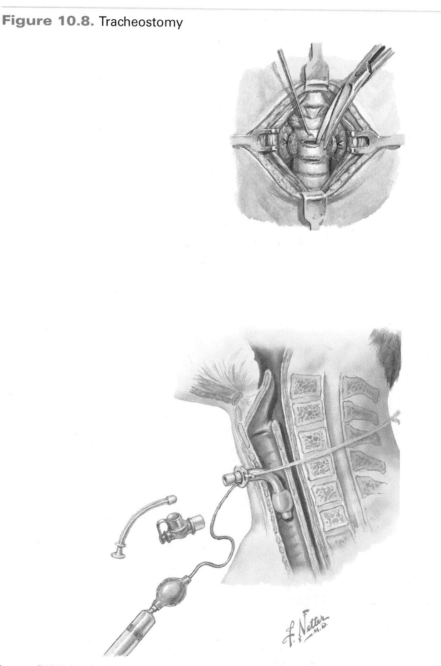

Key to Success

Note the differences at the end of the words trache*otomy* and trache*ostomy*. A tracheotomy procedure is an incision that allows access into the body cavity, whereas a tracheostomy is a connection established after the tube is inserted (as it connects the inside of the body cavity to the outside for drainage). Understanding the differences between these two suffixes (-*tomy* and -*stomy*) is imperative in understanding the procedure performed and, in some instances, which code to report for the procedure performed. The suffix -*tomy* means to make an incision, and -*stomy* means to make an opening from inside the body cavity to the outside.

There are two emergency tracheostomy codes that depend on the type of incision used to perform the procedure. A transtracheal incision cuts horizontally through the tracheal cartilage, while the cricothyroid membrane incision cuts vertically through the cricothyroid membrane at the upper end of the trachea.

The codes for tracheostomy are 31603, Tracheostomy, emergency procedure; transtracheal, and 31605, Tracheostomy, emergency procedure; cricothyroid membrane. Both are identified as emergency procedures; however, tracheostomies are also performed in nonemergent situations, when patients require long-term ventilation. For example, patients with severe brain injuries often need ventilation through a tracheostomy tube due to the presence of a large amount of secretions in the lungs and the inadequacy of natural breathing (Ahmadinegad 2011). When a tracheostomy is planned, the coder should report 31600, Tracheostomy, planned, or 31601, Tracheostomy, planned; younger than 2 years.

Moderate (Conscious) Sedation

Moderate (conscious) sedation is used during ED procedures to anesthetize patients during a medical or surgical procedure. Moderate sedation is a drug-induced depression of consciousness that still allows the patient to respond to commands and tactile stimulation. During moderate sedation, no additional interventions are required to maintain cardiovascular or respiratory function.

Moderate sedation codes (99151–99157) are based on the provider who performed the service, age of the patient, and time spent under sedation. There are three components of moderate sedation:

- *Preservice work.* This includes assessment of the patient's history, including experiences with sedation, drug allergies, a physical examination, a pre-sedation assessment, informed consent, and initial IV access and the administration of fluids (among other components).
- *Intraservice work.* This begins with the administration of the sedating agent(s) and ends when the procedure is complete and the administering physician ends personal face-to-face time with the patient. Intraservice work requires continuous face-to-face attendance of the physician and monitoring of the patient's response to the sedating agent.
- *Postservice work.* This component includes any additional face-to-face time, after the continuous face-to-face time during the procedure has ended. Such as monitoring the patient until he or she can safely be transferred from the

anesthesia or treatment area and readied for discharge. It is not included in the intraservice work time.

To select the correct code for a moderate sedation procedure, it is necessary to identify the intraservice work time involved in the procedure, as the code selection is based on the intraservice time only. Although the preservice and postservice work is included in the service, it is neither reported nor calculated into the moderate sedation time, as it is considered integral to the moderate sedation procedure. For example, if the total sedation time was 1 hour with 15 minutes of preservice work, 15 minutes of intraservice work, and 30 minutes of postservice work, then the coder would report 99152, Moderate sedation services provided by the same physician or other qualified healthcare professional performing the diagnostic or therapeutic service that the sedation supports, requiring the presence of an independent trained observer to assist in the monitoring of the patient's level of consciousness and physiological status; *initial 15 minutes of intraservice time*, patient age 5 years or older. Code 99152 reports 15 minutes of the intraservice work, which is the only item reported, even though the entire procedure took 1 hour.

Additional time over 15 minutes is reported with the appropriate add-on code to identify additional intraservice time in 15-minute increments. For example, if the intraservice work during the sedation required 45 minutes of time, then the codes reported would be 99152 (for the first 15 minutes), and 99153, Moderate sedation services provided by the same physician or other qualified healthcare professional performing the diagnostic or therapeutic service that the sedation supports, requiring the presence of an independent trained observer to assist in the monitoring of the patient's level of consciousness and physiological status; *each additional 15 minutes of intraservice time* ($\times$ 2 for the additional 30 minutes). In this example, if 45 minutes of time were spent on the service, it would be coded with 99152, 99153, and 99153 (or 99152 and 99153 $\times$ 2).

Incision and Drainage

Incision and drainage (I&D) is a procedure performed on an abscess or cyst that requires drainage. It consists of cutting into the skin above the cyst or abscess to allow for drainage of the pustular material. Emergency physicians may need to perform an I&D to drain a postoperative wound or skin infection. Codes selected for the incision and drainage (10040–10180) depend on the reason for the procedure, including acne surgery, abscess, pilonidal cyst, removal of a foreign body, hematoma, seroma, or other fluid collection, or postoperative wound infection. Codes are further divided based on whether the procedure was simple/single or complicated/multiple. For example, if an emergency physician performed an I&D on a single uncomplicated MRSA cyst on the buttock of a 25-year-old patient, the code reported would be 10060, Incision and drainage of abscess (eg, carbuncle, suppurative hidradenitis, cutaneous or subcutaneous abscess, cyst, furuncle, or paronychia); simple or single.

Foreign Body Removal

Sometimes related to an incision and drainage are foreign body removals. A **foreign body (FB)** is any unnatural object that is present inside the body or organ structure. FBs include materials that have been ingested (for example, a swallowed marble or coin), inhaled (such as an aspirated pill), purposefully inserted into a natural opening (such as a bead in a child's nose), or introduced through trauma (like a bullet from a gunshot wound) or injury (for instance, retained pieces of asphalt from a road rash incident or a splinter).

Accordingly, codes for FB removal cover procedures ranging from invasive surgery to remove deeply imbedded FBs, to removal of FBs requiring nothing more than forceps or a pair of tweezers. FB removals may be performed on natural body openings such as the ears, nose, and eyes or on the external structure of the body like the skin. More complex foreign body removals may be performed on the internal structures of the body, such as airways or the gastrointestinal tract. Code selection depends on the area from which the FB was removed, as well as the manner of the removal.

To find the code for a FB removal, search the CPT Index under the term *Removal* and refer to the subterm *Foreign Body*. Locate the site of the FB and available codes, and finally verify the code in the Tabular List. Codes listed in the Tabular may differ based on the complexity of the procedure or the technique used to remove the FB. For example, if an ED physician removed a bead from the nose of the patient via lateral rhinotomy (an incision into the side of the nose), the code reported would be 30320, Removal of foreign body, intranasal; by lateral rhinotomy.

Penetrating Wound Exploration

A **penetrating wound** is one that results from a trauma that pierces the skin and goes into the body's deeper structures, such as a stab or gunshot wound. Due to the life-threatening nature of this type of injury, patients with a penetrating wound are often brought to the ED for evaluation and treatment, which requires exploration of the penetrating wound to evaluate the damage caused by the injury. If severe damage is found, the patient may be transferred to the operating room for emergency surgery. If no significant damage is done, the ED physician may decide to repair the wound in the ED.

There are four codes for wound exploration, differentiated based on the area being explored (the neck, chest, abdomen/flank/back, or an extremity):

- 20100, Exploration of penetrating wound (separate procedure); neck
- 20101, Exploration of penetrating wound (separate procedure); chest
- 20102, Exploration of penetrating wound (separate procedure); abdomen/flank/back
- 20103, Exploration of penetrating wound (separate procedure); extremity

Wound exploration codes identify the surgical exploration, enlargement, and extension of the wound; debridement; removal of foreign body; and minimal ligation of blood vessels. If a major repair is done, the wound exploration code is not reported, as this would be included in the code for the major procedure (such as a major blood vessel repair). If this were the case, only the code for the major procedure would be reported, not the code for the wound exploration.

Lumbar Puncture

A **lumbar puncture**, also called a spinal tap, is a diagnostic procedure used to evaluate cerebrospinal fluid that surrounds the brain and spinal cord. Lumbar punctures are performed in the ED setting to diagnose conditions such as meningitis or subarachnoid hemorrhage, both of which can be life-threatening diseases. During the procedure, a needle is inserted into the spinal canal in the lumbar area, and a hollow tube is threaded into the space to obtain a sample of the cerebrospinal fluid (see figure 10.9).

There is one code for lumbar puncture when it is performed for diagnostic purposes: 62270, Spinal puncture, lumbar, diagnostic.

Figure 10.9. Lumbar puncture

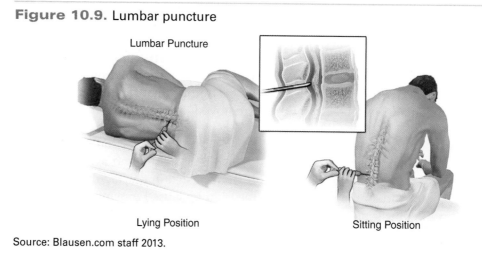

Lumbar Puncture

Lying Position   Sitting Position

Source: Blausen.com staff 2013.

Needle and Tube Thoracostomy

A **thoracostomy** is an opening created in the thoracic cavity, otherwise known as a chest tube. It acts as a drain for the thoracic cavity to drain blood, fluid, or air from around the lungs, heart, or esophagus. A thoracostomy can be performed by either a needle or a tube. In a needle thoracostomy, a hollow needle is directly inserted into an intercostal space (between the ribs) to allow for drainage. A tube thoracostomy consists of a trocar being placed between the ribs, through which a hollow tube is inserted into the chest and secured in place to allow for continuous drainage (USNLM 2019). A trocar is a surgical instrument with a long, pointed tube through which other instrumentation can be passed. Thoracostomies are performed in the ED to emergently treat patients suffering from **pneumothorax** (collapsed lung), **hemothorax** (blood in the pleural cavity), or **pleural effusion** (fluid buildup in the chest).

Codes for thoracostomies depend on the type of procedure performed (either by needle or tube), and the reason for the procedure.

- 32035, Thoracostomy; *with rib resection for empyema*, and 32036, Thoracostomy; *with open flap drainage for empyema*. These thoracostomies are performed specifically for empyema, a type of pleural effusion.

- 32551, Tube thoracostomy, includes connection to drainage system (eg, water seal), when performed, open (separate procedure). This code should be reported for any thoracostomy performed as a separate procedure for drainage of the pleural space (besides that done for empyema).

- 32554–32557, Thoracentesis, needle or catheter, aspiration of the pleural space. This range of codes identifies needle aspirations of the pleural cavity, performed with or without imaging guidance.

Additional Procedures

Additional procedures performed in the ED are noninvasive in nature and require external manipulation or therapy to an organ or body part. Remember that EDs still provide all the services performed by an urgent care clinic, including labs, x-rays and imaging services, and treatment of injuries. The next sections of this chapter discuss ED procedures such as reduction of dislocations, cardiopulmonary resuscitation, and control of nasal hemorrhage.

Dislocation Reduction

Dislocation reduction is the act of relocating a joint to its original location, in the case of joint dislocation or subluxation (partial dislocation). Depending on the joint and the patient, reductions may be performed under moderate sedation. If the joint is unable to be reduced into the socket successfully, then the patient would be admitted to the hospital so that the reduction could be performed surgically.

Codes for dislocation reduction depend on the site of the dislocation or subluxation, and whether the reduction was performed open or closed. An **open procedure** is one in which the skin is incised (or cut into) to perform the procedure. Open reductions are performed surgically, by cutting into the skin and surgically putting the joint back into place. A **closed procedure** is one in which the skin is not opened to perform the procedure. Closed reductions are performed without opening the skin; the healthcare provider manipulates the joint back into place externally.

To search for a dislocation reduction code, search for the term *Dislocation* in the Index, then locate the subterm for the body site of the dislocation and find the code for either open or closed reduction. Verify the code in the Tabular List.

Cardiopulmonary Resuscitation

Cardiopulmonary resuscitation, otherwise known as CPR, is a medical procedure that involves the healthcare provider repeatedly compressing a patient's chest in an attempt to circulate the blood and restore breathing to a patient who has suffered cardiac arrest (a stopping of the heart). CPR is continued until the patient is resuscitated or until the patient is declared deceased. CPR includes the use of chest compressions, breaths or breathing apparatus delivered to the patient, electronic defibrillation, or medications administered, such as epinephrine and lidocaine, as necessary.

There is one code for CPR: 92950, Cardiopulmonary resuscitation (eg, in cardiac arrest).

Control of Nasal Hemorrhage

Nasal packing is performed for uncontrollable hemorrhage from the nose (epistaxis or bloody nose). Nasal packing codes (30901–30906) are located in the Respiratory subsection of the CPT code book and depend on the type of packing performed. Anterior nasal hemorrhage control consists of either cauterization of the blood vessels or nasal packing materials (such as cotton balls, gauze, or nasal tampons) that are placed in the front of the nose to control the bleeding. Posterior control is the cautery of blood vessels or the packing of the posterior nasal cavity to control the hemorrhage (see figure 10.10).

Complete the exercises in There's a Code for That 10.2 to practice assigning procedure codes to ED services.

Emergency department procedures **10.2**

There's a Code for That

Read the following documentation and select the appropriate procedure and/or E/M codes.

1. A 4-year-old male patient seen in the ED with a FB in his nose. Mother reports that she was cooking breakfast when her son walked up to her with tears in his eyes and pointed to his nose. Small plastic brick toy was visible at the time,

(Continued on next page)

Figure 10.10. Control of nasal hemorrhage

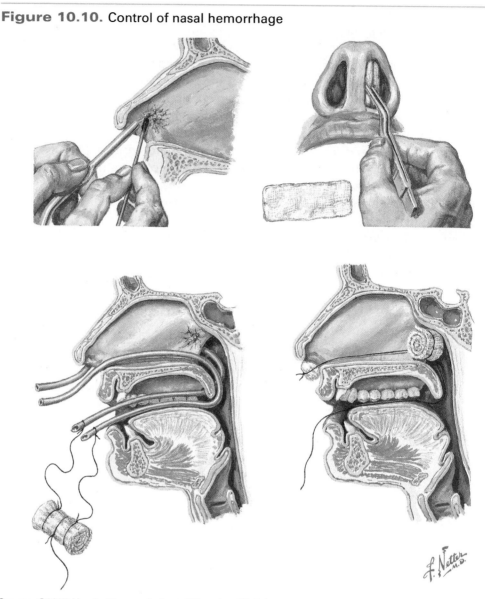

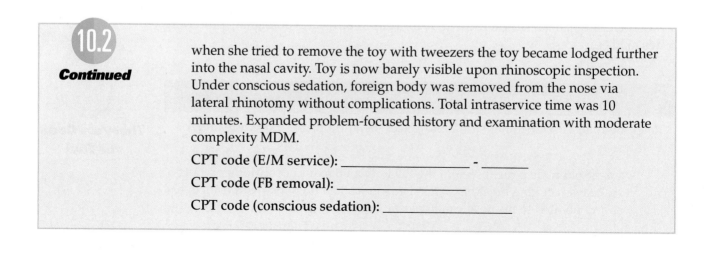

10.2

Continued

when she tried to remove the toy with tweezers the toy became lodged further into the nasal cavity. Toy is now barely visible upon rhinoscopic inspection. Under conscious sedation, foreign body was removed from the nose via lateral rhinotomy without complications. Total intraservice time was 10 minutes. Expanded problem-focused history and examination with moderate complexity MDM.

CPT code (E/M service): _____ - _____

CPT code (FB removal): _____

CPT code (conscious sedation): _____

2. Patient with severe anaphylactic reaction presented to the ER in respiratory distress. Endotracheal intubation performed.

   CPT code (intubation and injection): _____

3. Limited cautery of uncontrollable epistaxis.

   CPT code: _____

4. A 45-year-old male presents with multiple stab wounds in upper left shoulder and forearm from a bar fight. Penetrating wound exploration performed with extension of dissection and surgical exploration. No major damage was noted and wounds were repaired. (Note: because there were no major repairs performed, code only for the wound exploration).

   CPT code: _____

5. A 7-year-old female presents with severe headache and stiff neck. Mother reports that the symptoms came on suddenly and worsened over the course of the day. CSF obtained through lumbar puncture, tested positive for bacterial meningitis. Comprehensive history and examination with MDM of high complexity.

   CPT code (E/M service): _____ - _____

   CPT code (lumbar puncture): _____

Diagnostic Coding for Urgent Care and ED Services

The diagnosis code selected for the urgent care or ED service should identify the medical necessity for the service provided. Because patients may have a wide range of different conditions, signs, symptoms, or diagnoses, it is necessary to employ the entire ICD-10-CM code book while coding.

Key to Success

This section discusses coding for urgent care and ED services separately, although the conditions in this section may be seen in either setting depending on the circumstances.

Diagnostic Coding for Urgent Care Services

Coding for urgent care services requires a solid understanding of the differences between signs and symptoms and a definitive diagnosis and when to code for both, as well as the ability to code for infectious diseases. Injuries are also commonly seen in the urgent care center, the codes for which require detailed analysis of the healthcare documentation to extract all necessary details and select the required external cause codes.

Signs and Symptoms

Often when a patient seeks services at an urgent care clinic, it is due to a sudden-onset sign or symptom that happens when the patient's primary care provider is not available. Remember, when coding for signs and symptoms, if a definitive diagnosis is determined, then do not code for the related signs and symptoms. On the other hand, if a definitive diagnosis cannot be determined, then code only for the signs and symptoms. The only time it is necessary to code for both the signs and symptoms and a definitive diagnosis is when the signs and symptoms are not related to the definitive diagnosis.

When a patient presents to the clinic with signs and symptoms, diagnostic testing is usually performed to confirm the diagnosis. For example, if a patient presents with painful urination and a urinalysis confirms a urinary tract infection (UTI), then the patient's definitive diagnosis is a UTI. The confirmed diagnosis of the UTI is the only diagnosis code needed to support the medical necessity for the urinalysis procedure, and the painful urination code does not need to be reported.

If a definitive diagnosis has been determined but additional, *unrelated* signs or symptoms are also present, code for both the definitive diagnosis and the unrelated signs and symptoms. For instance, if a patient is diagnosed with a UTI but also has dizziness unrelated to the UTI diagnosis, the coder would report the UTI as well as the symptom of dizziness. Refer to figure 10.11 for a flowchart to help decide when it is appropriate to code for signs and symptoms versus a definitive diagnosis.

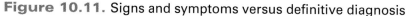

Figure 10.11. Signs and symptoms versus definitive diagnosis

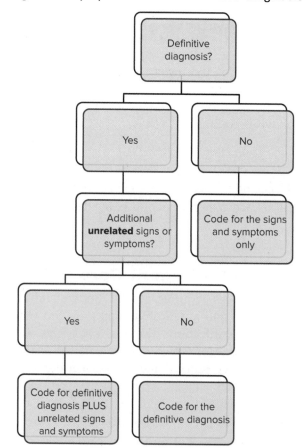

Infectious Diseases

Sometimes a diagnostic test for a sign or symptom results in a definitive diagnosis for an infectious disease. Infectious diseases are coded from chapter 1 (Certain Infectious and Parasitic Diseases) of the ICD-10-CM code book. Other conditions, while due to an infectious disease, may be coded from different chapters of the ICD-10-CM code book, such as respiratory conditions and ear infections.

Common infectious diseases seen in the urgent care setting are also commonly seen in the primary care setting, such as mononucleosis, streptococcal pharyngitis (strep throat), otitis media (ear infection), influenza, and conjunctivitis (pink eye). When coding for any type of infectious disease, if the specific pathogen is known (etiology), it should be identified with a code to identify the organism. Refer to chapter 4 (Learning the ICD-10-CM Code Book) for a discussion of etiology and manifestations including relevant OGCR.

The only exception to this is if a combination code exists that identifies the etiology and manifestation of the disease in one code. Combination codes include both the etiology (cause of the disease) and the manifestation (signs or symptoms of the disease) all in one code. For example, if a patient presents to the urgent care clinic complaining of fever with cough, chills, nausea, and headache, and it is confirmed that the patient has influenza, then the code for unspecified influenza should be used, J11.1, Influenza due to unidentified influenza virus with other respiratory manifestations. In this case, the one code (J11.1) identifies both the etiology (influenza, the infectious organism), as well as the manifestations of the disease (other respiratory manifestations).

If the specific influenza viral strain (etiology) is identified by the clinic, then it should be reported with the appropriate combination code to identify both the viral infection (influenza with other manifestation), and the specific infectious disease (etiology). For example, if the patient came into the office with a viral pneumonia and it was identified that the patient had influenza with pneumonia due to the novel influenza A virus, the appropriate code would be J09.X1, Influenza due to identified novel influenza A virus with pneumonia.

When there is no combination code to identify both the infectious organism (when known) and the etiology, the two conditions must be coded separately. For instance, if a patient is diagnosed with a lung abscess due to *Klebsiella pneumoniae* without pneumonia, the coder should report one code for the lung abscess, J85.2, Abscess of lung without pneumonia, and an additional code to identify the infectious organism, B96.1, Klebsiella pneuomoniae [K. pneumoniae] as the cause of disease classified elsewhere.

When identifying the etiology and manifestation of a disease with separate codes, select the "B" code for the infectious disease *as the cause of disease classified elsewhere.* This indicates that the infectious organism caused the manifestation identified by the other code. B codes are located in chapter 1 (Certain Infectious and Parasitic Diseases) of the ICD-10-CM code book in the section "Bacterial and viral infectious agents" (B95–B97). Beneath the category name in the ICD-10-CM code book, there is a note that these categories are for use as a supplementary or additional code to identify the infectious agent (etiology) of a disease classified elsewhere in the ICD-10-CM manual. This is an important category of codes to understand, as these codes are to be used only in conjunction with a primary code to identify the manifestation.

Sequencing of the two codes should be as indicated in the ICD-10-CM code book: the manifestation code is sequenced first, followed by the code to identify the etiology of the disease. Remember, as discussed in chapter 4, sequencing of these codes is guided by the notations in the Tabular List, including "code first" and "use additional code."

These notations tell coders when to sequence one code before another and in which situations.

When searching for an infectious disease in the ICD-10-CM code book, look up the main term *Infection, infected, infective*, and then find the subterm for the specific pathogen. If the pathogen has resulted in a manifestation that is coded elsewhere, be sure to select the subterm *as cause of disease classified elsewhere*, and then verify the code in the Tabular List.

Sexually transmitted infections (STIs) are also commonly seen in the urgent care setting. These include genital herpes, gonorrhea, chlamydia, trichomoniasis, syphilis, human papillomavirus (HPV), bacterial vaginosis, HIV/AIDS, and viral hepatitis. To search for a sexually transmitted disease in the ICD-10-CM code book, search for the name of the type of infection (such as *syphilis* or *trichomoniasis*) and then search for the subterm to identify the specific type of infection.

Injuries and External Causes

Injuries are often seen in the urgent care setting, especially since wait times are relatively short and most urgent care clinics have imaging services (such as x-rays) on-site. Thus, a patient with a possible fracture can be seen for a quick determination of the extent of the injury, receive initial treatment, and receive a referral for further treatment, if necessary. Also, some injuries like skin lacerations can be immediately repaired in the urgent care setting. Injuries commonly seen in the urgent care setting include muscle and joint sprains and strains, cuts and lacerations, minor burns, and fall injuries.

When a patient has multiple injuries, the coder should report one code for each injury, with the most severe injury sequenced first, followed by the less severe injuries. When coding for multiple injuries, remember:

Worst Comes First

External causes of injury codes are also common in ED encounters; each of these codes requires a solid understanding of the episode of service for the encounter and external causes of injury codes, discussed below.

External Causes of Injury

When coding for injuries, the healthcare provider needs to document the actual injury rather than a sign or symptom. For example, if a patient presents with wrist pain, an inconclusive x-ray is taken, and the healthcare provider documents suspected wrist fracture, the coder should report wrist pain (or another appropriate, documented sign or symptom) and *not* a code for a wrist fracture, as this diagnosis was not confirmed. Remember, coders cannot report a diagnosis that is *suspected, unconfirmed, rule-out,* or *questionable* in the outpatient setting (refer to the discussion of uncertain diagnoses in chapter 4 of this textbook).

When coding for any type of injury, it is necessary to include up to four codes for the external causes of the injury. As discussed in chapter 4, external cause codes are always sequenced *after* the codes for the primary medical condition (such as the injury suffered). External cause codes provide additional information surrounding the circumstances of the injury or illness but do not clearly identify the medical necessity for the service, so they have no impact on reimbursement. There are four possible external cause code categories, which should be ordered as follows.

- The *injury mechanism* is the manner in which the injury happened, such as kicked by a horse: W55.12XA, Struck by horse, initial encounter.
- The *activity* in which the patient was engaged when the injury happened, such as riding a horse: Y93.52, Activity, horseback riding.
- The *place of occurrence* is where the injury occurred, such as in a rodeo arena: Y92.39, Other specified sports and athletic area as the place of occurrence of the external cause.
- The *status* of the patient at the time of the activity, such as sport done for pay: Y99.0, Civilian activity done for income or pay.

These codes are meant to explain the circumstances surrounding an injury and are used by the patient's health insurance to determine whether a health insurance plan or other accident insurance plan, such as worker's compensation, needs to pay for the services provided to the patient. These codes are also used to collect data regarding certain types of injuries, such as dog bites or gunshot wounds.

Key to Success

The need to code for external causes depends on the state in which the healthcare services are provided. Some states do not require external cause codes, while other states mandate them. In some areas, it may be necessary to report external cause codes to certain payers who require them, whereas other payers will not process and may deny claims with external cause codes. It is imperative to understand the specific requirements for the encounter for which you are coding and report those codes accordingly. This textbook assumes that external causes are necessary to report, so as you read and come across an external cause described in the documentation, you should assign the appropriate code(s). Remember, external cause codes are always listed after the codes for the patient's medical condition(s); these codes are never sequenced first.

Identify the Encounter

When coding for injuries, a coder must identify the encounter for the injury (refer to chapter 4). Remember that the seventh character *A-initial* represents any encounter for which the patient is in active treatment. *D-subsequent* is when the patient is in the healing phase, and *S-sequela* is for a late effect, or sequela, of that condition. As most patients seen in the urgent care setting are experiencing acute conditions, the majority of the encounters will be *A-initial*. If, however, a patient received stitches in the urgent care clinic two weeks before returning for the removal of the stitches, then the return encounter would be *D-subsequent*.

For all initial encounters (ending with an *A*), it is necessary to identify all four external cause codes (if possible). For all encounters other than initial encounters, the coder needs to report only the external cause code for the injury mechanism, with either a *D-subsequent* or *S-sequela* seventh character, depending on the circumstances. See figure 10.12 for the OGCR related to coding for external causes of morbidity.

Figure 10.12. OGCR I.C.20

---

20. Chapter 20: External Causes of Morbidity (V00-Y99)

The external causes of morbidity codes should never be sequenced as the first-listed or principal diagnosis.

External cause codes are intended to provide data for injury research and evaluation of injury prevention strategies. These codes capture how the injury or health condition happened (cause), the intent (unintentional or accidental; or intentional, such as suicide or assault), the place where the event occurred the activity of the patient at the time of the event, and the person's status (e.g., civilian, military).

There is no national requirement for mandatory ICD-10-CM external cause code reporting. Unless a provider is subject to a state-based external cause code reporting mandate or these codes are required by a particular payer, reporting of ICD-10-CM codes in Chapter 20, External Causes of Morbidity, is not required. In the absence of a mandatory reporting requirement, providers are encouraged to voluntarily report external cause codes, as they provide valuable data for injury research and evaluation of injury prevention strategies.

a. General External Cause Coding Guidelines

1) Used with any code in the range of A00.0-T88.9, Z00-Z99

An external cause code may be used with any code in the range of A00.0-T88.9, Z00-Z99, classification that represents a health condition due to an external cause. Though they are most applicable to injuries, they are also valid for use with such things as infections or diseases due to an external source, and other health conditions, such as a heart attack that occurs during strenuous physical activity.

2) External cause code used for length of treatment

Assign the external cause code, with the appropriate 7th character (initial encounter, subsequent encounter or sequela) for each encounter for which the injury or condition is being treated. Most categories in chapter 20 have a 7th character requirement for each applicable code.

Most categories in this chapter have three 7th character values: A, initial encounter, D, subsequent encounter and S, sequela. While the patient may be seen by a new or different provider over the course of treatment for an injury or condition, assignment of the 7th character for external cause should match the 7th character of the code assigned for the associated injury or condition for the encounter.

3) Use the full range of external cause codes

Use the full range of external cause codes to completely describe the cause, the intent, the place of occurrence, and if applicable, the activity of the patient at the time of the event, and the patient's status, for all injuries, and other health conditions due to an external cause.

4) Assign as many external cause codes as necessary

Assign as many external cause codes as necessary to fully explain each cause. If only one external code can be recorded, assign the code most related to the principal diagnosis.

5) The selection of the appropriate external cause code

The selection of the appropriate external cause code is guided by the Alphabetic Index of External Causes and by Inclusion and Exclusion notes in the Tabular List.

6) External cause code can never be a principal diagnosis

An external cause code can never be a principal (first-listed) diagnosis.

7) Combination external cause codes

Certain of the external cause codes are combination codes that identify sequential events that result in an injury, such as a fall which results in striking against an object. The injury may be due to either event or both. The combination external cause code used should correspond to the sequence of events regardless of which caused the most serious injury.

8) No external cause code needed in certain circumstances

No external cause code from Chapter 20 is needed if the external cause and intent are included in a code from another chapter (e.g. T36.0X1- Poisoning by penicillins, accidental (unintentional)).

b. Place of Occurrence Guideline

Codes from category Y92, Place of occurrence of the external cause, are secondary codes for use after other external cause codes to identify the location of the patient at the time of injury or other condition.

Generally, a place of occurrent code is assigned only once, at the initial encounter for treatment. However, in the rare instance that a new injury occurs during hospitalization, an additional place of occurrence code may be assigned. No 7th characters are used for Y92.

Do not use place of occurrence code Y92.9 if the place is not stated or is not applicable.

c. Activity Code

Assign a code from category Y93, Activity code, to describe the activity of the patient at the time the injury or other health condition occurred.

An activity code is used only once, at the initial encounter for treatment. Only one code from Y93 should be recorded on a medical record.

The activity codes are not applicable to poisonings, adverse effects, misadventures or sequela.

Do not assign Y93.9, Unspecified activity, if the activity is not stated.

A code from category Y93 is appropriate for use with external cause and intent codes if identifying the activity provides additional information about the event.

d. Place of Occurrence, Activity, and Status Codes Used with other External Cause Code

When applicable, place of occurrence, activity, and external cause status codes are sequenced after the main external cause code(s). Regardless of the number of external cause codes assigned, there should be only one place of occurrence code, one activity code, and one external cause status code assigned to an encounter. However, in the rare instance that a new injury occurs during hospitalization, an additional place of occurrence code may be assigned.

e. If the Reporting Format Limits the Number of External Cause Codes

If the reporting format limits the number of external cause codes that can be used in reporting clinical data, report the code for the cause/intent most related to the principal diagnosis. If the format permits capture of additional external cause codes, the cause/intent, including medical misadventures, of the additional events should be reported rather than the codes for place, activity, or external status.

f. Multiple External Cause Coding Guidelines

More than one external cause code is required to fully describe the external cause of an illness or injury. The assignment of external cause codes should be sequenced in the following priority:

If two or more events cause separate injuries, an external cause code should be assigned for each cause. The first-listed external cause code will be selected in the following order:

External codes for child and adult abuse take priority over all other external cause codes.

See Section I.C.19., Child and Adult abuse guidelines.

External cause codes for terrorism events take priority over all other external cause codes except child and adult abuse.

External cause codes for cataclysmic events take priority over all other external cause codes except child and adult abuse and terrorism.

External cause codes for transport accidents take priority over all other external cause codes except cataclysmic events, child and adult abuse and terrorism.

Activity and external cause status codes are assigned following all causal (intent) external cause codes.

The first-listed external cause code should correspond to the cause of the most serious diagnosis due to an assault, accident, or self-harm, following the order of hierarchy listed above.

g. Child and Adult Abuse Guideline

Adult and child abuse, neglect and maltreatment are classified as assault. Any of the assault codes may be used to indicate the external cause of any injury resulting from the confirmed abuse.

For confirmed cases of abuse, neglect and maltreatment, when the perpetrator is known, a code from Y07, Perpetrator of maltreatment and neglect, should accompany any other assault codes.

See Section I.C.19. Adult and child abuse, neglect and other maltreatment

h. Unknown or Undetermined Intent Guideline

If the intent (accident, self-harm, assault) of the cause of an injury or other condition is unknown or unspecified, code the intent as accidental intent. All transport accident categories assume accidental intent.

1) Use of undetermined intent

External cause codes for events of undetermined intent are only for use if the documentation in the record specifies that the intent cannot be determined.

(Continued on next page)

Figure 10.12. *(Continued)*

i. Sequelae (Late Effects) of External Cause Guidelines

  1) Sequelae external cause codes

  Sequela are reported using the external cause code with the 7th character "S" for sequela. These codes should be used with any report of a late effect or sequela resulting from a previous injury.

  See Section I.B.10 Sequela (Late Effects)

  2) Sequela external cause code with a related current injury

  A sequela external cause code should never be used with a related current nature of injury code.

  3) Use of sequela external cause codes for subsequent visits

  Use a late effect external cause code for subsequent visits when a late effect of the initial injury is being treated. Do not use a late effect external cause code for subsequent visits for follow-up care (e.g., to assess healing, to receive rehabilitative therapy) of the injury when no late effect of the injury has been documented.

j. Terrorism Guidelines

  1) Cause of injury identified by the Federal Government (FBI) as terrorism

  When the cause of an injury is identified by the Federal Government (FBI) as terrorism, the first-listed external cause code should be a code from category Y38, Terrorism. The definition of terrorism employed by the FBI is found at the inclusion note at the beginning of category Y38. Use additional code for place of occurrence (Y92.-). More than one Y38 code may be assigned if the injury is the result of more than one mechanism of terrorism.

  2) Cause of an injury is suspected to be the result of terrorism

  When the cause of an injury is suspected to be the result of terrorism a code from category Y38 should not be assigned. Suspected cases should be classified as assault.

  3) Code Y38.9, Terrorism, secondary effects

  Assign code Y38.9, Terrorism, secondary effects, for conditions occurring subsequent to the terrorist event. This code should not be assigned for conditions that are due to the initial terrorist act.

  It is acceptable to assign code Y38.9 with another code from Y38 if there is an injury due to the initial terrorist event and an injury that is a subsequent result of the terrorist event.

k. External cause status

  A code from category Y99, External cause status, should be assigned whenever any other external cause code is assigned for an encounter, including an Activity code, except for the events noted below. Assign a code from category Y99, External cause status, to indicate the work status of the person at the time the event occurred. The status code indicates whether the event occurred during military activity, whether a non-military person was at work, whether an individual including a student or volunteer was involved in a non-work activity at the time of the causal event.

  A code from Y99, External cause status, should be assigned, when applicable, with other external cause codes, such as transport accidents and falls. The external cause status codes are not applicable to poisonings, adverse effects, misadventures or late effects. Do not assign a code from category Y99 if no other external cause codes (cause, activity) are applicable for the encounter.

  An external cause status code is used only once, at the initial encounter for treatment. Only one code from Y99 should be recorded on a medical record.

  Do not assign code Y99.9, Unspecified external cause status, if the status is not stated.

Source: CMS 2019b.

Complete the exercises in There's a Code for That 10.3 to practice assigning diagnosis codes to urgent care services.

10.3

There's a Code for That

Urgent care diagnoses

Read the following documentation and select the appropriate diagnosis code(s).

1. Patient with left knee pain presents to urgent care clinic after a wrestling injury. All x-rays performed were negative, suspect ligamentous injury. Refer to ortho for follow-up and further imaging.

ICD-10-CM code: _____ , _____

2. Patient seen for multiple lacerations. Following wounds were noted: simple wounds of right upper thigh, right hip, and abdomen. Intermediate wounds on right forearm, right shoulder, and forehead.

   ICD-10-CM codes: _____ , _____ , _____ ,

   _____ , _____ , _____

3. A 32-year-old female established patient seen for lymphadenopathy, sore throat, and hyperpyrexia. Lab tests performed included group A strep, influenza, and mono spot. Mono spot was positive for infectious mononucleosis.

   ICD-10-CM code: _____

4. X-ray performed on patient with severe cough, chest pain, and fever shows pneumonia infiltrates. Lab culture of sputum test positive for streptococcal pneumoniae.

   ICD-10-CM code: _____

5. Patient suffered impact injury during soccer practice at a local athletic field. She was practicing in her off-hours for a recreational soccer league. She was running toward another player when they collided and fell to the ground, after which two other players toppled over and fell on top of the patient. She is now complaining of chest pain and difficulty breathing. X-ray negative for any fracture or internal injuries. Impression: Contusion of right ribs.

   ICD-10-CM code (injury): _____

   ICD-10-CM codes (external causes): _____ , _____ ,

   _____ , _____

Diagnostic Coding for ED Services

Diagnoses for conditions seen in the ED setting typically revolve around life-threatening illnesses and injuries. These include cardiovascular conditions, skin infections, appendicitis, motor vehicle accidents, burns, sepsis, septicemia, and systemic inflammatory response syndrome (SIRS). Patients present to the ED for treatment with various conditions, some of which are true life-threatening emergencies, while others are simple problems that do not require any treatment. Coding diagnoses for ED services relies on the coder's ability to utilize the entire ICD-10-CM code book and read and interpret ICD-10-CM coding guidelines.

Cardiovascular Problems and Myocardial Infarctions

Chest pain, cardiac dysrhythmias, congestive heart failure, and myocardial infarctions are all conditions that may be seen in the ED setting.

Chest pain may be a symptom of an injury, such as a broken rib or soreness from a cough; or it may be more serious, such as an impending myocardial infarction or lower respiratory infection. This is why chest pain is commonly evaluated in the ED. Codes for chest pain identify the type of chest pain. If the chest pain is determined to be a symptom of a more definitive condition, such as myocardial infarction, then the myocardial infarction (or other definitive condition) should be coded, not the symptom of chest pain.

Other cardiovascular problems in the ED may include cardiac dysrhythmias and congestive heart failure, vascular diseases, and deep vein thromboses and pulmonary embolisms.

HCC

A **myocardial infarction (MI)**, otherwise known as a heart attack, is the death of a portion of the heart muscle due to lack of oxygen supply. Heart attacks vary in the site and type of the infarction, and codes depend on whether the MI is a STEMI (ST elevation myocardial infarction) or NSTEMI (non-STEMI), as well as if the MI is initial or subsequent.

Do not confuse a heart attack with cardiac arrest, which is the complete stoppage of the heart. In an MI, the heart may still be functioning for a period of time, depending on the severity of the infarction. This means that there is typically a window of time in which a patient experiencing a heart attack may still be treated before decompensation or death occurs. Furthermore, a patient having survived one heart attack may also experience another heart attack, either within a short period of time or years later. An initial MI (category I21) is the either the first MI or an MI that occurs more than 28 days (4 weeks) after an initial MI. For example, if the patient had a heart attack two years ago and presents to the ED today with a new heart attack, it would be coded with an I21 code to identify it as an initial MI.

A subsequent MI (category I22) is a heart attack that occurs within 28 days (4 weeks) of an initial MI. For example, if the patient that came in two weeks ago with a heart attack presents today with a different MI (an infarction of a different site), the MI for this encounter would be coded as a subsequent MI (I22). An additional code would be assigned to identify the initial MI. If the previous MI is older than 28 days, code I25.2, Old myocardial infarction, should be used to identify the previous MI. The old MI code may be used for any old MI, even if it occurred 10 years ago or more.

Figure 10.13. Acute versus subsequent MI flowchart

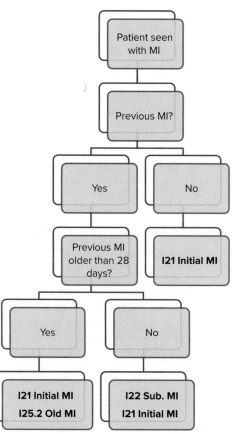

The flowchart in figure 10.13 identifies when an MI would be identified as either initial or subsequent, and the sequencing of each. Figure 10.14 provides the OGCR related to coding myocardial infarctions.

Figure 10.14. OGCR I.C.9.e

e. Acute myocardial infarction (AMI)

1) ST elevation myocardial infarction (STEMI) and non ST elevation myocardial infarction (NSTEMI)

The ICD-10-CM codes for type 1 acute myocardial infarction (AMI) identify the site, such as anterolateral wall or true posterior wall. Subcategories I21.0-I21.2 and code I21.3 are used for type 1 ST elevation myocardial infarction (STEMI). Code I21.4, Non-ST elevation (NSTEMI) myocardial infarction, is used for type 1 non ST elevation myocardial infarction (NSTEMI) and nontransmural MIs.

If a type 1 NSTEMI evolves to STEMI, assign the STEMI code. If a type 1 STEMI converts to NSTEMI due to thrombolytic therapy, it is still coded as STEMI.

For encounters occurring while the myocardial infarction is equal to, or less than, four weeks old, including transfers to another acute setting or a postacute setting, and the myocardial infarction meets the definition for "other diagnoses" (see Section III, Reporting Additional Diagnoses), codes from category I21 may continue to be reported. For encounters after the 4 week time frame and the patient is still receiving care related to the myocardial infarction, the appropriate aftercare code should be assigned, rather than a code from category I21. For old or healed myocardial infarctions not requiring further care, code I25.2, Old myocardial infarction, may be assigned.

2) Acute myocardial infarction, unspecified

Code I21.9, Acute myocardial infarction, unspecified, is the default for unspecified acute myocardial infarction or unspecified type. If only type 1 STEMI or transmural MI without the site is documented, assign code I21.3, ST elevation (STEMI) myocardial infarction of unspecified site.

3) AMI documented as nontransmural or subendocardial but site provided

If an AMI is documented as nontransmural or subendocardial, but the site is provided, it is still coded as a subendocardial AMI.

See Section I.C.21.3 for information on coding status post administration of tPA in a different facility within the last 24 hours.

4) Subsequent acute myocardial infarction

A code from category I22, Subsequent ST elevation (STEMI) and non-ST elevation (NSTEMI) myocardial infarction, is to be used when a patient who has suffered a type 1 or unspecified AMI has a new AMI within the 4 week time frame of the initial AMI. A code from category I22 must be used in conjunction with a code from category I21. The sequencing of the I22 and I21 codes depends on the circumstances of the encounter.

Do not assign code I22 for subsequent myocardial infarctions other than type 1 or unspecified. For subsequent type 2 AMI assign only code I21.A1. For subsequent type 4 or type 5 AMI, assign only code I21.A9.

If a subsequent myocardial infarction of one type occurs within 4 weeks of a myocardial infarction of a different type, assign the appropriate codes from category I21 to identify each type. Do not assign a code from I22. Codes from category I22 should only be assigned if both the initial and subsequent myocardial infarctions are type 1 or unspecified.

5) Other Types of Myocardial Infarction

The ICD-10-CM provides codes for different types of myocardial infarction. Type 1 myocardial infarctions are assigned to codes I21.0-I21.4.

Type 2 myocardial infarction (myocardial infarction due to demand ischemia or secondary to ischemic **im**balance) is assigned to code I21.A1, Myocardial infarction type 2 with the underlying cause **coded first**. Do not assign code I24.8, Other forms of acute ischemic heart disease, for the demand ischemia. **If** a type 2 AMI is described as NSTEMI or STEMI, only assign code I21.A1. Codes I21.0-I21.4 should only be assigned for type 1 AMIs.

Acute myocardial infarctions type 3, 4a, 4b, 4c and 5 are assigned to code I21.A9, Other myocardial infarction type.

The "Code also" and "Code first" notes should be followed related to complications, and for coding of postprocedural myocardial infarctions during or following cardiac surgery.

Source: CMS 2019b.

HCC Coding Corner

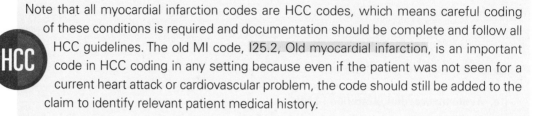

Note that all myocardial infarction codes are HCC codes, which means careful coding of these conditions is required and documentation should be complete and follow all HCC guidelines. The old MI code, I25.2, Old myocardial infarction, is an important code in HCC coding in any setting because even if the patient was not seen for a current heart attack or cardiovascular problem, the code should still be added to the claim to identify relevant patient medical history.

Sepsis, Septicemia, and SIRS

Sepsis, also referred to as septicemia or bacteremia, is a complication of an infection outside of the bloodstream, such as a tooth abscess or skin infection. Once a patient is deemed septic, the infectious organism has invaded the bloodstream and been carried throughout the blood to other sites of the body. This may result in acute organ dysfunction, in which case the patient is deemed to have severe sepsis that can result in septic shock and ultimately death.

Codes for sepsis identify the condition as either sepsis or severe sepsis. Severe sepsis is when the sepsis has caused any acute organ dysfunction or organ failure. The specific type of organ failure must also be identified in the documentation with a separate ICD-10-CM code. **Septic shock** is a severe drop in blood pressure caused by sepsis, which can lead to organ failure or death. If the sepsis is documented as occurring with septic shock, the coder should report the code for the septic shock.

Coding for sepsis requires multiple codes, depending on the condition.

- *Sepsis only.* To code for sepsis (or septicemia) without severe sepsis (no organ dysfunction), assign a code to identify the infectious organism, from category A40 or A41. For example, a patient with sepsis due to a group A streptococcal infection would be assigned code A40.0, Sepsis due to streptococcus, group A.

- *Severe sepsis (with organ dysfunction).* To code for severe sepsis, a minimum of three codes is required: one to identify the sepsis (septicemia code from category A40 or A41); one to identify the infection as severe sepsis, with or without septic shock (R65.2-); and a third code to identify the specific associated organ dysfunction (such as acute kidney failure N17.- or acute respiratory failure J96.0-). For example, a patient with severe sepsis due to Hemophilus influenza causing renal failure would be coded as follows: A41.3, Sepsis due to Hemophilus influenza, R65.2, Severe sepsis, and N17.9, Acute kidney failure, unspecified.

- **Systemic inflammatory response syndrome (SIRS)** is a noninfectious process, such as heatstroke or a traumatic injury. Although this condition is not due to an infectious process, it is coded similarly and from the same category as severe sepsis (R65). Coding for SIRS requires at least two codes: one for the underlying trauma or condition, and one to identify the SIRS, either with or without acute organ dysfunction (R65.10, Systemic inflammatory response syndrome (SIRS) of non-infectious origin without acute organ dysfunction, or R65.11, Systemic inflammatory response syndrome (SIRS) of non-infectious origin with acute organ dysfunction). An additional code should be reported to identify the acute organ dysfunction, if applicable. For example, a patient with SIRS due to heatstroke resulting in hepatic failure would be coded as follows: T76.0, Heatstroke and sunstroke, R65.11, Systemic inflammatory response syndrome (SIRS) of non-infectious origin with acute organ dysfunction, and K72. 00, Acute and subacute hepatic failure without coma.

Figure 10.15. OGCR I.C.1.d

---

d. Sepsis, Severe Sepsis, and Septic Shock

   1) Coding of Sepsis and Severe Sepsis

      (a) Sepsis

         For a diagnosis of sepsis, assign the appropriate code for the underlying systemic infection. If the type of infection or causal organism is not further specified, assign code A41.9, Sepsis, unspecified organism.

         A code from subcategory R65.2, Severe sepsis, should not be assigned unless severe sepsis or an associated acute organ dysfunction is documented.

        (i) Negative or inconclusive blood cultures and sepsis

           Negative or inconclusive blood cultures do not preclude a diagnosis of sepsis in patients with clinical evidence of the condition, however, the provider should be queried.

        (ii) Urosepsis

           The term urosepsis is a nonspecific term. It is not to be considered synonymous with sepsis. It has no default code in the Alphabetic Index. Should a provider use this term, he/she must be queried for clarification.

        (iii) Sepsis with organ dysfunction

           If a patient has sepsis and associated acute organ dysfunction or multiple organ dysfunction (MOD), follow the instructions for coding severe sepsis.

        (iv) Acute organ dysfunction that is not clearly associated with the sepsis

           If a patient has sepsis and an acute organ dysfunction, but the medical record documentation indicates that the acute organ dysfunction is related to a medical condition other than the sepsis, do not assign a code from subcategory R65.2, Severe sepsis. An acute organ dysfunction must be associated with the sepsis in order to assign the severe sepsis code. If the documentation is not clear as to whether an acute organ dysfunction is related to the sepsis or another medical condition, query the provider.

Source: CMS 2019b.

Sequencing of the codes involved in sepsis, severe sepsis, and SIRS depends on the coder's ability to identify and interpret coding guidelines in the ICD-10-CM code book. An excerpt of the sepsis coding guidelines is shown in figure 10.15. For sepsis, the code for septicemia should be sequenced before the code for severe sepsis, and the code for the acute organ dysfunction should follow the severe sepsis code. For SIRS, the code for the underlying condition or injury should be sequenced first, followed by the SIRS code and, finally, the code for the acute organ dysfunction (if applicable).

Appendicitis

Coding for appendicitis is markedly less difficult than coding for sepsis and SIRS, but because it is a common condition seen in the ED, it bears mention here. Right lower quadrant (RLQ) abdominal pain is a possible indicator of appendicitis that commonly results in an imaging procedure performed in the ED, such as an ultrasound or CT scan of the abdomen.

    Appendicitis is inflammation of the appendix that can be a life-threatening condition if the appendix ruptures, which can cause a systemic infection. Codes for appendicitis (K35–K37) identify the condition as either acute, chronic/recurrent, or unspecified. Acute appendicitis codes are divided depending on if any localized or generalized peritonitis (infection of the peritoneal cavity) is present, due to a rupture of the inflamed appendix, and with or without perforation, such as K35.30, Acute appendicitis with localized peritonitis, without perforation or gangrene.

Motor Vehicle Accidents

A motor vehicle accident (MVA) is an accident that involves any type of motor vehicle. Some MVAs occur with only one vehicle; others may involve multiple vehicles of different types, or a vehicle and a pedestrian or bicycle. When a patient is injured in an MVA, he or she is typically transported to the ED via ambulance. Injuries sustained in car accidents can range from nonexistent to the most severe, resulting in death.

Coding for an MVA requires one code for the actual injury sustained by the patient, such as a fracture, laceration, or whiplash injury. Additional codes that identify the circumstances surrounding the MVA should be included. Codes for MVAs are found in the following ICD-10-CM categories.

- Pedestrian injured in transport accident (V00–V09)
- Pedal cycle rider injured in transport accident (V10–V19)

Figure 10.16. Definitions related to transport accidents

NOTE   Definitions related to transport accidents:

(a) A transport accident (V00-V99) is any accident involving a device designed primarily for, or used at the time primarily for, conveying persons or goods from one place to another.

(b) A public highway [trafficway] or street is the entire width between property lines (or other boundary lines) of land open to the public as a matter of right or custom for purposes of moving persons or property from one place to another. A roadway is that part of the public highway designed, improved and customarily used for vehicular traffic.

(c) A traffic accident is any vehicle accident occurring on the public highway [i.e. originating on, terminating on, or involving a vehicle partially on the highway]. A vehicle accident is assumed to have occurred on the public highway unless another place is specified, except i the case of accidents involving only off-road motor vehicles, which are classified as nontraffic accidents unless the contrary is stated.

(d) A nontraffic accident is any vehicle accident that occurs entirely in any place other than a public highway.

(e) A pedestrian is any person involved in an accident who was not at the time of the accident riding in or on a motor vehicle, railway train, streetcar or animal-drawn or other vehicle, or on a pedal cycle or animal. This includes, a person changing a tire, working on a parked care, or a person on foot. It also includes the user of a pedestrian conveyance such as a babystroller, ice-skates, skis, sled, roller skates, a skateboard, nonmotorized or motorized wheelchair, motorized mobility scooter, or nonmotorized scooter.

(f) A driver is an occupant of a transport vehicle who is operating or intending to operate it.

(g) A passenger is any occupant of a transport vehicle other than the driver, except a person traveling on the outside of the vehicle.

(h) A person on the outside of a vehicle is any person being transported by a vehicle but not occupying the space normally reserved for the driver or passengers, or the space intended for the transport of property. This includes a person travailing on the bodywork, bumper, fender, roof, running board or step of a vehicle, as well as, hanging on the outside of the vehicle.

(i) A pedal cycle is any land transport vehicle operated solely by nonmotorized pedals including a bicycle or tricycle.

(j) A pedal cyclist is any person riding a pedal cycle or in a sidecar or trailer attached to a pedal cycle.

(k) A motorcycle is a two-wheeled motor vehicle with one or two riding saddles and sometimes with a third wheel for the support of a sidecar. The sidecar is considered part of the motorcycle. This includes a moped, motor scooter, or motorized bicycle.

(l) A motorcycle rider is any person riding a motorcycle or in a sidecar or trailer attached to the motorcycle.

(m) A three-wheeled motor vehicle is a motorized tricycle designed primarily for on-road use. This includes a motor-driven tricycle, a motorized rickshaw, or a three-wheeled motor car.

(n) A car [automobile] is a four-wheeled motor vehicle designed primarily for carrying up to 7 persons. A trailer being towed by the car is considered par of the car. It does not include a van or minivan - see definition (o)

(o) A pick-up truck or van is a four or six-wheeled motor vehicle designed for carrying passengers as well as property or cargo weighing less than the local limit for classification as a heavy goods vehicle, and not requiring a special driver's license. this includes a minivan and a sport-utility vehicle (SUV)

(p) A heavy transport vehicle is a motor vehicle designed primarily for carrying property, meeting local criteria for classification as a heavy goods vehicle in terms of weight and requiring a special driver's license.

(q) A bus (coach) is a motor vehicle designed or adapted primarily for carrying more than 10 passengers, and requiring a special driver's license.

(r) A railway train or railway vehicle is any device, with or without freight or passenger cars couple to it, designed for traffic on a railway track. This includes subterranean (subways) or elevated trains.

(s) A streetcar, is a device designed and used primarily for transporting passengers within a municipality, running on rails, usually subject to normal traffic control signals, and operated principally on a right-of-way that forms part of the roadway. This includes a tram or trolley that runs on rails. A trailer being towed by a streetcar is considered part of the streetcar.

(t) A special vehicle mainly used on industrial premises is a motor vehicle designed primarily for use within the building and premises of industrial or commercial establishments. This includes battery-powered airport passenger vehicles or baggage/mail trucks, forklifts, coal-cars in a coal min, logging cars and trucks used in mines or quarries.

(u) A special vehicle mainly used in agriculture is a motor vehicle designed specifically for use in farming and agriculture (horticulture), to work the land, tend and harvest crops and transport materials on the farm. This includes harvesters, farm machinery and tractor and trailers.

(v) A special construction vehicle is a motor vehicle designed specifically for use on construction and demolition sites. This includes bulldozers, diggers, earth levellers, dump trucks, backhoes, front-end loaders, pavers, and mechanical shovels.

(w) A special all-terrain vehicle is a motor vehicle of special design to enable it to negotiate over rough or soft terrain, snow or sand. Examples of special design are high construction, special wheels and tires, tracks, and support on a cushion of air. This includes snow mobiles, All terrain vehicles (ATV), and dune buggies. It does not include passenger vehicle designated as Sport Utility Vehicles (SUV).

(x) A water craft is any device designed for transporting passengers or goods on water. This includes motor or sail boats, ships, and hovercraft.

(y) An aircraft is any device for transporting passengers or goods in the air. This includes hot-air balloons, gliders, helicopters and airplanes.

(z) A military vehicle is any motorized vehicle operating on a public roadway owned by the military and being operated by a member of the military.

Source: CMS 2019b.

- Motorcycle rider injured in transport accident (V20–V29)
- Occupant of three-wheeled motor vehicle injured in transport accident (V30–V39)
- Car occupant injured in transport accident (V40–V49)
- Occupant of pick-up truck or van injured in transport accident (V50–V59)
- Occupant of heavy transport vehicle injured in transport accident (V60–V69)
- Bus occupant injured in transport accident (V70–V79)
- Other land transport accidents (V80–V89)

MVA codes are detailed codes that identify the person injured, how the injury happened, any other vehicles or objects involved in the accident, the person driving the transport vehicle, and the encounter (initial, subsequent, sequela). For example, if a patient suffered a whiplash injury while he was driving a car, when he accidentally hit the car in front of him in traffic because he was distracted by his cell phone, the ICD-10-CM code reported would be V43.52XA, Car driver injured in collision with other type car in traffic accident, initial encounter. Additional codes would be selected for the patient's other injuries as well as any other circumstances surrounding the event, such as the location of the accident and the patient status at the time of the accident.

To look for the code for an MVA, search in the External Cause of Injuries Index, located after the ICD-10-CM Main Index. Search under the term *Accident* and one of the subterms *traffic, nontraffic,* or *transport,* depending on the circumstances of the accident. See figure 10.16 for the definitions related to transport accidents.

Burns

The ICD-10-CM code book differentiates between burns and corrosions. **Burn codes** are for thermal burns that come from a heat source such as fire or hot appliance. This category also includes burns from electricity or radiation, with the exception of sunburns, which are coded elsewhere in category L55, Sunburn. **Corrosions** are burns due to chemicals. The guidelines are the same for coding either burns or corrosions.

Burns and corrosions codes (T20–T25) are classified by four factors:

- *Site:* This is the exact location of the burn. For multiple sites, one code should be reported for each individual burn, sequenced from most to least severe (worst comes first).

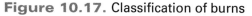

Figure 10.17. Classification of burns

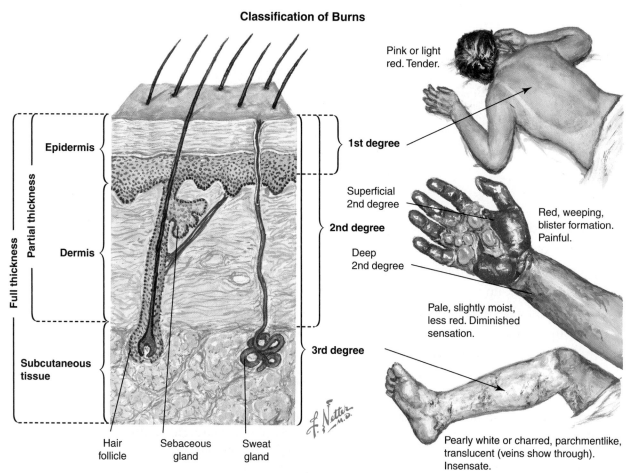

- *Depth:* Burns are classified by their depth—first degree (erythema), second degree (blistering), or third degree (full-thickness involvement), as illustrated in figure 10.17.
- *Extent:* The extent of a burn is measured by the total percentage of body surface covered by the burn. Body percentages are determined by the clinical staff treating the patient by two methods—the rule of nines and the Lund-Browder classification system, both shown in figure 10.18. The **rule of nines** divides the body's surface into percentages based on the number nine, with the groin area making up the remaining one percent of body surface. The **Lund-Browder classification** chart divides the body's surface into differing percentages, depending on the age of the patient. Because the child body is disproportionate to the adult body, the Lund-Browder classification system takes into account the varying percentage of certain body structures as the patient ages and the body becomes more proportionate to that of an adult. Although the clinical staff determines the extent of the burned area, coders must be able to identify the extent burned based on the documentation in the health record and assign the code(s) appropriately.
- *Agent:* The agent that caused the injury, which resulted in either a burn or a corrosion.

Because burns and corrosions are injuries, they all require a seventh character extension to identify the encounter and the identification of any external causes, when documented.

Figure 10.18. Extent of burn

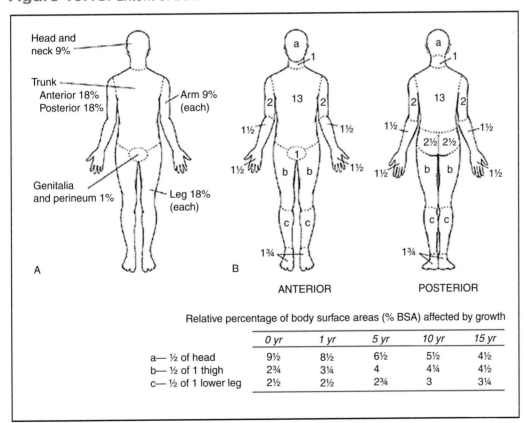

Relative percentage of body surface areas (% BSA) affected by growth

	0 yr	1 yr	5 yr	10 yr	15 yr
a— ½ of head	9½	8½	6½	5½	4½
b— ½ of 1 thigh	2¾	3¼	4	4¼	4½
c— ½ of 1 lower leg	2½	2½	2¾	3	3¼

(A) Rule of "nines"
(B) Lund-Browder diagram of estimating extent of burns

Source: HHS 2013.

Figure 10.19. OGCR I.C.19.d

d. Coding of Burns and Corrosions

The ICD-10-CM makes a distinction between burns and corrosions. The burn codes are for thermal burns, except sunburns, that come from a heat source, such as a fire or hot appliance. The burn codes are also for burns resulting from electricity and radiation. Corrosions are burns due to chemicals. The guidelines are the same for burns and corrosions.

Current burns (T20-T25) are classified by depth, extent and by agent (X code). Burns are classified by depth as first degree (erythema), second degree (blistering), and third degree (full-thickness involvement). Burns of the eye and internal organs (T26-T28) are classified by site, but not by degree.

1) Sequencing of burn and related condition codes

Sequence first the code that reflects the highest degree of burn when more than one burn is present.

a. When the reason for the admission or encounter is for treatment of external multiple burns, sequence first the code that reflects the burn of the highest degree.

b. When a patient has both internal and external burns, the circumstances of admission govern the selection of the principal diagnosis or first-listed diagnosis.

c. When a patient is admitted for burn injuries and other related conditions such as smoke inhalation and/ or respiratory failure, the circumstances of admission govern the selection of the principal or first-listed diagnosis.

2) Burns of the same anatomic site

Classify burns of the same anatomic site and on the same side but of different degrees to the subcategory identifying the highest degree recorded in the diagnosis (e.g., for second and third degree burns of right thigh, assign only code T24.311-).

3) Non-healing burns

Non-healing burns are coded as acute burns.

Necrosis of burned skin should be coded as a non-healed burn.

4) Infected Burn

For any documented infected burn site, use an additional code for the infection.

5) Assign separate codes for each burn site

When coding burns, assign separate codes for each burn site. Category T30, Burn and corrosion, body region unspecified is extremely vague and should rarely be used.

Codes for burns of "multiple sites" should only be assigned when the medical record documentation does not specify the individual sites.

6) Burns and Corrosions Classified According to Extent of Body Surface Involved

Assign codes from category T31, Burns classified according to extent of body surface involved, or T32, Corrosions classified according to extent of body surface involved, when the site of the burn is not specified or when there is a need for additional data. It is advisable to use category T31 as additional coding when needed to provide data for evaluating burn mortality, such as that needed by burn units. It is also advisable to use category T31 as an additional code for reporting purposes when there is mention of a third-degree burn involving 20 percent or more of the body surface.

Categories T31 and T32 are based on the classic "rule of nines" in estimating body surface involved: head and neck are assigned nine percent, each arm nine percent, each leg 18 percent, the anterior trunk 18 percent, posterior trunk 18 percent, and genitalia one percent. Providers may change these percentage assignments where necessary to accommodate infants and children who have proportionately larger heads than adults, and patients who have large buttocks, thighs, or abdomen that involve burns.

7) Encounters for treatment of sequela of burns

Encounters for the treatment of the late effects of burns or corrosions (i.e., scars or joint contractures) should be coded with a burn or corrosion code with the 7th character "S" for sequela.

8) Sequelae with a late effect code and current burn

When appropriate, both a code for a current burn or corrosion with 7th character "A" or "D" and a burn or corrosion code with 7th character "S" may be assigned on the same record (when both a current burn and sequelae of an old burn exist). Burns and corrosions do not heal at the same rate and a current healing wound may still exist with sequela of a healed burn or corrosion.

See Section I.B.10 Sequela (Late Effects)

9) Use of an external cause code with burns and corrosions

An external cause code should be used with burns and corrosions to identify the source and intent of the burn, as well as the place where it occurred.

Source: CMS 2019b.

Coding for burns requires at least two codes—one to identify the burn, as described previously, and another to identify the extent of the body surface, from category T31 or T32. Codes for body surface identify the *total body surface burned* and then the *percent involved in the third-degree burn.* Read the following example and selected codes.

A 40-year-old patient was lighting a trash fire in his yard with lighter fluid, when the fluid splashed back onto his pants and lit his clothes on fire. He suffered second degree burns on his right and left legs (18 percent body surface) and a third-degree burn on his right foot (1 percent body surface).

The codes selected for the injury would be the following:

- T24.291A, Burn of second degree of multiple sites of right lower limb, except ankle and foot, initial encounter
- T24.292A, Burn of second degree of multiple sites of left lower limb, except ankle and foot, initial encounter
- T25.321A, Burn of third degree of right foot, initial encounter
- T31.10, Burns involving 10–19% of body surface with 0% to 9% third degree burns

In this example, the first three burn codes identify the body sites and the degree of the burns. The fourth code identifies the total body surface involved (in this case, 19 percent) and the amount of the burn that was third degree (in this case 1 percent). See figure 10.19 for the OGCR related to coding burns and related conditions.

Complete the exercises in There's a Code for That 10.4 to practice assigning diagnosis codes to ED cases.

Emergency department diagnoses

10.4

There's a Code for That

Read the following documentation and select the appropriate diagnosis code(s).

1. Patient presents to the ED with acute STEMI of the circumflex coronary artery.

   ICD-10-CM code: _____

2. Patient presents to the ED with STEMI of the left anterior descending coronary artery. Patient had a STEMI of the left main coronary artery two months ago.

   ICD-10-CM codes: _____ , _____

3. Patient presents to ED in septic shock with acute kidney failure due to MRSA septicemia.

   ICD-10-CM codes: _____ , _____ , _____ ,

4. A 45-year-old male suffered second degree corrosive burns of both hands (including wrists) and arms in a work-related chemical spill. Total of 32 percent body surface burned. (Code for the burns only).

   ICD-10-CM codes: _____ , _____ , _____ ,

   _____

5. Patient presents to the ED complaining of RLQ pain for the last two days. Imaging reveals perforated appendicitis.

   ICD-10-CM code: _____

Putting It All Together: Coding for Urgent Care and ED Services

To select the correct codes for urgent care ED services, it is important to carefully read the documentation, then access each code book to find the procedure or service provided and the corresponding diagnosis or diagnoses to support the medical necessity for the service. Procedural codes for urgent care and ED services are found in the CPT code book, and diagnosis codes are found in the ICD-10-CM code book.

Determination of the correct codes relies on the answers to the following questions.

- What services were provided to the patient?
  - Was an E/M service provided?
    - For urgent care E/M encounters use the outpatient office E/M codes 99201 through 99215.
    - For emergency department E/M encounters use E/M codes 99281 through 99285.
  - Were any additional procedures performed, such as labs, x-rays, or other imaging services, or any additional medical or surgical procedures?
- Are there any applicable modifiers or add-on codes?
- Is there a definitive diagnosis for the encounter? If yes, this should be the first-listed diagnosis code. If not, then use the code for the signs or symptoms.
- For injuries, include codes to identify the external causes with the appropriate seventh character extension to identify the encounter.
- Follow all CPT and ICD-10-CM guidelines for selecting and sequencing codes. Remember, for injury diagnosis codes, sequence the codes for the more severe injury before the codes for the least severe injury.

The following vignette demonstrates how to select the appropriate diagnosis and procedure codes. Review the vignette, then complete the exercises in There's a Code for That 10.5 to practice coding for urgent care and ED services.

Michelle is coding for an urgent care encounter for a 60-year-old female new patient who presented to the clinic complaining of dizziness and slight nausea. She reports that she has recently just gotten over (two days ago) a sinusitis infection and head cold, for which she was on a Z-pack. Her last dose of antibiotics was two days ago. The physician assistant performed a detailed history and examination, with moderate complexity MDM, and diagnosed the patient with vestibular labyrinthitis, bilateral. Procedures performed in the clinic include a 50 mg IM injection of Phenergan (promethazine), and 12-lead ECG to rule out cardiac arrhythmia. Labs included cardiac enzymes (CK-MB, Myoglobin, Troponin), CBC (automated, complete), and blood glucose. CBC revealed slightly lowered WBC and RBC counts. Physician prescribed oral antihistamines and instructed patient to return as necessary if symptoms do not subside in one week.

First, Michelle asks herself: What did the healthcare provider do? The physician assistant performed an E/M encounter for a new patient in the urgent care setting, which she will code using the appropriate E/M encounter code from 99201 to 99205 with a modifier -25, to indicate that the E/M service was a significant, separately identifiable service from the procedures performed. The provider also administered a Phenergan injection, so she will need to code for the therapeutic injection as well as the substance, using a HCPCS code. Additional procedures included an ECG, a cardiac enzyme panel, a CBC, and a glucose test. Coding for the cardiac enzymes test requires that she select one code for each of the blood components that was tested for (to find these she goes to the Pathology and Laboratory, Chemistry entry in the Index and searches for each individual component). She selects the following codes:

- *99203-25, Level 3 office visit, new patient*

nergan
ction
{
- *96372, Therapeutic, prophylactic, or diagnostic injection (specify substance or drug); submuscular or intramuscular*
- *J2550, Injection, promethazine HCL, up to 50 mg*

- *93000, Electrocardiogram, routine ECG with at least 12 leads; with interpretation and report*

rdiac
zymes
{
- *82550, Creatine kinase (CK), (CPK); total*
- *82553, Creatine kinase (CK), (CPK); MB fraction only*
- *83874, Myoglobin*
- *84484, Troponin, quantitative*

- *85027, Blood count; complete (CBC), automated (Hgb, Hct, RBC, WBC and platelet count)*
- *82947, Glucose; quantitative, blood (except reagent strip)*

Now that she has the procedure codes, Michelle asks herself: Why did the physician assistant do it? In this case, the patient was diagnosed with vestibular labyrinthitis, which was the definitive diagnosis, so it includes the additional symptoms of dizziness and nausea. April searches under the term Labyrinthitis *in the Main Index of the ICD-10-CM code book, and references subcategory H83.0- for the code, and she chooses the following:*

- *H83.03, Labyrinthitis, bilateral*

She then rechecks the documentation to make sure she has coded everything for the encounter and reports the chosen codes on the claim for the service.

Coding for urgent care and emergency department services

10.5

There's a Code for That

Read the following documentation and select the appropriate CPT, HCPCS, and ICD-10-CM code(s).

1. Patient presents to the ED with right lower quadrant pain. Abdominopelvic CT (computed tomography) performed without contrast revealed acute unperforated appendicitis. After IV antibiotics administered in the ED, symptoms, WBC, and fever resolved satisfactorily and patient was discharged home, with a delayed (interval) appendectomy scheduled in 6 weeks. Comprehensive history and examination, with high complexity MDM in the ED setting. (Hint: do not code for the IV antibiotics or WBC).

   CPT codes: _____ , _____

   ICD-10-CM code: _____

(Continued on next page)

10.5

Continued

2. A 15-year-old male established patient presented to the urgent care clinic in the evening hours with moderate persistent asthma with acute exacerbation. Pulse oximetry revealed oxygen level of 89 percent, pressurized nebulizer treatment provided in the office. Provider performed an expanded problem-focused examination with moderate complexity MDM. Flu shot (IIV3) 0.5mL also administered in the office intramuscularly without counseling.

CPT codes: _____ - _____ , _____ ,

_____ , _____ , _____ ,

_____ , _____

ICD-10-CM code: _____

3. Patient received in the ED after MVA with traumatic pneumothorax. She was driving her pick-up truck when she began hydroplaning on a wet patch of road, hit a median, and flipped over, pinning her between her seat and the steering wheel. Tube thoracostomy performed in the ED and patient was transferred to the hospital for continued observation and treatment.

CPT codes: _____

ICD-10-CM code (code for the injury and the MVA only): _____ ,

_____

Case Study **Emergency Department Visit**

Emergency Department Treatment Log

PATIENT: Douglas Kaiser

DATE OF SERVICE: 11/14/20XX

SUBJECTIVE:
Patient c/o pain to right knee.
A noted onset of red, tender spot began yesterday on the medial aspect of the right knee. Since then the area of involvement has enlarged and he has noted an increase in stabbing pains, warmth, and mild swelling.
He denies any trauma to the knee area. No fever, chills, sweats, or open sores on the skin.
Has a history of cellulitis in the past. Negative past family history. Not currently on any medications. Allergic to all penicillins.

OBJECTIVE:
Afebrile, well-nourished, healthy appearing, alert, oriented and in no acute distress.
Physical examination of the right lower leg reveals right lower extremity (RLE) erythema, increased warmth to the skin, slight tissue edema, no lesions or wounds seen. Zero adenopathy.
Knee exam within normal limits, zero distal lesions.

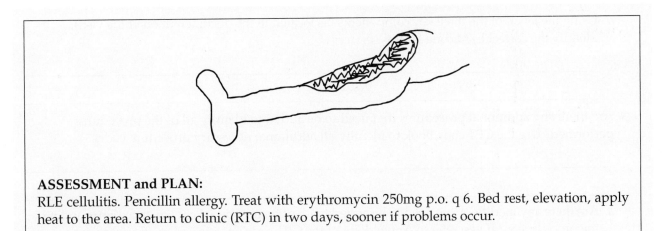

ASSESSMENT and PLAN:
RLE cellulitis. Penicillin allergy. Treat with erythromycin 250mg p.o. q 6. Bed rest, elevation, apply heat to the area. Return to clinic (RTC) in two days, sooner if problems occur.

SIGNED: Dr. Alejandro Jaramillo, MD

Use the following steps to select the appropriate codes for the case study.

1. Read the case study in full. As you read, look up any medical or procedural terms with which you are unfamiliar and use a medical dictionary or medical terminology text to define the unfamiliar terms.

2. Review the case study and answer the following question: *What did the doctor do?* In this case study, the documentation is in a simplified SOAP note format. Remember that the components of the SOAP note directly correspond to the key components of an E/M service. Answer the following questions to help you determine the correct E/M code.

   a. What is the place of service, type of service, and patient status?

   _____

   _____

   b. Identify the code range for this type of E/M service in the CPT code book.

   _____

   _____

   c. How many key components are necessary to select the level of service for this E/M type?

   _____

   _____

   d. Carefully review the documentation and determine the levels of the three key components of the E/M service.

      i. History:

      _____

      ii. Examination:

      _____

      iii. Medical Decision-Making:

      _____

e. Using the levels of the three key components (as located in the documentation of the visit), identify the correct E/M code for this service:

_____

_____

3. Are there any additional procedures that need to be added to identify all of the procedures performed? Use the CPT code book to identify all additional necessary procedure codes.

_____

_____

a. Are there any modifiers that need to be added to identify any special circumstance surrounding the procedure(s)? If yes, refer to Appendix A of the CPT code book to assign all appropriate modifiers.

_____

_____

4. Refer to the case study and answer the following question: *Why did the doctor do it?* To find the reason for the office visit, search for terms that will identify the medical condition. Then identify the patient's diagnoses.

a. _____

_____

b. _____

_____

5. Now that you have identified the patient's diagnoses, search the ICD-10-CM code book for the correct codes for these conditions. Follow these steps for each of the diagnoses identified.

a. Search the Main Index for the name of each condition and search through any applicable subterms and cross-references to locate the appropriate code.

i. _____

_____

ii. _____

_____

b. Verify the code(s) in the Tabular List. Locate the code(s) identified previously in the Tabular Listing of codes and refer to any applicable guidelines, notes, and symbols. Does the code selected correctly identify the patient's condition? If yes, list the code(s).

i. _____

_____

ii. _____

_____

c. Check the procedure note and ICD-10-CM guidelines and conventions to determine the correct sequencing of the diagnosis codes, if applicable. Correctly sequence the diagnosis codes.

_____

_____

6. Now that the procedure and diagnosis codes have been identified, list them on the CMS-1500 form template provided. Be sure to identify medical necessity for each service by correctly linking the procedure/supply and diagnosis codes. Refer to figure 3.6 for an example.

21. DIAGNOSIS OR NATURE OF ILLNESS OR INJURY Relate A-L to service line below (24E)			ICD Ind.	
A. _____	B. _____	C. _____	D. _____	
E. _____	F. _____	G. _____	H. _____	
I. _____	J. _____	K. _____	L. _____	

24. A. DATE(S) OF SERVICE From / To		B. PLACE OF SERVICE	C. EMG	D. PROCEDURES, SERVICES, OR SUPPLIES (Explain Unusual Circumstances) CPT/HCPCS | MODIFIER		E. DIAGNOSIS POINTER
MM DD YY / MM DD YY						
1						
2						
3						

HCC

End-of-Chapter Content

Instructions: Indicate whether the following statements are true or false (T or F). For false statements, rewrite the statement on the line below to make the statement true.

1. In an emergent situation, a patient is suffering from a life- or limb-threatening injury.

_____

_____

2. The place of service code is optional for healthcare claims.

_____

_____

3. Box 24.C of the CMS-1500 claim form is used to identify the place of service for the claim.

_____

_____

(Continued on next page)

(Continued)

4. Outpatient office E/M codes are used to report encounters in the urgent care setting.

_____

_____

5. A complete x-ray has at least the minimum number of views described in the CPT code for the complete service.

_____

_____

6. The professional component of an ECG consists of the healthcare provider reading and interpreting the test results.

_____

_____

7. Semi-permanent casts are often performed in the urgent care setting as a treatment for fractures until the patient can be seen by an orthopedist for definitive treatment.

_____

_____

8. There are three categories of complexity for would repair codes.

_____

_____

9. Coding for wound repair requires adding up the same lengths of the same sites and the same complexity.

_____

_____

10. An ED encounter is coded with inpatient observation codes from the E/M chapter.

_____

_____

Instructions: Choose the best answer.

1. In which of the following situations would a patient present to an urgent care clinic?
   a. After a severe car accident, having suffered traumatic, life-threatening injury
   b. When he has a high fever and his regular doctor is not available
   c. After falling from a tree and suffering a compound (open) fracture
   d. When he needs a routine physical examination

2. Which place of service code should be used for ED coding?
   a. 20
   b. 21
   c. 22
   d. 23

3. Which of the following is true regarding coding for urgent care and ED services?
   a. Only a small selection of CPT codes is used
   b. Many CPT codes are used, but not many ICD-10-CM codes
   c. It requires a good working knowledge of all sections of the CPT and ICD-10-CM code books
   d. E/M codes are the same for both settings

4. Which of the following type of procedures are used to determine the patient diagnosis for infectious diseases?
   a. X-rays and imaging services
   b. E/M encounters
   c. Surgical procedures
   d. Laboratory tests

5. Which of the following is a simple test that can diagnose a cardiac arrhythmia?
   a. Pulse oximetry
   b. Nebulizer treatment
   c. Electrocardiogram
   d. Incision and drainage

6. Which of the following describes an orthosis?
   a. An external device designed to immobilize a body part
   b. An internal device used to assist in surgical procedures
   c. A procedure to open airways allowing the patient to breathe more easily
   d. An injection of a therapeutic substance

7. Wound repairs are coded in which of the following?
   a. in
   b. cm
   c. mg
   d. mL

8. The time reported for moderate (conscious) sedation is for which component of the procedure?
   a. Preservice work
   b. Intraservice work
   c. Postservice work
   d. The entire procedure from start to finish

9. Which of the following is a procedure used to open the airways using instrumentation inserted into the mouth?
   a. Tracheostomy
   b. Tracheotomy
   c. Needle thoracotomy
   d. Endotracheal intubation

10. Codes for penetrating wound exploration include which of the following?
    a. Exploration and extension of the wound
    b. Major repair to blood vessels
    c. Repair of internal organs
    d. Extensive scar revision

11. When sequencing codes for injuries, which code should go first?
    a. The code for the least severe injury
    b. Sequencing does not matter
    c. The code for the most severe injury
    d. The codes should be sent on separate claims

12. Which of the following could cause systemic inflammatory response syndrome (SIRS)?

   a. An underlying infection
   b. A traumatic injury
   c. A routine physical examination
   d. Septicemia

Instructions: Answer the following question with the appropriate code(s) and modifier(s).

13. A 35-year-old male patient presents to the ED with anterior dislocation of left shoulder. He was wrestling (horseplay) while at work at a heavy truck body shop and his arm was twisted out of its socket by his opponent. He appears in good spirits but is in pain, and would like to undergo moderate sedation for the reduction procedure. Risks and benefits of the procedure explained. Moderate sedation was achieved using Ketamine, and the dislocation reduction took approximately 30 minutes due to difficulty in determining if the joint was back in place. E/M encounter involved comprehensive history and examination with high complexity MDM performed. (Tip: Moderate sedation does not count as an anesthesia service.)

CPT codes: _____ - _____ , _____ ,

_____ , _____

ICD-10-CM code: _____ , _____

References

Ahmadinejad, M., S. Karamouzian, and M. Lashkarizadeh. 2011. Use of Glasgow Coma Scale as an indicator for early tracheostomy in patients with severe head injury. *Tannafos* 10(1): 26–30. https://www.ncbi.nlm.nih.gov /pmc/articles/PMC4153128/.

American Medical Association (AMA). 2019. *CPT 2020 Professional Edition.* Chicago: AMA.

Blausen.com staff. 2013. Lumbar Puncture. Digital Image. Wikimedia Commons. https://en.wikipedia.org /wiki/Lumbar_puncture#/media/File:Blausen_0617 _LumbarPuncture.png.

Centers for Medicare and Medicaid Services (CMS). 2019a. CMS 1500. https://www.cms.gov/Medicare/CMS -Forms/CMS-Forms/CMS-Forms-Items/CMS1188854 .html.

Centers for Medicare and Medicaid Services (CMS). 2019b. ICD-10-CM Official Guidelines for Coding and Reporting FY 2020. https://www.cms.gov/Medicare /Coding/ICD10/Downloads/2020-Coding-Guidelines .pdf.

Hackethal, V. 2017 (August 16). Skip Pulse Oximetry in Bronchiolitis, Experts Say. https://www.medscape.com /viewarticle/884396.

US Department of Health and Human Services (HHS). 2013. Lund-Browder Chart. Radiation Emergency Medical Management. Digital Image. https://www.remm.nlm .gov/burns.htm.

US National Library of Medicine (USNLM) Medline Plus. 2019. Chest Tube Insertion. https://medlineplus.gov /ency/article/002947.htm.

Resources

Agency for Healthcare Research and Quality (AHRQ). 2014 (June). Healthcare Cost and Utilization Project Statistical Brief #174. https://www.hcup-us.ahrq.gov /reports/statbriefs/sb174-Emergency-Department -Visits-Overview.pdf.

American College of Emergency Physicians (ACEP). 2011. ED Facility Level Coding Guidelines. https://www.acep .org/administration/reimbursement/ed-facility-level -coding-guidelines/.

Journal of Urgent Care Medicine. 2008 (July). National Urgent Care Chart Survey. http://jucm.com/pdf /JUCM_Urgent_Care_Chart_Research.pdf.

University of Texas Health Science Center at Houston School of Public Health. 2011 (July). Top Twenty Primary Discharge Diagnoses in the Emergency Room in Harris County, Texas in 2009: Breakdown by Age and Payer Source. https://sph.uth.edu/content/uploads/2011/12 /Top-2009-ER-diagnoses-by-age-and-payer-source.pdf.

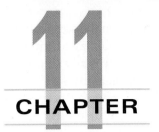

CHAPTER

Surgical Services

Learning Objectives

- Understand the basics of billing and coding for surgical services performed in the inpatient hospital, outpatient hospital, and ambulatory surgical center (ASC) settings
- Examine the basics of coding for surgical procedures from the CPT Surgery section

- Examine procedural codes, diagnosis codes, and guidelines for surgical services performed in the inpatient hospital, outpatient hospital, and ASC settings
- Determine and apply ICD-10-CM, CPT, and HCPCS codes to surgical services

Key Terms

Ablation
Admitting provider
Allograft
Ambulatory surgical center (ASC)
Appendectomy
Appendicitis
Autograft
Block
Cadaver donor
Cholangiography
Cholangitis
Cholecystectomy
Cholecystitis
Choledocholithiasis
Cholelithiasis
Code edit
Comorbid condition
Complication of care
Debridement
Destruction
Diagnostic procedure
Diaphragm

Endoscopy
Excised diameter
Excision
Global period
Global surgical package
Homograft
Incidental appendectomy
Incision
Introduction
Laparoscopy
Living donor
Manipulation
Margin
Mediastinum
Mohs micrographic surgery
National Correct Coding Initiative (NCCI)
Never events
Non-pressure ulcer
Outpatient
Outpatient hospital
Paring

Performing provider
Peritonitis
Postoperative diagnosis
Preoperative diagnosis
Pressure ulcer
Removal
Repair
Resection
Rhinoplasty
Robot-assisted surgery
Separate procedure
Shaving
Skin lesion
Skin ulcer
Stage
Surgical procedure
Therapeutic procedure
Transplantation
Unbundling
Xenograft

The complexities of coding in the surgical setting may be challenging for novice coders, but these skills are fundamental to understanding and being proficient in medical coding. A **surgical procedure** is any single, separate, systematic process upon or within the body that can be complete in itself; is normally performed by a physician, dentist, or other licensed practitioner; can be performed either with or without instruments; and is performed to restore disunited or deficient parts, remove diseased or injured tissues, extract foreign matter, assist in obstetrical delivery, or aid in diagnosis. Surgical procedures require a skilled practitioner to use manual and instrumental techniques to treat, investigate, or diagnose a patient's healthcare condition. Surgical procedures may also be performed to improve bodily function, change appearance, and repair body structures and organs.

Surgeries are, by definition, invasive procedures that usually involve breaking the skin in order to perform the procedure. Medical procedures, on the other hand, are less invasive, and rarely break the skin, if only minimally. Surgeries range from highly invasive and risky, such as transplant surgeries and internal organ repairs, to minimally or practically noninvasive procedure like wart cryosurgery. Thus, the settings in which surgeries are performed depend greatly on the *type* of surgery performed. This chapter discusses various types of surgeries and the different settings in which they are performed (inpatient hospital, outpatient hospital, and ambulatory surgical centers). It does not discuss minimally invasive surgeries that are often performed in the outpatient office setting like those performed in primary care, discussed in chapter 8 (Primary Care Services). This chapter also discusses the different surgical specialists who provide these services and the basics of coding for surgeries, including changes in the place of service and procedural and diagnostic coding for surgeries.

Surgical Billing and Coding Basics

Coding for surgical services requires a solid understanding of human anatomy and physiology, including medical terminology, the way surgical procedures are performed, and the terminology used to describe them. There are numerous settings in which surgeries are performed, determined by the complexity and riskiness of the procedure; there are also specific procedures approved for only certain settings. This chapter also addresses surgical coding and billing in general, as well as the different types of surgical specialists.

Surgical Settings

Given the various types of surgical procedures and the resources required to perform them, certain surgical procedures may be performed only in particular healthcare settings. Depending on the resources required and risks involved in performing the procedures, some minimally invasive surgeries, such as a biopsy, may be performed in the outpatient office setting. However, the majority of surgical procedures are performed in an inpatient hospital, outpatient hospital, or ambulatory surgical center.

Inpatient Hospital

Inpatients are patients who have been formally admitted to a hospital. Inpatient hospital surgeries typically involve a patient who has been admitted to a specific floor or unit, where they reside before or after the surgery. For example, a surgery patient may be admitted to a particular room in a hospital for preoperative evaluation and pre-procedural treatments, after which he or she is moved to the surgical suite or operating room where the surgery is performed. The patient then stays in the hospital until he or she has recovered from the surgery enough to be discharged either to the patient's home or to another facility, such as a rehabilitation hospital. The recovery process is usually at least overnight but can also be a longer period of time, lasting weeks or more. It depends on the type of surgery performed, the severity of the patient's condition, and any other comorbidities or complications that may develop.

When a surgery is performed in an inpatient facility, like an inpatient hospital, the doctor who performs the surgery reports the CPT code for the surgery, as well as any other procedural codes, such as E/M services; and the hospital facility reports the service the provider performed using ICD-10-PCS codes, which are inpatient procedural codes. This allows the healthcare provider to bill for the services he or she performed, such as a surgery or anesthesia service, and also allows the hospital to identify the service performed to justify the cost of the hospital resources for the patient while the services were being provided. Both the surgeon and the facility report ICD-10-CM (diagnosis) codes to identify the medical necessity for the service. This chapter discusses only the ICD-10-CM and CPT codes involved in performing surgical procedures, as would be billed by the performing surgeon. The inpatient facility (hospital) would report the ICD-10-CM and ICD-10-PCS codes involved in the procedure. Inpatient facility coding (using ICD-10-PCS codes) is discussed in chapter 20 (Inpatient Hospital Services) (see figure 11.1). Note, however, that the codes used to report procedures (either CPT/HCPCS or ICD-10-PCS) will depend on each individual facility. For example, some hospital outpatient facilities may report ICD-10-PCS codes, while others will report only CPT and HCPCS for procedures. The codes assigned depend on the manner in which the facility is credentialed with insurance payers and is yet another example of how flexibility is an important part of the profession of healthcare coding.

Figure 11.1. Facility inpatient versus professional outpatient coding

Codes Used to Identify	Inpatient Facility Services	Outpatient Professional Services
Diagnosis	ICD-10 **CM**	ICD-10 **CM**
Procedure	ICD-10 **PCS**	CPT
Supplies and Services	Hospital Service Codes	HCPCS
	↑	↑
	Reported by the hospital	**Reported by the surgeon**

When coding for services performed in the inpatient setting, like surgeries, it is easy to get confused between inpatient and outpatient coding. Inpatient facilities provide the room, board, equipment, and other supplies and services so the healthcare provider can perform the procedure, so the facilities bill for these items. They are like a medical hotel. The healthcare provider bills only for the service that he or she performed, such as a surgery or anesthesia service. Therefore, the codes reported by the healthcare provider are CPT codes that identify the specific procedures performed.

Inpatient hospital services reported by the physician (including observation stays and discharges) are billed with a special set of evaluation and management (E/M) codes, 99221 to 99239 (refer to chapters 7 and 8 for a discussion of E/M codes). These codes are used for a patient who has been formally admitted to a hospital as an inpatient, and a healthcare provider performs an E/M encounter with this patient. This healthcare provider does not have to be the **admitting provider** (the provider who admitted the patient to the hospital) nor the **performing** (or rendering) **provider** (the provider performing the surgery or other service), it can be any provider who performs an E/M encounter.

When billing for services provided in the inpatient hospital setting, it is necessary to use the place of service (POS) code 21, Inpatient Hospital, on the CMS-1500 form in box 24.B to identify that the procedure was performed in "a facility, other than psychiatric, which primarily provides diagnostic, therapeutic (both surgical and nonsurgical), and rehabilitation services by, or under, the supervision of physicians to patients admitted for a variety of medical conditions" (AMA 2019) (see figure 11.2).

Figure 11.2. CMS-1500 box 24.B: Place of service code 21-Inpatient Hospital

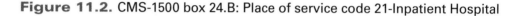
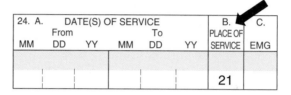

Source: CMS 2019a.

Outpatient Hospital

An **outpatient hospital** is a part of the hospital facility designed to treat patients who do not need to be admitted as an inpatient or require a bed for overnight care. It may be an actual part of the hospital or a separate building that provides outpatient services to patients such as diagnostic tests, screenings, and minor surgical procedures. An **outpatient** is a patient who has not been admitted as an inpatient but is still receiving services from the hospital facility. A patient who is staying in the main building of the hospital might be an outpatient because the physicians do not expect the patient to stay overnight or for an extended period of time, and thus he or she has not been formally admitted as an inpatient of the facility.

Because the patient has not been admitted and is considered outpatient, the E/M codes used to bill for these services are the same as those used for outpatient office encounters: 99201 to 99215 (first discussed in chapter 7). The place of service code indicates that the outpatient service was performed in the outpatient hospital setting, rather than the outpatient office setting (POS 11). Outpatient hospital codes are reported with POS code 22, On Campus-Outpatient Hospital. This POS location code is for "a portion of a hospital's main campus which provides diagnostic, therapeutic (both surgical and nonsurgical), and rehabilitation services to sick or injured persons who do not require hospitalization or institutionalization" (AMA 2019). See figure 11.3. Note that if the outpatient hospital is not part of the hospital's main campus, the correct POS code would be 19, Off Campus-Outpatient Hospital.

Figure 11.3. CMS-1500 box 24.B: Place of service code 22-On Campus Outpatient Hospital

Source: CMS 2019a.

Ambulatory Surgical Center (ASC)

An **ambulatory surgical center (ASC)** is an outpatient healthcare facility not affiliated with a hospital that specializes in diagnostic, preventive, and surgical procedures. As a well-equipped healthcare facility that can offer surgical interventions, ASCs perform surgical procedures outside of the hospital setting (either inpatient or outpatient). Often ASCs are owned by a group of physicians and some specialize in the type of services that are performed. For example, a group of ophthalmologists (eye surgeons) may open an ASC together in which they can perform surgical procedures on their own patients.

ASCs can thus provide the surgical services that a hospital can provide, but at a much lower cost to patients. This is because an ASC does not have to maintain the same overhead (in terms of staff and facility resources) that a large inpatient facility does. Furthermore, because an ASC can operate as an outpatient hospital, it may not have to charge the additional inpatient facility fees (ICD-10-PCS and hospital service codes, addressed in chapter 20 [Inpatient Hospital Services]) that an inpatient hospital charges. However, not *all* surgical procedures can be performed in the ASC setting, as only approved procedures may be safely performed at an ASC. Approved procedures are determined by the third-party payer according to the patient's insurance policy. ASCs do not have all the life-saving equipment and staff on hand (like a hospital) to handle large-scale operations that involve several medical and surgical specialists. Furthermore, because they are outpatient facilities, the procedures performed at the ASC must not require an overnight stay.

As an outpatient facility, the outpatient office E/M codes are used for evaluation and management encounters in the ASC setting (99201–99215). The place of service code indicates that the procedure took place in an ASC, rather than the outpatient office setting (POS 11); ASC codes are reported with POS 24, Ambulatory Surgical Center. This POS location code is for "a free-standing facility, other than a physician's office, where surgical and diagnostic services are provided on an ambulatory basis" (AMA 2019). See figure 11.4.

Figure 11.4. CMS-1500 box 24.B: Place of service code 24-Ambulatory Surgical Center

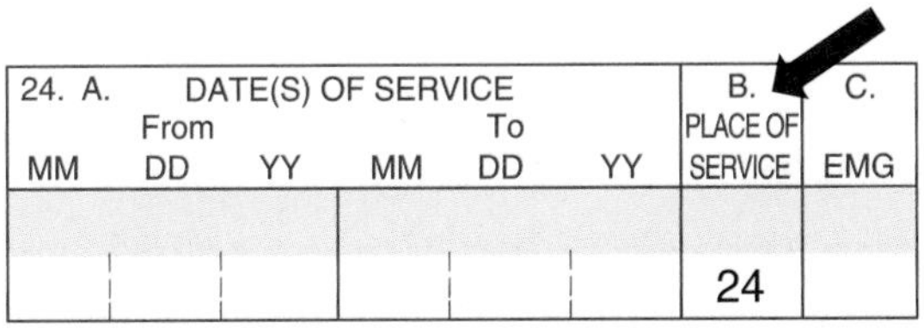

Source: CMS 2019a.

Approved Procedures by Site

Surgeries differ significantly depending on how invasive they are, how medically risky they are, how long they take, and what resources (staff, equipment) are required to perform the surgery. Therefore, certain healthcare settings are restricted to a set of approved procedures. Typically, these restrictions are set by third-party payers, who may or may not approve certain procedures at specific types of facilities depending on the facility's available resources. Other restrictions may be in place because of a lack of resources, such as the absence of an intensive care unit or the lack of available clinical staff (for example, a cardiothoracic surgeon in the area). Generally, inpatient hospitals are not restricted to a certain set of approved procedures because these facilities are equipped to perform more complex, resource-intensive surgeries (such as high-risk and trauma surgeries). That being said, if a hospital does not have the resources required to perform a complex or high-risk procedure (such as a heart transplant on a pediatric patient), the patient will likely be transferred to a hospital with the necessary resources.

Outpatient hospitals and ASCs may perform minor surgeries like biopsies, endoscopies, injections, cataract surgeries, arthrocentesis, hernia repair, tonsillectomies and adenoidectomies, arthroscopies, carpal tunnel and trigger release, and bunionectomies, as well as laparoscopic surgical procedures.

Services that may be provided by ASCs and outpatient clinics are also limited by payer regulations. For example, Medicare will not pay for just any service that is performed at an ASC; it must be included on the list of approved services in the ASC setting. These procedures have been determined by Medicare to not pose a significant safety risk, and they are not expected to result in an overnight stay following the procedure. For example, a surgical procedure performed at an ASC must meet the following criteria to be covered by Medicare:

- It must not pose a significant safety risk to the patient
- It cannot require an overnight stay or monitoring past midnight
- It cannot be reported using an unlisted services code (CMS 2017)

These criteria differ annually and from payer to payer, depending on the circumstances. It is always a good idea to verify if any planned service would be covered in the ASC setting with the patient's individual insurance policy.

ASC coding is also much more complicated than simply complying with a list of approved procedures. It requires an understanding of facility and professional fee coding, sometimes referred to as "pro-fee" coding, as ASCs typically perform both. The way an ASC bills for services depends on the way the ASC is set up. Some use the CMS-1500 form for outpatient billing and report CPT and HCPCS codes for services performed, whereas others use the UB-04 form for inpatient billing (discussed in chapter 20) and report ICD-10-PCS codes to identify the services performed. For the purposes of this chapter, it is assumed that the ASC reports ICD-10-CM, CPT, and HCPCS codes and bills services on the CMS-1500 claim form. ASCs also have a specific set of CPT modifiers to be used exclusively for the ASC setting. These modifiers are discussed later in this chapter.

Surgical Packages and Billing for Services

Imagine leaving a grocery store with a bag of groceries, inside of which is everything needed to make a specific recipe. At home, you use all of the ingredients together to make the dish. Coding for surgeries is similar to cooking a specific recipe. Instead of coding for each item—such as a preoperative evaluation and preparation, then an incision, then a surgical procedure, then the skin repair, followed by the postoperative evaluation, a two-week follow-up examination, and the removal of stitches or staples—the coder only reports *one* code that identifies all of these components (the recipe).

The **global surgical package** is a set of services included within a single code that identifies the surgery performed, other services integral to the procedure, and a specific amount of time after the surgery. The amount of time included in the surgical package is referred to as the **global period** and is defined by each individual insurance carrier. For example, Insurance A may have a 14-day global period for a specific procedure while Insurance B has a 20-day global period for the same procedure. It is important to verify the specific length of the global period with the insurance payer for each procedure performed on the patient. There are three types of global surgical packages that fit the Medicare definitions of each type of global period, depending on the type of surgical procedure performed.

- *Simple procedures, zero global period*. These are simple procedures, like an endoscopy, without any preoperative or postoperative procedures; the global period is only the day of the procedure.
- *Minor surgical procedures, 10-day global period*. For minor surgeries, such as wound repairs, the global period starts on the day of the procedure. This global period includes 11 total days (the day of the procedure and the additional 10-day global period).
- *Major surgical procedures, 90-day global period*. This type of surgery includes one day of preoperative care, so the global period starts the day before the surgery, unless the decision to perform the surgery was made on the day of the surgery. This global period includes 92 total days (the day before the procedure, the day of the procedure, and then the additional 90-day global period). An example of a major surgical procedure would be the insertion of a pacemaker or major organ transplant.

As a coder, it is important to understand surgical packages and what is included in the package because it impacts the modifiers and any additional services reported for the surgery. An E/M encounter that results in the decision for surgery should be reported with modifier -57, Decision for surgery, to identify it as a separate encounter that excludes it from the surgical package, so it is reimbursed separately.

Each surgical package includes a bundle of procedures, all identified by the one CPT code that is reported for the surgery:

- Pre-treatment (either the day before a major procedure or the day of a minor procedure)
- Preoperative care
- Surgical services including local infiltration or topical anesthesia, the surgery itself, immediate postoperative care, dictation of operative notes, and meetings or discussions with the patient or family and other physicians
- Evaluation of the patient in the recovery or post-anesthesia care unit (PACU)
- Writing orders for the patient
- Some surgeries also include conscious sedation in the global package
- Postoperative follow-up care (for up to 10 or 90 days, depending on the procedure)
- All services in the postoperative period, other than a return to the operating room (see figure 11.5) (CMS 2019b)

When a provider performs a surgery that includes a global period, every time the patient presents for a follow-up encounter with the provider who performed the surgery, the follow-up encounter is included in the code for the primary surgical service. For example, consider a patient who suffers a laceration and presents to an urgent care facility for stitches. The complex wound repair code (including the placement of the stitches) reported by the urgent care doctor has a 10-day global period. Therefore, all routine follow-up performed by the provider within 10 days of the original procedure, including the removal of the stitches, is included in the original wound repair code. In

Figure 11.5. Surgical package

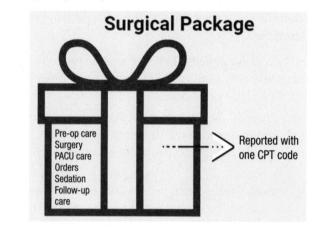

this case, when the patient presents for removal of uncomplicated stitches in the global period (10 days), the doctor removes those stitches without an expectation of payment for the removal. However, this does not mean that the urgent care doctor does not report any code at all. Rather, when a patient presents for routine care within the global period, code 99024, Postoperative follow-up visit, normally included in the surgical package, to indicate that an evaluation and management service was performed during a postoperative period for a reason(s) related to the original procedure, should be reported.

There are, however, important exceptions to this rule. If the patient in the previous example presents for removal of the stitches outside of the 10-day global period (on day 14, for example), then the provider may bill for the service using the appropriate code. Additionally, if the patient returns for an encounter *unrelated* to the surgery, or for a complication that requires a return to the operating room, then it may be billed separately, using the appropriate modifier. For example, if the patient returns to the urgent care office due to a urinary tract infection (not related to the original procedure), then this service may be billed separately. If this were the case, it would be important to append modifier -24, Unrelated evaluation and management service by the same physician or other qualified healthcare professional during a postoperative period, to the E/M code for the unrelated service. Additional modifiers that are important in breaking up the surgical package (to allow for separate payment of services not related to or in addition to the original surgical procedure) are modifier -78, Unplanned return to the operating/procedure room by the same physician or other qualified healthcare professional following initial procedure for a related procedure during the postoperative period, and modifier -79, Unrelated procedure of service by the same physician or other qualified healthcare professional during the postoperative period. Note that these three modifiers are important for payment of the service performed within the global period. If they are not appended to the CPT code, then it may be bundled into the code for the original surgical procedure and will not be paid separately.

When necessary, it is possible to separate the components of a surgical package and bill for only portions of the service using the appropriate modifier. Breaking up a surgical package is called **unbundling**, the practice of using multiple codes to bill for the individual steps in a single procedure rather than using a single code that includes all the steps of the comprehensive procedure. Unbundling may be considered unnecessary or improper coding, and codes that have been unbundled from a surgical package may be denied by the third-party payer. However, in some instances it may be necessary to report individual codes to identify procedures that are distinct from the primary surgical procedure. These individual services are referred to as separate procedures (refer to chapter 5, Learning the CPT and HCPCS Code Books), and are identified in the CPT code descriptions with the statement "separate procedure" in parentheses. As discussed in chapter 5, a **separate procedure** is one that is commonly part of another, more complex procedure, but may be performed independently or be otherwise unrelated to the procedure. For example, code 44850, Suture of mesentery (separate procedure), describes a procedure that is typically included within a more definitive procedure but may be reported even if no more definitive procedure was performed.

According to CPT guidelines, codes that are identified as separate procedures may be reported with a primary service when the separate procedure reports a service unrelated to or independent of the other procedure(s) performed. The separate procedure code should be appended with modifier -59, Distinct procedural service, to indicate that it was a distinct procedural service from the other procedure(s) performed. Separate procedure codes should be reported with a modifier -59 when they are performed at a different operative session, during a different procedure or surgery, in a different anatomical site or organ system, or with a separate incision, excision, lesion, or injury (AMA 2019). Refer to chapter 5 for a discussion of modifier -59 and when it may be necessary to use this modifier.

When reporting multiple surgeries or procedures performed on the same date, it may be necessary to check for code edits with the insurance payer. A **code edit** is an accuracy checkpoint in the claims-processing software that ensures all codes are valid and may be reported in conjunction with each other, and if any modifiers are necessary. An example of a code edit may be to check that a female procedure (like a hysterectomy) was performed only on a female patient.

CMS has instituted a national code editing system called **National Correct Coding Initiative (NCCI)** edits. NCCI was developed to promote national correct coding methodologies and to control improper coding leading to inappropriate payment in Part B Medicare claims. CMS developed its coding policies based on coding conventions defined in the CPT code book, national and local policies and edits, coding guidelines developed by national societies, analysis of standard medical and surgical practices, and a review of current coding practices (Casto 2019). NCCI edits are an important part of coding for surgical procedures because they identify when certain procedures may be reported together, when they may not be reported together, and when a modifier is required.

Surgical Specialties

The difference between a medical and surgical specialty is that a medical specialty performs noninvasive medical treatments and diagnostic evaluations, whereas a surgical specialty performs invasive surgical treatments and techniques. Remember that this is the difference between optometrists and ophthalmologists—optometrists perform procedures related to eyesight, such as refractions and prescription and fitting of contact lenses; and ophthalmologists treat the eyes (including performing surgery), such as the repair of a retinal detachment.

For most medical specialties, there is a corresponding surgical specialty. For example, there are pediatricians and pediatric surgeons. There are cardiologists and cardiothoracic surgeons. There are orthopedists and orthopedic surgeons. While both providers focus on the same medical specialty, surgeons receive additional training in surgical techniques and treatments. This chapter discusses surgical procedures, many of which are performed by surgical specialists.

The surgeries discussed in this chapter include those performed by colorectal, general, oral/maxillofacial, plastic and reconstructive, thoracic, vascular, bariatric, pediatric, burn/trauma and wound care, transplant, and foot and ankle surgeons. Orthopedic, neurological and spine, obstetrics and gynecology (OB/GYN), urology and nephrology, gastroenterology, and cardiovascular surgeries are discussed individually in later chapters.

Coding correctly for surgical procedures requires a thorough understanding of the Surgery section of the CPT code book, including how the Surgery subsections are organized and how to select and interpret CPT coding guidelines for surgical services.

Understanding Coding for Surgical Services

Understanding how to code for surgical procedures requires an in-depth understanding of the Surgery section of the CPT code book and its subsections, as well as the ability to interpret and apply CPT guidelines and rules. It also requires an understanding of the different types of surgical procedures.

Exploring the Surgery Subsections

There are 18 subsections in the Surgery section of the CPT code book, each one organized around a certain organ system or body area; they are listed as follows.

- General
- Integumentary
- Musculoskeletal
- Respiratory
- Cardiovascular
- Hemic and Lymphatic
- Mediastinum and Diaphragm
- Digestive
- Urinary
- Male Genital
- Reproductive System Procedures
- Intersex Surgery
- Female Genital
- Maternity Care and Delivery
- Endocrine System
- Nervous System
- Eye and Ocular Adnexa
- Auditory System

Each one of these subsections, organized by organ system/body area, contains a number of surgical procedures that are applicable to that specific body system. For example, the Integumentary subsection includes surgical procedures on the skin and accessory structures, such as excision of malignant lesions, skin grafting, burn debridement, and mastectomy procedures.

Each subsection is further subdivided into subheadings that combine surgeries performed on a specific body area or surgeries of the same type. Each subheading contains smaller groups of surgical procedures, called categories. For example, in figure 11.6 the Section name is *Surgery*, the subsection is the *Cardiovascular System*, the first subheading is *Heart and Pericardium*, and the first category is *Pericardium*.

Figure 11.6. Divisions of Cardiovascular subsection

Surgery
Cardiovascular System* (33016–37799)..216
The following is a listing of heading and subheadings that appear within the Cardiovascular System section of the CPT codebook. The subheadings or subsections denoted with asterisks (*) below have special instructions unique to that subsection. Where these are indicated, special "notes" or guidelines will be presented preceding those procedural terminology listings, referring to that subsection specifically.
Heart and Pericardium (33010–33999)...**216**
Pericardium*(33016–33050) 216
Cardiac Tumor (33120–33130) 216
Transmyocardial Revascularization (33140–33141)........216
Pacemaker or Implantable Defibrillator* (33202–33275).....217

Source: AMA 2019, 209.

Subsections of the Surgery section are all divided based on the specific types of procedures performed on each respective body area or organ system. For example, the Cardiovascular subsection is divided first by organ system (Heart and Pericardium, Arteries and Veins), and then by procedure type, specific organ, or condition (Pericardium, Cardiac Tumor, Transmyocardial Revascularization). The Musculoskeletal subsection, on the other hand, contains subheadings for organs (Hand and Fingers, Pelvis and Hip Joint), and subheadings by type of procedure (Application of Casts and Strapping, Endoscopy/Arthroscopy).

Understanding the way that these subsections are organized is integral to coding for surgical procedures. For example, a coder looking up a procedure performed to treat a cardiac tumor could refer to the table of contents at the beginning of the Cardiovascular subsection, find the subheading for Heart and Pericardium, and then find the category of codes for Cardiac Tumor (33120–33130) (see figure 11.6). Then the coder would refer to that code range to find the code.

Take the time to review the table of contents for each Surgery subsection in the CPT code book, as this will help with understanding the different types of procedures performed in these sections and how they are coded.

Key to Success

Do not overlook the organization of surgical subsections! It is easy to get lost in the CPT code book, especially if you are unfamiliar with the procedure you are looking up. When you are stuck, go back to the beginning of the subsection and look at the table of contents. Make a note of how the subsection is arranged, and find the section for the procedure you are searching for. Does this section of codes match the procedure code that you thought was right in the first place? If so, you are probably in the right place. If not, where did you go wrong?

Complete the exercises in There's a Code for That 11.1 to practice exploring the surgical subsections of the CPT manual.

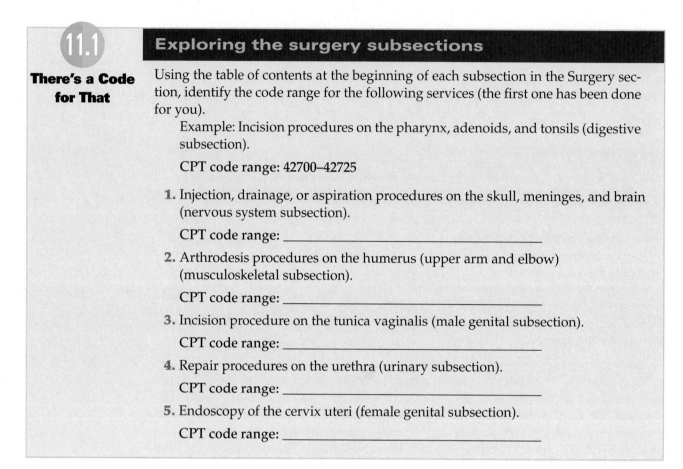

11.1

There's a Code for That

Exploring the surgery subsections

Using the table of contents at the beginning of each subsection in the Surgery section, identify the code range for the following services (the first one has been done for you).

Example: Incision procedures on the pharynx, adenoids, and tonsils (digestive subsection).

CPT code range: 42700–42725

1. Injection, drainage, or aspiration procedures on the skull, meninges, and brain (nervous system subsection).

   CPT code range: _____

2. Arthrodesis procedures on the humerus (upper arm and elbow) (musculoskeletal subsection).

   CPT code range: _____

3. Incision procedure on the tunica vaginalis (male genital subsection).

   CPT code range: _____

4. Repair procedures on the urethra (urinary subsection).

   CPT code range: _____

5. Endoscopy of the cervix uteri (female genital subsection).

   CPT code range: _____

Surgical Coding Guidelines

At the beginning of the surgery section in the CPT code book and in each of the Surgery subsections are important guidelines on how to use the codes in each of those sections. The guidelines at the beginning of the Surgery section apply to all the codes in that section (10021–69990). Additional guidelines are found within each subsection. In the Professional edition of the CPT code book, these guidelines are typically located on the green-shaded pages at the beginning of the Surgery section.

Guidelines at the beginning of the Surgery section include the CPT Description of Surgical Package, Follow-Up Care for Diagnostic Procedures, Follow-Up Care for Therapeutic Surgical Procedures, Supplied Materials, Reporting More Than One Procedure/Service, Separate Procedures, Unlisted Services or Procedures, Special Reports, Imaging Guidance, and Surgical Destruction. Coders should refer to these guidelines for definitions and instructions on assigning CPT codes in the Surgery section.

When guidelines are present in the Tabular List of codes (within a subsection), it is important to read through them before assigning a code, as these guidelines discuss when it is appropriate to report specific codes or use specific modifiers. Guidelines also offer descriptions of services and definitions of terms used in the code descriptions. See figure 11.7 for an example of guidelines found in the Surgery section.

Key to Success

It is easy to overlook guidelines in the CPT code book, but don't! These guidelines often define important terms and concepts, give important instructions on when to use (or not to use) specific codes, and provide general coding advice. If you see guidelines on the page of code, make sure you read them and take them into account before assigning any CPT code(s).

Any notes under a subheading (the heading in red in figure 11.7) pertain to all the codes within that subheading. All the notes under a category heading (the heading in blue in figure 11.7), pertain to all the codes in that category only. Any notes under individual codes or sets of codes (standalone and indented codes) pertain to the codes *above* the notes. For example, if an arthrotomy of the temporomandibular joint were done on both sides (bilaterally), the coder would need to report modifier -50 to identify it as a bilateral service (see parenthetical note under code 21010, Arthrotomy, temporomandibular joint, in figure 11.7).

Figure 11.7. Guidelines in the Surgery subsection

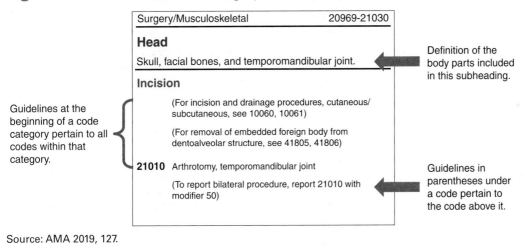

Source: AMA 2019, 127.

Key to Success

It is easy to overlook the parenthetical notes in the Tabular List of the Surgery section, but it is extremely important to read them and follow their instructions. If you have difficulty remembering that the notes are there, it might be a good idea to place a star, underline, or highlight important notes, so you do not forget them.

Types of Surgical Procedures

Categories of codes in the Surgery subsections are groups of procedures that are similar in nature. They are all procedures that use the same instrumentation, surgical technique, or treat a specific condition. Some of these categories are used across all of the subsections of surgical codes. For example, the category Excision is found in all the subsections. The Excision category groups together all of the surgical procedures performed to excise a specific organ, body part, or foreign body.

The following procedures include the common surgical categories found in the CPT Surgery section. Note that this is not an all-inclusive list, these are only the most common surgical categories. Additional categories of codes are specific to the subsection in which they appear and may not be found anywhere else in the CPT code book. For example, the Incision and Drainage category is listed in the Integumentary subsection, but not in the Cardiovascular subsection.

- *Incision.* An **incision** is a cut made on a body part or organ. Codes found within an incision category include incision and drainage (I&D) codes and surgical incision codes for exploration, removal of foreign bodies, biopsies, or other surgical service. For example, code 39000, Mediastinotomy with exploration, drainage, removal of foreign body, or biopsy; cervical approach, is an incision code. Note that sometimes an entire category is reserved for Incision and Drainage codes, and I&D codes are excluded from the Incision category.

- *Excision.* An **excision** is the surgical removal of an organ, body tissue, lesion, or other body part or foreign object. Note that any excision code is an *open* removal, using a scalpel. For example, an open biopsy of an intranasal lesion includes cutting into the nose to excise the tissue sample (see code 30100, Biopsy, intranasal). On occasion, the term **resection** is used to identify the excision of tissue. In CPT coding, *resection* is the removal of all or part of an organ or body tissue. For example, a resection of the small intestine would be an excision of a portion of tissue from the small intestine (see code 44202, Laparoscopy, surgical; enterectomy, resection of small intestine, single resection and anastomosis). Note that the definition of resection in ICS-10-PCS coding differs from this definition used in CPT coding. When learning ICD-10-PCS coding, resection refers to the complete removal of an organ, rather than just a portion (as is sometimes the case in CPT coding).

- *Introduction.* An **introduction** is the insertion of a device, object, or substance into a body part or organ. Introduction codes may sometimes be classified as Injections, in which a therapeutic or diagnostic substance is injected into the patient. An example of an introduction code is 58300, Insertion of intrauterine device (IUD).

- *Removal.* A **removal** is taking out a device, object, or substance from a body part or area. Because removal procedures are sometimes related or performed in conjunction to introduction procedures, some removal codes are included in the same category of codes for introduction procedures—for example, 58301, Removal of intrauterine device (IUD).

- *Repair.* A **repair** is a procedure performed to return an organ or body part to its original function, or to improve functioning or improve a cosmetic outcome. For example, a rhinoplasty is performed to repair the shape and/or function of the nose, and it may also be done for cosmetic purposes. See code 30400, Rhinoplasty, primary; lateral and alar cartilages and/or elevation of nasal tip.

- *Destruction.* A **destruction**, or **ablation**, is a procedure that destroys tissue. It may be done in several different ways including laser surgery, electrosurgery, cryosurgery, chemosurgery, surgical curettement, radiocautery, radiofrequency ablation, or tissue volume reduction. Note that an ablation differs from an excision, as no tissue remains after a destruction procedure because the tissue is destroyed during the procedure. An excision, however, preserves the tissue but removes it from the body (in this way, many biopsies are excision procedures because the tissue is not destroyed). An example of a destruction procedure is 54050, Destruction of lesion(s), penis (e.g., condyloma, papilloma, molluscum contagiosum, herpetic vesicle), simple; chemical (this is a destruction of penile tissue using chemical destruction).

- *Other Procedures.* The Other Procedures category of codes often lists a specific type of repair or a range of different types of procedures that do not belong in any other category. For example, nasal packing codes are in the Other Procedures category of codes in the Nose subheading of the Respiratory System subsection (see codes 30901–30999).

- *Endoscopy.* An **endoscopy** is a procedure performed with the aid of an endoscope. This device has a small camera attached to the end of a long, thin, lighted tube, which is inserted through a natural opening or stoma. The healthcare provider can maneuver the endoscope through a body passage, such as the gastrointestinal tract, to see inside the organ for diagnostic or therapeutic services. The endoscopy is named after the body passageway that is viewed during the procedure. For example, a bronchoscopy is an endoscopic examination of the bronchus, and a cystoscopy is an endoscopic examination of the urinary bladder. Figure 11.8 displays the use of a bronchoscope to perform an endoscopic examination of the bronchus and lungs, which would be coded with 31622, Bronchoscopy, rigid or flexible, including fluoroscopic guidance, when performed; diagnostic, with cell washing, when performed (separate procedure).

Figure 11.8. Bronchoscopy

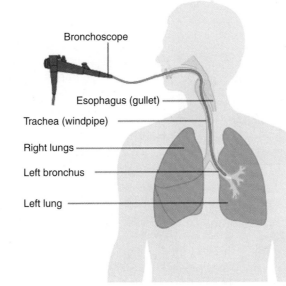

Source: Cancer Research UK 2014.

Endoscopes are highly specialized instruments and may be used in numerous procedures, such as biopsies and removal of foreign bodies. When coding for endoscopies, it is important to keep in mind that there are three components to endoscopy coding—approach, extent, and surgical versus diagnostic services.

- *Approach*. When coding for an endoscopy, it is necessary to select the code for the correct approach to the procedure. Coders should ask themselves: Where was the endoscope inserted? Note that not all endoscopy codes differ by approach, so this may not always impact code selection.

- *Extent*. The code used to identify the endoscopy differs based on how far the endoscope was inserted in the patient. For example, an endoscopy inserted through the mouth, through the pharynx and larynx, and then stopped at the trachea would be considered a tracheoscopy. If it was inserted all the way into the bronchus, then it would be considered a bronchoscopy. Coders should ask themselves: How far did the endoscopy go? Code to the furthest extent of the endoscopy.

- *Surgical versus diagnostic services*. Endoscopic procedures can be either diagnostic or surgical. A *diagnostic* endoscopy is one that is performed to determine a diagnosis. A *surgical* procedure is one that is performed to treat a diagnosis. Some endoscopy codes are purely diagnostic, whereas others describe an endoscopic procedure in which a surgical treatment was performed, like the removal of a foreign body, biopsy, or placement of a stent. When an endoscopy is done to determine a diagnosis and a surgical procedure is performed during the same endoscopy, then the coder should only report the surgical endoscopy. (More on the difference between diagnostic and surgical, or therapeutic, procedures is discussed in the next section of this chapter). If a

Figure 11.9. Surgical endoscopic procedures

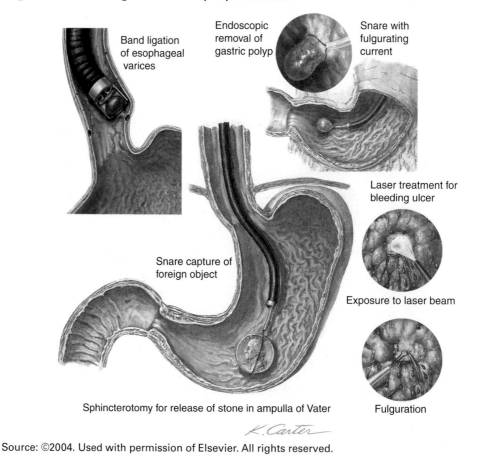

Band ligation of esophageal varices

Endoscopic removal of gastric polyp

Snare with fulgurating current

Laser treatment for bleeding ulcer

Snare capture of foreign object

Exposure to laser beam

Sphincterotomy for release of stone in ampulla of Vater

Fulguration

K. Carter

surgical endoscopy is performed, code only for the surgical procedure and not the diagnostic endoscopy as well, as the surgery code includes the diagnostic service. When multiple surgical procedures are performed during the same endoscopy, append modifier -51, Multiple procedures, to the codes for the additional procedures performed. Note that modifier -51 is not approved for use by the outpatient hospital (the facility) but may be reported on the physician's claim for the service. (See figure 11.9 for illustrations of surgical endoscopic procedures.)

A variety of surgical procedures can be performed endoscopically. If a surgical procedure is performed during the endoscopy, report the code for the surgical procedure, not the diagnostic procedure. Use one code for each surgical procedure performed, with additional codes appended with modifier -51.

- *Laparoscopy.* A **laparoscopy** is similar in nature to an endoscopy, as it uses a lighted scope that is inserted into the body through several small incisions to perform a diagnostic or therapeutic procedure. In this procedure, a fiber-optic laparoscope is inserted through the skin of the abdominal wall, after which air is injected into the abdominal cavity so the surgeon can see and access the internal organs (see figure 11.10). Although they have the same suffix (-*scopy*), do not confuse a laparoscopic procedure with an endoscopic procedure, as they are two different types of services. Laparoscopic procedures are less invasive than and provide alternatives to open surgeries. When coding for any type of surgery, pay close attention to whether it was performed openly or laparoscopically.

Figure 11.10. Laparoscopy

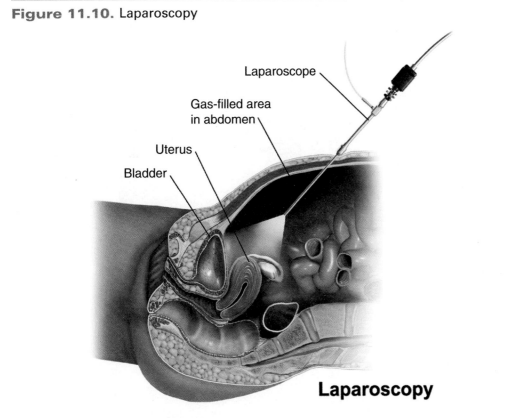

Laparoscopy

A laparoscopic examination of the peritoneum.
Source: Blausen.com staff 2014.

Open procedures are found in the Excision category of codes, while laparoscopic procedures are found in the Laparoscopy category of codes. For example, see 51990, Laparoscopy, surgical; urethral suspension for stress incontinence.

A technologically advanced and increasingly utilized type of laparoscopic procedure is robotic-assisted surgery, performed with the aid of a robot with miniature instruments controlled by the surgeon (see figure 11.11). Robotic surgeries allow a maximum range of motion and precision and help in reducing surgeon fatigue. When coding for a procedure that was performed via robotic-assisted surgery, such as a robotic-assisted laparoscopic hysterectomy, the coder should select the code for the laparoscopic version of the procedure, and append modifier -22, Increased procedural services (more on this modifier in the next section of this chapter). An additional HCPCS code may also be used to identify the service performed with the help of a robotic surgical system: S2900, Surgical techniques requiring use of robotic surgical system. This code should be reported in addition to the code for the primary procedure. However, note that this code is not considered payable by Medicare, and it is unlikely to be reimbursed by a third-party payer. Thus, it is likely to be reported to justify any additional charges (as identified by modifier -22) for the procedure.

Figure 11.11. Robotic-assisted surgery

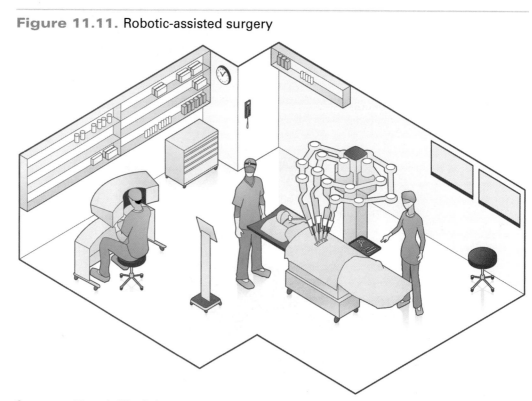

Source: mathisworks/iStockphoto.com.

Key to Success

Laparoscopic procedures are minimally invasive. They are performed using several small incisions into the body cavity, through which instruments are inserted to perform the surgical procedure (a closed procedure). Any procedure performed laparoscopically ending with the suffix -*scopy* (or -*scopic*) is located under the Laparoscopy category in the CPT code book. Open procedures that involve a direct incision into the body cavity through which the surgeon performs the procedure using his or her hands, scalpels, and other tools (an open procedure) are located in the Incision, Excision, Removal, or Repair categories (among others). Keep this important distinction in mind when coding for surgical services. Any procedural description ending in -*scopy* should be coded as a laparoscopic procedure, *not* an open procedure (see figure 11.12 for more surgical terminology). Note that endoscopic procedures also end with the suffix -*scopy*, so these should also be differentiated from open procedures.

- *Transplantation*. A transplantation procedure removes a damaged, diseased, or otherwise nonfunctioning organ from the body and replaces it with a donated organ in its place. Often the new organ is from a donor (either a live or cadaver donor), and sometimes the original organ is left in place. Only a handful of organs in the human body may be transplanted, so the Transplantation category is not found in each of the Surgery subsections. For example, liver transplantations are found in codes 47133 to 47147.

- *Manipulation*. Manipulation is manually moving one body part into its original location or into another location. For example, an orthopedist may manually move a fractured radius back into its original location before placing a cast on the outside of the arm to immobilize the extremity. The majority of all manipulation codes are located in the Musculoskeletal System subsection, but a few other manipulation categories are found elsewhere in the Surgery section. See code 27275, Manipulation, hip joint, requiring general anesthesia, as an example of a manipulation code.

Figure 11.12. Surgical terminology

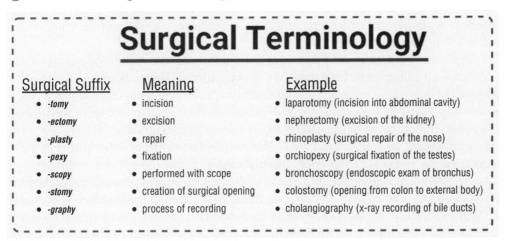

Key to Success

There are a number of additional categories of codes found in the Surgery subsections, so as you learn more about surgical coding and become more familiar with surgeries and the CPT codes they represent, you will notice more categories of procedures. When you encounter a category of codes for a procedure for which you are unfamiliar, search for any guidelines that may describe the procedure and use a medical dictionary and other reference items to obtain more information about the procedures in that category. This textbook introduces the beginning coder to some of these procedures, but as medicine and surgical techniques evolve, these categories are sure to change. Being flexible and knowing how to access and use your resources is a helpful way to stay ahead of these changes.

The next section of this chapter discusses the actual CPT codes for surgical services, as well as related diagnosis codes for many different surgical specialties.

Procedural and Diagnostic Coding for Surgical Services

Coding for surgeries requires an understanding of the difference between diagnostic and therapeutic procedures and preoperative and postoperative diagnoses, as well as the ability to correctly report any complication or comorbidities. It further requires the ability to interpret precise procedural descriptions and report them accurately, with the appropriate modifier (if necessary) and a diagnosis code or codes that fully support the medical necessity for the service.

Therapeutic versus Diagnostic Procedures

Procedures can be either therapeutic or diagnostic. A **diagnostic procedure** is performed to determine a diagnosis. For example, a diagnostic bronchoscopy is performed to determine if there is a medical condition in the bronchus or lungs. A **therapeutic procedure** is performed to treat a diagnosis. For example, if a bronchoscopy were performed to remove a foreign body, it would be considered a therapeutic procedure because it treated the medical condition (removal of the foreign body). A surgical procedure is an invasive procedure and may be performed to determine a diagnosis or to treat a diagnosis.

In some cases, a diagnostic procedure is transformed into a therapeutic procedure. For example, if a diagnostic bronchoscopy was performed due to hemoptysis (coughing up blood) to determine the cause of the condition, and then it was found that a foreign body was present in the bronchus and removed, then the definitive procedure was therapeutic (the removal of the foreign body to treat the diagnosis).

It is important to understand the difference between diagnostic and therapeutic procedures, as some surgical code descriptions include these terms. Although the difference between diagnostic and therapeutic procedures is present throughout the CPT code book, the difference between these two types of procedures is especially important when coding for endoscopies. Endoscopy codes are divided based on if the procedure was diagnostic or therapeutic (identified as surgical in the CPT code set). For example, compare codes 31231, Nasal endoscopy, *diagnostic,* unilateral or bilateral (separate procedure), and 31237, Nasal endoscopy, *surgical;* with biopsy, polypectomy or debridement (separate procedure).

Pay attention to this type of difference between CPT code descriptions in the Surgery section. Any procedure that is performed to determine a diagnosis is a diagnostic procedure; any procedure performed to treat a known diagnosis is a surgical (therapeutic) procedure. If the diagnosis is determined during the diagnostic procedure and it is then transformed into a therapeutic procedure, select the code for the therapeutic (or surgical) service.

Preoperative and Postoperative Diagnoses

When a diagnostic procedure is performed and converted into a therapeutic procedure, it is likely done because a medical condition was encountered during the diagnostic procedure and treated at that time. In this case, the preoperative diagnosis was either for a medical screening, or sign or symptom, and the postoperative diagnosis was a definitive diagnosis—the condition that required treatment. Therefore, there are two diagnoses—the preoperative and postoperative diagnoses.

A **preoperative diagnosis** is the diagnosis given to the patient at the beginning of a procedure. For example, if a patient is coughing up blood and requires a bronchoscopy, then the preoperative diagnosis is hemoptysis. The **postoperative diagnosis** is the definitive medical condition of the patient either diagnosed or treated during the procedure. For example, if the bronchoscopy discovers a foreign body in the bronchus that was the cause of the hemoptysis, then the postoperative diagnosis is foreign body in the bronchial tube, rather than hemoptysis. In this case, the coder would only assign the code for the postoperative diagnosis (foreign body), rather than the preoperative diagnosis (hemoptysis).

Sometimes the preoperative and postoperative diagnoses are the same, and other times they are different. When these two diagnoses differ, the postoperative diagnosis is the one that should be reported on the claim as the medical necessity for the service. According to the guidelines for outpatient surgical coding, the postoperative diagnosis is the most definitive, which is why it should be reported, rather than the preoperative diagnosis (see figure 11.13).

Using the given example, the preoperative diagnosis for the patient coughing up blood would be R04.2, Hemoptysis, and the postoperative diagnosis would be T17.508A, Unspecified foreign body in bronchus causing other injury, initial encounter. The diagnosis code reported for the procedure would be the latter code, as illustrated in figure 11.14.

In this example, the hemoptysis code would not be reported because it is a symptom of the definitive diagnosis (the foreign body). However, if there were additional, unrelated signs, symptoms, or comorbid conditions or complications, then those should be reported in addition to the primary diagnosis.

Figure 11.13. OGCR IV.N

> **N. Ambulatory Surgery**
>
> For ambulatory surgery, code the diagnosis for which the surgery was performed. If the postoperative diagnosis is known to be different from the preoperative diagnosis at the time the diagnosis is confirmed, select the postoperative diagnosis for coding, since it is the most definitive.

Source: CMS 2019c.

Figure 11.14. Preoperative versus postoperative diagnosis

> PREOPERATIVE DIAGNOSIS: Hemoptysis
> POSTOPERATIVE DIAGNOSIS: FB in bronchus
> ICD-10-CM Code: T17.508A, Unspecified foreign body in bronchus causing other injury, initial encounter

Complications and Comorbidities

As previously mentioned in this chapter, the surgical process from admission to discharge can sometimes be brief and last less than 24 hours, or it can be long and last days, weeks, or more. This all depends on the patient's comorbid conditions and any complications of care.

A comorbid condition is a chronic or long-term condition that presents along with another chronic or long-term condition; for example, diabetes mellitus and epilepsy. Comorbidities can make recovery from a surgery more difficult or lengthy. When a patient presents with multiple comorbid conditions, each condition should be represented with an individual ICD-10-CM code, with the diagnosis code for the condition that required treatment sequenced first.

An additional consideration for diagnosis coding in the surgical setting is complications of care. A complication of care is a condition that occurs as a result of the medical care or surgery. For example, an organ transplant may result in the body rejecting the transplanted organ. This would be a complication of the transplant. To report a condition as a complication of care, the documentation must clearly identify the cause and effect relationship between the surgery (or medical treatment provided) and the resulting complication. If there are any questions about the relationship, the coder should ask the healthcare provider for clarification (see figure 11.15).

Figure 11.15. OGCR I.B.16

> **16. Documentation of Complications of Care**
> Code assignment is based on the provider's documentation of the relationship between the condition and the care or procedure, unless otherwise instructed by the classification. The guideline extends to any complications of care, regardless of the chapter the code is located in. It is important to note that not all conditions that occur during or following medical care or surgery are classified as complications. There must be a cause-and-effect relationship between the care provided and the condition, and an indication in the documentation that it is a complication. Query the provider for clarification, if the complication is not clearly documented.

Source: CMS 2019c.

Codes for complications of care are found in each respective body system chapter in the ICD-10-CM code book and are often listed as either intraoperative (during the procedure) or postprocedural (after the procedure) complications. For example, code E89.0, Postprocedural hypothyroidism, is listed in chapter 4 (Endocrine, Nutritional and Metabolic Diseases) of the code book, and is the result of a medical procedure.

Coding for complications of care are listed in various areas of the ICD-10-CM code book and identify complications that may result from surgical procedures throughout the body. When searching for a complication of care, search for the term *Complication* in the ICD-10-CM Index, and then refer to either the specific body system, type of procedure, or resulting medical condition. There are many pages of subterms and cross-references under the term *Complication*, so it is important to pay attention to the main entries and follow all subterms and cross-references carefully.

Key to Success

When searching through long lists of main terms, subterms, and cross-references in the ICD-10-CM Main Index, pay attention to the lines on the far side of each column. These help to orient coders to the main terms and indented terms. It may also be helpful to use a ruler or straightedge to keep track of the subterms and indentations.

For example, prosthetic left knee joint instability in a patient who underwent a knee transplant two years ago may be coded as a complication of the previous knee joint prosthesis. In this case, the coder would look up *Complication* in the Index, then refer to the subterm *joint prosthesis,* then *mechanical,* and then the specific type of mechanical problem—in this case *instability,* which refers the coder to the code T84.02-. Once the code is identified, it needs to be verified in the Tabular List, and all necessary characters added to make a valid code. In this case, code options identify the laterality and specific joint. The correct code for this example would be T84.023A, Instability of internal left knee prosthesis, initial encounter. Figure 11.16 lists the additional OGCR related to complications of care.

Surgery Modifiers

There are numerous CPT modifiers that are applicable for surgical services, an additional set of modifiers that are designed specifically for ASC and outpatient hospital use, and others that are used to report never events. For this reason, knowing the modifiers applicable to surgical services is especially important for accurately reporting surgical procedures and optimizing payment for them.

CPT Modifiers

CPT modifiers that are applicable to surgical services include the following:

- Modifier -22, Increased procedural services. This modifier should be used when the work required to perform a service was above and beyond that which is typically required. The documentation for the service must clearly identify why the service was considered increased, by describing the additional time, intensity, technical difficulty, severity of the patient's condition, or physical or mental effort involved in the procedure. It may also be necessary to include a special report in addition to the claim to identify the nature, extent, and need for any additional time, effort, or equipment necessary to complete the service. The special report should justify the use of modifier -22.

- Modifier -47, Anesthesia by surgeon. This modifier should be appended to the code for the medical procedure to indicate that the anesthesia was administered directly by the surgeon who performed the procedure. Modifier -47 should be appended to the anesthesia code (discussed in the following chapter), rather than the code for the surgical procedure.

- Modifier -50, Bilateral procedure. This modifier should be appended to the code for a primary procedure when that procedure was performed bilaterally (on both sides), and the CPT code description is for a unilateral procedure. If the code for the primary procedure was for a unilateral service, and that procedure was performed bilaterally, then modifier -50 should be appended to the procedure code to identify it as bilateral. For example, code 69210, Removal impacted cerumen requiring instrumentation, unilateral, is a unilateral code. If this procedure was performed on both ears (bilaterally), then it would be reported as follows: 69210-50. If, on the other hand, the CPT code descriptor notes that it is either unilateral or bilateral, and the procedure was performed bilaterally, then modifier -50 would not need to be appended to the code for the service.

- Modifier -51, Multiple procedures. This modifier is used when a provider performs multiple procedures of the same type. For example, if a podiatry surgeon performs a partial ostectomy on two metatarsal heads, then he would report code 28288, Ostectomy, partial, exostectomy or condylectomy, metatarsal head, each metatarsal head, twice, with the second code appended with

Figure 11.16. OGCR I.C.19.g

g. Complications of care

1) General guidelines for complications of care

(a) Documentation of complications of care

See Section I.B.16. for information on documentation of complications of care.

2) Pain due to medical devices

Pain associated with devices, implants or grafts left in a surgical site (for example painful hip prosthesis) is assigned to the appropriate code(s) found in Chapter 19, Injury, poisoning, and certain other consequences of external causes. Specific codes for pain due to medical devices are found in the T code section of the ICD-10-CM. Use additional code(s) from category G89 to identify acute or chronic pain due to presence of the device, implant or graft (G89.18 or G89.28).

3) Transplant complications

(a) Transplant complications other than kidney

Codes under category T86, Complications of transplanted organs and tissues, are for use for both complications and rejection of transplanted organs. A transplant complication code is only assigned if the complication affects the function of the transplanted organ. Two codes are required to fully describe a transplant complication: the appropriate code from category T86 and a secondary code that identifies the complication.

Pre-existing conditions or conditions that develop after the transplant are not coded as complications unless they affect the function of the transplanted organs.

See I.C.21. for transplant organ removal status.

See I.C.2. for malignant neoplasm associated with transplanted organ.

(b) Kidney transplant complications

Patients who have undergone kidney transplant may still have some form of chronic kidney disease (CKD) because the kidney transplant may not fully restore kidney function. Code T86.1- should be assigned for documented complications of a kidney transplant, such as transplant failure or rejection or other transplant complication. Code T86.1- should not be assigned for post kidney transplant patients who have chronic kidney (CKD) unless a transplant complication such as transplant failure or rejection is documented. If the documentation is unclear as to whether the patient has a complication of the transplant, query the provider.

Conditions that affect the function of the transplanted kidney, other than CKD, should be assigned a code from subcategory T86.1, Complications of transplanted organ, Kidney, and a secondary code that identifies the complication.

For patients with CKD following a kidney transplant, but who do not have a complication such as failure or rejection, *see section I.C.14. Chronic kidney disease and kidney transplant status.*

4) Complication codes that include the external cause

As with certain other T codes, some of the complications of care codes have the external cause included in the code. The code includes the nature of the complication as well as the type of procedure that caused the complication. No external cause code indicating the type of procedure is necessary for these codes.

5) Complications of care codes within the body system chapters

Intraoperative and postprocedural complication codes are found within the body system chapters with codes specific to the organs and structures of that body system. These codes should be sequenced first, followed by a code(s) for the specific complication, if applicable.

Complication codes from the body system chapters should be assigned for intraoperative and postprocedural complications (e.g., the appropriate complication code from chapter 9 would be assigned for a vascular intraoperative or postprocedural complication) unless the complication is specifically indexed to a T code in chapter 19.

Source: CMS 2019c.

modifier -51, as follows: 28288, and 28288-51. This modifier indicates to the payer that the procedure was performed multiple times. Insurance will usually pay 100 percent for the primary procedure, and then reduce the amount of payment for the second or subsequent procedures, paying at a downward scale of 75 percent, 50 percent, and 25 percent. The exact amount of reimbursement depends on the agreement with the insurance payer. Note that this modifier should not be used with add-on codes, E/M codes, physical medicine or rehabilitation, or provision of supplies such as vaccines. Note that modifier -51 is not approved for use by the outpatient hospital facility. It may only be reported by an independent provider billing for services performed.

- Modifier -52, Reduced services. This modifier should be used to identify that a procedure was partially reduced or eliminated at the discretion of the healthcare provider. For example, if a code description is for a bilateral service, but only the unilateral service was performed, then the code for the full procedure would be reported with modifier -52.

- Modifier -53, Discontinued procedure. This modifier should be used to identify that a procedure was discontinued due to extenuating circumstances that threaten the well-being of the patient. For example, if a patient undergoing a procedure becomes hypotensive or experiences respiratory distress, and the procedure is discontinued, the normal procedure code would be reported with modifier -53.

Modifiers -52 and -53 are very similar, but are used in two very different situations, so be careful! Modifier -52 is used when the procedure is not completed to the full extent of the code description, based on the provider's judgment. Modifier -53 is used **MOD** when the procedure is discontinued due to the patient's health or other extenuating circumstance that threatens the well-being of the patient.

- Modifier -54, Surgical care only. This modifier should be used when the provider performs only the *surgical* portion of a service. It is used to break up the surgical package so that the provider is only paid for the portion of the procedure performed; in this case the surgery itself, about 70 percent of the charge (depending on the insurance). For example, a general surgeon working in an emergency department may perform only the surgical portion of an appendectomy, which involves only the incision and removal of the appendix in the operating room.

- Modifier -55, Postoperative management only. This modifier should be used when the provider performs only the *postoperative* portion of the service. Like modifier -54, it is used to break up the surgical package so that the provider is only paid for the portion of the procedure that was performed; in this case the postoperative management of the patient, about 20 percent of the charge (depending on the insurance). For example, if a physician in an emergency department had to complete the postoperative follow-up of an appendectomy patient because the general surgeon was unable to, then the appendectomy procedure would be reported with a modifier -55 (the surgeon would report his or her portion of the procedure with the same appendectomy code appended with modifier -54).

- Modifier -56, Preoperative management only. This modifier should be used when the provider performs only the *preoperative* portion of the service. Like modifiers -54 and -55, it is used to break up the surgical package so that the provider is only paid for the portion of the procedure that was performed; in this case the preoperative management of the patient, about 10 percent of the charge (depending on the insurance). For example, if one provider completed the preoperative evaluation and preoperative preparation of a surgical appendectomy patient, but was called out to perform a different procedure and a different provider performed both the surgical and postoperative portions of the service, then he or she would report the appendectomy procedure appended with modifier -56. (See figure 11.17 for an example of how these modifiers may impact payment).

- Modifier -62, Two surgeons. This modifier should be used when a procedure is performed by two surgeons. In this case, each surgeon would report the procedure, both appended with modifier -62, and each would only get paid for half of the service performed.

- Modifier -63, Procedure performed on infants less than 4 kg. This modifier should be appended to any service performed on a neonate or infant who weighs less than 4 kg. It is used to identify the increased complexity and work required for patients of this size. Note that it may only be reported with codes within the range 20010 to 69990, and cannot be used on E/M, anesthesia, radiology, pathology and laboratory, or medicine services. Some surgical codes are exempt from the use of modifier -63, which are listed in Appendix F of the CPT code book. Parenthetical notes are also included throughout the CPT code book for surgical codes that are exempt from this modifier.

Figure 11.17. Example of modifiers -54, -55, and -56 impacting payment

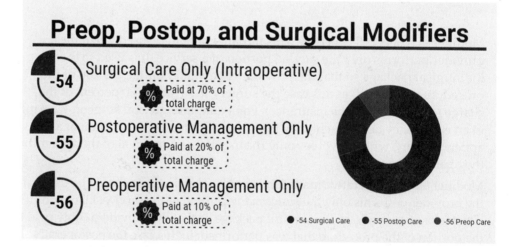

- Modifier -66, Surgical team. This modifier should be used when a team of surgeons perform a highly complex medical procedure. These surgeries require the concomitant services of several providers, often of different medical specialties, with the addition of other highly trained personnel or complex equipment. Each participating healthcare provider should report the code for the procedure appended with modifier -66. In terms of payment, each provider receives payment for the service according to a predetermined agreement made between the surgeons and the insurance company.

- Modifier -76, Repeat procedure or service by same physician or other qualified healthcare professional. This modifier should be used when a procedure or service is repeated by the same healthcare provider after the original procedure or service. For example, if an endoscopy is performed twice in one day by the same healthcare provider, both procedures would be reported by the same physician, with the second procedure appended with the modifier. Note that this modifier should not be used with E/M services.

- Modifier -77, Repeat procedure by another physician or other qualified healthcare professional. This modifier should be used when a procedure or service is repeated in the same day, but performed by a different healthcare provider. For example, if an endoscopy was performed in the morning by one provider, and then the same procedure is performed by a different provider later in the day, this subsequent procedure would be reported with the modifier -77.

- Modifier -78, Unplanned return to the operating/procedure room by the same physician or other qualified healthcare professional following initial procedure for a related procedure during the postoperative period. This modifier should be used when a procedure is performed in an operating room or surgical suite, and is an unplanned procedure following the initial procedure, related to the original procedure. It is used when a patient experiences a complication after the primary procedure and must return to the operating room or surgical suite for an additional procedure. The subsequent procedure should be appended with modifier -78. This modifier may also be used to identify a circumstance when a patient is within the global period but requires a return to the operating room due to a complication or other problem related to the original procedure, as discussed previously in this chapter.

- Modifier -79, Unrelated procedure or service by the same physician or other qualified healthcare professional during the postoperative period. This modifier is used to indicate that the procedure performed is unrelated to the primary surgical procedure. It is used while the patient is within the global package timeframe for the primary procedure, and allows reimbursement for the unrelated procedure. If this modifier is not used for the unrelated procedure, then it will be considered part of the surgical package for the primary procedure and will not be paid separately.

- Modifier -80, Assistant surgeon. This modifier is used to indicate that the procedure is performed by an assistant surgeon. This occurs when one surgeon assists another surgeon in the performance of a procedure, and the assisting surgeon is present for most of the procedure. The primary operating surgeon would report the procedure without a modifier, and the assistant surgeon would report the procedure with modifier -80 to indicate that he or she was the assistant surgeon for the procedure.

- Modifier -AS, Physician assistant, nurse practitioner, or clinical nurse specialist services for assistant at surgery. This modifier is essentially the same as modifier -80, except that it is used when the assistant surgeon is a mid-level provider such as a physician assistant (PA), clinical nurse specialist (CNS), or nurse practitioner (NP). Note that this is a HCPCS modifier, and it is not listed in the CPT code book. Instead it is found in the modifiers listing in the HCPCS code book.

- Modifier -81, Minimum assistant surgeon. This modifier is similar to modifier -80, but is used when the assistant surgeon is only present for a relatively short period of time and provides only minimal assistance to the primary surgeon. The primary surgeon would report the service without a modifier, and the minimum assistant surgeon would report the service with modifier -81.
- Modifier -82, Assistant surgeon (when qualified resident surgeon not available). This modifier is used in teaching hospitals and should be used when a qualified resident surgeon is not available to assist at surgery, and minimal assistance at surgery is required. The assistant surgeon would report the procedure code with modifier -82.

MOD Note that there are four codes that identify when a surgeon assisted at surgery: 80, 81, 82, and AS. These modifiers are used by the surgeon who performed the assistance and are paid at a reduced amount. For example, appending modifier -82 to a service reported to Medicare might mean that the payment is only 16 percent of the full-service amount. Modifier -62, Two surgeons, and modifier -66, Surgical team, also identify circumstances where more than one surgeon performs a procedure, but here they are working together rather than assisting one primary surgeon. In these cases, payment for the services performed is usually predetermined between the surgeons and insurance providers prior to the surgery.

These modifiers should be used for medical procedures used in the inpatient hospital setting. Procedures performed in the outpatient hospital or ASC setting have a different set of applicable modifiers.

ASC or Hospital Outpatient Modifiers

There are several modifiers that are used specifically for services performed in the ASC or outpatient hospital settings. Although some of them are similar to those used for inpatient services, there are a handful of completely separate modifiers that are used specifically for services in these settings. The list of ASC modifiers is located in Appendix A of the CPT code book.

Note that not all ASC modifiers are listed here, only those that are significantly different than those described in the previous section (CPT modifiers).

- Modifier -27, Multiple outpatient hospital E/M encounters on the same date. This modifier should be used when the patient receives multiple E/M encounters on the same date of service, performed in different outpatient hospital settings. The E/M services may be performed by either the same or two different healthcare providers, but the E/M encounters both must be performed at different outpatient settings. For example, if a patient had an E/M encounter and then endoscopy performed in an ASC for trouble swallowing in the morning, and then had to go to the emergency department later in the day where another E/M procedure was performed, then the E/M encounter would be appended with modifier -27.
- Modifier -73, Discontinued outpatient hospital/ambulatory surgical center (ASC) procedure prior to the administration of anesthesia. This modifier should be used to identify that a procedure was discontinued due to extenuating circumstances that threaten the well-being of the patient, and that the procedure

was discontinued *prior* to the administration of anesthesia. This includes local, regional block, or general anesthesia.

- Modifier -74, Discontinued outpatient hospital/ambulatory surgical center (ASC) procedure after administration of anesthesia. This modifier is very similar to modifier -73, except that it is used to identify that a procedure was discontinued due to extenuating circumstances *after* administration of the anesthesia (local, regional block, or general), or after the procedure was started (incision was made, intubation started, or scope inserted).

Note that modifiers -73 and -74 are both very similar to modifier -53, Discontinued procedure, which is used for physician billing. The difference (besides that fact that these modifiers may only be used in the outpatient hospital or ASC setting), is that they describe *when* the procedure was discontinued—either before or after the administration of anesthesia or the beginning of the procedure.

The existence of these ASC and outpatient hospital modifiers is one of the reasons why ASC coding and billing is so different from other traditional coding and billing. Coding for ASC and outpatient hospital services requires more insight into the special nature of the outpatient/inpatient relationship, and specific knowledge on how each individual facility charges for services. For example, some ASCs may be classified as outpatient facilities, in which case they would report outpatient codes only. On the other hand, some ASCs may be affiliated with an inpatient hospital, in which case they may be required to report inpatient codes (such as ICD-10-PCS) as well as outpatient (CPT) codes. This all depends on each individual ASC and the way in which the facility is organized.

Never Events

In rare instances a mistake is made in treatment that is erroneously performed by the healthcare provider. These are called **never events,** a term coined in 2001 by Ken Kizer of the National Quality Forum (NCF) to identify serious errors in medical treatment that should never happen (AHRQ 2019). Never events are classified as the following: surgery performed on the wrong body part, surgery performed on the wrong patient, and wrong surgery performed on the patient. These are rare events that are not considered payable by the insurance company. Because the healthcare provider made the error in treatment, he or she is expected to write off the cost of that treatment. It may not be charged to either the patient or the patient's third-party payer. To report a never event, the procedure code should be appended with the appropriate HCPCS modifier:

- PA, Surgical or other invasive procedure on wrong body part
- PB, Surgical or other invasive procedure on wrong patient
- PC, Wrong surgery or other invasive procedure on patient

Never events may happen in either the inpatient or the outpatient setting, and no matter the setting they are not reimbursable services. This includes services performed by other providers during the same visit that are related to the never event. However, after the patient has been discharged, any medically necessary services are covered by the patient's third-party payer, regardless of whether or not they are related to the never event.

Complete the exercises in There's a Code for That 11.2 to test your knowledge of surgical modifiers.

Surgical modifiers

Read the description of the surgical procedure and assign the appropriate modifier for the case (code only for the modifier, not the procedure performed).

1. Patient was sedated and prepped and colonoscope was inserted for screening examination. Ten minutes into the procedure, the patient began experiencing respiratory distress. Procedure was discontinued, and the colonoscope was removed. Patient was awoken and placed under observation.

   Modifier: _____

2. Surgeon destroyed three malignant lesions using cryosurgery: one on the left arm, one on right leg, and one on right foot.

   Modifier: _____

3. Dr. A performed an exploratory laparotomy on the patient, but was unable to perform the postoperative care and follow-up services, as he was called out to an emergency. Dr. B was called in to perform the postoperative care. Which modifier should be appended to Dr. B's service?

   Modifier: _____

4. In the ASC setting, a surgical procedure was discontinued due to extenuating medical circumstances after patient anesthesia was administered.

   Modifier: _____

5. Surgical procedure was begun but was quickly discontinued when it was discovered that the procedure had been started on the wrong patient.

   Modifier: _____

6. Complex surgical procedure performed by team of surgeons consisting of an oral maxillofacial surgeon, a plastic reconstructive surgeon and neurosurgeon.

   Modifier: _____

Coding for Surgical Services

The surgeries discussed in this section include those performed by general, transplant, plastic and reconstructive, and burn and trauma surgeons, and include skin, general, and transplant surgeries. Additional surgical procedures are discussed throughout the rest of this text within their respective specialties, such as orthopedic, female genital, neurological and spine, and such. Note, however, that the surgeries described in this chapter may be performed by many different types of surgical specialists. Additionally, some surgeries may be performed by primary care practitioners or urgent care providers (such as removal of lesions or wound repair).

These surgeries may be performed in several different settings—from inpatient hospital to outpatient hospital, as well as ambulatory surgical center. Some procedures (such as excision or destruction of lesions) may also be performed in the outpatient office setting. The setting in which the procedure is performed depends on the complexity of the surgery, the training of the performing provider, whether the patient needs

mass or tumor. Note that codes in category C50 do not include malignancies on the skin of the breast. Category C50, Malignant neoplasms of breast, includes codes for the deeper structures of the breast, rather than of the skin of the breast. This is an important distinction, as neoplasms of the skin are reported with different codes. In addition to the breast cancer code, report a supplementary code to identify the patient's estrogen receptor status, if known (Z17.0, Estrogen receptor positive status [ER+], or Z17.1, Estrogen receptor negative status [ER-]). If the patient has already undergone a mastectomy procedure, which removes the breast tissue, then the appropriate code from category Z90.1-, Acquired absence of breast and nipple, should be reported. For example, a patient that is status post right mastectomy would be coded with Z90.11, Acquired absence of right breast and nipple.

Key to Success

The difference between the skin of the breast and the deeper structures of the breast is an important distinction when coding, as it will change the subsection or chapter of code used to report the condition or the procedure. If the malignancy is on the *skin* of a structure or body part, this is different than it being *in* the body part. For example, the excision of a skin lesion on the leg is different than the excision of a lesion in the deep tissues of the leg.

   Rhinoplasties may also be performed by plastic and reconstructive surgeons. A rhinoplasty is the surgical repair or revision of the nose, either for cosmetic or functional and medical purposes. Codes for rhinoplasties are located in the Respiratory system subsection under the Repair category (30400–30630). Note that these procedures do involve the deeper structures of the nose, and not just the skin on the outside of the nose.

   Skin flap, graft, and tissue transfer procedures may be performed by dermatologists, wound specialists, or plastic and reconstructive surgeons. These procedures place a portion of skin or synthetic skin substitute over a damaged or diseased area of skin for repair. Skin replacement procedures include the surgical preparation of the graft site, which may include cleaning, debridement, extension of the wound surface, or removal of nonviable tissue. After the site is prepared, a skin graft is placed on the area for repair and anchored into place. Skin grafts and replacements may be temporary or permanent depending on the type of graft or wound and the patient's individual healing process.

   Depending on the circumstance, different graft substances may be used to complete the procedure. An autograft is a skin graft from a different site from the patient's own body. An allograft is a skin graft from tissue from a donor. A xenograft is a skin graft made from a different species (commonly pig skin). A homograft is a skin graft taken from a donor of the same species. Autografts and allografts are both homografts, except that an autograft is from the patient and an allograft is from a donor of the same species. Because allografts and xenografts are made from tissues that are recognized as foreign by the patient's body, they will eventually be rejected. Therefore, these two types of skin grafts are temporary and must eventually be replaced with an autograft.

   Coding for skin flaps and tissue transfers is complex and requires an understanding of the type of flap, graft, or tissue transfer; site of the procedure; size of the graft or skin replacement; and any additional procedures performed. They include the following:

   • Adjacent Tissue Transfer or Rearrangement (14000–14350). Tissue transfers or rearrangements are not technically skin grafts, although they do use a portion of the patient's own skin to cover a defect area. These procedures involve rearranging an area of tissue to cover an area that needs to be covered. This is done by incising the tissue in a specific pattern and stretching it over the defect. The size of the skin transfer or rearrangement is based on the size of the primary defect (for example, a 1.5 cm wound), plus the size of the secondary defect (a 3 cm advancement flap created), which are added to calculate the total skin defect size (1.5 cm primary defect + 3 cm secondary defect = 4.5 cm total defect size). Codes for adjacent tissue transfers *include* the excision of a defect or lesion, and the excision of a benign (11400–11446) or malignant (11600–11646) lesion should not be coded separately. Coding for these procedures relies on the site and size (measured in square centimeters) of the tissue transfer or rearrangement (see figure 11.21).

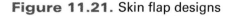

Figure 11.21. Skin flap designs

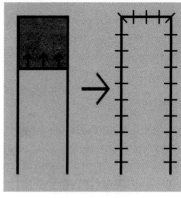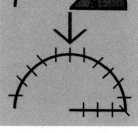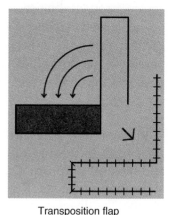

Advancement flap	Rotation flap	Transposition flap
Source: Taylornate 2011a.	Source: Taylornate 2011b.	Source: Taylornate 2011c.

- Skin Replacement Surgery (15002–15278). Skin replacement surgeries include free grafts of skin and skin substitutes, used to cover a defect in the skin. A free graft is one that has been completely removed from the surrounding tissue and does not remain connected to any type of blood supply but is completely excised from the donor site and placed on the site of the graft. Before a skin graft can be placed on a site, the site must be prepared to receive the graft. This surgical preparation of the area includes excision of an open wound, burn eschar, scar, or incisional release of scar contracture. In some cases, after the site is prepared, it may be closed using adjacent tissue transfer (described previously) or complex repair codes. Surgical preparation codes (15002–15005) are not to be used for debridement of tissue, wound management, or for the removal of nonviable tissue in a chronic wound (such as venous or diabetic wounds). Codes for autografts, tissue cultured autografts, and skin substitute grafts (15040–15278) identify the application of skin grafts. Code selection requires the identification of the type of graft used, such a split-thickness, dermal autograft, or full-thickness, as well as the site and size of the graft. A split-thickness graft is one in which the epidermis and only part of the dermis is used for the graft. A dermal autograft is a skin graft from a donor. A full-thickness skin graft is one in which the epidermis and the entire thickness of the dermis is included in the graft. Pay close attention to the add-on codes in this selection of codes. These codes may be added to the code for the primary procedure and should total the full size of the graft that was performed. Multiple add-on codes may be necessary. For example, if a patient received a 200 sq cm tissue cultured skin autograft of the trunk, the codes would be as follows:

- 15150, Tissue cultured skin autograft, trunk, arms, legs; *first 25 sq cm or less*
- 15151, Tissue cultured skin autograft, trunk, arms, legs; *additional 1 sq cm to 75 sq cm*
- 15152, Tissue cultured skin autograft, trunk, arms, legs; *each additional 100 sq cm, or each additional 1% of body area of infants and children, or part thereof*

Code 15150 accounts for the first 25 sq cm; 15151 accounts for the next 75 sq cm, which together with the previous code equals 100 sq cm. The last code, 15152, accounts for the remaining 100 sq cm. So, the correct reporting of a 200 sq cm tissue cultured skin autograft would be 15150, 15151, and 15152 (25 cm + 75 cm + 100 cm = 200 cm).

- Flaps (Skin and/or Deep Tissues) (15570–15738). Skin and deep tissue flaps identify planned, staged procedures that may be completed over a period of time. This is because either the procedure is delayed, or the tissue is formed into a tube and kept connected to a blood supply and slowly walked to the recipient site. This allows the skin graft to stay viable as it is slowly maneuvered into place over a period of time. Codes for skin and deep tissue grafts are identified based on the service performed—either the formation of the graft (direct or tubed pedicle), delay or sectioning of the flap, or transfer of the flap. When assigning these codes, pay attention to the type of tissue used in the procedure and the site of the graft. Codes identify the recipient site, not the donor site.

- Other Flaps and Grafts (15740–15777). These codes identify a range of other skin flaps and grafts that do not fit into any other category. For example, 15758, Free fascial flap with microvascular anastomosis, is a free graft (not attached to a blood supply) of fascia connected at the graft site with microvascular anastomosis. Code selection requires identification of the type of graft as well as any additional services performed.

Burn Surgeries and Wound Treatments

Wounds may be complex, non-healing, chronic, or necrotizing; and wound treatment surgeries and procedures are closely monitored, staged services that may require various elements before the wound is ultimately healed. Procedures to treat burns, open wounds, and chronic wounds may include repair or grafting, as discussed previously, or other special procedures like debridement, burn and pressure ulcer treatment, and wound care management services.

- **Debridement** is the removal of dead, diseased, infected, or otherwise nonviable tissue from a wound to improve the healing ability of the area. After debridement of a wound, only healthy tissue is left remaining, and bandaged or treated to promote healing. Codes for debridement (11000–11047) rely not only on the size of the wound, but on the depth of the debridement. When coding for a debridement, select the code for the deepest level of tissue removed during the debridement session such as skin, subcutaneous tissue muscle fascia, muscle, or bone. Note that some of the debridement codes report a specific site or type of skin condition, while others do not. Debridement of nails are reported with codes 11720 and 11721, depending on the number of nails debrided. Note that these debridement codes are not to be used for the debridement of burn wounds.

- Active Wound Care Management codes (97597–97610) report debridement of dermal or epidermal tissue only, as well as wound care procedures including negative pressure wound therapy services. These codes are not to be used with debridement codes from the Integumentary subsection (11042–11047) nor are they to be used to report the debridement of burn wounds.

- Burns, Local Treatment codes (16000–16036) refer to the treatment of the burned surface only, and include the application of materials such as dressings to the wound. These codes do not, however, include any other necessary related medical services such as E/M encounters or skin grafting or replacement (both are reported separately). Code selection requires the identification of the percentage of body surface involved in the burn and the depth of the burn. The CPT code book relies on the Lund-Browder Classification for burn percentages, as discussed in chapter 10 (Urgent Care and Emergency Department Services). Burn debridement codes are classified as first-degree, second-degree (partial thickness), or as an escharotomy (to treat full-thickness, third-degree burns).

- Pressure Ulcers (Decubitus Ulcers). These codes (15920–15999) identify the treatment of pressure, or decubitus, ulcers. Code selection relies on the site of the ulcer and additional removal such as an ostectomy (removal of bone) and type of closure (when identified). Note that these codes are only to be used with pressure ulcers and not with wounds identified as non-pressure or venous ulcers. Treatment of non-pressure ulcers, such as venous ulcers, is coded with the appropriate debridement, skin closure, or skin flap code, as applicable.

Diagnostic Coding for Burns and Skin Ulcers

Diagnostic codes for repairs of the skin should detail the area and extent of the wound, burn, or ulcer. Diagnostic coding for burns is discussed in chapter 10 (Urgent Care and Emergency Department Services). Remember, burn codes identify the *site* of the burn, the *extent* of the burn, the *depth* of the burn, and the *agent* that caused the burn.

A **skin ulcer** is an open wound on the skin that may be caused by infection, pressure, or venous problems. When coding for ulcers of the skin, coders must be able to identify that the ulcer is indeed on the skin, and not in any underlying structures or organs. For example, a stomach ulcer or corneal ulcer are both located in those organs (the stomach and the cornea of the eye, respectively). There are two main types of skin ulcers—pressure and non-pressure. A **pressure ulcer**, also known as a bedsore or decubitus ulcer, is an ulcer that has occurred on the skin because of prolonged pressure on the skin, which causes reduced blood flow and oxygen to the tissue, and ultimately death of the tissue in that area. They most commonly develop on areas with an underlying bone such as heels, ankles, hips, and tailbone (see figure 11.22.) A **non-pressure ulcer** is an ulcer on the skin caused by anything other than pressure, such as one caused by atherosclerosis of the extremities (and loss of blood circulation), chronic venous hypertension, diabetes mellitus, postthrombotic syndrome, postphlebitic syndrome, or varicose veins. They are often chronic problems that are difficult to heal.

Diagnostic coding for skin ulcers requires the healthcare provider to identify the ulcer as either pressure or non-pressure. Codes further identify the site of the ulcer such as heel, ankle, or thigh, as well as the laterality of the condition. Pressure ulcers are located in category L89, Pressure ulcer. For pressure ulcers, the severity of the ulcer should be identified by stage or depth, as follows:

- Stage 1: skin changes limited to persistent focal edema
- Stage 2: with abrasion, blister, partial thickness skin loss involving epidermis and/or dermis

- Stage 3: full-thickness skin loss involving damage or necrosis of subcutaneous tissue
- Stage 4: with necrosis of soft tissues through to underlying muscle, tendon, or bone
- Pressure-induced deep-tissue damage

Figure 11.22. Pressure ulcer sites

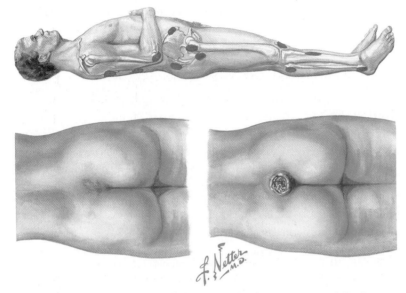

First Image: Common sites of pressure ulcers, which occur on areas with underlying bone.
Second image: Inflammation around the sacrum. Third image: A sacral pressure ulcer.
Source: ©2017. Used with permission of Elsevier. All rights reserved.

In some cases, an ulcer cannot be staged, such as when it is covered with a skin graft or covered with eschar tissue. In this case, the coder should report the *unstageable* option. Any associated gangrene should also be identified using code I96, Gangrene, not elsewhere classified. The gangrene code should be sequenced before the code for the pressure ulcer.

Non-pressure ulcers are located in category L97, Non-pressure chronic ulcer of lower limb, not elsewhere classified, and L98.4, Non-pressure chronic ulcer of skin, not elsewhere classified. Coding for non-pressure ulcers is similar to coding for pressure ulcers due to the fact that codes identify the site of the ulcer, the severity of the ulcer in terms of depth, and whether the condition presents with or without necrosis:

- Limited to breakdown of skin
- With fat layer exposed
- With necrosis of muscle
- With necrosis of bone
- Muscle involvement without evidence of necrosis
- Bone involvement without evidence of necrosis
- Other specified severity
- Unspecified severity

Figure 11.23. OGCR I.C.12

---

12. Chapter 12: Diseases of the Skin and Subcutaneous Tissue (L00-L99)

a. Pressure ulcer stage codes

1) Pressure ulcer stages

Codes in category L89, Pressure ulcer, identify the site and stage of the pressure ulcer.

The ICD-10-CM classifies pressure ulcer stages based on severity, which is designated by stages 1-4, **deep tissue pressure injury**, unspecified stage and unstageable.

Assign as many codes from category L89 as needed to identify all the pressure ulcers the patient has, if applicable.

See Section I.B.14 for pressure ulcer stage documentation by clinicians other than patient's provider.

2) Unstageable pressure ulcers

Assignment of the code for unstageable pressure ulcer (L89.--0) should be based on the clinical documentation. These codes are used for pressure ulcers whose stage cannot be clinically determined (e.g., the ulcer is covered by eschar or has been treated with a skin or muscle graft) and pressure ulcers that are documented as deep tissue injury but not documented as due to trauma. This code should not be confused with the codes for unspecified stage (L89.--9). When there is no documentation regarding the stage of the pressure ulcer, assign the appropriate code for unspecified stage (L89.--9).

3) Documented pressure ulcer stage

Assignment of the pressure ulcer stage code should be guided by clinical documentation of the stage or documentation of the terms found in the Alphabetic Index. For clinical terms describing the stage that are not found in the Alphabetic Index, and there is no documentation of the stage, the provider should be queried.

4) Patients admitted with pressure ulcers documented as healed

No code is assigned if the documentation states that the pressure ulcer is completely healed **at the time of admission.**

5) Patients admitted with pressure ulcers documented as healing

Pressure ulcers described as healing should be assigned the appropriate pressure ulcer stage code based on the documentation in the medical record. If the documentation does not provide information about the stage of the healing pressure ulcer, assign the appropriate code for unspecified stage.

If the documentation is unclear as to whether the patient has a current (new) pressure ulcer or if the patient is being treated for a healing pressure ulcer, query the provider.

For ulcers that were present on admission but healed at the time of discharge, assign the code for the site and stage of the pressure ulcer at the time of admission.

6) Patient admitted with pressure ulcer evolving into another stage during the admission

If a patient is admitted to an inpatient hospital with a pressure ulcer at one stage and it progresses to a higher stage, two separate codes should be assigned: one code for the site and stage of the ulcer on admission and a second code for the same ulcer site and the highest stage reported during the stay.

7) Pressure-induced deep tissue damage

For pressure-induced deep tissue damage or deep tissue pressure injury, assign only the appropriate code for pressure-induced deep tissue damage (L89.--6).

b. Non-Pressure Chronic Ulcers

1) Patients admitted with non-pressure ulcers documented as healed

No code is assigned if the documentation states that the non-pressure ulcer is completely healed **at the time of admission**.

2) Patients admitted with non-pressure ulcers documented as healing

Non-pressure ulcers described as healing should be assigned the appropriate non-pressure ulcer code based on the documentation in the medical record. If the documentation does not provide information about the severity of the healing non-pressure ulcer, assign the appropriate code unspecified severity.

If the documentation is unclear as to whether the patient has a current (new) non-pressure ulcer or if the patient is being treated for a healing non-pressure ulcer, query the provider.

For ulcers that were present on admission but healed at the time of discharge, assign the code for the site and severity of the non-pressure ulcer at the time of admission.

3) Patient admitted with non-pressure ulcer that progresses to another severity level during the admission

If a patient is admitted to an inpatient hospital with a non-pressure ulcer at one severity level and it progresses to a higher severity level, two separate codes should be assigned; one code for the site and severity level of the ulcer on admission and a second code for the same ulcer site and the highest severity level reported during the stay.

See Section I.B.14 for pressure ulcer stage documentation by clinicians other than patient's provider.

Source: CMS 2019c.

The underlying cause of the ulcer should also be documented with causal language—for example, "non-pressure ulcer of the right heel *due to* atherosclerosis of the lower extremities." This clearly shows that the ulcer is a result of the atherosclerosis. In this case, two codes should be selected: one for the underlying cause (atherosclerosis of the extremities), and one for the non-pressure ulcer (category L97 code).

Note that most skin ulcer codes are HCC codes, and so the documentation of these conditions should be as specific as possible, as should code selection. See figure 11.23 for the OGCR related to coding pressure ulcers.

Complete the exercises in There's a Code for That 11.4 to practice assigning diagnosis and procedure codes for skin flaps and wound treatments.

Diagnostic and procedural coding for skin flaps and wound treatments

11.4

There's a Code for That

Read the description of the procedure and assign the appropriate ICD-10-CM and/or CPT codes.

1. Excision of 2.5 cm benign nevus on the anterior abdomen of a 54-year-old male patient. Wound site covered with 5.0 cm advancement flap.

   CPT code: _____

   ICD-10-CM code: _____

2. Debridement of second degree burn on left lower leg (8 percent of body surface).

   CPT code: _____

   ICD-10-CM code: _____

3. Excision of stage 4 sacral pressure ulcer with involvement of bone. Partial ostectomy performed and excision site was covered with skin flap closure.

   CPT code: _____

   ICD-10-CM code: _____

General Surgery

General surgery is a medical specialty that focuses on surgical procedures all over the human body, with an emphasis on the abdominal area, including procedures on the esophagus, stomach, small and large intestines, liver, pancreas, and the gallbladder and bile ducts. General surgeons may also perform surgeries on the thyroid gland, peripheral vascular conditions, hernias, soft tissue and traumatic injuries, and conditions affecting the skin and breast. The exact procedures that a general surgeon performs depend on his or her level of expertise, interest, and regional resources. For example, a general surgeon working in the same vicinity as a surgical endocrinologist is less likely to perform a thyroidectomy than a general surgeon working in a region in which there are no other surgical specialists more qualified to perform the procedure.

Coding for general surgery requires an overall knowledge of surgical procedures and how to report them with CPT codes. Furthermore, depending on the specialized training or interests of the general surgeon, he or she might specialize in certain types of procedures. Typically, general surgeons focus on surgeries of the abdomen, including appendectomy, cholecystectomy, herniorrhaphy, and other procedures performed on the mediastinum and diaphragm and the abdomen, peritoneum, and omentum.

Mediastinum and Diaphragm

The mediastinum is the area in the thorax in between the lungs. It is the compartment that contains the heart and great vessels, esophagus, trachea, phrenic and cardiac nerves, thoracic duct, thymus, and chest lymph nodes (see figure 11.24). Procedures on the mediastinum are limited, as this structure is a compartment for other organs in the chest. They are located in the Mediastinum and Diaphragm subsection (39000–39499) and include mediastinotomy (an incision into the mediastinum for exploration or drainage), resection (excision) of a mediastinal cyst or tumor, and mediastinoscopy with biopsy (when performed). Note that because the mediastinum is located in the thoracic cavity, in close vicinity to the heart and lungs, procedures on this area are more likely to be performed by a thoracic surgeon.

Figure 11.24. Mediastinum and diaphragm

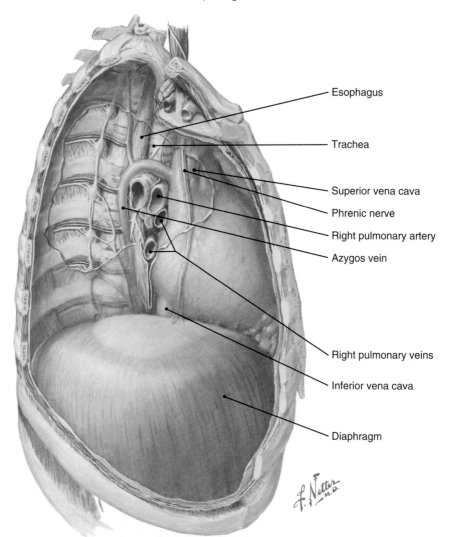

Esophagus

Trachea

Superior vena cava

Phrenic nerve

Right pulmonary artery

Azygos vein

Right pulmonary veins

Inferior vena cava

Diaphragm

The **diaphragm** is a muscle that lies underneath the thoracic cavity, separating the heart and lungs from the abdominal contents. This muscle also performs an important function in breathing as it contracts and expands, allowing the lungs to draw in and expel air. Procedures performed on the diaphragm are limited as well. They are located in the Mediastinum and Diaphragm subsection (39000–39599). They include repair of lacerations or diaphragmatic hernias, imbrication for eventration (a procedure to reshape an abnormally elevated diaphragm), and resection of diaphragmatic tumors.

Appendectomy and Appendicitis

Appendicitis is a problem that is commonly treated surgically by removing the appendix, a procedure often performed by general surgeons in the inpatient hospital setting. **Appendectomy** (removal of the appendix) codes are straightforward:

- 44950, Appendectomy. This procedure is performed on a patient with **appendicitis**, an inflammation of the appendix. If left untreated, an inflamed appendix may rupture, causing a dangerous infection of the peritoneal cavity. This code may also be used to report an **incidental appendectomy**, which is performed in addition to a primary procedure in the abdomen. For example, a surgeon performing a **cholecystectomy** (removal of the gallbladder) may choose to also perform an incidental appendectomy at the time of the primary procedure (the cholecystectomy) as a preventive procedure to prevent future appendicitis and the need for another surgery. Incidental appendectomies are usually not coded, as they are minor procedures. However, if it is necessary to report an incidental appendectomy that was performed along with a primary procedure, append modifier -52, Reduced services, to the code for the appendectomy and the code for the primary procedure.

- 44955, Appendectomy; *when done for indicated purpose at time of other procedure (not as separate procedure)*. In some instances, when a surgeon is performing an abdominal procedure, he or she may notice that the appendix is inflamed or calcified, and perform an appendectomy at the time of the primary procedure. In this case, the appendix is not removed as an incidental procedure but rather due to an *"indicated purpose"* at the time of the primary procedure. Note that this is an add-on code that should be used in addition to the code for the primary procedure. When reporting this procedure code, the diagnosis code for the "indicated purpose" is needed to identify that the appendectomy was medically necessary.

- 44960, Appendectomy; *for ruptured appendix with abscess or generalized peritonitis*. This appendectomy code is to report the removal of an appendix that has already ruptured or resulted in generalized **peritonitis** (infection within the peritoneal cavity).

- 44970, Laparoscopy, surgical, appendectomy. This code should be used for an appendectomy that was performed laparoscopically and may be performed in the hospital outpatient setting.

Diagnosis codes for conditions of the appendix are located in categories K35 to K38, Diseases of the Appendix. Codes should identify the condition as Acute appendicitis (K35), Other appendicitis (K36), or Unspecified appendicitis (K37). Codes for acute appendicitis further identify if the appendix has ruptured and resulted in peritonitis. If peritonitis is present, coders should identify the peritonitis as either generalized or localized peritonitis. The code for unspecified appendicitis (K37) should only be used when the documentation does not identify the appendicitis as either acute (K35) or chronic/recurrent (K36). Additional codes for diseases of the appendix (category K38) identify conditions of the appendix, which may or may not require removal of the appendix, such as hyperplasia, diverticulum, and fistula of the appendix.

Cholecystectomy, Cholelithiasis, and Cholecystitis

Cholecystitis is the inflammation of the gallbladder and is usually related to a complication of stones in the gallbladder—a condition called cholelithiasis. A **cholecystectomy** is a procedure performed to remove the gallbladder, commonly done in the inpatient setting. Codes for cholecystectomies identify the type of removal (laparoscopic or open/excisional) and any additional procedures performed along with the removal of the gallbladder.

- Laparoscopic procedures (47562–47579) are less invasive procedures that involve the use of thin instruments inserted through small incisions, aided by the use of a video camera, and may be performed in the outpatient hospital setting.

- Open/Excisional procedures (47600–47715) are more invasive and are likely to be performed in the inpatient hospital setting.

Note that many of these code descriptions include **cholangiography**, which is an examination of the bile ducts used to identify an obstruction. A cholangiography may be performed in addition to a cholecystectomy to detect any further obstructions that may require an additional procedure.

Obstructions in the gallbladder and bile ducts are commonly caused by **cholelithiasis**, the presence of gallstones. **Choledocholithiasis** is the presence of one of more gallstones in the common bile duct. If the bile duct is obstructed by the gallstones, it may result in **cholecystitis**—an inflammation of the gallbladder. This is a painful condition that may require surgical removal of the gallbladder (cholecystectomy), as described previously. See figure 11.25 for an illustration of both conditions.

Figure 11.25. Cholelithiasis and choledocholithiasis

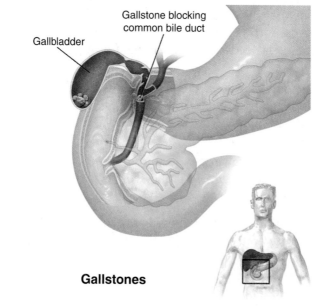

Gallstones

Source: BruceBlaus 2015.

Diagnosis codes for gallstone and biliary tract conditions (K80, K81, K82, K83) identify the condition as either the presence of calculi (lithiases), including the location of the calculus (the gallbladder or the bile ducts), or that the gallstones have resulted in an inflammation of the gallbladder (cholecystitis). Cholecystitis may also present without the presence of gallstones.

Cholelithiasis (K80) codes require careful reading of the components included in the codes (see figure 11.26). Reporting the correct code relies on identification of the following:

- *The location of the stone*, either the gallbladder, bile ducts, or both the gallbladder and bile ducts.

- *The presence or absence of cholecystitis or cholangitis* (inflammation of the bile ducts). Identify whether the condition presents with cholecystitis, without cholecystitis, with cholangitis, without cholangitis, or without cholangitis and cholecystitis. Note that if the patient has cholecystitis due to cholelithiasis, documentation should specify that the patient has both conditions. If the patient has acute cholecystitis without cholelithiasis, report code K81.0.

- *The acuity of the condition*. If cholecystitis or cholangitis is present, it should be identified as acute, chronic, or acute and chronic.

- *The presence or absence of obstruction* (with or without obstruction).

Figure 11.26. Cholelithiasis code components

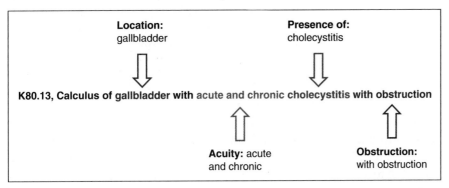

Abdomen, Peritoneum, and Omentum, and Herniorrhaphy

The last heading in the Gastrointestinal subsection in the CPT code book includes codes for procedures performed on the Abdomen, Peritoneum, and Omentum (49000–49999). Unlike the rest of the procedures in the gastrointestinal subsection, these codes identify procedures that are performed on the structures within the abdomen or on the abdomen itself. They include exploratory, drainage, and lavage of the peritoneal cavity; biopsy; excision and destruction of tumors within the peritoneal cavity; removal of peritoneal foreign bodies and insertion and removal of devices or obstructive material; and herniorrhaphies (repair of hernias).

There are four components to repair of hernia procedure codes (49491–49659), for hernioplasty, herniorrhaphy, and herniotomy). Note that not all of these components are present in every hernia code.

- *Type.* The type of hernia identifies the area or structures involved in the herniation. They include inguinal, lumbar, femoral, incisional/ventral, epigastric, umbilical, and spigelian.
- *Recurrence.* Hernias may be identified as either initial (the first instance of the hernia) or recurrent (the hernia has recurred more than once in the same location).
- *Clinical presentation.* The clinical presentation of the hernia identifies it as either reducible (meaning that the structure can be easily moved back into its original location), or incarcerated/strangulated (meaning that the structure cannot be moved back into its original location). Incarcerated or strangulated hernias may be dangerous, leading to restriction of blood flow, death of the structure, or gangrene.
- *Age of the patient.* Some hernia codes differ based on the age of the patient. If the code description does not describe the patient's age, then this component will not change the code selection.

Note that codes for the repair of diaphragmatic hernias (39503–39541) are located in the diaphragm subsection of the CPT code book.

Diagnosis codes for hernias are in categories K40 to K46 and contain many of the same components of hernia procedure codes.

- *Type of hernia.* These include inguinal (K40), femoral (K41), umbilical (K42), ventral (K43), diaphragmatic (K44), other (K45), and unspecified abdominal hernia (K46).
- *Laterality.* Inguinal and femoral hernias should be identified as either unilateral (one sided) or bilateral (both sides). Note that codes for unilateral hernias do not specify the side of the hernia, just that it presents unilaterally.
- *Recurrence.* Hernias should be specified as either recurrent or not. If the documentation does not specify that the hernia is recurrent, then select the code for the "not specified as recurrent" option.
- *Presence of obstruction.* Codes identify whether the hernia is obstructed or not, as with or without obstruction. Note that in procedural coding for hernia repairs the clinical terminology is incarcerated or strangulated, whereas in diagnostic coding the terminology is obstructed. They should be used for the same condition.
- *Presence of gangrene.* The presence of gangrene should also be identified. Note that gangrene may present with or without obstruction.

When coding for hernias and hernia repairs, it is important to make sure that the hernia diagnosis code matches the procedure, so that it fully supports the medical necessity for the service. For example, if the coder selected diagnosis code K40.21, Bilateral inguinal hernia, without obstruction or gangrene, recurrent, with procedure code 49555, Repair recurrent femoral hernia; reducible, the service would be considered not medically necessary and would not be paid. This is because the types of hernia do not match; the diagnosis code identifies the condition as an inguinal hernia, while the procedure code identifies the hernia as a femoral hernia.

Complete the exercises in There's a Code for That 11.5 to practice identifying the procedure and diagnosis codes for general surgery procedures.

Coding for general surgery

11.5

Read the description of the procedure and assign the appropriate ICD-10-CM and/or CPT codes.

There's a Code for That

1. Herniorrhaphy with hydrocelectomy performed on 4-year-old male patient with initial, reducible inguinal hernia.

   CPT code: _____

   ICD-10-CM code: _____

2. Cholecystectomy without cholangiography performed laparoscopically on 30-year-old female patient with cholelithiasis and acute cholecystitis without obstruction.

   CPT code: _____

   ICD-10-CM code: _____

3. Laparoscopic appendectomy completed on a 60-year-old male patient with ruptured appendix with localized peritonitis.

   CPT code: _____

   ICD-10-CM code: _____

Transplant Surgery

Transplant surgeries may be performed by a healthcare specialist trained in a specific field of medicine (such as a cardiovascular surgeon), or one who specializes in transplants specifically (a cardiac transplant specialist). Any type of transplant is a complex, major procedure, and as such is performed in the inpatient hospital setting. Organs and tissues that can be transplanted include the heart, lungs, intestines, islet cells (from the pancreas), kidneys, liver, pancreas, corneas, thymus, stomach, testis, bone, skin, stem cells, and hands. However, some of these procedures are rare (such as hand transplants) and performed only in specialized settings with trained surgeons and clinical technicians. In these infrequent cases, it may be necessary to use the unlisted services code to report the procedure performed, or a combination of codes to report each service performed.

Transplants that have a specific set of transplant codes in the CPT code book include the heart (33927–33945), intestines (included in the range 44100–44160), liver (47133–47147), lung (32850–32856), pancreas (48550–48556), and kidney (50300–50380). When coding for transplant procedures, there are three components of the procedure that should be clearly identified and reported for the service performed.

- *Removal of the donated organ.* This includes the harvesting of the organ from the donor. In some cases, the donor of the organ is a cadaver donor (brain dead patient from whom organs are being harvested), or the donor may be a living donor (when the organ being donated is one that can be harvested from a living patient).
- *Backbench work to prepare the organ.* Backbench work involves the preparation of the organ for transplantation, including dissection of the organ from soft tissues and preparation of the valves and vessels for transplantation.

- *Transplantation of the organ.* Transplantation of the donated organ may include the removal of the recipient's organ(s) prior to the transplantation, or not. Once the recipient area is prepared for the organ transplantation, then the transplantation code identifies the placement of the organ in the patient, with or without the removal of the recipient's organ.

The coder should report only the service that was performed by his or her provider. For example, if the provider performed a cadaver donor pneumonectomy (removal of the lungs), and then the lungs were transported to another facility for the transplant, performed by a different surgeon, then the coder would only report the code for the removal of the donated organ, 32850, Donor pneumonectomy(s) (including cold preservation), from cadaver donor.

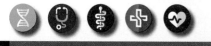

Putting It All Together: Coding for Surgical Services

When coding for surgical services, keep in mind that multiple procedure codes may be necessary to report the service fully. Do not code for services that are included in the surgical package or the code description for the primary procedure. See figure 11.27 for steps to coding for surgical services.

Figure 11.27. Steps to coding for surgical services

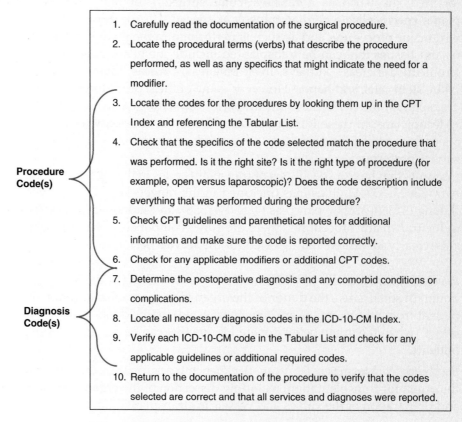

1. Carefully read the documentation of the surgical procedure.
2. Locate the procedural terms (verbs) that describe the procedure performed, as well as any specifics that might indicate the need for a modifier.

Procedure Code(s)

3. Locate the codes for the procedures by looking them up in the CPT Index and referencing the Tabular List.
4. Check that the specifics of the code selected match the procedure that was performed. Is it the right site? Is it the right type of procedure (for example, open versus laparoscopic)? Does the code description include everything that was performed during the procedure?
5. Check CPT guidelines and parenthetical notes for additional information and make sure the code is reported correctly.
6. Check for any applicable modifiers or additional CPT codes.

Diagnosis Code(s)

7. Determine the postoperative diagnosis and any comorbid conditions or complications.
8. Locate all necessary diagnosis codes in the ICD-10-CM Index.
9. Verify each ICD-10-CM code in the Tabular List and check for any applicable guidelines or additional required codes.
10. Return to the documentation of the procedure to verify that the codes selected are correct and that all services and diagnoses were reported.

The following vignette demonstrates how to select the appropriate diagnosis and procedural codes for a surgical service.

Robert is coding for a surgical service performed in the inpatient setting. He reads through the procedural note as follows to find the correct diagnosis and procedure codes:

Procedure: *Excision subcutaneous nodules anterior pelvic wall*

Procedure in detail: *The patient was met in the pre-operative holding area and the surgical site and the procedure were confirmed. The patient was then brought to the operating room and positioned in the supine position on the operating table. After patient induction of general anesthesia, the lower abdomen was prepped and draped in a sterile fashion. Local anesthetic was infiltrated into the dermis of the C-section scar. The entire scar was incised. Palpation revealed 3 masses in the subcutaneous fat. They were excised in toto using Bovie cautery, as follows: 1 cm soft tissue tumor, 2 cm soft tissue tumor, 1.5 cm soft tissue tumor. The masses did not invade the anterior rectus fascia. Electrocautery was used for hemostasis. Sponge and needle counts were confirmed. The wound was irrigated with saline and hemostasis was confirmed. Scarpa's fascia was approximated using 2-0 vicryl. 3-0 vicryl was used to approximate the deep side of the dermis. 4-0 nylon Monocryl was used in a subcuticular fashion to close the incision. The incision was dressed with Dermabond. The patient was extubated and transferred to the recovery room having tolerated the procedure well.*

Robert first asks himself: What did the doctor do? In this case the provider excised three soft tissue tumors from the anterior pelvic wall. Robert searches for the Main term Excision *in the Main Index, then finds the subterm* tumor, *and then* abdominal wall, *which leads him to the code range 22900 to 22903. He then refers to this code range and selects code 22902, Excision, tumor, soft tissue of abdominal wall, subcutaneous; less than 3 cm. Because there were three tumors excised, each of which were less than 3 cm, he reports this code three times, as follows:*

- *22902 × 3, Excision, tumor, soft tissue of abdominal wall, subcutaneous; less than 3 cm*

Now that Robert has the procedure code, Robert asks himself: Why did the doctor do it? In this case, the indication for the procedure was for subcutaneous nodules of the anterior pelvic wall. Robert searches the Main Index of the ICD-10-CM code book for Tumor, *but cannot find a subterm for abdominal wall. Instead, he refers to the cross reference to* see also Neoplasm, by site, *and refers to the entry for benign neoplasm of the abdominal wall in the Table of Neoplasms. He selects the following code:*

- *D23.5, Other benign neoplasm of sin and trunk*

Now that he has both the procedure and diagnosis codes for the service, Robert rechecks the documentation to make sure he has coded everything and reports the chosen codes for the surgery.

Case Study | **Excision of Benign Lesions**

PATIENT: Ryan Curtis

PROCEDURE: Lesion excision, removal of skin tags on neck

INDICATIONS: Benign neoplasm of skin, Acrochordon

PROCEDURE NOTE:
Verified correct patient and sites. Sites marked, Consent form signed, 3 areas on his back were anesthetized locally with 2% lidocaine with epinephrine, prepped and draped in sterile fashion. Following verification of anesthetic effect, lesions were removed in their entirety in elliptical fashion. Lesions were as follows: left upper back 11 mm lesion excised. Wound was closed with a single subdermal stitch of 4-0 Vicryl, +3 superficial simple sutures with Prolene. Left mid-back 13 mm lesion excised. Wound was closed with single subdermal stitch of 4-0 Vicryl, +3 subdermal simple sutures with 3-0 Prolene. Left lower back 13 mm lesion excised. Wound was closed single subdermal stitch of 4-0 Vicryl, +3 subdermal simple sutures with 3-0 Prolene. Good hemostasis. No complications. Wounds cleaned and dressed with bacitracin, Telfa, and Tegaderm. Aftercare instructions given, follow-up for suture removal in 14 days. Follow up sooner if develop signs/symptoms of a wound infection. Specimens forwarded to the lab for pathological analysis. Patient will be contacted with results.

Eight pedunculated acrochordons removed from around the base of the neck. Skin cleaned with alcohol pad. Acrochordons grasped with smooth forceps and removed sharply at the base with scissors. Band-aids applied.

ESIMATED BLOOD LOSS: Minimal

COMPLICATIONS: None, patient tolerated the procedure well

SIGNED: Dr. Topher Crawley, MD

Use the following steps to select the appropriate codes for the case study.

1. Read through the case study and answer the question: *What did the doctor do?* In this case study, identify the name of the procedure.

   _____

   _____

2. Now that you have identified the procedure, locate the code for the procedure in the CPT code book.

   a. Search the Index for the procedure and search through the options.

b. Refer to the codes listed in the Tabular section and identify the correct code range.

_____

_____

c. In the listing of codes, check for any guidelines, important definitions, or parenthetical notes. Select the appropriate codes and list them here.

_____

_____

d. Are there any additional procedures that need to be added to identify all of the procedures performed? If yes, follow the previous steps to identify the codes for the additional procedures.

_____

_____

e. Are there any modifiers that need to be added to identify any special circumstance surrounding the procedure(s)? If yes, refer to Appendix A of the CPT code book to assign all appropriate modifiers.

_____

_____

3. Now that the procedure(s) and modifier(s) have been identified, review the case study and answer the following question: *Why did the doctor do it?*

_____

_____

4. Now that you have the name of the patient's diagnoses, search the ICD-10-CM code book for the correct codes for these conditions. Follow these steps for each of the diagnoses identified.

a. Search the Main Index for the name of each condition and search through any applicable subterms and cross-references to locate the appropriate code.

i. _____

_____

ii. _____

_____

b. Verify the code in the Tabular List. Locate the code identified previously in the Tabular Listing of codes and refer to any applicable guidelines, notes, and symbols. Does the code selected correctly identify the patient's condition? If yes, list the code here.

i. _____

_____

ii. _____

_____

c. Check the procedure note and ICD-10-CM guidelines and conventions to determine the correct sequencing of the diagnosis codes, if applicable. Correctly sequence the diagnosis codes.

_____

_____

5. Now that the procedure and diagnosis codes have been identified, list them on the CMS-1500 form. Be sure to correctly link the procedure and diagnosis codes. Remember to add the number of units as necessary.

21. DIAGNOSIS OR NATURE OF ILLNESS OR INJURY Relate A-L to service line below (24E)			ICD Ind.	22. RESUBMISSION CODE
A.	B.	C.	D.	
E.	F.	G.	H.	23. PRIOR AUTHORIZATION NU
I.	J.	K.	L.	

24. A. DATE(S) OF SERVICE		B. PLACE OF SERVICE	C. EMG	D. PROCEDURES, SERVICES, OR SUPPLIES (Explain Unusual Circumstances) CPT/HCPCS · MODIFIER	E. DIAGNOSIS POINTER	F. $ CHARGES	G. DAYS OR UNITS
From MM DD YY	To MM DD YY						
1							
2							
3							

End-of-Chapter Content

Instructions: Indicate whether the following statements are true or false (T or F). For false statements, rewrite the statement on the line below to make the statement true.

1. An invasive procedure rarely involves breaking the skin in order to perform the procedure.

_____

_____

2. An inpatient is one that has been formally admitted to a hospital.

_____

_____

3. POS code 21 would be used to report services performed in the inpatient hospital setting.

_____

_____

4. Outpatients in a hospital must be confined to the outpatient unit and may never stay in the main building of the hospital.

_____

_____

5. E/M codes 99201 to 99215 should be used for encounters in the ASC setting.

_____

_____

6. A minor surgical procedure typically includes a 90-day global period.

_____

_____

7. Surgical procedures are found in the Medicine section of the CPT code book.

_____

_____

8. An excision is an open procedure.

_____

_____

9. A therapeutic procedure is one that is performed to treat a diagnosis.

_____

_____

10. Modifier -47 should be appended to the code for an anesthesia procedure that was performed by an anesthesiologist.

_____

_____

Instructions: Match the terms with the appropriate descriptions.

1. _____ Incision

2. _____ Excision

3. _____ Introduction

4. _____ Removal

5. _____ Repair

6. _____ Destruction

7. _____ Endoscopy

8. _____ Laparoscopy

9. _____ Transplantation

10. _____ Manipulation

A. The insertion of a device, object, or substance into a body part or organ

B. Procedure to destroy tissue, also known as ablation

C. Taking out a device, object, or substance from a body part or area

D. Manually moving a body part into its original location or into another location

E. A cut made on a body part or organ

F. Procedure performed to return an organ or body part to its original function, to improve function, or to improve cosmetic appearance

G. Procedure that uses a lighted scope, inserted through incisions into the body to perform a diagnostic or therapeutic procedure

H. The surgical removal of an organ, body tissue, lesion, or other body part or foreign object

I. Removal of a damaged, diseased, or nonfunctioning organ and replacing it with a donated organ

J. Procedure performed with the aid of an endoscope inserted through a natural opening or stoma

Instructions: Choose the best answer.

1. Which of the following is a noninvasive, nonsurgical procedure?
   a. Cryosurgery
   b. Organ transplant
   c. Nebulizer treatment
   d. Internal organ repair

2. In which setting would a major or risky surgery be performed?
   a. Inpatient hospital
   b. Outpatient hospital
   c. Ambulatory surgical center
   d. Outpatient office

3. Which set of E/M codes are used for hospital inpatient E/M encounters?
   a. 99201–99215
   b. 99217–99226
   c. 99221–99239
   d. E/M services are not billed for inpatients

4. What does ASC stand for?
   a. Acute setting for care
   b. Ambulatory surgical care
   c. Ambulatory surgical center
   d. Acute surgery center

5. Which of the following is a facility in which the patient would remain overnight?
   a. Urgent care clinic
   b. Ambulatory surgical center
   c. Inpatient hospital
   d. Office

6. Which of the following rules apply to procedures performed at an ASC?
   a. The procedure cannot pose a significant safety risk to the patient
   b. The procedure may be emergent or life threatening in nature
   c. The procedure must involve an overnight stay for the patient
   d. The procedure may be performed anywhere, including in the physician's office

7. How many days are included in the global period for a major surgical procedure?

   a. 10 days
   b. 90 days
   c. 30 days
   d. 45 days

8. Where can the guidelines for CPT surgical codes be found?

   a. At the beginning of the Surgery section
   b. Within each subsection of medicine codes
   c. Before specific codes located in parentheses
   d. After the diagnosis description

9. A robot-assisted surgery is which type of procedure?

   a. Laparoscopy
   b. Endoscopy
   c. Excision
   d. Introduction

10. If the pre- and postoperative diagnoses differ, which diagnosis should be reported to identify the medical necessity for the procedure?

    a. The preoperative diagnosis
    b. Both preoperative and postoperative diagnoses
    c. The postoperative diagnosis
    d. Neither—send in a special report to explain the lack of ICD-10-CM code

11. A surgical procedure was performed by a team of two surgeons. Each of the surgeons had an equal share of responsibility in the procedure. Which modifier should be appended to the procedure?

    a. -62
    b. -82
    c. -66
    d. -AS

12. Each layer of skin excised in Mohs surgery is referred to as a what?

    a. Block
    b. Specimen
    c. Stage
    d. Lesion

13. Which of the following grafts would come from a donor of a different species?

    a. Autograft
    b. Allograft
    c. Xenograft
    d. Homograft

Instructions: Answer the following questions with the appropriate code(s) and modifier(s).

1. Healthy liver was harvested from a 32-year-old female patient declared brain dead.

   CPT code: _____

2. Transplantation of kidney, without recipient nephrectomy.

   CPT code: _____

3. Cholangiography reveals choledocholithiasis with acute cholecystitis, with obstruction. Emergent cholecystectomy performed at the same session.

   CPT code: _____

   ICD-10-CM code: _____

4. Debridement of all five toenails on the left foot and three toenails on the right foot due to onychomycosis.

   CPT code: _____

   ICD-10-CM code: _____

5. A 42-year-old female with malignant neoplasm of the right upper outer breast underwent lumpectomy procedure of the right breast with axillary lymphadenectomy.

   CPT code: _____

   ICD-10-CM code: _____

References

Agency for Healthcare Research and Quality (AHRQ). 2019 (September). Never Events. https://psnet.ahrq.gov /primers/primer/3/never-events.

American Health Information Management Association (AHIMA). 2017. *Pocket Glossary of Health Information Management and Technology*, 5th ed. Chicago: AHIMA.

American Medical Association (AMA). 2019. *CPT® 2020 Professional Edition*. Chicago: AMA.

Blausen.com staff. 2014. Laproscopy. Digital Image. Wikimedia Commons. https://commons.wikimedia .org/wiki/File:Blausen_0602_Laparoscopy_02.png.

BruceBlaus. 2015. Gallstones.png. Digital Image. Wikimedia Commons. https://commons.wikimedia.org/wiki /File:Gallstones.png.

Cancer Research UK. 2014. Diagram Showing a Bronchoscopy. Digital Image. Wikimedia Commons. https://commons.wikimedia.org/wiki/File:Diagram _showing_a_bronchoscopy_CRUK_053.svg.

Centers for Medicare and Medicaid Services (CMS). 2019a. CMS 1500. https://www.cms.gov/Medicare/CMS -Forms/CMS-Forms/CMS-Forms-Items/CMS1188854 .html.

Centers for Medicare and Medicaid Services (CMS). 2019b. (July 25). Medicare Claims Processing Manual Chapter 12, Physicians/Nonphysician Practitioners. https:// www.cms.gov/Regulations-and-Guidance/Guidance /Manuals/downloads/clm104c12.pdf.

Centers for Medicare and Medicaid Services (CMS). 2019c. ICD-10-CM Official Guidelines for Coding and Reporting FY 2020. https://www.cms.gov/Medicare /Coding/ICD10/Downloads/2020-Coding-Guidelines .pdf.

Centers for Medicare and Medicaid Services (CMS). 2017. Ambulatory Surgical Centers (Rev. 3939, 12-22-17). Chapter 14 in *Medicare Claims Processing Manual*. https:// www.cms.gov/Regulations-and-Guidance/Guidance /Manuals/Downloads/clm104c14.pdf.

National Cancer Institute (NCI). 1985a. Kaposi's Sarcoma. Digital image. National Cancer Institute. https:// visualsonline.cancer.gov/details.cfm?imageid=2168.

National Cancer Institute (NCI). 1985b. Melanoma. Digital image. Wikimedia Commons. https://commons .wikimedia.org/wiki/File:Melanoma.jpg.

Nelson, Kelly. 2012a. Skin Cancer, Basal Cell Carcinoma, Superficial. Digital image. National Cancer Institute. https://visualsonline.cancer.gov/details .cfm?imageid=9236.

Nelson, Kelly. 2012b. Skin Cancer, Squamous Cell Carcinoma, Leg. Digital image. National Cancer Institute. https://visualsonline.cancer.gov/details .cfm?imageid=9249.

Taylornate. 2011a. Advancement flap.svg. Digital image. Wikimedia Commons. https://commons.wikimedia .org/wiki/File:Advancement_flap.svg.

Taylornate. 2011b. Rotation flap.svg. Digital image. Wikimedia Commons. https://commons.wikimedia .org/wiki/File:Rotation_flap.svg.

Taylornate. 2011c. Transposition flap.svg. Digital image. Wikimedia Commons. https://commons.wikimedia .org/wiki/File:Transposition_flap.svg.

Resources

American Academy of Professional Coders (AAPC). 2014 (October 15). Coding Robot-assisted Surgery. https:// www.aapc.com/blog/28266-coding-robot-assisted -surgery/.

American Association of Oral and Maxillofacial Surgeons (AAOMS). 2013. Ambulatory Surgical Center Coding and Billing. http://www.aaoms.org/images/uploads /pdfs/asc_coding_and_billing.pdf.

Casto, A.B., ed. 2019. *ICD-10-CM Code Book: 2020*. Chicago: AHIMA.

Centers for Medicare and Medicaid Services (CMS). 2018 (September). Global Surgery Booklet. https:// www.cms.gov/Outreach-and-Education/Medicare -Learning-Network-MLN/MLNProducts/downloads /GlobalSurgery-ICN907166.pdf.

Centers for Medicare and Medicaid Services (CMS). 2005 (January 14). Pub. 100–04 Medicare Claims Processing. https://www.cms.gov/Regulations-and-Guidance /Guidance/Transmittals/downloads/R434CP.pdf.

Chrysopoulo, M.T. 2017 (August 7). Tissue Flap Classification. https://emedicine.medscape.com /article/1284474-overview#a1.

Smith, G.I. 2019. *Basic Current Procedural Terminology and HCPCS Coding, 2020*. Chicago: AHIMA.

CHAPTER 12

Anesthesia and Pain Management Services

Learning Objectives

- Understand the basics of billing and coding within the specialty of anesthesia and pain management services
- Examine procedural codes and guidelines for anesthesia and pain management services
- Examine diagnosis coding and medical necessity for anesthesia and pain management services
- Determine and apply ICD-10-CM, CPT, and HCPCS codes to anesthesia and pain management services

Key Terms

Acupuncture
Analgesia
Anesthesia services
Anesthesiology
ASA crosswalk
Base units
Cervicalgia
Chronic pain
Conversion factor (CF)
Electrodiagnostic studies
Electromyography (EMG)
Enthesopathy
Epidural steroid injection

Facet joint injection
Fibromyalgia
General anesthesia
Integrative medicine
Interventional pain procedures
Kyphoplasty
Local anesthesia
Lumbago
Moderate (conscious) sedation
Modifying factors
Monitored anesthesia care (MAC)
Myalgia
Myositis

Nerve condition study (NCS)
Occipital nerve block
Osteoarthritis
Pain management services
Peripheral nerve stimulation
Physical status modifier
Qualifying circumstance CPT codes
Radiculopathy
Radiofrequency nerve ablation
Regional anesthesia
Sciatica
Spinal cord stimulation (SCS)
Time units

Anesthesia and pain management specialties both aim to reduce sensation (usually the sensation of pain); however, **anesthesia services** are procedures that create analgesia—the absence of pain—and are provided for a brief amount of time in order to facilitate a medical procedure, such as a surgery. Unlike anesthesia procedures, which are performed as part of a medical or surgical procedure to anesthetize the patient, **pain management services** are given as a treatment for chronic pain in patients who are not undergoing any type of surgical procedure. Pain management services are often aimed at reducing discomfort for patients suffering from chronic pain. **Chronic pain** is the constant or long-term sensation of pain that may be due to postoperative complications, past injuries, or nerve conditions. Pain management procedures are designed to improve quality of life for patients by alleviating chronic pain. The goal of pain management is not to cure the pain or underlying cause of the pain but to treat or reduce the pain to a level considered manageable by the patient.

This chapter discusses both anesthesia and pain management coding. The intricacies of anesthesia billing and its impact on the codes reported for anesthesia services are examined first, followed by a discussion of pain management basics. The chapter concludes with an overview of how procedural and diagnostic coding are applied for both specialties.

Anesthesia Billing and Coding Basics

Anesthesiology is the healthcare specialty of relieving patient pain before, during, and after surgery. The aim of anesthesia services is to provide **analgesia**, or the inability to feel pain. Anesthesiologists perform the majority of their services in the inpatient hospital, outpatient hospital, or ambulatory surgery center (ASC) settings in which patients are undergoing invasive, painful surgeries.

Anesthesia coding is quite different from medical evaluation and management (E/M) or surgical procedure coding. Instead of coding for the procedure performed by the doctor, anesthesia codes identify the anesthesia service provided while the doctor was performing the procedure. Anesthesia codes do not specify the exact substance administered to induce anesthesia or the specifics of the anesthesia service itself. Rather, anesthesia codes identify the surgical procedure the patient was undergoing that necessitated the anesthesia in the first place. Anesthesia codes are located in a special (Anesthesia) section of codes in the CPT code book. Furthermore, billing for anesthesia services requires a special calculation to determine how much to charge for the service performed, depending on the circumstances surrounding each particular service. Pain management, on the other hand, is more similar to surgical and healthcare coding, as it uses codes from the Surgery section of the CPT code book. Pain management procedures are more like surgical interventions that treat either the cause of the pain (such as removing a herniated disc) or the symptom of pain (such as an injection of anesthetic into a joint or nerve).

Beginning coding professionals must understand the basics of anesthesia services, including how services are billed, how the services are coded, and the difference between anesthesia and pain management procedures.

There are three main types of providers that may provide anesthesia services—anesthesiologists, anesthesiology assistants (AAs), and certified registered nurse anesthetists (CRNAs). Anesthesiologists are medical doctors who specialize in anesthesiology. AAs are similar to physician assistants (PAs), in that they have completed a graduate program in medical training with an emphasis in anesthesia.

CRNAs, on the other hand, are registered nurses (RNs) who have completed a graduate program with an emphasis in anesthesia. AAs and CRNAs are both mid-level providers who are able to perform anesthesiology procedures only under the supervision of an anesthesiologist. It is important to understand the differences between anesthesiology providers, as the codes billed may differ depending on which provider performed the service (discussed later in this chapter).

Billing for anesthesia services is further complicated by the varying nature of anesthesia procedures. Anesthesia services are performed in a number of different ways, such as by the intravenous or inhaled administration of drugs or other substances to induce unconsciousness and analgesia. The anesthesiologist is the practitioner who determines which type of anesthesia is best according to the patient's specific needs and what is needed for the surgical or medical procedure. The anesthesiologist administers the anesthesia and monitors the patient during the surgical procedure to ensure that the anesthesia is working and the patient's vital signs are stable. See figure 12.1 for an illustration of these differences in coding.

Figure 12.1. Anesthesiology and surgery coding

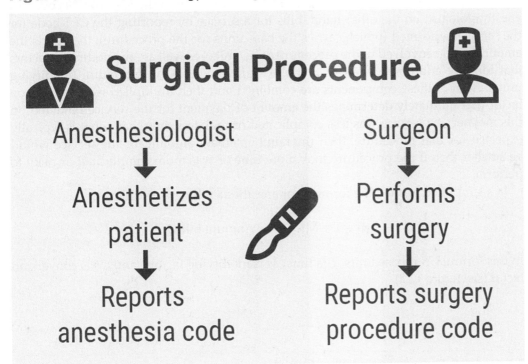

The actual anesthesia service, including the time spent on the service, varies greatly depending on the patient, the medical procedure, and any complications that may occur during the surgery. For example, an anesthesiologist administering anesthesia to a patient for a routine appendectomy may spend less time monitoring the patient during the anesthesia procedure than if the surgeon were performing a complicated appendectomy that took an inordinate amount of time, or if the patient were very young or very old. The following sections of this chapter discuss the unique nature of billing and coding for anesthesia services, which combine many elements including the basic service, the time it took to perform the service, and any modifying factors involved in the service. This chapter also discusses the detailed documentation requirements for anesthesia services.

Billing and Coding for Anesthesia Services

Billing for anesthesia services is not as simple as reporting a specific CPT code and linking to an ICD-10-CM code to identify the medical necessity for the service. These two items are still required, but additional information is needed to bill for anesthesia services appropriately.

Correct billing of anesthesia services is based on three things: base units, time units, and modifying factors. Base units are numerical values given to each anesthesia service, time units identify the amount of time spent on the anesthesia service, and modifying factors identify any additional complications or extra work needed to perform the procedure. These three components are combined according to each anesthesia service and multiplied by a conversion factor—a dollar amount—to calculate the amount of payment for the anesthesia service. Although CMS annually publishes a conversion factor for anesthesia services, this conversion factor may vary across insurance policies and often changes from year to year. The conversion factor determines the dollar amount billed per service.

Billing for anesthesia services is vastly different from typical billing for medical or surgical services. For example, a primary care physician bills for a preventive medical examination by submitting the CPT code along with the ICD-10-CM code. An anesthesiologist, on the other hand, bills for a service by reporting the CPT code for the service performed (which carries the base units for the procedure), then adds the amount of time involved in the procedure (time units), as well as any modifying factors that identify additional work or complexity involved in the procedure (modifying units). Each of these components are combined and then multiplied by a conversion factor that ultimately determines the amount of payment for the service rendered. In this manner, if a service was less complicated or took less time than what is typically expected for that procedure, then the reimbursement amount for the service would be smaller than if the procedure took more time or was more complicated or risky to perform.

In a simplified format, the formula for anesthesia billing is as follows:

$$(B + T + M) \times CF = \text{Amount billed}$$

In this formula, B is base units, T is time, M is modifying factors, and CF is conversion factor (see figure 12.2).

Figure 12.2. Anesthesia billing formula

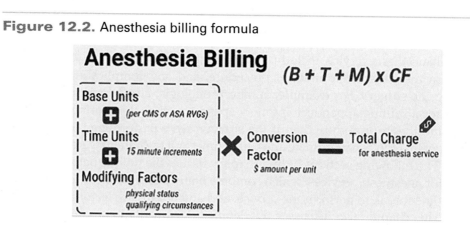

Base Units

Base units, a set of numerical values created and maintained by the American Society of Anesthesiologists (ASA), give each anesthesiology service a numerical relative value in relation to how complicated or risky a procedure is, and are used to set the relative cost of each procedure. The higher the base values for an anesthesia procedure, the higher the charge for that procedure; the lower the base units, the lower the charge for the procedure. Base unit values assigned by CMS range from 0 for unlisted procedures, to 2 for add-on codes, to 30 for more complex procedures (00796, Anesthesia for all intraperitoneal procedures in upper abdomen including laparoscopy; liver transplant [recipient]) (CMS 2018).

A simple procedure may be assigned 1 base unit, a moderate procedure may be assigned 3 base units, and a complicated procedure may be assigned 5 base units. So, a more complicated or risky procedure holds more value (in terms of billing) than a simpler procedure, and anesthesiologists may be reimbursed more for complex procedures and less for simpler procedures. For example, CPT code 00524, Anesthesia for closed chest procedures; pneumocentesis, is assigned 4 base units. Code 00528, Anesthesia for closed chest procedures; mediastinoscopy and diagnostic thoracoscopy not utilizing 1 lung ventilation, is assigned 8 units, as this is a more complex closed chest procedure than the pneumocentesis. Code 00529, Anesthesia for closed chest procedures; mediastinoscopy and diagnostic thoracoscopy utilizing 1 lung ventilation, is assigned 11 base units, as this procedure is more complex than the mediastinoscopy without lung ventilation.

Base unit values are published on the CMS website each year for reference (see figure 12.3); note that these base unit values were last updated in 2018. Base unit values

Figure 12.3. CMS anesthesia base units

Code	2018 Base Unit
00100	5
00102	6
00103	5
00104	4
00120	5
00124	4
00126	4
00140	5
00142	4
00144	6
00145	6
00147	4
00148	4
00160	5
00162	7
00164	4
00170	5

Source: Adapted from CMS 2018.

are also published in the American Society of Anesthesiologists Relative Value Guide (ASA RVG), which contains more than 300 CPT codes, all of which have a relative value assigned. When billing for services covered by Medicare, coders should refer to the base units published by CMS. However, some commercial payers use the base unit values published by the ASA. Therefore, coders should use the ASA RVG when coding for commercial payers (unless otherwise stated by the contract with the payer) to determine the base unit values for procedures performed, and use the Medicare base unit values when coding claims for Medicare patients.

Though base unit values are reviewed and updated by either CMS or the ASA on an annual basis, this sometimes results in little to no changes in these values. For example, figure 12.3 shows the 2018 base unit values published by Medicare. These values have not been changed since they were published in 2018. The services included in the base unit are

- All usual anesthesia services, such as the determination of the anesthesia dose and substance, preparation of the patient and administration of the anesthesia, and monitoring during the procedure (except the time involved in the procedure and any modifying factors)
- Usual pre- and postoperative visits
- Administration of fluids or blood products
- Interpretation and monitoring of noninvasive monitoring procedures, such as ECG, temperature, blood pressure, oximetry, capnography, and mass spectrometry (AMA 2019)

Base unit values do not include the placement of arterial, central venous, or pulmonary arterial catheters or the use of transesophageal echocardiography (TEE) (among other procedures, as discussed in the following Procedural Coding section). Any additional procedures (other than those identified previously) are included in the base units for the anesthesia service reported and may not be reported separately.

When coding for anesthesia services, knowing the base unit value of each procedure is important. When anesthesia is provided to a patient undergoing more than one procedure, only the anesthesia procedure with the *highest* base units should be billed. Therefore, to correctly report the service(s) provided, anesthesia coders must know and understand the base values of each of the services performed by the provider for whom they bill.

For example, if the surgeon is performing a liver transplant and an appendectomy, only the anesthesia for the liver transplant should be reported, because it has the higher number of base units. According to CMS, the base unit values for an appendectomy (code 00790, Anesthesia for intraperitoneal procedures in upper abdomen including laparoscopy; not otherwise specified) are 7, whereas the base unit values for a patient receiving anesthesia for a liver transplant (code 00796, Anesthesia for intraperitoneal procedures in upper abdomen including laparoscopy; liver transplant (recipient)) are 30. In this case, the base unit values for the liver transplant procedure outweigh those for the appendectomy procedure, so only the liver transplant anesthesia code should be reported. The anesthesia service for the appendectomy would be included in the base units for the more complex procedure (liver transplant). Any additional procedures that the provider performed above and beyond either anesthesia service may be reported separately.

Complete the exercises in There's a Code for That 12.1 to test your understanding of base unit values.

Base unit values

Using the following table, identify either the number of base unit values for the given anesthesia code, or determine which anesthesia code should be reported.

Code	Units	Code	Units	Code	Units	Code	Units
00100	5	00164	4	00222	6	00470	6
00102	6	00170	5	00300	5	00472	10
00103	5	00172	6	00320	6	00474	13
00104	4	00174	6	00322	3	00500	15
00120	5	00176	7	00326	7	00520	6
00124	4	00190	5	00350	10	00522	4
00126	4	00192	7	00352	5	00524	4
00140	5	00210	11	00400	3	00528	8
00142	4	00211	10	00402	5	00529	11
00144	6	00212	5	00404	5	00530	4
00145	6	00214	9	00406	13	00532	4
00147	4	00215	9	00410	4	00534	7
00148	4	00216	15	00450	5	00537	7
00160	5	00218	13	00452	6	00539	18
00162	7	00220	10	00454	3	00540	12

Source: Adapted from CMS 2018.

1. Which anesthesia service holds the highest number of base units: 00454 or 00402? _____

2. The surgeon performed a radical mastectomy of the bilateral female breasts, with internal mammary node dissection. Which anesthesia code would be reported for the service: 00404 or 00406? _____

3. The surgeon performed multiple intracranial procedures while the patient was under anesthesia, including a craniotomy for evacuation of hematoma (00211) and a cranioplasty of depressed skull fracture (00215). Which anesthesia service should be reported?

   CPT code: _____

4. The surgeon performed a bronchoscopy (00520) as well as a biopsy of the soft tissue of the accessory sinuses (00164). Which anesthesia code should be reported?

   CPT code: _____

Time

The time units for anesthesia services identify the duration of the procedure, from the beginning of the anesthesia service until the patient is released to a postoperative or post-anesthesia care unit (PACU). Time units are based on the standard time measurements in guidelines determined by either the ASA or per the patient's third-party payer. The anesthesia time starts when the anesthesiologist (or AA or CRNA) begins to prepare the patient for the anesthesia service. This can take place in the operating room or other designated area. The time calculated does not include a preoperative evaluation performed by the anesthesiologist, which may be completed before the patient is even in the operating suite, but varies depending on when the provider performing the medical procedure begins the service—for example, the moment the provider starts an intravenous line, begins to place monitors on the patient, administers sedation, or begins to physically prepare the patient for the anesthesia service in any other manner and remains in constant attendance.

Anesthesia time ends when the anesthesiology provider has transferred care of the patient to a postoperative area or PACU. The end time never occurs in the operating room. The time reported is continuous, encompassing the entire time of the service from start to finish.

Time is reported in 15-minute increments, so a service that lasted 60 minutes would total 4 time units (60 minutes divided by 15-minute increments = 4 units). Any additional time less than 7.5 minutes should be rounded down and not counted in the total time reported, and any additional time over 7.5 minutes should be rounded up to the next unit. For example, if the provider spent 67 minutes on the service (60 minutes = 4 time units, plus 7 extra minutes), the total time units reported would be 4. On the other hand, if the provider spent 68 minutes on the service (60 minutes = 4 time units, plus 8 extra minutes) the total time units reported would be 5.

These are the standard time ASA and AMA reporting guidelines. However, keep in mind that Medicare has different time reporting rules, as other insurance carriers might. For example, Medicare requires that the total time spent on a procedure be divided by 15, and then the units reported in increments of one decimal point. For example, 5 minutes total would be 0.3 units (5 minutes divided by 15 = 0.3 units), 6 minutes would be 0.4 units (6 minutes divided by 15 = 0.4 units), and so on. For the purposes of this textbook, time reported should be in full integers, rounding down anything under 7.5 minutes and rounding up anything over 7.5 minutes, according to ASA/AMA guidelines. Time units are entered in box 24.G on the CMS-1500 claim form (see figure 12.4).

Time units are yet another example of how the intricacies of billing affect the coding of claims, and how understanding the differences between payer guidelines and requirements is an integral part of correctly reporting codes and additional information entered on claims.

Figure 12.4. Time units in box 24.G

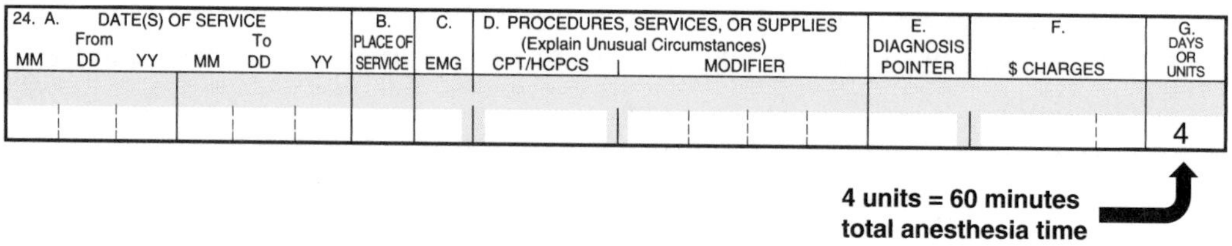

4 units = 60 minutes total anesthesia time

Source: CMS 2019a.

Modifying Factors

Modifying factors are similar to CPT modifiers in that they provide additional information to the anesthesia procedure description and describe an anesthesia procedure that was more complex, or required additional skill to complete, than it would have been if performed on a normal, healthy patient. Modifying factors come in two forms: CPT modifiers, called physical status modifiers, which are appended to the CPT code for the anesthesia service; and qualifying circumstances codes, which are supplementary CPT codes that may be reported in addition to the anesthesia service codes to identify further complexity involved in the anesthesia procedure. Modifying factors are published as part of the CPT code set and may be updated annually. They assign additional units to the base and time units for the procedure according to a preset amount per modifying factor. The exact number of additional units or values assigned to the modifying factor depend on the values assigned by the patient's insurance payer. For example, some insurance plans may assign additional units to qualifying circumstances codes, while others bundle these codes into the primary service and do not provide any additional payment.

Physical Status Modifiers

Physical status modifiers are appended to the end of the anesthesia procedure code for a given service to identify the physical status of the patient and capture any additional complexity that may be present due to the patient's physical condition. Physical status modifiers begin with the letter *P* and end with a number (1 through 6), and identify the physical status of the patient as follows:

- P1, A normal, healthy patient. For example, a healthy non-smoking patient with minimal or no alcohol use.

- P2, A patient with mild systemic disease. A patient with a mild systemic disease, without any functional limitations, such as a current smoker (without problems); social drinker; pregnant without complications; mild obesity (BMI between 30 and 40); or controlled diabetes or hypertension.

- P3, A patient with severe systemic disease. A patient that has one or more moderate or severe diseases with functional limitations, such as uncontrolled or poorly controlled diabetes or hypertension; morbid obesity (BMI over 40); hepatitis; alcohol abuse or dependence; an end-stage renal disease (ESRD) patient undergoing dialysis; an implanted pacemaker; a premature infant; a myocardial infarction (MI) more than three months ago; or history of cerebrovascular accident (CVA/stroke) or transient ischemic attack (TIA).

- P4, A patient with severe systemic disease that is a constant threat to life. A patient who has a moderate or severe condition with functional limitations (as described previously), which presents a constant threat to life, such as recent MI (less than three months ago); CVA/stroke; TIA; coronary atherosclerosis; sepsis; or ESRD not undergoing regularly scheduled dialysis.

- P5, A moribund patient who is not expected to survive without the operation. A patient whose medical condition presents an immediate threat to life and, as such, must undergo immediate operation. For example, ruptured aneurysm, massive traumatic injury, or intracranial bleeding.

- P6, A declared brain-dead patient whose organs are being removed for donor purposes. This patient has been declared brain dead and is receiving anesthesia during the procedures to harvest internal organs for donation. (ASA 2019)

For example, the anesthesia service code for a patient with controlled diabetes would be appended with modifier -P2, A patient with mild systemic disease. Alternatively, the anesthesia procedure code for a patient with uncontrolled diabetes, stage 5 chronic kidney disease, and hypertension would be appended with - P3, A patient with severe systemic disease. Physical status modifiers usually hold a unit value that should be added to the total units for the anesthesia service. However, this depends on the patient's insurance payer. For example, some insurance policies assign additional *time* units for physical status modifiers, rather than additional *base* units. This is yet one more reason why coders must be vigilant about the patient's insurance payer when entering codes for claims. Figure 12.5 shows examples of unit values for physical status modifiers.

Figure 12.5. Physical status modifier unit values

Physical Status Modifier	Unit Value
P1	0
P2	0
P3	1
P4	2
P5	3
P6	0

Qualifying Circumstances

Qualifying circumstances CPT codes are add-on codes that should be used in addition to the code for the anesthesia service (as well as any applicable physical status modifier). They describe services that are particularly difficult due to the extraordinary condition of the patient, notable operative conditions, or unusual risk factors. They are all designated add-on codes that must be reported with the primary code for the anesthesia service and may never be reported alone. Qualifying circumstance codes are listed in the CPT code book in the guidelines at the beginning of the Anesthesia section. They are as follows:

- 99100, Anesthesia for patient of extreme age, younger than 1 year and older than 70. This code identifies patients who are either very young or very old; it should be used in addition to the code for the anesthesia service. However, pay attention to the code description for anesthesia services, as some describe a procedure on a pediatric patient. When this is the case, the add-on code to identify the patient as of extreme young age is not necessary. For example, code 00326, Anesthesia for all procedures on the larynx and *trachea in children younger than 1 year of age*, already identifies the patient as under the age of 1 year, so the qualifying circumstance code 99100 is not necessary.

- 99116, Anesthesia complicated by utilization of total body hypothermia. Hypothermia may be induced for some anesthesia procedures because of its ability to protect the heart and brain during certain procedures. When hypothermia is induced during the procedure, this qualifying circumstance code should be used, except if the code for the anesthesia procedure includes hypothermia in the code description (such as 00563, Anesthesia for procedures on heart pericardial sac, and great vessels of chest; with pump oxygenator *with hypothermic circulatory arrest*).

- 99135, Anesthesia complicated by utilization of controlled hypotension. Hypotension (low blood pressure) is used during surgical procedures to reduce the need for blood transfusions and to help with patient outcomes by reducing bleeding as well as helping to maintain a bloodless surgical field.

- 99140, Anesthesia complicated by emergency conditions (specify). A procedure is considered an emergency when a delay in treatment would lead to an increased threat to the patient's life or limb. The specific emergency conditions must be clearly identified in the documentation for the procedure.

More than one qualifying circumstance code may be used, if necessary, to fully describe the circumstances of the anesthesia service. For example, anesthesia for a pneumocentesis on a 9-month-old patient complicated by emergency conditions would be coded as follows: 00524, Anesthesia for closed chest procedures; pneumocentesis, plus 99100, Anesthesia for patient of extreme age, younger than 1 year and older than 70, and 99140, Anesthesia complicated by emergency conditions.

Each qualifying circumstance code holds a unit value that should be added to the rest of the units for the procedure. For example, the 9-month-old undergoing a pneumocentesis procedure would have an additional unit value added for the qualifying circumstance code 99100, and an additional two unit values for the qualifying circumstances code 99140. Note again that the exact amount of values added by each qualifying circumstance code depends on the insurance payer. Some third-party payers bundle qualifying circumstance codes into the payment for the anesthesia procedure, while others may add only one extra value point per qualifying circumstance code. Yet others use a scale in which each qualifying circumstance code holds a unique value. Figure 12.6 shows an example of the unit values of qualifying circumstance codes.

Medicare does not take into account modifying factors, and it does not pay for any additional work (as identified by modifying factor units) for anesthesia procedures. Medicare accounts only for the base and time units for each procedure.

Figure 12.6. Qualifying circumstance unit values

Qualifying Circumstance Code	Unit Value
99100	1
99116	5
99135	5
99140	2

Conversion Factor

Once the units for the procedure have been totaled, this number must be multiplied by the conversion factor (CF) rate, which is the dollar amount per unit for the reimbursement of anesthesia services. The conversion factor depends on the insurance payer being billed, so it is important to understand which payer is being billed for the service when calculating the amount of payment expected from the insurance. The dollar amount is negotiated in a private contract between the anesthesia office and the insurance payer. For example, the conversion factor between an anesthesia provider and a third-party payer may be negotiated to a dollar amount of $25.00 per unit value.

Medicare, on the other hand, has an annually published conversion factor used to calculate anesthesia payment amounts for each service. Medicare CFs change according to the region in which the anesthesia service was billed, creating a discrepancy in payments depending on where the anesthesia procedure was performed. See figure 12.7 for an excerpt of the 2020 CMS conversion factors for anesthesia services. Note that the CF for services provided in Alabama is 21.16, whereas the CF for services performed in Alaska is 30.86. An anesthesia provider in Alaska would be paid almost $10.00 more per unit than an anesthesia provider in Alabama (CMS 2019b).

Figure 12.7. Selected CMS conversion factors for anesthesia services, 2020

Locality	Locality Name	National Anes CF of 22.2016
00	ALABAMA	21.16
01	ALASKA	30.86
00	ARIZONA	21.70
13	ARKANSAS	20.66
54	BAKERSFIELD	22.63

Source: Adapted from CMS 2019b.

Documentation of Anesthesia Services

Documentation for anesthesia services should include the details of the pre-anesthesia evaluation, the record of the intraoperative or procedural anesthesia (in a time-based record of events), and a record of the post-anesthesia transfer of care and end time of the procedure. Anesthesia health records are complicated forms that include numerous details. Figure 12.8 depicts an example of a paper anesthesia record.

Pain management is a healthcare specialty similar to anesthesia. Both categories of procedure are performed to reduce or eliminate sensation; however, pain management is less complicated in terms of reimbursement and more complicated in terms of CPT coding.

Pain Management Billing and Coding Basics

Pain management is a specialty in which healthcare providers employ various procedures to improve the quality of life and ease the suffering of patients with chronic pain.

It is a unique specialty, because it is a treatment-based—not cure-based—healthcare specialty. In other words, pain management treats the symptom of pain and not the underlying cause of the pain. However, some pain management procedures may be focused on eliminating the causes of pain, such as performing a spinal surgery to decompress a pinched nerve or herniated disc. In many instances, there is no possible cure for the chronic pain, making pain management the only option patients have to live a normally functioning life.

Because pain management is a long-term process, billing for pain management may be complicated by payer requirements and approvals for procedures that may be done only once per specified timeframe. For example, radiofrequency ablation, a procedure performed to treat chronic pain, may be allowed only once a year by the patient's insurance company. However, it may be necessary to perform the procedure more often than every 12 months. When this is the case, the provider's office may request a prior authorization for the procedure from the patient's insurance. If the insurance does not authorize the procedure, the patient must either pay for the service out of his or her pocket or go without the service until the 12 months has passed. At the very

Figure 12.8. Paper anesthesia record

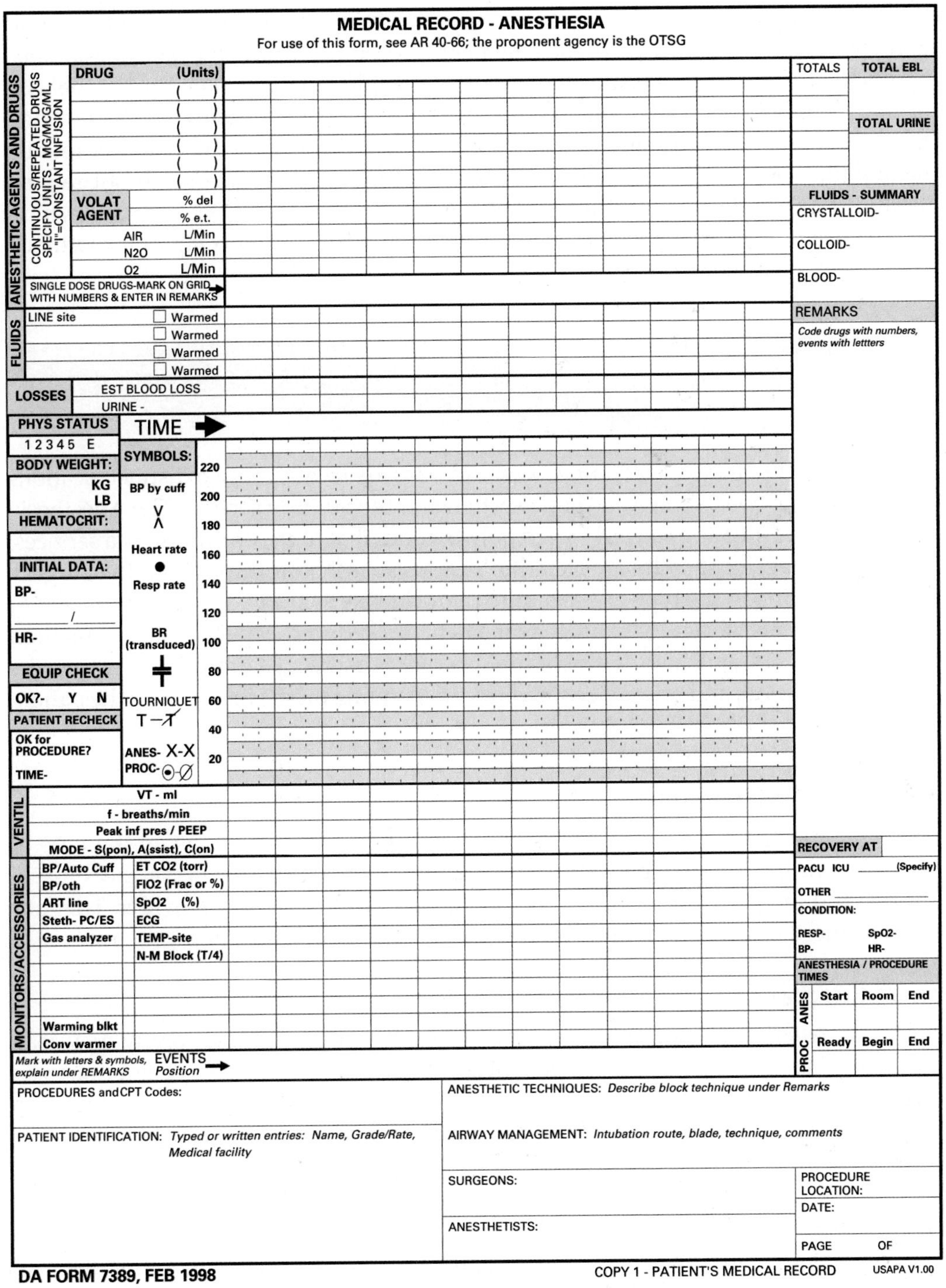

MEDICAL RECORD - ANESTHESIA

For use of this form, see AR 40-66; the proponent agency is the OTSG

ANESTHETIC AGENTS AND DRUGS

CONTINUOUS/REPEATED DRUGS SPECIFY UNITS - MG/MCG/ML, "I"=CONSTANT INFUSION

DRUG (Units)

( )
( )
( )
( )
( )
( )

VOLAT AGENT % del
% e.t.

AIR L/Min
N2O L/Min
O2 L/Min

SINGLE DOSE DRUGS-MARK ON GRID WITH NUMBERS & ENTER IN REMARKS

TOTALS | TOTAL EBL

TOTAL URINE

FLUIDS - SUMMARY

CRYSTALLOID-

COLLOID-

BLOOD-

REMARKS

Code drugs with numbers, events with lettters

FLUIDS

LINE site
☐ Warmed
☐ Warmed
☐ Warmed
☐ Warmed

LOSSES EST BLOOD LOSS
URINE -

PHYS STATUS
1 2 3 4 5 E

TIME

BODY WEIGHT:
KG
LB

HEMATOCRIT:

INITIAL DATA:
BP-
/
HR-

EQUIP CHECK
OK?- Y N

PATIENT RECHECK
OK for PROCEDURE?
TIME-

SYMBOLS:
BP by cuff
V
Λ
Heart rate
●
Resp rate
BR (transduced)
TOURNIQUET
T—T
ANES- X-X
PROC- ⊙-Ø

220
200
180
160
140
120
100
80
60
40
20

VENTIL
VT - ml
f - breaths/min
Peak inf pres / PEEP
MODE - S(pon), A(ssist), C(on)

MONITORS/ACCESSORIES
BP/Auto Cuff | ET CO2 (torr)
BP/oth | FIO2 (Frac or %)
ART line | Sp02 (%)
Steth- PC/ES | ECG
Gas analyzer | TEMP-site
N-M Block (T/4)
Warming blkt
Conv warmer

Mark with letters & symbols, explain under REMARKS EVENTS Position

RECOVERY AT
PACU ICU ______ (Specify)
OTHER ______
CONDITION:
RESP- Sp02-
BP- HR-

ANESTHESIA / PROCEDURE TIMES

ANES: Start | Room | End

PROC: Ready | Begin | End

PROCEDURES and CPT Codes:

ANESTHETIC TECHNIQUES: *Describe block technique under Remarks*

PATIENT IDENTIFICATION: *Typed or written entries: Name, Grade/Rate, Medical facility*

AIRWAY MANAGEMENT: *Intubation route, blade, technique, comments*

SURGEONS:

PROCEDURE LOCATION:

DATE:

ANESTHETISTS:

PAGE OF

DA FORM 7389, FEB 1998 COPY 1 - PATIENT'S MEDICAL RECORD USAPA V1.00

Source: APD 1998.

least, this means that billers and coders in pain management need to be careful about what procedure is being performed, whether or not it is a payable procedure, and if it needs a prior authorization from the patient's insurance.

Unlike anesthesia procedures, pain management services are reported with procedure codes from the Surgery section of the CPT code book. Anesthesia procedure codes identify the procedure performed on the patient that necessitated the anesthesia.

Pain management procedures are performed by the healthcare provider and codes reflect the actual procedure performed. Sometimes a patient may require anesthesia during the surgical procedure, in which case the pain management provider would report the codes for the pain management procedure while the anesthesiologist reports the CPT code for the anesthesia service provided to the patient during the pain management procedure. Because pain management codes are surgical CPT codes, they may be reported like any other surgical or medical service. They do not require the identification of base units, time units, or modifying factors, and do not rely on anesthesia conversion factors. Rather, they are paid on the medical fee schedule typical for all other healthcare specialties. Coding for other healthcare specialties is discussed throughout the rest of this textbook.

Procedural Coding for Anesthesia and Pain Management Services

Anesthesia and pain management procedure codes are located in two distinct locations in the CPT code book—the Anesthesia section and the Surgery section. The Anesthesia section of the CPT code book is devoted only to codes that represent anesthesia services, and pain management codes are found in various subsections throughout the Surgery section according to the type of procedure performed.

Coding for anesthesia or pain management procedures depends on the method of analgesia used and how it was administered. Some codes are dependent on the patient's condition, and code selection differs depending on the reason why the patient was treated.

Types of Anesthesia

There are four main types of anesthesia, the usage of which depends on the type of surgery performed, the expected duration of the surgery, the health of the surgery patient, and the preferences of the patient and the anesthesiology provider. The four types of anesthesia are moderate, local, regional, and general sedation.

Moderate (Conscious) Sedation

Moderate (conscious) sedation is a type of anesthesia given either orally or via an injection. This method allows the patient to be sedated but awake so he or she can respond to commands if necessary. Moderate sedation is discussed in further detail in chapter 10 (Urgent Care and Emergency Department Services). Moderate (conscious) sedation is coded with CPT codes 99151 through 99157.

Local Anesthesia

Local anesthesia blocks a small amount of nerves using an injection or a topical cream or spray that numbs a specific portion of the body. It is usually initiated by the healthcare provider performing the procedure, rather than an anesthesiologist. For example, a provider can inject an anesthetic cream into a patient's skin to allow for excision of a lesion of the chest without the patient experiencing any pain. Local anesthesia is often used for minor surgeries or to perform small wound repairs. Patients receiving local anesthesia may also receive moderate sedation at varying levels to help them relax and induce drowsiness, and to make the injection of the local anesthetic and ensuing procedure more tolerable. Once the procedure is complete, local anesthesia is allowed to gradually wear off until the patient regains full sensation. This process may take a few hours or up to a day, depending on the type of anesthesia administered and procedure performed.

There is no CPT code for the administration of local anesthesia, as this service is bundled into the payment for the surgical procedure. However, if the patient did receive moderate sedation in addition to the local anesthesia, the moderate sedation may be coded.

Regional Anesthesia

Regional anesthesia employs an injection to block a large amount of nerves, numb a more extensive body area, and prepare the patient for an extensive surgery or procedure. Regional anesthesia is commonly used for procedures involving the lower part of the body—on the legs, during vaginal delivery and cesarean sections, or during urogenital surgery. Regional anesthesia may entail a single injection of anesthetic or may be a continuous administration of an anesthetic through a catheter or tube that is left in place throughout a surgical procedure or hospital stay. Codes for regional anesthesia are located in the Surgery section of the CPT manual.

Common regional anesthesia procedures are spinal and epidural injections. A sedative may also be used with regional anesthesia to help the patient relax and better endure the injection of the regional anesthetics. Once the procedure is complete, the regional anesthesia is stopped (as in the case of an epidural) and allowed to gradually wear off until the patient has regained full sensation and function of the body area that was anesthetized.

In both local and regional anesthesia, the patient is awake and aware of the procedures. Moderate sedation is used to help the patient relax and undergo the procedure by reducing the patient's level of consciousness. Local and regional anesthesia procedure codes are found in the Surgery section of the CPT code book, as they are considered surgical procedures in which the anesthesiologist must actually perform the injection of the anesthetic substance into the patient. However, if the regional anesthesia service was performed in order to anesthetize the patient to facilitate a *different* healthcare procedure, the appropriate code from the Anesthesia section of the CPT code book is assigned. To find anesthetic injections in the CPT code book, search for the term *Injection*, and then *Anesthetic Agent*, and find the subterm for the area being anesthetized. For nerve injections, search for the term *Injection*, and then *Nerve*, and find the subterm for *Anesthetic*.

General Anesthesia Care

General anesthesia is the administration of a substance that results in a complete loss of consciousness in order to produce analgesia to facilitate a surgical or other healthcare procedure (Palmetto 2013). It may be given intravenously, inhaled through a mask, or administered both intravenously and by inhalation. It results in the patient being completely unconscious, with no memory of the surgical procedure when they wake up. General anesthesia is the riskiest form of anesthesia because the patient is rendered completely unconscious, requiring close monitoring of breathing and heart rate. As such, it is only used for procedures that cannot be performed with either local or regional anesthetic or moderate sedation. Patients may also be sedated before the general anesthesia is administered.

Monitored anesthesia care (MAC) is a similar procedure that produces analgesia in a patient and may be performed along with or in lieu of general anesthesia. MAC is an anesthesia service that is consists of a conscious sedation, control of patient anxiety, and pain control. MAC services result in a more rapid post-anesthesia recovery, which makes MAC services suitable for outpatient procedures (Das and Ghosh 2015). MAC services are similar to moderate sedation (refer to chapter 10), however, a MAC provider must be a qualified anesthesiologist because he or she must be ready to convert to a full general anesthesia service in the case of an adverse event. In moderate sedation, the healthcare provider performing the anesthesia service is the provider performing the procedure, not a certified anesthesiologist provider. Both general anesthesia and MAC services are reported with codes from the Anesthesia section of the CPT code book.

General anesthesia results in the need to assist the patient's respiration to ensure adequate ventilation, which is done via an oral airway (a small plastic tube that keeps the airway open by keeping the tongue in place so that it does not cover the epiglottis) or with a mask that fits over the nose and mouth. Due to its reliability in ensuring adequate breathing, endotracheal intubation is commonly used to assist the patient's breathing during the surgical procedure and is often used in procedures that are lengthy or if the patient is receiving large amounts of anesthesia.

Throughout the general anesthesia procedure, the patient's vital signs are closely monitored by the anesthesiologist. This includes the patient's heart rate, blood pressure, and blood oxygen levels, which are recorded continuously in the provider's documentation of the entire procedure. Once the procedure is complete, the anesthesiologist reverses the anesthesia using a medicinal agent, which stops the effects of the anesthesia, allowing the patient to wake up and regain sensation; the patient is taken to the post-anesthesia care unit. General anesthesia services are reported with CPT codes 00100 through 01999. They can be found by searching under the term *Anesthesia* in the CPT Index. Figure 12.9 illustrates the differences among types of anesthesia.

Figure 12.9. Types of anesthesia

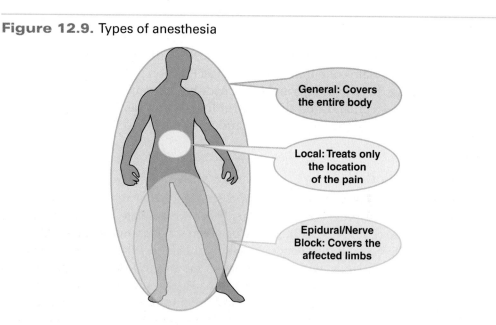

Understanding the different types of anesthesia services is integral to coding for them appropriately, as the different types of anesthesia services are located in different sections of the CPT code book.

Procedural Coding for Anesthesia Services

Anesthesia services are reported with codes 00100 to 01999. Note that not all anesthesia procedures are included in this code range, as some local and regional injections are located in the Surgery section codes.

As with the other five sections of the CPT code book, the Anesthesia section begins with a selection of guidelines applicable to anesthesia codes. These guidelines provide important information on anesthesia services and code descriptions, as well as guidelines for time reporting, supplied materials, separate or multiple procedures, and special reports (special reports are discussed in detail in chapter 5 [Learning the CPT and HCPCS Code Books]). For example, coders with questions on how time is reported for anesthesia codes may refer to the guidelines at the beginning of the Anesthesia section to read the CPT guidelines related to time reporting: "Time for anesthesia procedures may be reported as customary in the local area. Anesthesia time begins when the anesthesiologist begins to prepare the patient for the induction of anesthesia in the operating room (or in an equivalent area) and ends when the anesthesiologist is no longer in personal attendance, that is, when the patient may be safely placed under postoperative supervision" (AMA 2019). This section also includes the anesthesia physical status modifiers and qualifying circumstances add-on codes for reference.

Key to Success

The beginning of each section in the CPT code book begins with a selection of important guidelines applicable to all of the codes in that section. This is a good place to write notes, reminders, and other codes or modifiers that are important for this section of codes. This is especially a beneficial strategy to help you succeed in taking certification exams. Most exams will allow you to write notes and highlight important items in the code books, as long as you do not tape anything to the pages or write down sample test questions. Ask your instructor or check the website for the certification exam for which you are preparing to see what you are allowed to write in your books.

Coding for anesthesia services can be a bit confusing because the codes are different than surgical, medical, or E/M codes. However, it is easier to find the correct CPT codes for anesthesia codes once you know how they work.

The anesthesia section of the CPT code book is divided by body area or condition. For example, the first subheading is Head, then Neck, then Thorax (Chest Wall and Shoulder Girdle). Under these headings is a list of the anesthesia services for patients undergoing a procedure on those respective body areas. For example, under the subheading Head, the first code, 00100, Anesthesia for procedures on salivary glands, including biopsy, covers any anesthesia service performed on a patient undergoing any kind of procedure on his or her salivary glands (including a biopsy).

In this way, anesthesia codes are not too much more complicated than surgical or medical CPT codes; they just require a change of thinking. When coding for anesthesia services, coders must identify the main procedure that the surgeon performed. The anesthesia provider is not performing the surgery on the salivary glands, just anesthetizing the patient for the procedure, and the anesthesia code is what the anesthesiologist reports. The surgeon reports the code for the procedure performed using a CPT code from elsewhere in the CPT manual and bills it separately (refer to figure 12.1).

Note that there are four subsections at the end of the Anesthesia section that describe anesthesia procedures performed for specific conditions or specific types of procedures. Rather than a particular body system, these three sections describe anesthesia procedures for specific types of procedures that may occur throughout the body: Radiological Procedures (01916–01936), Burn Excisions or Debridement (01951–01953), Obstetric (01958–01969), and Other Procedures (01990–01999).

When a patient is anesthetized and the healthcare provider performs more than one procedure, the anesthesiologist should report only the anesthesia code representing the most complex procedure, represented by the highest number of base units (as discussed previously). For example, if the patient received a liver transplant and an appendectomy in the same operative session, then the anesthesiologist would only report one anesthesia code—in this case code 00796, Anesthesia for intraperitoneal procedures in upper abdomen including laparoscopy; liver transplant, and *not* report code 00840, Anesthesia for intraperitoneal procedures on lower abdomen including laparoscopy; not otherwise specified (for the appendectomy). When determining which code to report (the most complex procedure), report the code with the highest base units, as determined by ASA RVG or CMS RVG.

The American Society of Anesthesiologists (ASA) also publishes a valuable tool in anesthesia coding, the **ASA Crosswalk**—a book that bridges all applicable CPT surgical and therapeutic procedure codes to the appropriate anesthesia codes. The crosswalk lists the CPT surgical or therapeutic code, and then crosswalks, or maps, the surgical code to the appropriate anesthesia code to report the procedure. This is helpful for anesthesia coders, as they can look up the surgical CPT code for the procedure performed by the surgeon, and the book refers the them to the anesthesia code that should be reported for the accompanying anesthesia service. For example, code 44970, Laparoscopy, surgical, appendectomy, would crosswalk to anesthesia code 00840, Anesthesia for intraperitoneal procedures on lower abdomen including laparoscopy; not otherwise specified. The crosswalk is a valuable resource for anesthesia coders to ensure that the anesthesia code selected is appropriate for the surgical procedure performed.

Key to Success

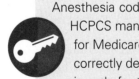

Anesthesia coding requires additional resources other than the ICD-10-CM, CPT, and HCPCS manuals. These are the relative value guides (both ASA and CMS versions, for Medicare patients) and the anesthesia crosswalk. These resources help coders correctly determine the base units per procedure and identify the correct anesthesia code for the medical procedure performed.

When coding for anesthesia services, there are a number of HCPCS modifiers that may be appended depending on the provider of the anesthesia service. It may also be necessary to report additional procedures that were performed along with the anesthesia service.

Anesthesia Providers and Modifiers

There are three providers that are qualified to perform an anesthesia service: anesthesiologists, anesthesiology assistants (AA), and certified registered nurse anesthetists (CRNA). Anesthesiologists are medical doctors who may perform services at their own discretion, whereas AAs and CRNAs are mid-level providers who must work under the supervision of an anesthesiologist. CRNAs may perform services without the constant attendance of an anesthesiologist, but an anesthesiologist must be on-site (in the building) during procedures to assist if necessary. It is necessary to identify the provider of anesthesia service using the appropriate HCPCS modifier:

- AA, Anesthesiology services performed personally by anesthesiologist
- AD, Medical supervision by a physician; more than four concurrent anesthesia procedures
- QK, Medical direction of two, three, or four concurrent anesthesia procedures involving qualified professionals
- QY, Medical direction of one certified registered nurse anesthetist (CRNA) by an anesthesiologist
- QX, CRNA service: with medical direction by a physician
- QZ, CRNA service: without medical direction by a physician

Modifier -AA should be used to identify that the service was provided directly by the anesthesiologist. Modifiers -AD, -QK, and -QY should be used by an anesthesiologist to report that he or she supervised the anesthesiology procedure performed by an AA or CRNA. The mid-level provider bills for his or her service using the same anesthesia code appended with -QX to indicate that the anesthesiologist supervised the procedure. When this happens, both the supervising anesthesiologist and the CRNA performing the procedure receive a percentage of the anesthesia reimbursement. Modifier -QZ is used when the CRNA performs the anesthesia service without the supervision of an anesthesiologist (see figure 12.10).

Figure 12.10. Anesthesia provider modifiers

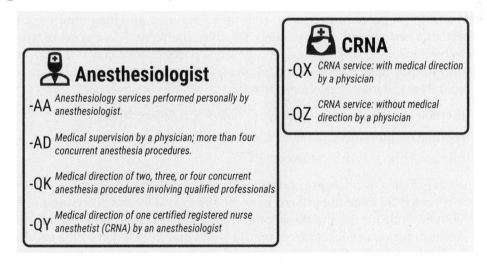

Additional modifiers used for anesthesia services include:

- G8, Monitored anesthesia care (MAC) for deep complex, complicated, or markedly invasive surgical procedure
- G9, Monitored anesthesia care for patient who has history of severe cardiopulmonary condition
- QS, Monitored anesthesia care service

These modifiers all report specific circumstances in which monitored anesthesia care is administered by an anesthesiologist, in some cases to help justify why the sedation was performed by an anesthesiologist, rather than the physician.

MOD

Multiple modifiers might be necessary in order to correctly report anesthesia services. For example, a modifier may be required to identify the provider of service as the anesthesiologist, -AA; another modifier may be needed to identify the service as monitored anesthesia care, -QS; and yet another modifier may identify the patient's status as having a severe systemic disease, -P3. Coding correctly for anesthesia services requires identification of all the factors involved in reporting these services correctly: identification of the procedure code, identification of the provider of service, identification of the patient's physical status, the amount of time involved in the procedure, and whether any qualifying circumstances were involved. Remember that sometimes multiple qualifying circumstance codes may be necessary too!

Additional Procedures and Bundled Services

There are many procedures bundled into the anesthesia service that may not be coded elsewhere. These include

- the administration of fluids and/or blood
- usual monitoring services (patient vitals, temperature, blood pressure, ECG/EKG [93000–93010], oxygen level, capnography, and mass spectrometry)

When these procedures are performed with the anesthesia service they are considered part of the service and cannot be reported elsewhere. The anesthesiologist may perform additional procedures throughout the service, such as cardiopulmonary resuscitation, interpretation of lab tests, blood transfusions, bronchoscopy, or laryngoscopy. Several additional procedures may be considered bundled into the primary code for the anesthesia service and not separately payable. Therefore, it is a good practice to always check insurance policy regarding which services may or may not be reported separately for payment. However, the following additional procedures are commonly paid separately and may be necessary to report in certain circumstances.

- Insertion of central venous catheter (36555–36558, 36568, 36569)
- Insertion of intra-arterial catheter (36620–36625)
- Insertion of Swan-Ganz catheter (93503)

When any of these services are performed in addition to the anesthesia service, they may be reported by appending them with modifier -59, Distinct procedural service, along with the code for the anesthesia procedure. Catheters are commonly inserted to allow for the infusion of substances or products and may be inserted by the anesthesia provider before or during the anesthesia procedure. In order for the anesthesia provider to be able to code for the catheter (or line) placement, it must have been performed by the anesthesia provider (and not the healthcare provider) and the procedure must be fully documented with a diagnosis to identify the medical necessity for the service.

In addition to the list given, any procedures that are performed to control postoperative pain may also be coded in addition to the code for the primary anesthesia service. Note that these procedures are performed only when the original procedure is complete and the patient has fully recovered from the anesthesia and operation, but still requires anesthesia services for pain management. These include

- Epidural spinal injections (62320–62323 for single injections, 62324–62327 for continuous infusion or intermittent bolus). For subsequent daily hospital management of postoperative pain, report code 01996, Daily hospital management of epidural or subarachnoid continuous drug administration. Do not calculate time units for code 01996; instead report one unit per day.
- Nerve blocks. Codes for nerve blocks are based on the nerve being blocked and identify either a single injection or continuous infusion by catheter. The nerve being blocked must be identified in the documentation (brachial plexus, sciatic nerve, femoral nerve, lumbar plexus).

Do not include the time for performing the given procedure within the total anesthesia time. These codes are reported in addition to the anesthesia service, appended with modifier -59. Note that these procedures are separately reportable for *postoperative pain management only*. Postoperative pain management is anesthesia provided to the patient after the surgery or procedure is performed and the patient has been transferred to the postoperative unit, but still requires some sort of anesthesia service to control pain in the postoperative period. This means that the procedure has been completed, including the original anesthesia service, but the patient is still in pain and needs additional pain management procedures in order to manage his or her comfort level.

Complete the exercise in There's a Code for That 12.2 to practice assigning procedure codes to anesthesia services.

Procedural coding for anesthesia services

12.2

There's a Code for That

Read the following documentation and select the appropriate CPT code for the anesthesia service. Remember to include the appropriate modifier(s) for physical status and anesthesia provider, as well as any qualifying circumstances code(s).

1. Anesthesiologist provided anesthesia for diagnostic arthroscopy on right knee joint of a normal, healthy patient.

   CPT code: _____ - _____ , -_____

2. CRNA (under direct supervision by anesthesiologist) provided anesthesia for open osteotomy of humerus on a patient with uncomplicated pregnancy.

   CPT code: _____ - _____ , -_____

3. Without supervision by anesthesiologist, CRNA provided physiological support for the harvesting of a declared brain-dead patient.

   CPT code: _____ - _____ , -_____

4. Anesthesiologist provided anesthesia for a 76-year-old male patient receiving a coronary artery bypass graft with pump oxygenator. Patient has poorly controlled diabetes and has a history of MI approximately one year ago.

   CPT codes: _____ - _____ , -_____ , _____

Procedural Coding for Pain Management Services

Pain management procedure codes are located in the Surgery section of the CPT code book, mostly in the Nervous System subsection. There are many different pain management methods, which depend on the type of practitioner, and his or her specialty and level of interest. Methods include electrodiagnostic studies to help find the cause of the pain, integrative medicine like acupuncture and yoga, interventional pain procedures, muscle and joint injections, peripheral nerve stimulation, and spinal cord stimulation.

Electrodiagnostic Studies

Electrodiagnostic studies are a way of measuring the electrical activity in muscles and nerves, and can help diagnose the cause or specific area from which pain is originating. There are two types of electrodiagnostic studies—electromyography and nerve conduction study.

Electromyography (EMG) evaluates the condition of muscle and nerves to determine the cause of pain, such as a pinched nerve or a diseased muscle. Electromyography codes may be found in the range 95860 through 95872, and in other locations in the CPT code book. To find the code for the EMG service performed, access the CPT Index and search for the term *Electromyography*, then refer to the type of EMG (fine wire, needle, surface), and the subterm for the area being evaluated (cranial nerve supplied muscle, extremities, face and neck muscles) (Mount Sinai Hospital n.d.a).

A **nerve conduction study (NCS)** is a test that activates nerves and gauges their responses as a way of determining if there is a problem with the functioning of the nerve. Nerve conduction tests are often performed alongside EMG evaluations to provide a complete picture of the patient's nerves and to determine the cause of the patient's pain. Codes for NCS (95905–95913) identify the number of studies performed. Examples include code 95907, Nerve conduction studies; 1–2 studies, or 95912, Nerve conduction studies, 11–12 studies (Mount Sinai Hospital n.d.a).

Key to Success

Remember that Appendix J (Electrodiagnostic Medicine Listing of Sensory, Motor, and Mixed Nerves) includes a summary of sensory, motor, and mixed nerves with the appropriate nerve conduction study (NCS) code. Write a reminder next to codes 95905 to 95913 in the CPT Tabular List to refer to Appendix J if you need help assigning codes to specific nerves.

Integrative Medicine

Integrative medicine consists of complementary and alternative therapies that may be used to treat chronic pain. Integrative medicine combines traditional healthcare treatments with alternative therapies such as acupuncture, yoga, cupping, and nutritional integration. **Acupuncture** is an ancient method of treating a variety of ailments like headaches, low back pain, anxiety, inflammation, constipation, insomnia, joint pain, nerve pain, stress, and tinnitus. The practice of acupuncture consists of inserting thin, flexible needles into specific areas of the body to restore the body's balance and relieve discomfort. Medical acupuncture codes (97810–97814) are based on time spent with the patient performing the procedure, and whether or not the procedure was performed with electrical stimulation.

Interventional Pain Procedures

Interventional pain procedures are a range of different procedures that use invasive interventions to treat the patient's pain. They include epidural injections, medial branch blocks and facet joint injections, radiofrequency nerve ablations, joint injections, occipital nerve blocks, and kyphoplasty.

Epidural Steroid Injections

An **epidural steroid injection** is a minimally invasive procedure that can treat pain in the neck, shoulders, arms, back, buttocks, and legs, resulting from irritation of spinal nerves due to conditions such as herniated discs, degenerative disc disease, and arthritis (Mount Sinai Hospital n.d.b). Note that an epidural steroid injection is an injection of long-lasting corticosteroid, which is an anti-inflammatory agent and *not* an anesthetic substance. An anesthetic substance can be injected through an epidural site, but this is usually done as part of an anesthesia procedure, or to alleviate postoperative pain (see figure 12.11).

Figure 12.11. Epidural injection

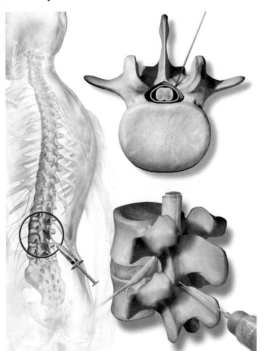

Source: Blausen.com staff 2013a.

When coding for epidural injections, know the substance involved, the site of the epidural injection (cervical, thoracic, lumbar, or sacral), and whether or not imaging guidance was used. Imaging guidance is the use of imaging, such as x-ray, CT scan, ultrasound, or fluoroscopy during the procedure to help guide the surgeon. For example, code 62320, Injection(s), of diagnostic or therapeutic substance(s) (eg, anesthetic, antispasmodic, opioid, steroid, other solution), not including neurolytic substances, including needle or catheter placement, interlaminar epidural or subarachnoid, cervical or thoracic; without imaging guidance, identifies the substance involved, *diagnostic or therapeutic substance not including neurolytic substance*; the site of the injection, *cervical or thoracic*; and if imaging guidance was used, *without imaging guidance*. When the procedure is performed without imaging guidance, the healthcare provider injects the area without the use of any imaging services to help see the exact injection site.

To find the code for an epidural injection, search for the term *Epidural* in the CPT Index, then reference the type of epidural procedure. For epidural anesthesia procedures, reference the main term *Epidural Anesthesia* in the CPT Index.

Medial Branch Nerve Blocks and Facet Joint Injections

Facet joint injections are injections made into the facet joint of the vertebra (see figure 12.12) that are used to treat pain coming from the small joints of the spine. Injections made into this area deliver low doses of long-lasting corticosteroids or local anesthetics directly to the source of the pain (the joint) to alleviate discomfort. Medial nerves connect to the facet joints and are injected concurrently with the facet joint injection (Mount Sinai Hospital n.d.b).

Figure 12.12. Facet joints of the vertebra

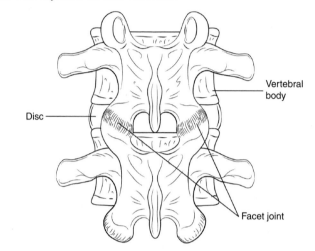

Vertebral body

Disc

Facet joint

Source: ©AHIMA

Codes for facet joint injections (64490–64495) are based on the area of the injection—either cervical or thoracic, or lumbar or sacral. Add-on codes identify additional levels of the vertebra that were injected. Refer to figure 12.13, which identifies the individual vertebrae of the spinal column as well as level of the spine. A level is each individual vertebral level injected. For example, the injections at the first level might be L2 to L3, a second level L3 to L4, and a third level L4 to L5. Code 64493, Injection(s), diagnostic or therapeutic agent, paravertebral facet (zygapophyseal) joint (or nerves innervating that joint) with image guidance (fluoroscopy or CT), lumbar or sacral; *single level*, for the first level injected (L2 to L3), and then the add-on codes for the second level and then the other add-on code for the third (or any other additional) level: 64494, Injection(s), diagnostic or therapeutic agent, paravertebral facet (zygapophyseal) joint (or nerves innervating that joint) with image guidance (fluoroscopy or CT), lumbar or sacral; *second level*, and 64495, Injection(s), diagnostic or therapeutic agent, paravertebral facet (zygapophyseal) joint (or nerves innervating that joint) with image guidance (fluoroscopy or CT), lumbar or sacral; *third and any additional level(s)* (see figure 12.14). Note that the add-on code 64495 may only be reported once per day, even if the provider performed more than three facet joint injections.

If the facet joint injection was performed bilaterally, append modifier -50, Bilateral procedure to each injection that was performed bilaterally.

Radiofrequency Nerve Ablations

Radiofrequency nerve ablation is a procedure used to treat back and neck pain by using a controlled heat source to disable nerves responsible for causing pain. The procedure is performed using a small needle with a heated tip placed near the nerve causing

Figure 12.13. Levels of the spine

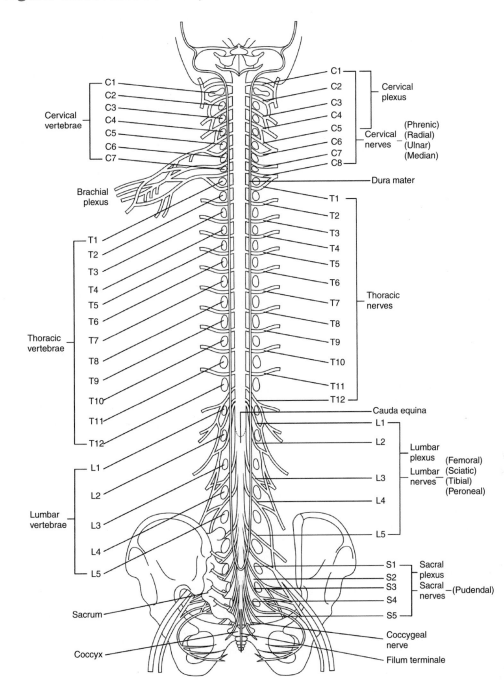

Source: ©AHIMA.

Figure 12.14. Facet joint injection coding

CPT Code	Facet Joint Injected
64493	L2 to L3
64494	L3 to L4
64495	L4 to L5

the pain, to disrupt the nerve's ability to send a pain signal (Mount Sinai Hospital n.d.b).

Codes for radio frequency nerve ablation are found under the section of codes titled Destruction by Neurolytic Agent (e.g., Chemical, Thermal, Electrical, or Radiofrequency), Chemodenervation (64600–64681). To find the correct code, it is necessary to identify the area or nerve destroyed by the procedure. Be careful to read parenthetical notes and guidelines in this section of codes to ensure correct code selection. For example, code 64616, Chemodenervation of muscle(s); neck muscle(s), excluding muscles of the larynx, unilateral (eg, for cervical dystonia, spasmodic torticollis), is followed by important guidelines located in parentheses after the code: *For bilateral procedure, report 64616 with modifier 50;* and *for chemodenervation guided by needle electromyography or muscle electrical stimulation, see 95873, 95874. Do not report more than one guidance code for any unit of 64616.*

Joint Injections

A joint injection is an injection of a therapeutic substance, such as corticosteroid, local anesthetics, or hyaluronan, into a joint to relieve pain caused by painful joint conditions such as osteoarthritis, synovitis, or inflammatory arthritis.

Coding for joint injections requires the identification of the joint, the substance injected, and whether or not the procedure was performed with ultrasound or imaging guidance. Note that joint injection codes are included in the Musculoskeletal System subsection of the CPT code book, not the Nervous System subsection. This is because the injections are given directly into the patient's affected joint. To search for the code, refer to the main term *Injection* in the CPT Index, then find the subterm for either the area of the injection, such as *Joint, Nerve,* or *Trigger Point* (a small, tight area of muscle tissue), or the type of substance injected, such as *Anesthetic Agent,* as applicable.

Occipital Nerve Blocks

An **occipital nerve block** is an injection directly into the greater and lesser occipital nerves, used to treat headaches and migraines (Mount Sinai Hospital n.d.b). There is one code for occipital nerve block, 64405, Injection(s), anesthetic agent(s) and/or steroid; greater occipital nerve.

Key to Success

Turn to code 64405, Injection(s), anesthetic agent(s) and/or steroid; greater occipital nerve, in your CPT code book. Note that this code is located with the subheading for Extracranial Nerves, Peripheral Nerves, and Autonomic Nervous System, and in the category of codes that identify procedures on the facial, vagus, and phrenic nerves (among others). These are all *peripheral* nerves located in the cranium. They are not part of the *central* nervous system. Keep this in mind when coding for services performed on nerves in the cranial and cervical area. Even though they are close to the central nervous system in distance, they are still part of the peripheral nervous system.

Kyphoplasty

A **kyphoplasty** is a treatment for vertebral compression fractures and the pain they cause. In this procedure, a balloon is threaded through an incision in the back, to the site of the compression fracture, where it is slowly inflated to push the compressed bone back into place. Once in place, cement is injected into the area to hold the bone in the proper position. This is a more invasive procedure than most injections for pain management, and is usually done in an operating room under general anesthesia (Mount Sinai Hospital n.d.b).

Kyphoplasty codes, 22513 to 22515, identify the site of the procedure—either lumbar or thoracic. The add-on code 22515 should be used for each additional thoracic or lumbar vertebral body involved in the procedure. For example, if the provider performed a kyphoplasty on two lumbar vertebrae, then the codes selected would be 22514, Percutaneous vertebral augmentation, including cavity creation (fracture reduction and bone biopsy included wen performed), using mechanical device (eg, kyphoplasty), 1 vertebral body, unilateral or bilateral cannulation, inclusive of all imaging guidance; *lumbar*, and 22515, Percutaneous vertebral augmentation, including cavity creation (fracture reduction and bone biopsy included when performed), using mechanical device (eg, kyphoplasty), 1 vertebral body, unilateral or bilateral cannulation, inclusive of all imaging guidance; *each additional thoracic or lumbar vertebral body*.

Peripheral Nerve Stimulation

Peripheral nerve stimulation is a way to help treat pain that results from traumatic injury or dysfunction of the peripheral nerves. The procedure is performed by placing small electrodes next to peripheral nerves to ensure that the correct nerves have been identified for the procedure. Once the nerves causing the pain are found, the trial leads are removed and a neurostimulator is placed, with permanent leads and a small battery pack, to continuously stimulate the nerves and relieve pain (Mount Sinai Hospital n.d.c).

Codes for peripheral nerve stimulation procedures are in the range for Neurostimulators (Peripheral Nerve) (64553–64595). Code selection relies on the procedure performed (such as percutaneous implantation through a small incision in the skin, an open incision for implantation, revision or replacement of the device, or complete removal of the device) and the nerve involved in the procedure (cranial, peripheral, and such).

Once the device is in place, it may be necessary to analyze the functioning of the neurostimulators and program the stimulator for optimal function. These services are reported with codes from the Medicine section, Neurostimulators, Analysis-Programming (95970–95982). These codes identify the nerves treated by the neurostimulators and various services related to the analysis and programming of the neurostimulator.

Spinal Cord Stimulation

Spinal cord stimulation (SCS) is similar to peripheral nerve stimulation, except this procedure is performed on the spinal nerves. Once the exact spinal nerves causing the pain are identified, a permanent battery and lead wires are placed to alleviate pain. Spinal cord stimulation can also be programmed with a remote control to work at certain times, such as when the patient is walking, and then turn the leads off before lying down for bed (Mount Sinai Hospital n.d.c).

Codes for spinal cord stimulation are also similar to those for peripheral nerve stimulation. Codes in the range for Neurostimulators (Spinal) (63650–63688) identify the procedure performed (percutaneous implantation, laminectomy for implantation, removal, or revision), as well as any imaging guidance (fluoroscopy).

The decision to treat chronic pain using any one of these surgically invasive procedures is based on a number of factors and must be medically necessary. Diagnostic coding for anesthesia services requires the indication for the operation and indications of medical necessity for any additional procedures performed during the anesthesia session. Pain management, on the other hand, relies on more specific diagnoses that must be placed in a specific order to identify the reason why the patient was seen for pain management, and to justify the pain management procedure with an indication of medical necessity for the service.

Complete the exercises in the There's a Code for That 12.3 to practice reporting procedure codes for pain management services.

12.3

There's a Code for That

Procedural coding for pain management services

Read the following documentation and select the appropriate CPT code for the pain management service.

1. Needle EMG of the thoracic paraspinal muscles.

   CPT code: _____

2. Thoracic epidural anesthesia injection with fluoroscopic guidance.

   CPT code: _____

3. Radiofrequency ablation of bilateral cervical spinal and accessory nerves with electrical stimulation for guidance on a patient with chronic migraine.

   CPT codes: _____ , _____

4. Laminectomy performed to gain open access to the spinal column, and electrode plate with simple receiver is placed in the epidural space for spinal neurostimulation.

   CPT code: _____

Diagnosis Coding for Anesthesia and Pain Management Services

Diagnostic coding for anesthesia procedures must identify the medical necessity for the procedure performed, for which the patient was placed under anesthesia. Pain management diagnosis coding is a bit more complicated, as it requires an indication for medical necessity for the pain management procedure (that is, the diagnosis of pain), as well as the underlying diagnosis for what is causing the pain, if known. There are also a number of guidelines that identify the correct reporting of pain diagnoses.

Diagnostic Coding for Anesthesia Services

Diagnostic coding for anesthesia procedures requires the identification of the indication for the procedure(s) performed. In other words, anesthesiologists do not diagnose patients; they rely on the documentation of the diagnosis from the healthcare provider performing the procedure. In this case, diagnostic coding for anesthesia services is relatively straightforward. Remember, if the preoperative and postoperative diagnoses for a patient differ from each other, select the postoperative diagnosis as the diagnosis code for the service.

The only exception to this is if the patient experiences some kind of medical condition or reaction to the anesthesia, for which the anesthesiologist has to perform additional procedures, such as inserting an arterial catheter or transesophageal echocardiography.

If the patient has a reaction to the anesthesia procedure, the appropriate complication of anesthesia code should be reported. These include

- T88.2---, Shock due to anesthesia
- T88.3---, Malignant hyperthermia due to anesthesia
- T88.4---, Failed or difficult intubation
- T88.5, Other complications of anesthesia:
    o T88.51--, Hypothermia following anesthesia
    o T88.52--, Failed moderate sedation during procedure
    o T88.53--, Unintended awareness under general anesthesia during procedure
    o T88.59--, Other complications of anesthesia

For any of the code categories T88.2, T88.3, or T88.5, use an additional code for adverse effect to identify the drug administered. For example, if a patient was administered ketamine, a drug used in moderate sedation, and the drug wore off and the patient regained full consciousness during the procedure, code T88.52XA, Failed moderate sedation during procedure, initial encounter, should be reported, as well as code T41.295A, Adverse effect of other general anesthetics, initial encounter.

Do not confuse complications of anesthesia codes with *history* of complications to anesthesia codes. A history code identifies a condition that the patient reports having experienced in the past, but which he or she is not currently experiencing. For example, if the patient had been anesthetized in the past (either moderate sedation or general anesthesia), and the anesthesia did not work as intended, then one of the following codes would be reported: Z92.83, Personal history of failed moderate sedation, or Z92.84, Personal history of unintended awareness under general anesthesia. These codes should be used if the patient has a personal history of these reactions, but is not currently experiencing said reaction.

Diagnostic Coding for Pain Management Procedures

Coding for pain management is slightly more complicated than coding for anesthesia services due to the numerous guidelines that govern code selection and sequencing for pain management procedures. This sequencing of codes for anesthesia and pain management conditions is important. Remember to check for notes in the ICD-10-CM Tabular List to *use additional code*, *code first*, and *code also*. When you see *use additional code*, report the additional code *after* the code you are referencing. When you see *code first*, report the additional code *before* the code you are referencing. When you see *code also*, you can place the additional code either before or after the code you are referencing, depending on the circumstances of the encounter.

Additional diagnoses that may require pain management procedures also include acute and chronic pain, post-thoracotomy and postprocedural pain, neoplasm related pain, and additional relevant diagnoses.

Acute and Chronic Pain

Chronic pain is the constant or long-term sensation of pain and, among other causes, may be a result of postoperative complications, past injuries, or nerve conditions. Acute pain is the short-term sensation of pain, which may last from just moments to a matter of months and is typically due to an injury, soft tissue damage, or acute condition. Correctly coding for acute and chronic pain relies on close reading of the guidelines pertaining to these conditions, as well as the reason for the patient's healthcare encounter (to treat the underlying cause of the pain or to treat the pain itself). When a patient presents with the symptom of pain, such as right knee pain, and there is no definitive diagnosis, the coder should report the unspecified code for the pain—code M25.561, Pain in right knee. (Find the code for knee pain, reference the term *pain* in the ICD-10-CM Index, and then the site of the pain.)

However, if the knee pain is identified as acute, chronic, post-thoracotomy/postprocedural, or neoplasm-related, an additional code from category G89, Pain, not elsewhere classified, should be reported in addition to the knee pain code. So, if the condition was chronic right knee pain due to a traumatic injury, then two codes would be needed to identify the condition: M25.561, Pain in right knee, and G89.21, Chronic pain due to trauma. (Note that sequencing of these two codes will depend on the circumstances of the encounter). If the patient's pain is a *symptom* of an underlying condition, such as osteoarthritis, and the patient is being seen for a treatment of the underlying condition, then it is not necessary to use a code from category G89 to identify the pain and the underlying condition. In this case, it would only be necessary to assign the code for the definitive condition (osteoarthritis).

However, if the patient has an underlying condition that is causing the pain (like osteoarthritis), and the patient is being seen for treatment of the pain (rather than the underlying condition), then a code from category G89 should be reported, and sequenced before the code for the underlying condition. For example, if the patient is being seen for a pain management procedure (an injection of the knee joint) due to chronic pain in the knee from osteoarthritis, then the codes selected should be as follows:

1. G89.29, Other chronic pain

2. M25.561, Pain in right knee

3. M17.11, Unilateral primary osteoarthritis, right knee

In this example, remember that the patient is being seen for pain management, so the additional codes to identify the acuity and the specific site of the pain are necessary, in addition to the code for the underlying condition (see figure 12.15).

Figure 12.15. Sequence of diagnosis codes for pain management

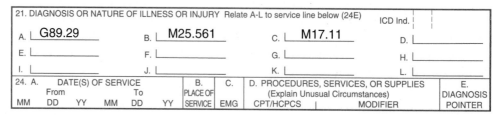

Source: CMS 2019a.

According to OGCR, the only time a code from category G89 should be sequenced first is if the patient is being seen for a pain management procedure, intended to treat the patient's pain. If the treatment is aimed at the underlying condition, then the code for the underlying condition should be coded first (see figure 12.16). For example, if the patient is being seen for medication management of osteoarthritis, then the primary code for the encounter would be M17.11, Unilateral primary osteoarthritis, right knee. The codes for chronic pain and knee pain would not be assigned, as these are included in the primary diagnosis of osteoarthritis of the knee.

Figure 12.16. OGCR I.C.6.b through I.C.6.b.ii

---

b. Pain-Category G89

1) General coding information

Codes in category G89, Pain, not elsewhere classified, may be used in conjunction with codes from other categories and chapters to provide more detail about acute or chronic pain and neoplasm-related pain, unless otherwise indicated below.

If the pain is not specified as acute or chronic, post-thoracotomy, post procedural, or neoplasm-related, do not assign codes from category G89.

A code from category G89 should not be assigned if the underlying (definitive) diagnosis is known, unless the reason for the encounter is pain control/management and not management of the underlying condition.

When an admission or encounter is for a procedure aimed at treating the underlying condition (e.g., spinal fusion, kyphoplasty), a code for the underlying condition (e.g., vertebral fracture, spinal stenosis) should be assigned as the principal diagnosis. No code from category G89 should be assigned.

(a) Category G89 Codes as Principal or First-Listed Diagnosis

Category G89 codes are acceptable as principal diagnosis or the first-listed code:

- When pain control or pain management is the reason for the admission/encounter (e.g., a patient with displaced intervertebral disc, nerve impingement and severe back pain presents for injection of steroid into the spinal canal). The underlying cause of the pain should be reported as an additional diagnosis, if known.

- When a patient is admitted for the insertion of a neurostimulator for pain control, assign the appropriate pain code as the principal or first-listed diagnosis. When an admission or encounter is for a procedure aimed at treating the underlying condition and a neurostimulator is inserted for pain control during the same admission/encounter, a code for the underlying condition should be assigned as the principal diagnosis and the appropriate pain code should be assigned as a secondary diagnosis.

(b) Use of Category G89 Codes in Conjunction with Site Specific Pain Codes

(i) Assigning Category G89 and Site-Specific Pain Codes

Codes from category G89 may be used in conjunction with codes that identify the site of pain (including codes from chapter 18) if the category G89 code provides additional information. For example, if the code describes the site of the pain, but does not fully describe whether the pain is acute or chronic, then both codes should be assigned.

(ii) Sequencing of Category G89 Codes with Site-Specific Pain Codes

The sequencing of category G89 codes with site-specific pain codes (including chapter 18 codes), is dependent on the circumstances of the encounter/admission as follows:

- If the encounter is for pain control or pain management, assign the code from category G89 followed by the code identifying the specific site of pain (e.g., encounter for pain management for acute neck pain from trauma is assigned code G89.11, Acute pain due to trauma, followed by code M54.2, Cervicalgia, to identify the site of pain).

- If the encounter is for any other reason except pain control or pain management, and a related definitive diagnosis has not been established (confirmed) by the provider, assign the code for the specific site of pain first, followed by the appropriate code from category G89.

Source: CMS 2019c.

Post-thoracotomy and Postprocedural Pain

Post-thoracotomy and postprocedural pain is not reported if the pain is experienced immediately after surgery because of the procedure. However, if the pain remains

Figure 12.17. OGCR I.C.6.3

---

3) Postoperative Pain

The provider's documentation should be used to guide the coding of postoperative pain, as well *as Section III. Reporting Additional Diagnoses and Section IV. Diagnostic Coding* and *Reporting in the Outpatient Setting.*

The default for post-thoracotomy and other postoperative pain not specified as acute or chronic is the code for the acute form.

Routine or expected postoperative pain immediately after surgery should not be coded.

(a) Postoperative pain not associated with specific postoperative complication

Postoperative pain not associated with a specific postoperative complication is assigned to the appropriate postoperative pain code in category G89.

(b) Postoperative pain associated with specific postoperative complication

Postoperative pain associated with a specific postoperative complication (such as painful wire sutures) is assigned to the appropriate code(s) found in Chapter 19, Injury, poisoning, and certain other consequences of external causes. If appropriate, use additional code(s) from category G89 to identify acute or chronic pain (G89.18 or G89.28).

Source: CMS 2019c.

---

and requires treatment, then codes from category G89 may be reported to identify the condition (see figure 12.17).

There are two scenarios for which there are guidelines for reporting post-thoracotomy or postprocedural pain:

- If the pain is not related to any specific postoperative complication, then use the appropriate pain code from category G89. For example, pain in the knee three months after a knee joint prosthesis insertion, would not be reported as postprocedural pain, as the pain is experienced after the healing phase of the prosthesis insertion surgery is complete.

- If the postoperative pain is associated with any specific complication, such as painful wire sutures, then report the code for the complication. Coders may also report a code from category G89, if it is necessary to identify the pain as acute or chronic.

Neoplasm-Related Pain

Code G89.3, Neoplasm-related pain (acute) (chronic), should be reported when any pain is documented because of a cancer, primary or secondary malignancy, or tumor. For example, pain due to an osteosarcoma (cancer of the bone) of the lower leg would be reported with the appropriate ICD-10-CM pain code (site specific), as well as the G89 code for the neoplasm-related pain. When a patient presents for a pain management encounter for the treatment of the pain, sequence the neoplasm-related pain code first, with an additional code to identify the malignancy.

When the patient presents for treatment of the malignancy, then the code for the malignancy should be sequenced first, with an additional code to identify the neoplasm-related pain, if necessary. In this case, it is not necessary to include an additional code to identify the specific site of the pain (see figure 12.18).

Additional Diagnoses for Pain Management

There are numerous underlying causes of pain, ranging from psychological factors to underlying diseases (such as osteoarthritis) to traumatic injuries. Many of the pain management procedures discussed are used to treat musculoskeletal conditions, such as osteoarthritis, muscle pain and inflammation, back pain and sciatica, and spinal and intervertebral disc disorders.

Figure 12.18. GCR I.C.6.5

---

5) Neoplasm Related Pain

Code G89.3 is assigned to pain documented as being related, associated or due to cancer, primary or secondary malignancy, or tumor. This code is assigned regardless of whether the pain is acute or chronic.

This code may be assigned as the principal or first-listed code when the stated reason for the admission/encounter is documented as pain control/pain management. The underlying neoplasm should be reported as an additional diagnosis. When the reason for the admission/encounter is management of the neoplasm and the pain associated with the neoplasm is also documented, code G89.3 may be assigned as an additional diagnosis. It is not necessary to assign an additional code for the site of the pain.

See Section I.C.2 for instructions on the sequencing of neoplasms for all other stated reasons for the admission/ encounter (except for pain control/pain management).

Source: CMS 2019c.

Osteoarthritis

Osteoarthritis is a degenerative condition of the joints that results from wear and tear of the cartilage between joints; and causes pain, swelling, and problems with range of motion of the joint. Diagnosis codes for osteoarthritis are found in categories M15 through M19, Osteoarthritis, and depend on the identification of the type and site of the condition, including laterality. For example, M19.171, Post-traumatic osteoarthritis, right ankle and foot, identifies the type of osteoarthritis, *post-traumatic*; the site, *ankle and foot*; and the laterality, *right*.

Muscle Pain and Inflammation

Muscle pain and inflammation can take many forms, such as enthesopathies, myositis, and myalgias.

An **enthesopathy** is an inflammation of the tendon or ligament at the site of attachment to the bone that causes pain, tenderness, stiffness, and swelling. Enthesopathies include ankylosing spondylitis (inflammation of the joints of the spine), plantar fasciitis (which results in pain in the heel and bottom of the foot), and Achilles tendinitis.

Myositis is an inflammation of the muscle that can be caused by an infection, injury, medicine, or a chronic disease, and causes muscle weakness and pain, along with other symptoms.

Myalgia is muscle pain, which may be a symptom of many medical conditions including overuse of the muscle, overstretching, infection, or disease process. **Fibromyalgia** (M79.7, Fibromyalgia) is a myalgia that is characterized by chronic, full-body pain, with a sensitivity to pressure. Fibromyalgia also causes fatigue, problems sleeping, memory problems, restless leg syndrome, numbness or tingling, and other psychological factors such as depression and anxiety.

When coding for muscle pain and inflammation, identify the specific type of condition (tendinitis, spondylosis, fasciitis, fibromyalgia), and then the specific site, if necessary. For paired organs, report the code for the correct laterality of the condition. For spinal conditions, it is necessary to identify the specific site of the condition according to spinal region, as follows: occipito-atlanto-axial, cervical, cervicothoracic, thoracic, thoracolumbar, lumbar, lumbosacral, sacral and sacrococcygeal, or multiple sites in the spine. Refer to figure 12.13 for an illustration of these areas of the spine. Note that ICD-10 diagnosis codes may combine two areas of the spine, such as lumbosacral. In this case, the code identifies that the medical condition exists in both of those areas (for example, M54.17, Radiculopathy, lumbosacral region).

Back Pain and Sciatica

Back pain is typically experienced at a specific area along the spine, such as **cervicalgia** (neck pain), M54.2, Cervicalgia, or **lumbago** (low back pain), M54.5, Low back pain.

Sciatica (M54.3-) is a combination of pain, numbness, and weakness along the sciatic nerve from the lower back area, radiating to the buttocks and the leg. It is usually caused by a lower back problem putting pressure on the sciatic nerve.

Diagnosis codes for back pain identify the specific region of the pain. Codes for sciatica identify the laterality of the condition. Note that there is an additional subcategory of codes for lumbago with sciatica (M54.4-) that should be used when a patient experiences both conditions concurrently. Also note that if any of these conditions are due to an intervertebral disc disorder, then the coder should report the code for the disc disorder that includes the symptoms of pain or sciatica.

Intervertebral Disc Disorders

Intervertebral disc disorders are common causes of pain due to spinal issues. They include intervertebral disc deterioration, herniation, and prolapse of an intervertebral disc. These problems can cause chronic or radiating pain, numbness, tingling, and loss of strength and range of motion of movement; and can also result in **radiculopathy**, a nerve-related pain (see figure 12.19 for an illustration of a herniated disc causing a pinched nerve).

Codes for intervertebral disc disorders (M50 and M51) identify the region (and in some cases the exact vertebra) involved in the pain, as well as any additional conditions that may present with the disc disorder like sciatica pain, radiculopathy, or myelopathy. For example, code M50.123, Cervical disc disorder at C6-C7 level with radiculopathy,

Figure 12.19. Clinical manifestations of lumbar disc herniation

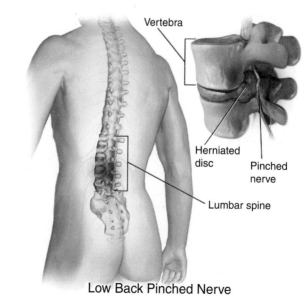

Source: Blausen.com staff 2013b.

identifies the general area of the spine (*cervical*), in addition to the specific vertebrae involved (*C6-C7*), as well as the manifestation of the condition (*radiculopathy*).

Complete the exercises in There's a Code for That 12.4 to practice identifying diagnosis codes for anesthesia and pain management services.

Diagnostic coding for anesthesia and pain management services

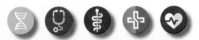

There's a Code for That

12.4

Read the following documentation and select the appropriate ICD-10-CM diagnosis code(s) for the anesthesia or pain management service.

1. Patient undergoing open herniorrhaphy manifested malignant hyperthermia due to inhalation anesthesia.

   ICD-10-CM codes: _____ , _____

2. Patient undergoing inhaled anesthesia for open repair of open traumatic femur shaft fracture of the right leg.

   ICD-10-CM code: _____

3. Patient with ankylosing spondylitis of the thoracolumbar spine presents for management of his chronic pain.

   ICD-10-CM code: _____ , _____

4. A 45-year-old male presents with lumbago and sciatica due to thoracic disc prolapse.

   ICD-10-CM code: _____

5. Interstitial myositis of the left shoulder.

   ICD-10-CM code: _____

Putting It All Together: Coding for Anesthesia and Pain Management Services

In order to select the correct codes for an anesthesia or pain management service, it is important to carefully read the documentation then access each code book to find the procedure or service provided and the corresponding diagnosis or diagnoses to support the medical necessity for the service. Procedural codes for anesthesia services are found in the Anesthesia section of the CPT code book, and diagnosis codes are found in the ICD-10-CM code book. Some anesthesia services may also be found in the Surgery section of the CPT code book, such as postoperative epidurals or pain management procedures. Pain management procedures are found in the Surgery section of the CPT code book.

Determining the correct codes relies on the answers to the following questions.

- What service was provided to the patient—was it an anesthesia service or pain management service?

- For anesthesia services, you need the following information:
  - The base unit values for the anesthesia service
  - The time spent on the anesthesia service
  - Any applicable modifying factors:
    - Physical status of the patient
    - Qualifying circumstances surrounding the service
  - Were any additional services performed that are not included in the anesthesia service, such as TEE or PICC line insertion? (If so, code for the additional service with modifier -59.)
  - Add any applicable HCPCS modifiers to identify the provider of the anesthesia service or any specific circumstances surrounding the service.
  - For pain management procedures, check coding guidelines for any applicable add-on codes or modifiers for additional or bilateral procedures.
- What is the primary condition being treated?
  - In anesthesia coding, this is the reason why the patient is having the procedure.
  - For pain management encounters, pay close attention to the sequencing of the diagnosis codes (remember to check the coding guidelines in the ICD-10-CM code book).
- Are there any additional diagnoses that need to be included to justify the medical necessity of the services?

The following vignette demonstrates how to select the appropriate diagnosis and procedure codes. After reviewing the vignette, complete the exercises in There's a Code for That 12.5 to practice coding for anesthesia and pain management services.

Sandra is completing the coding for an anesthesia case for a patient that received anesthesia services related to the delivery of her child. The normal, healthy patient, at 39 weeks' gestation, was brought into the delivery room and labor was induced at 0850 hours. The patient's labor progressed until the anesthesiologist was called into perform an epidural for management of the patient's pain at 1500 hours. After the administration of the epidural, the patient's labor progressed less rapidly, and eventually the patient was taken for cesarean section due to prolonged second stage of labor. The patient's epidural was transferred to epidural anesthesia for cesarean section, after which a single live born child was delivered without further incident. After the procedure was complete, epidural was removed and care of the patient was transferred to the delivery nurse. Total time for the epidural for labor was 3.5 hours (210 minutes), and the total time for the cesarean anesthesia was 30 minutes.

First, Sandra asks herself: What did the anesthesiologist do? The anesthesiologist performed an neuraxial labor anesthesia (epidural) procedure for a planned vaginal delivery, which was converted to a cesarean delivery. She looks up the procedures in the CPT Index under the main term Anesthesia, *then references the subterm* Neuraxial, *and then* Cesarean Delivery, *and finds two codes: 01968 and 01969. Code 01968 is for anesthesia for cesarean delivery, and code 01969 is for cesarean hysterectomy, so in this case the correct code is 01968 as no hysterectomy was performed. Sandra notes that 01968 is an add-on code, and according to the parenthetical note in the CPT code book should be used in conjunction with 01967, to identify the anesthesia for the planned vaginal delivery.*

- *01967, Neuraxial labor analgesia/anesthesia for planned vaginal delivery*
- *01968, Anesthesia for cesarean delivery following neuraxial labor analgesia/anesthesia*

Now, Sandra needs to identify the base units for the anesthesia service. She refers to the CMS RVGs for anesthesia services and determines that the base units for 01967 are 5 and the base units for 01968 are 2 (see figure 12.20).

Figure 12.20. Base unit values for CPT range 01967 through 01991

CPT code	Base Unit Value
01967	5
01968	2
01969	5
01990	7
01991	3

Now she needs to determine the time units that she will report for the service. Time units for the patient's insurance company are reported in 15-minute increments, and the total time spent on the epidural service was 210 minutes, so she reports 14 units (210 minutes divided by 15-minute increments = 14 units), which is reported for CPT code 01967. The total time spent for the cesarean anesthesia was 30 minutes, which would be reported with 2 units on procedure code 01968.

Finally, Sandra needs to identify any modifying factors for the anesthesia service. In this case, the patient was a normal, healthy patient, so she can append physical status modifier -P1, A normal healthy patient. No qualifying circumstances are relevant and need to be reported on the claim. She will also add modifier -AA, Anesthesia service performed personally by anesthesiologist, to indicate that the procedure was performed personally by the anesthesiologist.

Sandra also needs to calculate the amount of money to charge for the service, so she must add all of the units for the service and multiply them by the conversion factor for the area in which the procedure was performed. The anesthesia was performed in Arizona, so she refers to the CMS locality-adjusted conversion factor tables (accessed via the CMS website). The conversion factor is 21.80 (see figure 12.21), and she enters this amount in the charges for the claim.

Figure 12.21. Calculating anesthesia charges

CPT code	Base Units	Time Units	Modifying Factors	Conversion Factor	Total Charge Amount
01967	5	14	0	$21.80	$1,456.00
01968	2	2	0	$21.80	$ 87.20

Her calculations are as follows: $(B + T + M) \times CF$ = Total charge amount

Now that Sandra has the procedure codes, modifiers, and the charge amount, she needs to identify the ICD-10-CM code(s) for the diagnosis. She asks herself: Why did the doctor do it? In this case, the patient was anesthetized for a cesarean section, which was necessary due to prolonged second stage of labor. Sandra finds this by searching under the term Delivery *in the ICD-10-CM Index, and then references the subterm* complicated by, *and then* prolonged labor, *and finds the code for second stage, O63.1. When a delivery occurs, an additional code should also be reported to identify the outcome of the delivery, in this case a single live born infant, Z37.0, as well as the weeks of gestation, Z3A.39.*

- *O63.1, Prolonged second stage (of labor)*
- *Z37.0, Single live birth*
- *Z3A.39, 39 weeks gestation of pregnancy*

Sandra enters the codes and charges on the claim and reviews the claim to ensure everything was entered correctly (see figure 12.22).

Figure 12.22. Reporting anesthesia services

21. DIAGNOSIS OR NATURE OF ILLNESS OR INJURY Relate A-L to service line below (24E)				ICD Ind.		22. RESUBMISSION CODE		ORIGINAL REF. NO.		
A. 063.1	B. Z37.1	C. Z3A.39	D.							
E.	F.	G.	H.			23. PRIOR AUTHORIZATION NUMBER				
I.	J.	K.	L.							

24. A. DATE(S) OF SERVICE						B. PLACE OF SERVICE	C. EMG	D. PROCEDURES, SERVICES, OR SUPPLIES (Explain Unusual Circumstances) CPT/HCPCS	MODIFIER	E. DIAGNOSIS POINTER	F. $ CHARGES	G. DAYS OR UNITS	H. EPSDT Family Plan	I. ID. QUAL.	J. RENDERING PROVIDER ID. #
From MM	DD	YY	To MM	DD	YY										
1 XX	XX	XX	XX	XX	XX			01967	AA P1		1456.00	14		NPI	
2 XX	XX	XX	XX	XX	XX			01968	AA P1		87.20	2		NPI	

Source: CMS 2019a.

Key to Success

Coding for anesthesia services may or may not require performing the calculations to add the base units, time units, modifying factors, and then multiplying the sum by the conversion factor. Many anesthesia electronic health record systems have these functions built in, so the calculations are performed automatically. However, is it still important to understand these calculations, as not all anesthesia providers have the same software, and you may find yourself in the rare situation in which these calculations must be done by hand.

12.5 Coding for anesthesia and pain management services

There's a Code for That

Read the following documentation and select the appropriate CPT and ICD-10-CM code(s) for the anesthesia or pain management service.

1. A 78-year-old female experiencing chronic pain underwent balloon kyphoplasty to repair vertebral compression fractures at the T5 and T6 levels.

   CPT codes: _____ , _____

   ICD-10-CM code: _____

2. Anesthesia administered by CRNA without anesthesiologist supervision for patient undergoing kyphoplasty of the T5 and T6 vertebrae for compression fractures at those levels in a 78-year-old female with mild hypertension.

   CPT codes: _____ - _____ - _____ , _____

   ICD-10-CM code: _____

3. Anesthesia provided for 4-year-old female receiving heart and lung transplant for myxoma of the heart, CHF, and cardiomyopathy, which are a constant threat to her life.

   CPT codes: _____ - _____

   ICD-10-CM code: _____

4. Bilateral facet joint injections with fluoroscopic guidance of the C6, C7, and C8 vertebrae performed on 48-year-old male with chronic pain in the neck, bilateral shoulders, and bilateral arms.

   CPT codes: _____ - _____ , _____ - _____ ,

   _____ - _____

   ICD-10-CM codes: _____ , _____ , _____ ,

   _____ , _____ , _____

Case Study Flexible Sigmoidoscopy with Anesthesia

PATIENT: Lawrence Egbert

PROCEDURE: Flexible sigmoidoscopy with anesthesia

PREOPERATIVE DIAGNOSIS: History of rectal cancer, status post colon resection, rectal incontinence

POSTOPERATIVE DIAGNOSIS: History of rectal cancer, status post colon resection, rectal incontinence

FINDINGS: Anastomotic stenosis

ESTIMATED BLOOD LOSS: Minimal

DRAINS: None

DISPOSITION: Awakened from anesthesia and taken to recovery room in stable condition, having suffered no untoward event.

COMPLICATIONS: None

TECHNIQUE: After informed consent was obtained, this patient with mild systemic disease was placed in the left lateral position. General anesthesia was administered by anesthesia. A timeout was performed and the patient and procedure were confirmed. A digital rectal exam was performed. Fibrosis was noted at the anastomosis. No masses were palpable. This was followed by flexible sigmoidoscopy. The endoscope was introduced through the anastomosis and up to the sigmoid colon. The quality of prep was poor with heavy stool burden in the sigmoid and rectal area. This was irrigated to visualize the anastomosis. A posterior recess was noted consistent with patient's history of perirectal sinus that had healed well. No evidence of recurrent malignant disease was noted.

A guidewire was then passed through the scope into the sigmoid colon and the scope was withdrawn. The anastomotic area was then dilated using Savary dilators starting at 45 French dilating it up to 60 French. The dilators were removed and a repeat endoscopy was performed. There is no evidence of injury or bleeding from the anastomosis. No evidence of perforation was noted. The procedure was terminated and patient was taken to the recovery room in stable condition. There were no immediate complications and the estimated blood loss was minimal.

SIGNED: Dr. Topher Crawley, MD

Use the following steps to select the appropriate codes for the case study.

1. Read through the case study and answer the question: *What did the doctor do?* Remember that for this case, you are coding only for the anesthesia performed that facilitated the procedure. In this case study, identify the name of the procedure.

_____

_____

2. Now that you have identified the procedure, determine the type of anesthesia that was administered by the anesthesiologist, in addition to any applicable physical status or qualifying circumstances.

_____

_____

3. Locate the code for the anesthesia procedure in the CPT code book.
   a. Search the Index for the procedure and search through the options.
   b. Refer to the codes listed in the Tabular section and identify the correct code range.

   _____

   _____

   c. In the listing of codes, check for any guidelines, important definitions, or parenthetical notes. Select the appropriate code and list it here.

   _____

   _____

   d. Identify all necessary physical status modifiers and qualifying circumstance codes and add them here.

   _____

   _____

4. Now that the procedure(s) and modifier(s) have been identified, review the case study and answer the following question: *Why did the doctor do it?*

_____

_____

5. Now that you have identified the patient's diagnoses, search the ICD-10-CM code book for the correct codes for these conditions. Follow these steps for each of the diagnoses identified.

   a. Search the Main Index for the name of each condition and search through any applicable subterms and cross-references to locate the appropriate code.

   i. _____

   _____

   ii. _____

   _____

   iii. _____

   _____

   iv. _____

   _____

   b. Verify the code in the Tabular List. Locate the code identified previously in the Tabular Listing of codes and refer to any applicable guidelines, notes, and symbols. Does the code selected correctly identify the patient's condition? If yes, list the code here.

   i. _____

   _____

   ii. _____

   _____

   iii. _____

   _____

   iv. _____

   _____

   c. Check the procedure note and ICD-10-CM guidelines and conventions to determine the correct sequencing of the diagnosis codes, if applicable. Correctly sequence the diagnosis codes.

   _____

   _____

6. Now that the procedure and diagnosis codes have been identified, list them on the CMS-1500 form. Be sure to correctly link the procedure and diagnosis codes. Remember to add the number of units as necessary. For this case study, do not calculate the time, base units, or modifying factors. Assign only the ICD-10-CM and CPT codes to the claim, with correct code linkage.

21. DIAGNOSIS OR NATURE OF ILLNESS OR INJURY Relate A-L to service line below (24E) ICD Ind.				22. RESUBMISSION CODE
A.	B.	C.	D.	
E.	F.	G.	H.	23. PRIOR AUTHORIZATION NU
I.	J.	K.	L.	

24. A. DATE(S) OF SERVICE From / To MM DD YY MM DD YY	B. PLACE OF SERVICE	C. EMG	D. PROCEDURES, SERVICES, OR SUPPLIES (Explain Unusual Circumstances) CPT/HCPCS MODIFIER	E. DIAGNOSIS POINTER	F. $ CHARGES	G. DAYS OR UNITS
1						
2						
3						

End-of-Chapter Content

Instructions: Indicate whether the following statements are true or false (T or F). For false statements, rewrite the statement on the line below to make the statement true.

1. Analgesia is the inability to feel pain.

2. The modifier used for services provided by anesthesiology assistants is -AA.

3. Coders may use the CMS or ASA RVG to find the base units for anesthesia services.

4. When an anesthesiologist provides an anesthesia service for more than one procedure at the same operative session only one anesthesia code is billed—the one with the highest base units.

5. Physical status modifiers describe a particularly difficult anesthesia service due to the condition of the patient, notable operative conditions, or unusual risk factors.

_____

_____

6. Pain management specialists employ various procedures to improve the quality of life for patients suffering from chronic pain.

_____

_____

7. Anesthesia services are located in the Surgery section of the CPT code book.

_____

_____

8. Anesthesia codes identify the general procedure performed by the surgeon for which the patient was anesthetized.

_____

_____

9. Medical acupuncture may be performed for pain management purposes but these services may not be coded on the health record.

_____

_____

10. A peripheral nerve stimulation device is implanted directly in the spinal column for pain management.

_____

_____

Instructions: Choose the best answer.

1. Which of the following components takes into account how long an anesthesia procedure took to complete, from start to finish?

   a. Base units
   b. Time units
   c. Physical status
   d. CPT code

2. Which of the following is the correct formula for calculating the amount billed for anesthesia services?

   a. $B + T + CF = M$
   b. $(B + T + M) = CF$
   c. $CF \times (B + T + M)$
   d. $B + T + M + CF$

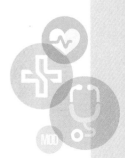

3. Which of the following units takes into consideration the relative value for each anesthesia service?

   a. Base
   b. Time
   c. Physical status modifiers
   d. Conversion factor

4. Time units for most commercial payers are reported in increments of how many minutes?

   a. 1 minute
   b. 7.5 minutes
   c. 30 minutes
   d. 15 minutes

5. Which physical status modifiers would be used for a patient with a severe systemic disease that is a constant threat to life?

   a. P6
   b. P5
   c. P4
   d. P3

6. Which qualifying circumstance code should be reported for a patient who received anesthesia under controlled hypothermia?

   a. 99100
   b. 99116
   c. 99135
   d. 99140

7. How many unit values are assigned for qualifying circumstance code 99140?

   a. 1
   b. 2
   c. 5
   d. 4

8. Which type of anesthesia blocks a small amount of nerves using an injection, topical cream, or spray?

   a. Local
   b. Regional
   c. General
   d. Moderate (conscious) sedation

9. In which of the following types of anesthesia is the patient completely unconscious?

   a. Local
   b. Regional
   c. General
   d. Moderate (conscious) sedation

10. Which of the following anesthesia codes should be appended to a service performed by a CRNA with anesthesiologist supervision?

    a. -AA
    b. -QY
    c. -QZ
    d. -QX

11. Which of the following pain management procedures uses invasive interventions to treat the patient's pain?

    a. Integrative medicine
    b. Electrodiagnostic studies
    c. Medical management
    d. Interventional pain procedures

12. Which type of pain management procedure injects a steroid or anesthetic directly into the patient's spinal joints?

    a. Epidural steroid injections
    b. Facet joint injections
    c. Trigger point injections
    d. Occipital nerve blocks

13. A patient with a history of failed anesthesia underwent a surgical procedure under general anesthesia. Which of the following ICD-10-CM diagnosis codes should be assigned?

    a. Z92.83
    b. T88.53
    c. T88.4
    d. Z92.84

14. A patient with neoplasm-related pain presented for a pain management procedure. Which code should be sequenced as the first-listed diagnosis?

    a. The code for the neoplasm
    b. The code for acute pain
    c. The code for the pain management procedure
    d. The code for chronic pain

Instructions: Answer the following questions with the appropriate code(s) and modifier(s).

1. An anesthesiologist performed anesthesia for a patient with ESRD on a regular dialysis schedule, receiving a kidney transplant. The patient was transferred to the PACU and care transferred to PACU nurse. Two hours later, anesthesiologist was called back in to perform a single injection epidural without imaging guidance in the thoracic area, to manage the patient's postprocedural pain.

   CPT codes: _____ - _____ , - _____ ,

   _____ - _____

   ICD-10-CM codes: _____ ,

   _____ , _____

2. A 65-year-old female with idiopathic peripheral neuropathy presented for monthly acupuncture treatment. 30 minutes of medical acupuncture with 20 needles provided without electrical stimulation.

   CPT codes: _____ , _____

   ICD-10-CM code: _____

References

American Medical Association (AMA). 2019. *CPT 2020 Professional Edition*. Chicago: AMA.

American Society of Anesthesiologists (ASA). 2019 (October 23). ASA Physical Status Classification System. https://www.asahq.org/standards-and-guidelines/asa-physical-status-classification-system.

Army Publishing Directorate (APD). 1998 (February 1). DA Form 7389: Medical Record - Anesthesia. https://armypubs.army.mil/pub/eforms/DR_a/pdf/A7389.pdf.

Blausen.com staff. 2013a. Blausen 0354 EpiduralSteroidInjection.png. Digital image. Wikimedia Commons. https://commons.wikimedia.org/wiki/File:Blausen_0354_EpiduralSteroidInjection.png.

Blausen.com staff. 2013b. Blausen 0484 HerniatedLumbarDisc.png. Digital image. Wikimedia Commons. https://commons.wikimedia.org/wiki/File:Blausen_0484_HerniatedLumbarDisc.png.

Centers for Medicare and Medicaid Services (CMS). 2019a. CMS 1500. https://www.cms.gov/Medicare/CMS-Forms/CMS-Forms/CMS-Forms-Items/CMS1188854.html.

Centers for Medicare and Medicaid Services (CMS). 2019b (October 29). Locality-Adjusted Anesthesia Conversion Factors as a result of the CY 2020 Final Rule. https://www.cms.gov/Medicare/Medicare-Fee-for-Service-Payment/PhysicianFeeSched/Downloads/2020-Anesthesia-Conversion-Factors.zip.

Centers for Medicare and Medicaid Services (CMS). 2019c. ICD-10-CM Official Guidelines for Coding and Reporting FY 2020. https://www.cms.gov/Medicare/Coding/ICD10/Downloads/2020-Coding-Guidelines.pdf.

Centers for Medicare and Medicaid Services (CMS). 2018. 2018 Anesthesia Base Units by CPT Code. https://www.cms.gov/Medicare/Medicare-Fee-for-Service-Payment/PhysicianFeeSched/Downloads/2018-Anesthesia-BaseUnits-CPT.zip.

Das, S. and S. Ghosh. 2015 (January-March). Monitored anesthesia care: An overview. *Journal of Anaesthesiology Clinical Pharmacology* 31(1): 27–29. https://www.ncbi.nlm.nih.gov/pmc/articles/PMC4353148/.

Mount Sinai Hospital. n.d.a. Electromyography. https://www.mountsinai.org/health-library/tests/electromyography.

Mount Sinai Hospital. n.d.b. Interventional Pain Procedures Under X-Ray Guidance. http://www.mountsinai.org/patient-care/service-areas/pain-management/pain-management-services/interventional-spinal-procedures-under-x-ray-guidance.

Mount Sinai Hospital. n.d.c. Peripheral Nerve Stimulation. http://www.mountsinai.org/patient-care/service-areas/pain-management/pain-management-services/peripheral-nerve-stimulation.

Palmetto GBA. 2013 (July). Anesthesia Billing Guide. https://engage.ahima.org/HigherLogic/System/DownloadDocumentFile.ashx?DocumentFileKey=9af2a07d-26e1-4694-b1de-a4c59d0dbc30.

Resources

abeo. 2016 (February 15). Specialty Tip #15 Anesthesiology. http://abeo.com/wp-content/uploads/2016/02/15-ICD10_SpecialtyTips_Anesthesiology.pdf.

Centers for Medicare and Medicaid Services (CMS). 2019. Physicians/Nonphysician Practitioners (Rev. 4339, 07-25-19). Chapter 12 in *Medicare Claims Processing Manual*. https://www.cms.gov/Regulations-and-Guidance/Guidance/Manuals/Downloads/clm104c12.pdf.

Mount Sinai Hospital. n.d. Pain Management Services and Treatments. http://www.mountsinai.org/patient-care/service-areas/pain-management/pain-management-services.

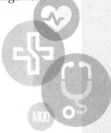

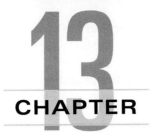

CHAPTER

Radiology and Imaging Services

Learning Objectives

- Understand the basics of billing and coding for independent radiology and imaging centers
- Examine procedural codes and guidelines for independent radiology and imaging services
- Examine diagnosis coding and medical necessity for independent radiology and imaging services
- Determine and apply ICD-10-CM, CPT, and HCPCS codes to independent radiology and imaging services

Key Terms

Anterior

Antero-posterior

Axial plane

Computed tomography (CT)

Contralateral

Contrast material

Coronal plane

Distal

Doppler ultrasound

Global radiology service

Imaging services

Independent radiology and imaging center

Inferior

Ipsilateral

Lateral

Lateral (view)

Magnetic resonance imaging (MRI)

Mammography

Medial

Nuclear medicine

Oblique

Pleural effusion

Posterior

Postero-anterior

Professional component (PC)

Projection

Proximal

Pulmonary edema

Radiologic guidance

Radiological supervision and interpretation (S&I)

Radiologist

Radiology services

Sagittal plane

Superior

Technical component (TC)

Transverse plane

Ultrasound

X-ray

Radiology and imaging services are medical procedures that use various techniques to view the inner structures of the body for diagnostic or therapeutic purposes. **Radiology services**, which include x-rays and CT scans, use radiation to produce images of the inside of the body, such as bones and organs. **Imaging services** is a more inclusive term used for the wide array of types of techniques used to produce images of the inside of the body, including radiology services, ultrasounds, fluoroscopy, and nuclear imaging.

This chapter discusses radiology and imaging techniques including basics of radiology and imaging services, billing for radiology and imaging procedures, and substantiating radiology and imaging services with the appropriate diagnosis codes.

Radiology and Imaging Basics

When coding for radiology services, knowledge of the different settings and providers, components of the services, and the medical terminology—including the terms used for body plans, body positions, movement, and projections of radiology services—is important. Coders must also remember the importance of the professional and technical components of radiology procedures, and that they must bill only for the portion of the service performed by each healthcare provider.

Radiology and Imaging Settings and Providers

Radiology and imaging services are performed in various healthcare settings—independent facilities that focus on only imaging procedures, inpatient and outpatient hospitals, or individual clinics that use certain imaging services relevant to their specialty services.

An **independent radiology and imaging center** is an office that specializes only in radiology and imaging techniques. These offices receive requests from physicians to perform a specific imaging service or services on a patient, and then send the result of the imaging study to the requesting provider. For example, if a patient went to her primary care provider (PCP) and complained of pelvic pain, the PCP might choose to have an ultrasound of the patient's abdomen performed to rule out ovarian cysts. In some cases, depending on the type of provider and resources, an in-house ultrasound machine to perform the imaging may be available. If not, then the provider would likely send the patient to an imaging center that would perform the imaging service. The imaging center would receive the request from the patient's PCP, perform the ultrasound, and then send a written report of the findings to the PCP. This report may be provided through an electronic health record (EHR) system, emailed, or faxed. Often, depending on the type of imaging service performed, the actual images from the service are also sent with the report of the findings via the EHR system, emailed, or saved to a data storage device for transport to the requesting provider.

Radiology services may also be performed in the facility setting (inpatient or outpatient hospital). In these settings, the imaging or radiology service is often performed for an acute problem or as part of a surgical procedure. For example, a patient complaining of severe abdominal pain that presents to the emergency department may have an ultrasound of the abdomen done to rule out appendicitis. In the outpatient setting, imaging guidance may be used to help lead an outpatient surgical procedure; for example, fluoroscopic guidance used during a facet joint injection for the administration of a corticosteroid for pain management.

Some healthcare specialist offices may invest in their own imaging equipment so that certain radiology or imaging studies may be performed directly in the office. For example, a maternal-fetal healthcare specialist may invest in a number of ultrasound machines so that patients can receive ultrasounds in the office and the results are read immediately. Orthopedists also often have x-ray equipment so they can diagnose patient conditions and the healing status of fractures.

When a healthcare office has its own imaging equipment, the images produced are typically read by the ordering physician. For example, the maternal-fetal healthcare specialist orders an ultrasound for a high-risk patient and then reads the ultrasound results, or the orthopedist reads the x-rays and determines if a fracture is present or not. However, when the ordering provider is not present, the image is usually read by a radiologist.

A **radiologist** is a medical doctor who specializes in the diagnosis and treatment of medical conditions using radiology and imaging techniques. These include x-rays, ultrasounds, computed tomography (CT), magnetic resonance imaging (MRI), nuclear medicine, and positron emission tomography (PET) scans. Radiologists are further trained in radiation safety, protection, and the effects of radiation on the human body, as well as imaging techniques and interpretation of imaging studies.

A radiology technician is the staff member trained to perform the imaging procedure. This person has received specialized training in how to operate the imaging machine, such as x-ray or ultrasound machine, and knows how to position the patient at the optimum angle for the image so the radiologist can get a clear view of the body area, organ, or other internal component involved in the imaging service. Radiology technicians are usually certified in their field of expertise and have completed formal schooling such as diagnostic medical sonography or radiology technician program.

These differences become significant when coding for radiology services, as there are two components to imaging procedures—the technical component and the professional component.

Components of Radiology Services

In any typical imaging service—such as an ultrasound, x-ray, or MRI scan—a technician uses the appropriate machine to take images of the patient, according to the directions of the ordering provider. Once these images are captured, the radiologist or ordering provider reads the images to determine the patient's diagnosis. This doctor then provides a written report of the findings of the imaging service (for instance, a fracture, gallstones, or tumor).

There are two components to an imaging services, each capturing a portion of the service provided (figure 13.1). The **technical component (TC)** of a service includes the equipment, supplies, clinical personnel, and any other costs needed to perform the imaging procedure. For example, the technical component of an x-ray would include the x-ray machine, any supplies used to take the x-ray, and the salary for the x-ray technician who captured the image.

The **professional component (PC)** of a service includes the professional supervision, interpretation, and written report of the findings from the imaging service. For example, the professional component of an x-ray would be the radiologist reading the x-ray and determining that a fracture is present (interpreting the results), and then submitting a written report of his or her findings to the ordering provider.

Billing for imaging services depends on the portion of the service that was provided by the office. For example, if an ultrasound were performed at an imaging center and the images were sent directly to the ordering doctor without interpretation, the imaging center would bill only for the *technical* component of the service—because only the technical component was provided (machine and any supplies used, and the

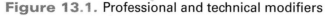

Figure 13.1. Professional and technical modifiers

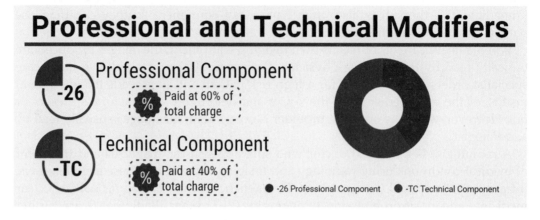

clinical staff required to operate the machine and perform the ultrasound). The doctor receiving the images, however, would bill only for the *professional* component of the service (interpretation of the images and a written report of the findings). In this way, imaging centers, radiologists, and any other provider who performs and reads imaging services can divide the components of an imaging service, and bill only for the portion of the service they performed.

Billing for either of these portions is done by adding the appropriate modifier to the CPT code for the radiology procedure. Modifier -26, Professional component, is used to indicate that only the professional component of the procedure was performed. So, using the previous example, an ultrasound was performed and sent to the provider's office, who then read, interpreted, and delivered a written report of the findings. The CPT code reported by the provider's office would be appended with modifier -26 to indicate that only the professional component of the service was performed.

Billing for the technical component of the procedure is done by appending modifier -TC, Technical component, to the code. In the previous example, the imaging center performing the ultrasound would report the CPT code for the ultrasound procedure, appending it with modifier -TC to indicate that only the technical part of the procedure was performed. Modifier -TC should only be used when the reporting facility owns the equipment and pays for the performance of the imaging service, as well as the salary for the clinical staff needed to perform the service. However, there may be a caveat to the reporting of modifier -TC and imaging services for some types of healthcare settings. For example, in the inpatient hospital setting, if the inpatient hospital facility performed the radiology procedure, then this would be reported not with a CPT code but rather with an ICD-10-PCS code to identify the procedure performed, as discussed in chapter 20 (Inpatient Hospital Services). In the outpatient hospital setting (submitting professional fee codes), the third-party payer may assume that the hospital owns the radiology equipment, and so the use of modifier -TC is not necessary (Verhovshek 2015). As with other areas of healthcare coding, it is necessary to check with payer policy to ensure that the patient's insurance accepts modifier -TC and verify the rate at which they pay for the service.

Using either of these modifiers divides the CPT code into two parts—one technical and one professional—so the provider who performed the service can bill for that portion of the service. Appending either of these modifiers indicates that the reimbursement for the procedure is broken into two parts. The exact amount depends on the insurance but usually performing the technical component of the procedure pays more than performing the professional component of the procedure. For example, the technical component of the procedure might pay 60 percent of the allowable amount of payment for the code, whereas the professional component might pay 40 percent of the allowable amount of payment for the code. Note, however, that these payment percentages depend on the third-party payer for the service.

When a provider performs both the technical and professional components of a code, it is not necessary to append any modifier to the code. For example, if the ultrasound is performed in the office of an obstetrician where the practice owns the ultrasound machine, pays the clinical staff to perform the procedure, and also pays the doctor to read the ultrasound and interpret the results, then the practice would bill for *each* component of the imaging service (both professional and technical). In this case, the same CPT code would be reported, once per date of service, *without any modifiers*. This is called billing for the **global radiology service**. A global radiology service is the performance of both components of the procedure—professional and technical—by the same facility. Billing for the global service requires simply the reporting of the CPT code for the service, appended without either the -26 or -TC modifier (see figure 13.2 for an illustration of the components of a radiology service).

Figure 13.2. Components of radiology services

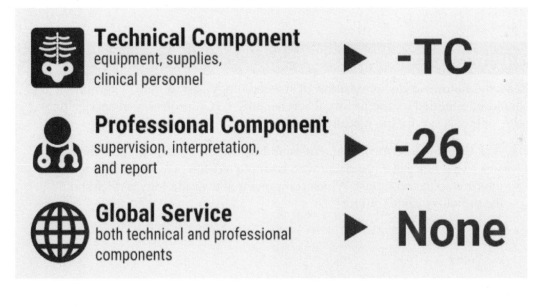

Technical Component
equipment, supplies, clinical personnel
▶ **-TC**

Professional Component
supervision, interpretation, and report
▶ **-26**

Global Service
both technical and professional components
▶ **None**

Key to Success

Think about surgery billing and global surgery packages discussed in chapter 11 (Surgical Services). A global surgical package includes all of the little procedures needed to perform the surgery. Billing for the global radiology service is very similar. When *neither* the -26 nor the -TC modifiers are used, it indicates that the provider performed the global radiology procedure, which included both the professional and technical components of the service.

Services that include both the professional and technical components are found in sections other than the Radiology section of the CPT code book. Some codes in the

Medicine section as well as the Pathology and Laboratory sections also identify either component of the code. For example, code 93005, Electrocardiogram, routine ECG with at least 12 leads; tracing only, without interpretation and report, is a Medicine section code that identifies only the technical components of the procedure (tracing only without interpretation and report). On the other hand, code 93010, Electrocardiogram, routine ECG with at least 12 leads; interpretation and report only, identifies only the professional component of the service (interpretation and report only). Neither of these codes requires either modifier -26 or -TC because the component is identified in the code description. It is important to pay close attention to code descriptions, as some identify either portion of the service performed with different codes, rather than needing to use modifier -TC or -26. The wording to look out for here is **radiological supervision and interpretation (S&I)**, which is the professional component of the study, and includes the supervision of the radiology service as well as interpretation of the results. For example, code 74445, Corpora cavernosography, *radiological supervision and interpretation*, already describes the procedure as the professional component. It is not necessary to include modifier -26 with this code, as this code *only* applies for the professional component.

Complete the exercises in There's a Code for That 13.1 to practice identifying the components of a radiology service.

13.1

There's a Code for That

Radiology components

Read the following documentation of the radiology service and determine if it should be reported as the technical service only (-TC), professional service only (-26), or global service (no modifier).

1. A chest x-ray is performed at a freestanding radiology center. The films are sent to the office of a physician who is employed at a private practice for interpretation and report. Which component of the radiology service should the radiology center bill for?

   a. Technical
   b. Professional
   c. Global

2. A chest x-ray is performed at a freestanding radiology center. The films are sent to the office of a physician who is employed at a private practice for interpretation and report. Which component of the radiology service should the physician that reads the report bill for?

   a. Technical
   b. Professional
   c. Global

3. A spinal x-ray is performed at an orthopedic clinic that employs the physician who reads and interprets the x-ray films. Which component will the orthopedic clinic bill for?

   a. Technical
   b. Professional
   c. Global

4. A hospital performs an abdominal imaging service for a patient with severe abdominal pain. A physician who is not employed by the hospital reads the images and determines that the patient has a ruptured appendix. Which component would the physician bill for?

a. Technical
b. Professional
c. Global

5. An imaging center performs a series of scans on a patient with suspected cancer. The in-house radiologist reads the scans and determines that there are a number of metastases present throughout the body. Which component would the imaging center bill for?

a. Technical
b. Professional
c. Global

Medical Terminology for Radiology and Imaging Procedures

Reporting the correct radiology code requires a solid knowledge of the basic directional terms, planes of the body, and projection terminology. These terms help coding professionals to understand the documentation of the radiology or imaging service so that the correct CPT code may be reported for the service.

Basic Directional Terms

Basic directional terms are often used to describe the general direction of a body part or area. Although these terms are useful in coding across all healthcare specialties, they are especially important when coding for radiological procedures. For example, diagnosis coding relies frequently on identification of the exact location of the condition, such as of the proximal arm versus the distal arm. Radiology and imaging service coders must be able to decipher the provider's documentation, which may include these terms, to determine which code should be reported for the service. They include:

- **Anterior:** situated toward the front of the body (such as the face or the breasts)
- **Posterior:** situated toward the back of the body (such as the buttocks or heels)
- **Superior:** toward the top of the body (the head)
- **Inferior:** toward the bottom of the body (the feet)
- **Medial:** toward the midline of the body (the belly button)
- **Lateral:** away from the midline of the body (the sides)
- **Proximal:** toward the center of the body (the upper arm)
- **Distal:** away from the body (the fingertips)
- **Ipsilateral:** the same side of the body (the right upper and lower extremities)
- **Contralateral:** the opposite side of the body (the right arm and the left arm)

Planes of the Body

The planes of the body are imaginary lines that dissect the body into sections. Just as with directional terms, the planes of the body are often used in health record documentation to identify the general area of a medical condition or procedure and include the following (see figure 13.3).

- The axial plane is a horizontal line perpendicular to the long axis of the body that divides the body into superior and inferior portions (top and bottom halves). The axial plane is also known as the transverse plane, or transaxial plane.
- The sagittal plane is a vertical line that divides the body into right and left halves.
- The coronal plane is also a vertical line but divides the body into anterior and posterior halves (front and back).

Projection

The projection of an imaging service is the direction in which the imaging rays pass through the body. For example, an x-ray machine is positioned at the front of the body, and the ray passes in through the anterior (the front of the body) and out through the posterior (the back of the body). The projection of an imaging service is also known as the view, so if there are two projections during an imaging service, this means the service consisted of two views and include:

- Antero-posterior (AP), which passes through the front to the back of the body
- Postero-anterior (PA), which passes through the back to the front of the body
- Lateral, which passes from one side of the body to the other (for example, from the right to the left)
- Oblique, which passes through the body at a diagonal angle

Figure 13.3. Planes of the body and basic directional terms

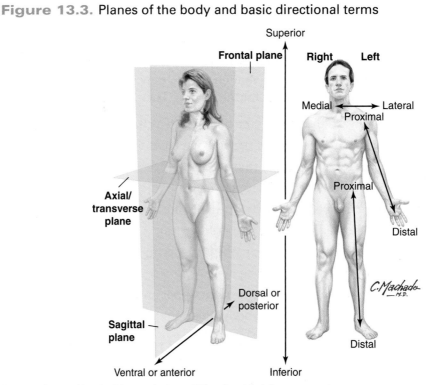

Key to Success

Knowing basic directional terms, planes of the body, and terms for projections is an important part of being able to decipher a health record and determine the correct procedure or diagnosis code. As you read through procedural notes or descriptions of surgical or radiology procedures, it helps to picture the procedure in your mind as the steps of the procedure are being described in the documentation. Knowing the planes of the body, directional terms, and projections is a good place to start.

Procedural Coding for Radiology and Imaging Services

Procedural coding for radiology and imaging services requires an understanding of how the Radiology section of the CPT code book is organized, the different types of imaging services included in the Radiology section, guidelines for coding radiology services, including how to code for contrast material, and modifiers used in radiology coding.

All radiology and imaging services are located in the Radiology section of the CPT code book, which is organized first by the type of radiology service provided and then subcategorized by the area that was included in the study, or the specific type of study or service provided. These services include diagnostic radiology services, diagnostic ultrasound, radiologic guidance, mammography, bone and joint studies, radiation oncology, and nuclear medicine. It is also important to understand the modifiers other than -26 and -TC that are used in radiology coding.

Diagnostic Radiology Services

The first and largest subsection of the Radiology section of the CPT code book is Diagnostic Radiology (Diagnostic Imaging) (70010–76499). This section includes codes for a number of different radiology and imaging services, arranged by general body area. Codes for several different imaging studies may be listed within each body area, such as radiologic examinations, special imaging studies, magnetic resonance imaging, and computed tomography scans. Diagnostic radiology services also include the administration of contrast materials.

Radiologic Examination (X-ray)

An x-ray examination is a form of imaging that produces a beam of x-rays, a form of electromagnetic radiation, that pass through the body. As the rays pass through the body, denser objects, like bones, absorb less of the radiation than less dense objects like internal organs or blood vessels. The rays that are not absorbed are captured behind the image, creating a negative image of the dense structures within the body (see figure 13.4). The human body is made up of many structures of varying densities, which makes x-ray imaging a painless and noninvasive method for diagnosing a range of medical conditions such as fractures, pneumonia, cysts, and tumors (NIBIB 2016). Code descriptions in the CPT code book refer to x-rays as radiologic examinations.

Figure 13.4. Posteroanterior chest x-ray

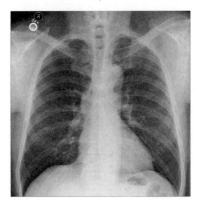

Key to Success

Do not be surprised when you do not see any CPT codes for "x-rays." Code descriptions in the CPT code book refer to x-rays as radiologic examinations. For example, code 72100, Radiologic examination, spine, lumbosacral; 2 or 3 views, is for an x-ray of the lumbosacral spine. On the other hand, health record documentation may read that the patient received an x-ray or radiographic examination of the spine. In this case, the coder must realize that an x-ray or radiographic examination in the health record is the same procedure described in the CPT code description as a radiologic examination.

Codes for x-rays often describe the number of views included in the procedure. A view is the angle at which the x-ray was taken. Multiple x-ray angles help to diagnose a medical condition with certainty. So, if a patient with a possible wrist fracture received an anteroposterior x-ray, a lateral x-ray, and an oblique x-ray of the wrist, then the x-ray of the wrist entailed three views (anteroposterior, lateral, and oblique).

When searching for the code for an x-ray in the CPT code book, reference either the term *X-ray* or *Radiology* in the Index, and then locate the subterm for the type of procedure and the area that was viewed in the procedure. In this case, if the patient had an x-ray of the wrist, the coder should reference the subterm *Wrist*, which leads to code range 73100 to 73110. Code options include 73100, Radiologic examination, wrist; *2 views*, or 73110, Radiologic examination, wrist; *complete, minimum of 3 views*. In this example, the x-ray consisted of three views, so the correct code would be 73110. If the x-ray had only consisted of one or two views, then the correct code would be 73100. Note that code 73110 describes a complete x-ray of the wrist, with a minimum of three views. This means that if more than three views were taken, such as five or six views, the correct code would still be 73110, as it describes a *minimum* of three views.

Key to Success

Notice that when you are searching for an x-ray in the Index, you can look up the term "x-ray," but when you verify the code(s) in the Tabular List, they are all listed as "Radiologic examinations." Don't let this confuse you! X-rays and radiologic examinations are the same procedure.

Special Radiological Studies

There are a number of special radiological studies listed in the Diagnostic Radiology subsection of the CPT code book. These are a special set of x-rays used to diagnose specific medical conditions. They are found throughout the Diagnostic Radiology section, and instead of describing an x-ray of a specific body area or organ, they are listed by the name of the study itself. For example, a dacryocystography is a radiologic examination of the lacrimal sacs and associated structures within the orbital area of the eyes. It is performed by injecting a contrast material into the nasolacrimal ducts and then a series of x-rays are taken. To look up a special radiological study, search for the term directly in the CPT Index (in this case the coder should look up *Dacryocystography*).

Key to Success

If you are coding for a special radiological study and you are having problems locating the code, use a medical dictionary and your knowledge of anatomy and physiology to determine the body area or organ system involved in the study. Then use this information to search for the radiologic examination of that particular body part, or scan through the table of contents for the Diagnostic Radiology subsection of codes.

Note that in this example, and for many special radiological studies, the code describes the *radiological supervision and interpretation* of the study: 70170, Dacryocystography, nasolacrimal duct, *radiological supervision and interpretation*. In this case, the imaging study is performed by injecting a contrast material into the patient's nasolacrimal ducts, and then taking the x-ray images. The entire procedure would be reported with two codes: one for the injection and one for the x-ray supervision and interpretation. The injection is coded in the appropriate surgery section of the CPT code book (in this case 68850, Injection of contrast medium for dacryocystography).

The coder should report *only* the portion of the service that was performed by their healthcare provider. For example, if both the injection and the imaging study were performed by the same physician, then both codes should be reported. If the two components were performed by different providers, then each provider should code only for the service that he or she performed. Note that because the x-ray code in this example identifies the radiological supervision and interpretation of the study, modifier -26 should not be appended to the code to identify the professional component.

Computed Tomography (CT)

A **computed tomography (CT)**, also known as computed axial tomography (CAT) scan is an imaging study that combines x-ray images from different angles to produce a virtual cross-section of the area being studied. CT scans are noninvasive and painless procedures, which may be used to diagnose patients suffering from acute traumatic events or patients with acute symptoms such as chest or abdominal pain, or difficulty breathing. It is also often used to create images of the chest, head, abdomen, and pelvis, because it can provide a cross-sectional view of all types of body tissues (see figure 13.5).

Codes for CT scans are located in the Diagnostic Radiology subsection of codes and are usually listed after radiologic examination codes in each respective body area. Code selection depends on the site of the CT scan and whether or not any contrast material was used. For example, code 72192, Computed tomography, pelvis; without contrast material, identifies the area of the study (pelvis), as well as whether or not contrast material was used (without contrast material).

Figure 13.5. Axial CT scan of the head

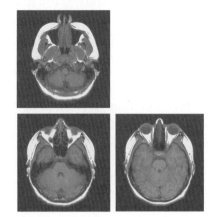

Magnetic Resonance Imaging (MRI)

Magnetic resonance imaging (MRI) is a form of imaging that uses strong magnetic fields and radio waves to produce detailed images of the anatomy and physiology of the internal structures of a patient's body and can be used to diagnose a range of medical conditions. MRI images include more detail of vascular structures and soft tissues than those produced by x-ray imaging. MRI studies are noninvasive and painless and may be used to diagnose neurologic conditions like dementia and cerebrovascular diseases, cardiovascular conditions, cancer staging, and assessment of joint diseases, and countless other conditions (see figure 13.6).

Figure 13.6. MRI of a lumbosacral herniated disc

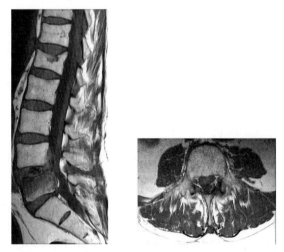

Codes for MRI studies are located in the Diagnostic Radiology subsection, usually listed after radiologic examination and computed tomography scan codes. Code selection depends on the site of the MRI, and whether or not any contrast material was used. For example, code 72198, Magnetic resonance angiography, pelvis, with or without contrast material(s), identifies the site of the study (pelvis) and whether contrast material was used (with or without contrast).

Contrast Materials

Contrast material, or contrast medium, is a substance that is injected into the patient to enhance the contrast of certain structures in the body while performing x-rays and imaging procedures. Contrast material may be given to the patient orally, rectally, or via injection, depending on the imaging procedure and intent of the study. For example, some imaging studies of the gastrointestinal tract may require a swallowed contrast material, and an x-ray of the lung may require an inhaled contrast material. However, note that according to CPT guidelines, only contrast that is given intravascularly (into a blood vessel), intra-articularly (into a joint), or intrathecally (into the spinal canal) counts as "with contrast" for CPT code selection. In other words, if the contrast material is not given via an injection, it does not count as contrast for the purposes of code assignment. This is due to the fact that the administration of the contrast material (as built into the code description) is only reported when it requires the physician's skill to do so.

Key to Success

If you forget what exactly counts as "contrast" for a radiology procedure, remember to refer to the pages before the radiology section of the CPT code book. In this area, you will find a heading for "Administration of Contrast Materials" that describes exactly what constitutes a contrast material and when to code (or not code) for the contrast material.

The use of contrast material produces images that may be more or less detailed in certain areas and, as a result, it is common that diagnostic radiology studies may be performed with contrast, without contrast, or with and without contrast, depending on the needs of the study. When coding for contrast, there are three code options:

- without contrast
- with contrast
- without contrast material(s) followed by contrast material(s) and further sequences

This last option identifies procedures that are performed with and without contrast. The imaging study is done without contrast material first, then contrast material is administered, and then the imaging study is performed again. Figure 13.7 shows an abdominal imaging CT with varying stages of contrast material. The top left image shows the abdominal CT without contrast and the other three images show varying stages of the contrast material working its way through the organs and abdominal structures.

When a contrast agent is used, it is also necessary to report the contrast material used with the appropriate supply code (HCPCS code). These HCPCS codes identify the specific contrast material used. Codes for contrast materials can be found in the Supplies for Radiology Procedures (Radiopharmaceuticals) (A9500–A9700) and in Contrast (Q9951–Q9983) in the HCPCS code book. For example, if an MRI of the brain was performed with and without contrast (contrast material used was Gadolinium), the codes reported would be 70553, Magnetic resonance (e.g., proton) imaging, brain (including brain stem); without contrast material followed by contrast material(s) and further sequences, and A9579, Injection, gadolinium-based magnetic resonance contrast agent, not otherwise specified (NOA), per ml.

Figure 13.7. Contrast in abdominal imaging

CTs Demonstrating Time Sequence from Organs Without Contrast to Clearance of Contrast By Kidneys

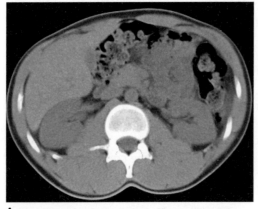

A. Noncontrast CT study. Note the subtle differences between the shades of grey in the solid viscera. Blood vessels in the liver are not well seen.

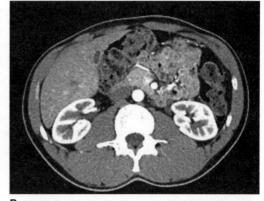

B. Arterial phase image. After 30 seconds of the injection, the contrast is predominantly in the arteries, which are seen as white rounded and linear structures.

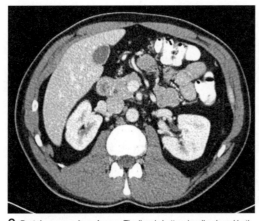

C. Portal-venous phase image. The liver is better visualized, and both the portal veins and the hepatic veins are opacified *(white)*. Contrast has also reached both the renal cortex and the medulla.

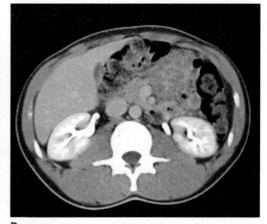

D. Contrast clearance by the kidneys and ureters at approximately 120 seconds. Contrast in the organs is "washing out" and is excreted by the kidneys. The renal calices, renal pelvis, and ureters become white with the concentrated contrast.

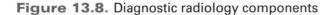

Figure 13.8 shows the multiple components of coding for diagnostic radiology services. Complete the exercises in There's a Code for That 13.2 to practice assigning codes for diagnostic radiology procedures.

Figure 13.8. Diagnostic radiology components

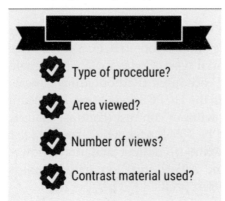

Type of procedure?

Area viewed?

Number of views?

Contrast material used?

Diagnostic radiology procedures

13.2

There's a Code for That

Read the following documentation of the Diagnostic Radiology service and identify the correct Radiology procedure code(s).

1. CT of the abdomen with oral contrast.

   CPT code: _____

2. CT of the abdomen and pelvic without contrast.

   CPT code: _____

3. Antero-posterior and lateral radiographs of the chest taken on a patient with atypical chest pain.

   CPT code: _____

4. X-ray of the cervical spine, antero-posterior, lateral, and both oblique views were obtained.

   CPT code: _____

5. MRI of the right shoulder with 100 ml low osmolar contrast.

   CPT code: _____

   HCPCS code: _____ x _____

6. Physician was called into ED to read x-ray films of patient involved in MVA. Films included complete x-ray of left ankle and complete x-ray examination of left foot.

   CPT codes: _____ - _____ , _____ - _____

Diagnostic Ultrasound

The next subsection of codes in the Radiology section of the CPT code book is Diagnostic Ultrasound (76506–76999), which includes codes for ultrasound evaluations. The format of this subsection is similar to the Diagnostic Radiology subsection, as codes are listed according to body area. An **ultrasound**, also known as a sonogram, uses high-frequency sound waves through the use of a transducer applied to a specific area of the body. The sound waves bounce off internal structures in the body, creating an image on a computer screen. Ultrasounds are noninvasive, painless, and do not require the patient to undergo any type of radiation; and are commonly used to view the real-time structure and movement of the internal organs of the body, as well as blood vessels and blood flow. Ultrasounds can be specialized using 3D technology, which transforms the sounds waves into a 3D image projected to the computer screen. A **Doppler ultrasound** is a special technique that uses color-coded mapping during the ultrasound procedure that allows the viewer to see oxygenated and de-oxygenated blood flow through body organs in real time (see figure 13.9) (NIBIB 2017).

Codes for ultrasound studies identify the type of ultrasound technique used, the area viewed in the study, and whether the study was limited or complete. There are a number of different ultrasound techniques. In some cases, the ultrasound technique impacts code selection. For example, code 76511, Ophthalmic ultrasound, diagnostic; quantitative A-scan only, identifies an A-scan of the eyes, whereas code 76512, Ophthalmic ultrasound, diagnostic; B-scan (with or without superimposed

Figure 13.9. Ultrasound imaging

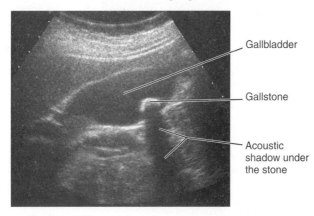

Gallbladder

Gallstone

Acoustic shadow under the stone

A. Ultrasound image of a gallstone. Note the bright echogenicity of the stone and the lack of echoes beneath the stone. The gallbladder is otherwise anechoic because it is filled with fluid.

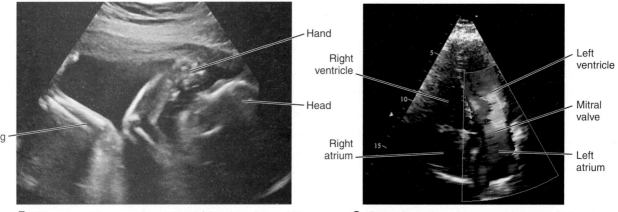

Hand

Right ventricle

Head

Leg

Left ventricle

Mitral valve

Right atrium

Left atrium

B. Ultrasound image of a second-trimester fetus. Ultrasound is used to monitor prenatal development, detect congenital defects, and determine sex.

C. Color Doppler ultrasound image of blood flowing from left atrium into the left ventricle. By convention, red color is blood flowing toward the transducer on the skin; blue is flow away from the transducer.

non-quantitative A-scan), identifies a B-scan that may or may not be performed with an A-scan. On the other hand, code 76800, Ultrasound, spinal canal and contents, does not identify the type of scan that was used to perform the imaging procedure. Ultimately, if the type of scan is not listed in the code description (as in the spinal canal ultrasound), then it does not impact code selection. The types of scans are as follows:

- A-mode scan produces a one-dimensional ultrasonic measurement.
- M-mode scan produces a one-dimensional ultrasonic measurement with tracing of the amplitude and velocity of echo-producing structures.
- B-scan ultrasounds include a two-dimensional ultrasound scan, which produces a two-dimensional display.
- Real-time scan produces a two-dimensional display along with movement in real-time.

- Doppler ultrasound evaluates the integrity of vascular structures and blood flow. Note that the Doppler imaging that is included in ultrasound codes is for anatomic structure identification in conjunction with the ultrasound. For Doppler studies that evaluate the vascular structures using both color and spectral, Doppler is separately reportable using Noninvasive Vascular Diagnostic Studies codes (93880–93990).

When coding for pelvic ultrasounds, note the difference between codes for Obstetrical pelvic ultrasounds (76801–76828) and those for non-obstetrical ultrasound (76830–76857). Obstetrical ultrasounds are performed on the fetus in a pregnant female patient, and codes depend on the type of ultrasounds and any additional procedures performed. Non-obstetrical ultrasounds are performed on the pelvic of non-pregnant females and males. Note also that there are a number of add-on codes through this section to identify each additional gestation for patients with a multiple pregnancy. If the ultrasound is performed with 3D imaging, report the service with either 76376, 3D rendering with interpretation and reporting of computed tomography, magnetic resonance imaging, ultrasound, or other tomographic modality with image postprocessing under concurrent supervision; not requiring postprocessing on an independent workstation, or 76377, 3D rendering with interpretation and reporting of computed tomography, magnetic resonance imaging, ultrasound, of other tomographic modality with image postprocessing under concurrent supervision; requiring image postprocessing on an independent workstation, in addition to the obstetric ultrasound code.

Radiologic Guidance

The next subsection in the Radiology section of the CPT code book is Radiologic Guidance (77001–77022). **Radiologic guidance** procedures are performed together with an invasive or minimally invasive procedure to help guide the provider performing the procedure to the correct anatomical location. There are three types of radiologic guidance: fluoroscopic, computed tomography (CT), and magnetic resonance (MR) guidance. Code selection depends on the type of guidance performed and the primary surgical procedure. Fluoroscopic guidance codes are all add-on codes that should be used in conjunction with the code for the primary surgical procedure. For example, code 77003, Fluoroscopic guidance and localization of needle or catheter tip for spine or paraspinous diagnostic or therapeutic injection procedures (epidural or subarachnoid), is an add-on code for fluoroscopic guidance.

Because guidance procedures are performed in conjunction with another procedure, there are many parenthetical notes (discussed first in chapter 5 [Learning the CPT and HCPCS Code Books]) in this section of codes that identify when each code may or may not be used in conjunction with the code for the surgical procedure. For example, in parentheses under code 77003 is a list of the surgical codes that it may be reported with: *(Use 77003 in conjunction with 61050, 61055, 62267, 62270, 62272, 62273, 62280, 62281, 62282, 62284, 64510, 64517, 64520, 64610)*. It also identifies specific codes with which 77003 may not be reported: *(Do not report 77003 in conjunction with 62320, 62321, 62322, 62323, 62324, 62325, 62326, 62327)*.

Mammography

The next subsection contains codes for Breast, Mammography studies (77046–77067). **Mammography**, or a mammogram, is an x-ray image of the breast used to diagnose breast conditions such as tumors or fibrocystic diseases (see figure 13.10). Note that even though a mammography is a diagnostic x-ray procedure, it is located in its own special subsection of codes.

Figure 13.10. Mammographic imaging

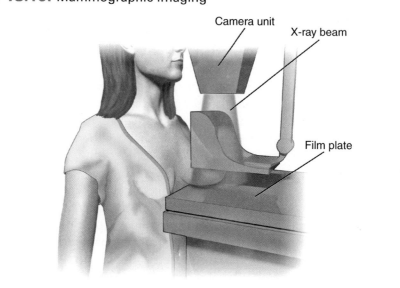

Mammogram

Source: Blausen.com staff 2014.

Code selection depends on the specific type of procedure and if the mammography was bilateral or unilateral. It is important to note the difference between a diagnostic mammography (77065–77066) and a screening mammography. A diagnostic mammography is performed when a patient has some sort of clinical sign or symptom, such as a lump in the breast or nipple discharge. A screening mammography (77067) is performed on a regular basis when no symptoms are present to detect early changes in the breast, which may indicate breast cancer. This is a preventive examination and is typically covered by most insurance companies, as long as it is performed according to schedule.

A number of mammography codes include the use of computer-aided detection (CAD), a recognition software used to decrease the rates of false-negatives in mammography studies, and this increases the detection of breast cancer via mammography. Codes for both diagnostic and screening mammographies include CAD when performed—for example, 77065, Diagnostic mammography, including computer-aided detection (CAD) when performed; unilateral (Castellino 2005).

Bone and Joint Studies

The next subsection of the Radiology section of the CPT code book is for Bone/Joint Studies (77071–77086). These are special studies on the bones and joints designed to help diagnose conditions of the bones, such as osteoporosis, as well as specialized studies for bone age, bone growth, and bone tumors. For example, code 77072, Bone age studies, and 77073, Bone length studies (orthoentgenogram, scanogram), both identify different types of bone studies.

Radiation Oncology

The next subsection of the Radiology section of the CPT code book is unique from the others in this section. Whereas the majority of Radiology codes are used to diagnose medical conditions, Radiation Oncology codes (77261–77799) are used to treat oncological conditions. These codes identify services to manage, plan, and deliver radiation treatments to patients with cancer.

Because radiation oncology is performed on patients with cancer and metastatic diseases, it is better discussed within the specialty context of Hematology and Oncology (see chapter 18, under the Hematology and Oncology section). This section of codes is mentioned only in passing in this chapter.

Nuclear Medicine

Nuclear medicine is the practice of using small radioactive elements that are introduced into the patient through an intravenous injection. These elements are designed to travel to a specific organ or type of tissue. Then their radioactive emissions are captured with a nuclear medicine scan, such as a positron emission tomography (PET) or single-photon emission computerized tomography (SPECT) scan, to produce a detailed image of the patient's internal structures and organs. These images can help locate and diagnose the metabolic rates of cancerous tumors and the functioning of internal organs or body tissues (see figure 13.11).

Figure 13.11. Nuclear medicine imaging

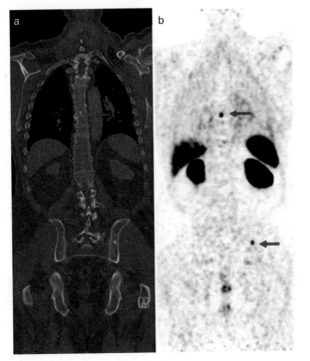

Source: Rauscher et al. 2016.

Codes for nuclear medicine studies depend on the body area or organ involved in the study, the extent of the study (limited area, multiple areas, whole body), and special nature of the test, such as with or without vascular flow, or with or without intrinsic factor. When coding for nuclear medicine procedures, pay close attention to the code descriptions, as multiple codes that differ from each other only slightly may exist within the same body area. For example, code 78700, Kidney imaging morphology, has four different variations of the same procedure indented beneath it, including *with vascular flow* (78701), *with vascular flow and function, single study without pharmacological intervention* (78707), *with vascular flow and function, single study, with pharmacological intervention (e.g., angiotensin converting enzyme inhibitor and/or diuretic)* (78708), *with vascular flow and function, multiple studies, with and without pharmacological intervention (e.g., angiotensin converting enzyme inhibitor and/or diuretic)* (78709).

Modifiers in Radiology Coding

There are a handful of modifiers used in radiology coding that identify special aspects of the procedure and that may have a significant impact on reimbursement.

- Modifiers -26, Professional component, and -TC, Technical component, identify the professional and technical components of a radiological service, as previously discussed in this chapter.

- Modifiers -LT, Left side, and -RT, Right side, identify the laterality of the radiology procedure, and are used for imaging procedures that may be done on either side of the body, such as x-ray of the elbow (right or left).

- Modifier -52, Reduced services, may be used in the case of radiology services when a radiology service is not completed to the full extent of the code description. For example, if an x-ray code described a minimum of three views but only one view was completed, it may be necessary to report the service with modifier -52 to identify that it was a reduced service (not completed to the full extent of the code description).

- Modifier -59, Distinct procedural service, may also be necessary when additional imaging services are performed on different sites.

- Modifier -76, Repeat procedure or service by same physician or other healthcare professional, and modifier -77, Repeat procedure or service by another physician or healthcare professional, may be necessary to append to services that were repeated. For example, an x-ray was taken to diagnose a dislocated shoulder that the surgeon then reduced back into the joint, and an additional x-ray was taken to ensure that the shoulder joint was properly back in place. Modifiers -76 and -77 are discussed in more detail in chapter 11.

Complete the exercises in There's a Code for That 13.3 to practice assigning codes for radiology procedures.

13.3 Radiology procedures

There's a Code for That

Read the following documentation of the Radiology service and identify the correct Radiology procedure code(s).

1. Complete renal ultrasound, suspect kidney stones.

CPT code: _____

2. Nuclear medicine parathyroid scan with SPECT.

CPT code: _____

3. Follow-up pelvic ultrasound on patient with PCOS.

   CPT code: _____

4. Complete osseous survey of the axial and appendicular skeleton.

   CPT code: _____

5. Bilateral MRI of breasts.

   CPT code: _____

6. SPECT scan of liver with measurement of vascular flow.

   CPT code: _____

Diagnosis Coding for Radiology and Imaging Services

Diagnosis coding for radiology services depends on whether it is a diagnostic imaging service performed to determine a diagnosis, or if the patient already has a diagnosis and the image is used to determine healing status, tumor progression or remission, or fetal growth, for example. Signs and symptoms are commonly coded, especially when an imaging procedure is performed and a definitive diagnosis cannot be determined. When diagnoses are definitively determined, they may include a variety of lung conditions, breast conditions, uterine fibroids or cysts, gallstones, and kidney stones. Fracture coding is also important in reporting radiology procedures correctly.

Diagnostic Imaging Services

Diagnostic imaging services are performed to determine a diagnosis. In many cases, a patient has suffered an injury or illness or is experiencing symptoms that may indicate an internal medical condition, such as a fracture or pneumonia. Diagnostic imaging services are requested by an ordering physician who has determined that an imaging study is necessary in order to definitively determine the patient's diagnosis. The radiologist receives the orders, performs the imaging procedure, and reads the images and determines the diagnosis, if possible. In some cases, it is not possible to determine a diagnosis, while a definitive diagnosis is easily known in other cases.

Images with No Definitive Diagnosis

Just as in coding for physical examinations and office visits in which no definitive diagnosis is determined, the coder should only report the signs or symptoms that prompted the imaging service. For example, if a patient with a severe productive cough receives a chest x-ray to rule out pneumonia, and the x-ray results do not clearly show that pneumonia is present, then the coder must only report the sign or symptom that prompted the x-ray procedure (the cough).

In many cases, the radiologist may write that a specific condition is "suspected," "possible," "questionable," or that it needs to be "ruled-out." If any of these questionable terms are present, then the questionable diagnosis must not be coded. Again, only the signs or symptoms that prompted the imaging service in the first place can be coded. Sometimes, the provider who orders the imaging service (the ordering physician) will identify a diagnosis for the imaging service order. For instance, if the patient received a chest x-ray for shortness of breath and the radiologist's impression of the x-ray was "suspected pleural effusion," then the code that should be reported for the case would be shortness of breath. The pleural effusion was only suspected and was not determined as the diagnosis; therefore, it cannot be coded. If necessary, query the healthcare provider regarding the patient's diagnosis (as mentioned in chapters 4 and 5) before reporting the diagnosis code.

Common signs and symptoms that require imaging services are chest pain, limb pain, abdominal pain, joint pain, and cough. Remember, when coding for pain it is necessary to search for the term *pain* in the ICD-10-CM Index and then the specific site of the pain.

Images with a Definitive Diagnosis

When an imaging service is ordered and a definitive diagnosis is determined, the coder should report the definitive diagnosis and not the signs or symptoms of the disease. Common diagnoses that may be seen on x-rays include conditions of the lungs, breast conditions, and the presence of stones in the urinary tract (including the kidneys) and gallbladder and bile ducts.

Conditions of the Lungs

Imaging services such as x-rays and CTs are commonly used to diagnose a number of different conditions affecting the lungs and pleura. These include:

- Pneumonia (J12–J18). Most pneumonia codes identify the infectious organism or specific type of pneumonia. If this information is known, then code to the highest level of specificity for the code. If no other information is known other than the fact that pneumonia is present, use the unspecified version of the code: J18.9, Pneumonia, unspecified organism.
- Pleural effusion (J90–J91). **Pleural effusion** is a collection of fluid in the pleural space between the pleural sac, which lines the lung, and the lung itself. This fluid places pressure on the lung and does not allow it to expand completely, causing shortness of breath or chest pain. Pleural effusion is found in a range of

Figure 13.12. Pleural effusion on x-ray and CT

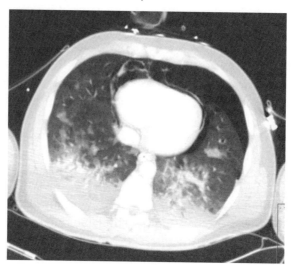

Source: Konijn et al. 2008.

conditions—cardiovascular and pulmonary conditions, inflammatory diseases, and malignancies (see figure 13.12). When coding for pleural effusions, if the cause of the condition is known, use category J91, Pleural effusion in conditions classified elsewhere, and further specify if the effusion is due to a malignancy or other condition classified elsewhere. An additional code should be used to identify the underlying condition (either the malignancy or the underlying condition coded elsewhere). If the underlying cause of the effusion is not known, use the unspecified code J90, Pleural effusion, not elsewhere classified.

- Pulmonary edema (J81). **Pulmonary edema** is a fluid collection in the lungs themselves caused by heart failure, myocardial infarction, cardiac ischemia, and other heart problems, as well as sepsis and severe anemia. Symptoms of pulmonary edema include respiratory fatigue, chest pain, and cough. Codes for pulmonary edema identify the condition as either acute (J81.0, Acute pulmonary edema) or chronic (J18.1, Chronic pulmonary edema). According to the Tabular note at the beginning of chapter 10 (Diseases of the Respiratory System), if the patient has any known history or current use of tobacco or tobacco products, an additional code should be selected to identify the tobacco use or history, as necessary. These include Z77.22, Contact with and (suspected) exposure to environmental tobacco smoke (acute) (chronic), P96.81, Exposure to (parental) (environmental) tobacco smoke in the perinatal period, Z87.891, Personal history of nicotine dependence, Z57.31, Occupational exposure to environmental tobacco smoke, F17.-, Tobacco dependence, or Z72.0,Tobacco use. If the pulmonary edema is due to chemical exposure, radiation, drowning, high altitude, or other external agent, do not use the code from category J81. Search for the term *Edema* in the ICD-10-CM Index, then refer to the subterm *lung*, and then the appropriate type of pulmonary edema. Be sure to verify the code in the Tabular List.

- Abnormal findings that are not otherwise classified can be reported with codes from category R91, Abnormal findings on diagnostic imaging of lung. These include the presence of a solitary pulmonary nodule, or other nonspecific finding of lung field.

Additional lung conditions such as pulmonary nodules, embolisms, and cysts or tumors may also be found using imaging techniques. These codes can be found by referencing the Main Index of the ICD-10-CM code book and following the main terms, subterms, and cross references, then verifying the code in the Tabular List.

Conditions of the Breasts

Breast imaging studies may be useful in finding a number of different breast conditions. These include cysts, malignancies, fibrocystic changes, hematomas, lipomas, and mastitis (see figure 13.13). Many breast disorders are coded within categories N60 to N65, Disorders of breast, including mammary dysplasia (cysts and fibrocystic changes), inflammatory disorders of the breast (mastitis and abscess), hypertrophy, lump in breast, and other disorders (signs and symptoms of the breast).

When an imaging study of the breast is done due to a lump in the breast and a tumor is found, it is not possible to determine whether or not the lump is malignant from the imaging study alone. A biopsy of the lump must be performed in order to identify if the lump is benign or malignant. Remember, if a diagnostic imaging study cannot determine the definitive diagnosis, then code only for the sign or symptom. If the patient already has a diagnosis of either a benign or malignant neoplasm of the breast and the imaging study is done to determine the location or growth or decline of the tumor, then report the code for the diagnosis that has already been determined.

There are two codes to report that a patient presented for a breast imaging study to screen for breast malignancies. Z12.31, Encounter or screening mammogram for malignant neoplasm of breast, should be used when a patient presents for a screening mammogram. Screening mammograms are a common breast imaging procedure and are performed as a preventative service when the patient has no symptoms, such as a breast lump. If a patient presents for a screening mammogram and no abnormalities are present, report code Z12.31. If an abnormality is present, then report the code for the screening mammogram first, followed by the code for the abnormality, such as a mass or lump. Code Z12.39, Encounter for other screening for malignant neoplasm of breast, should be used when an imaging service other than a mammogram is used to perform the breast screening. Note that these two screening codes should only be used when the patient presents for a routine screening.

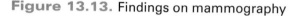

Figure 13.13. Findings on mammography

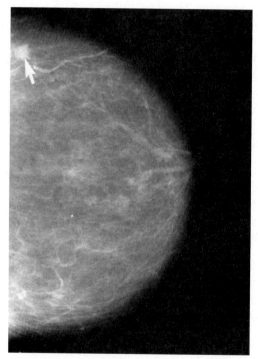

Source: National Cancer Institute 1991.

If a breast abnormality is found on a diagnostic imaging of the breast, the finding should be reported with a code from category R92, Abnormal and inconclusive findings of diagnostic imaging of breast. These include mammographic microcalcification, mammographic calcification, and inconclusive mammogram (dense breasts), or other abnormal or inconclusive finding.

Cholelithiasis and Nephrolithiasis

Imaging services are commonly used to find stones in the gallbladder and bile ducts as well as in the kidneys. Coding for cholelithiasis, or gallstones, requires detailed reading of the code descriptions to ensure that the code selected correctly reports the documented condition (for example, K80.60, Calculus of gallbladder and bile duct with cholecystitis, unspecified, without obstruction). For a refresher on coding for cholelithiasis, refer to chapter 10 (Urgent Care and Emergency Department Services).

A nephrolithiasis, otherwise known as kidney stone, is also diagnosed with the use of imaging, such as x-ray or CT scan. Coding for nephrolithiasis is decidedly simpler than coding for cholelithiasis, as codes rely on the site of the stone (for example, code N20.1, Calculus of ureter). Category N20, Calculus of kidney and ureter, includes codes for calculus of the kidney, calculus of the ureter, calculus of both kidney and ureter, and unspecified urinary calculus.

Fracture Coding

When a patient presents to a healthcare provider with a possible fracture, an x-ray is usually ordered to confirm if indeed a fracture is present, determine exactly which bone or bones are fractured, and identify the clinical aspects of that fracture. Coding for fractures is complicated and reporting the correct code depends on a number of factors.

Orthopedic specialists (bone doctors, also called orthopedists or orthopods) are trained to diagnose, treat, and manage the healing of fractures. As such, orthopods are more likely to perform diagnostic imaging for fractures, read the images, and specify the patient's exact type of fracture. Orthopedic services are discussed in chapter 15 (Orthopedic Services), with a more thorough discussion of fracture diagnosis coding. At the very least, diagnosis codes for fractures identify the site of the fracture (the specific bone that is fractured), the laterality, whether the fracture is open (pierces the skin) or closed (does not pierce the skin), and the encounter (initial, subsequent, or sequela). For example, note how each of these details are provided in code S42.001A, Fracture of unspecified part of *right clavicle, initial encounter* for *closed fracture*.

To search for a fracture in the Index, look up the term *Fracture*, and then refer to the section for either pathological or traumatic fractures. Pathological fractures are caused by a disease process, such as osteoporosis. Traumatic fractures are caused by a traumatic injury, such as a fall. Then find the subterm for the site of the fracture. Follow all additional subterms and cross-references, and verify the code in the Tabular List. All fracture codes are seven-character codes, which means that a seventh character should be assigned to identify the encounter for the fracture. For a refresher of seventh-character extensions, refer to chapter 4 (Learning the ICD-10-CM Code Book).

Complete the exercises in There's a Code for That 13.4 to practice assigning diagnostic codes for radiology procedures.

Diagnostic coding for radiology procedures   13.4

There's a Code for That

Read the following documentation of the radiology service and identify the correct diagnosis code(s).

1. Complete renal ultrasound, suspect kidney stones in patient with flank pain.

   ICD-10-CM code: _____

2. Patient with hypercalcemia received parathyroid SPECT scan. Impression: probable parathyroid adenoma of the upper pole of the left thyroid bed.

   ICD-10-CM code: _____

(Continued on next page)

13.4

Continued

3. Encounter for bilateral screening mammogram revealed lump in left breast. Patient has a significant family history of breast cancer.

   ICD-10-CM codes: _____ , _____ , _____

4. Impression from renal ultrasound: calculus of kidney and ureter.

   ICD-10-CM code: _____

5. A 56-year-old patient with congestive heart failure presents for x-ray of the chest. Patient is experiencing shortness of breath, chest pain, and a feeling of fullness in the chest. X-ray positive for acute pulmonary edema.

   ICD-10-CM code: _____ , _____

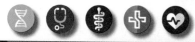

Putting It All Together: Coding for Radiology and Imaging Services

Coding correctly for radiology and imaging services requires an understanding of the different types of studies, coding components for each type of code, an understanding of the professional and technical components of each service, and how to differentiate between a service that has a definitive diagnosis and one that does not.

Determination of the correct codes relies on the answers to the following questions.

- What type of imaging procedure was performed (x-ray, MRI, CT, ultrasound)?
- What body area, organ, or organ system was visualized by the imaging procedure?
  - How many views were included in the procedure?
  - Was contrast material used?
  - Was the procedure limited or complete?
  - Was the procedure bilateral or unilateral? If unilateral, which side was imaged?
- Which component should you code for?
  - Code for the global fee (no modifiers) if the office owns the imaging equipment, and the provider also works for the same clinic.
  - Code for the technical component (modifier -TC) if the clinic or facility owns the equipment but does not employ the healthcare provider who read the films.
  - Code for the professional component (modifier -26) if the provider interpreted and provided a report for images that were produced by an independent facility.
- Were there any additional procedures or imaging services that should be coded as well?
  - If so, check for the need for modifiers.

- Is there a definitive diagnosis for the imaging service?
    - If yes, then code the definitive diagnosis.
    - If no, then code for the signs, symptoms, or abnormal finding code.
    - If the image is for a screening service, report the screening diagnosis code.

The following vignette demonstrates how to select the appropriate diagnosis and procedure codes. After reviewing the vignette, complete the exercises in There's a Code for That 13.5 to practice diagnostic and procedural coding for radiology and imaging services.

Bethany is a recent graduate from a medical billing and coding program and she just landed a job in a local independent radiology and imaging center. Now that Bethany is ready to begin coding in her position at the imaging center, she remembers that she needs to ask herself two questions: What did the doctor do? and Why did the doctor do it? She is coding the following imaging report.

Study Name: Mammography
Description: Diagnostic mammography of the right female breast with computer-aided detection (CAD)
Clinical indication: Lump in right breast
Image Report: 1.5 cm mass on right breast seen in the right upper outer quadrant, consistent with ductal carcinoma in situ. Recommend ultrasound-guided biopsy of lump to confirm diagnosis.
Impression: 1.5 cm mass in right breast

First, Bethany asks herself: What did the doctor do? In this case, the procedure was a diagnostic mammography of the right female breast with computer-aided detection. There were no additional procedures performed. Also, there is no mention of whether only the professional component or the technical components were performed, so she will code for the global service, without modifiers. She refers to the CPT Index and finds the term Mammography, *and then with* Computer-Aided Detection (CAD), *which leads her to the code range 77065 to 77067. She turns to this section in the Tabular List of codes and determines that her correct imaging code is:*

77065-RT, Diagnostic mammography, including computer-aided detection (CAD), when performed; unilateral

Note that Bethany appended modifier -RT to the code to indicate the laterality of the procedure.

Now that she has her procedure code, she asks herself: Why did the doctor do it? In this case, the clinical indication, which is the reason why the imaging study was performed, was due to a lump in the breast. This is different than the imaging report that indicates the findings are consistent with ductal carcinoma in situ. However, the impression at the end of the report, which is the final impression that the radiologist got from the study, was a 1.5 cm mass in the right breast. Bethany remembers that she can only code for a definitive diagnosis, so she cannot code for the ductal carcinoma in situ. The provider wrote that the findings were "consistent with" ductal carcinoma in situ, not that the patient has ductal carcinoma in situ. In this case, she must code for the signs or symptoms, which is the lump/mass in the right breast. She looks up the term lump *in the ICD-10 Index, and the cross-reference is to* see Mass. *She then refers to the term* Mass *in the Index, and then* Breast, *which refers her to code N63. She verifies the code in the Tabular and codes to the highest level of specificity to identify the exact location of the lump, and assigns the correct code:*

> N63.11, *Unspecified lump in the right breast, upper outer quadrant*

She then rechecks the documentation to make sure she has coded everything for the encounter, and reports the chosen codes on the claim for the service.

13.5
There's a Code for That

Diagnostic and procedural coding for radiology and imaging services

Read the following documentation and assign the appropriate CPT, HCPCS, and ICD-10-CM code(s) for the encounter.

1. Study: X-ray of left foot

   Indication: Pain

   Technique: Three views

   Findings: Bones of the foot are intact, no stress fractures noted. Mild swelling is noted along the dorsal aspect of the foot.

   Impression: No acute fracture or injury noted.

   CPT code: _____ - _____

   ICD-10-CM codes: _____

2. MRI of the internal auditory canals with and without contrast material. Contrast administered was 50 mL of Gadavist (gadobutrol). Patient has right-sided hearing loss and a clinical history of acoustic neuroma. Impression from today's study: Slight increase in right cerebellopontine angle mass compatible with vestibular schwannoma.

   CPT code: _____ , _____ × _____

   ICD-10-CM codes: _____ , _____

3. CT of the abdomen without contrast and CT of the pelvis with contrast on patient with abdominal pain. Patient's clinical history is significant for post-cholecystectomy 8 months ago. Impression: CT of the abdomen and pelvis is without findings to explain the patient's symptoms. Post-cholecystectomy.

   CPT code: _____

   ICD-10-CM codes: _____ , _____

Case Study | **Radiological Examination of Right Lower Extremity**

PATIENT: Roberta Weiss

ORDERING PROVIDER: Susan Alameda, DO

XR TIB-FIB-LOWER LEG-RIGHT

Findings: AP and lateral views of the right tibia and fibula compared to previous scan from initial injury three weeks ago.

The cortical irregularity at the proximal metaphysis of the fibula now has disruption of the cortex and a band of sclerosis with mild periosteal reaction consistent with a healing fracture. No displacement of angulation. Postsurgical changes at the ankle are stable.

IMPRESSION: Healing fibular fracture

SIGNED: Dr. Gene I. Kim, MD

Use the following steps to select the appropriate code(s) for the case study.

1. Read through the case study and answer the question: *What did the doctor do?* In the case study, identify the name of the imaging procedure.

   _____

   _____

2. Now that you have the name of the procedure, locate the code for the procedure in the CPT code book.
   a. Search the Index for the procedure and search through the options.
   b. In the listing of codes, check for any guidelines, important definitions, or parenthetical notes. Select the appropriate code and list it here.

   _____

   _____

   c. Are there any modifiers that need to be added to identify any special circumstance surrounding the procedure(s)? If yes, refer to Appendix A of the CPT code book to assign all appropriate modifiers.

   _____

   _____

3. Now that the procedure(s) and modifier(s) have been identified, review the case study and answer the following question: *Why did the doctor do it?*

_____

_____

4. Now that you have the name of the patient's diagnoses, search the ICD-10-CM code book for the correct codes for these conditions. Follow these steps for each of the diagnoses identified.

a. Search the Main Index for the name of each condition and search through any applicable subterms and cross-references to locate the appropriate code.

_____

_____

b. Verify the code in the Tabular List. Locate the code identified previously in the Tabular Listing of codes and refer to any applicable guidelines, notes, and symbols. Does the code selected correctly identify the patient's condition? If yes, list the code here.

_____

_____

5. Now that the procedure and diagnosis codes have been identified, list them on the CMS-1500 form.

21. DIAGNOSIS OR NATURE OF ILLNESS OR INJURY Relate A-L to service line below (24E) ICD Ind.				22. RESUBMISSION CODE
A. L_____ B. L_____ C. L_____ D. L_____				
E. L_____ F. L_____ G. L_____ H. L_____				23. PRIOR AUTHORIZATION NU
I. L_____ J. L_____ K. L_____ L. L_____				

24. A. DATE(S) OF SERVICE		B. PLACE OF SERVICE	C. EMG	D. PROCEDURES, SERVICES, OR SUPPLIES (Explain Unusual Circumstances) CPT/HCPCS	MODIFIER	E. DIAGNOSIS POINTER	F. $ CHARGES	G. DAYS OR UNITS
From MM DD YY	To MM DD YY							
1								
2								
3								

HCC

End-of-Chapter Content

Instructions: Indicate whether the following statements are true or false (T or F). For false statements, rewrite the statement on the line below to make the statement true.

1. Radiology services may be performed in the inpatient or outpatient settings.

_____

_____

2. Radiological supervision and interpretation is the professional component of a procedure.

_____

_____

3. Modifier -26 is used to identify the global radiology service.

_____

_____

4. When a provider performs both the technical and professional components of a service, do not append a modifier.

_____

_____

5. The plane of an imaging service is the direction in which the imaging rays pass through the body.

_____

_____

6. MRI uses strong ultrasonic waves to produce detailed images of the internal structures of the patient.

_____

_____

7. Contrast material may be injected intravenously, intrathecally, or intra-articularly.

_____

_____

8. There is no difference between obstetric and non-obstetric pelvic ultrasound codes.

_____

_____

9. When a definitive diagnosis is not determined by the imaging procedure, it is ok to report the probable diagnosis.

_____

_____

10. Pleural effusion is fluid buildup within the lungs themselves.

_____

_____

Instructions: Match the terms with the appropriate descriptions.

1. _____ Anterior		A.	Away from the body
2. _____ Posterior		B.	The same side of the body
3. _____ Superior		C.	Toward the midline of the body
4. _____ Inferior		D.	Toward the top of the body
5. _____ Medial		E.	Toward the back of the body
6. _____ Lateral		F.	The opposite side of the body
7. _____ Proximal		G.	Toward the center of the body
8. _____ Distal		H.	Away from the midline of the body
9. _____ Ipsilateral		I.	Toward the front of the body
10. _____ Contralateral		J.	Toward the bottom of the body

Instructions: Choose the best answer.

1. Which type of medical doctor specializes in the diagnosis and treatment of medical conditions using radiology and imaging techniques?

   a. Imaging technician
   b. Radiologist
   c. Inpatient hospitalist
   d. Certified radiological supervisor

2. A physician on-call read an x-ray report for a study that was performed at the hospital. Which component of the radiology service was performed?

   a. Professional
   b. Technical
   c. Global
   d. None, this would not be billable

3. Which component of a radiology service represents the equipment, supplies, and clinical staff that took the image?

   a. Professional
   b. Technical
   c. Global
   d. Both professional and technical components

4. Which modifier is used to identify the global radiology service?

   a. -26
   b. -TC
   c. -GB
   d. No modifier

5. Which plane of the body is a vertical line that divides the body into anterior and posterior halves?

   a. Axial
   b. Transverse
   c. Sagittal
   d. Coronal

6. Which subsection of the Radiology section contains codes for PET and SPECT scans?

   a. Diagnostic Radiology
   b. Radiologic Guidance
   c. Ultrasound
   d. Nuclear Medicine

7. Which imaging type combines a number of x-ray images to produce a virtual cross-section of the area being studied?

   a. X-ray
   b. CT
   c. MRI
   d. PET

8. When coding for a radiology service that was performed with and without contrast, how is the service reported?

   a. Use the code for with contrast
   b. Use the code for without contrast
   c. Use the code for without contrast followed by with contrast
   d. Use one code for with contrast, and another code for without contrast

9. Which imaging technique allows the viewer to see blood flow through body organs in real time?

a. Doppler ultrasound
b. Nuclear imaging
c. Radiologic guidance
d. MRI

10. What type of imaging service is performed on a scheduled basis as a preventative measure to rule out breast cancer?

a. Diagnostic mammogram
b. MRI of the breast
c. Screening mammogram
d. Screening ultrasound of the breast

11. Which modifier should be used when multiple x-rays were performed by the same doctor on the same site on the same day?

a. -59
b. -77
c. -76
d. No modifier would be necessary

Instructions: Answer the following questions with the appropriate code(s) and modifier(s).

1. Diagnostic mammogram on a female patient with a lump in her right breast confirmed the presence of fibroadenosis of the right breast.

CPT code: _____

ICD-10-CM code: _____

2. Diagnostic x-ray examination of the right clavicle confirms displaced fracture (closed fracture, initial encounter).

CPT code: _____

ICD-10-CM code: _____

3. Clinical indication: Left neck and shoulder pain × 2 months

Contrast material: None

Technique: MRI of the cervical spine

Findings: Moderate narrowing of disc space from C4–5 with spondylosis.

Impression: Spondylosis of the cervical spine with radiculopathy

CPT code: _____

ICD-10-CM code: _____

4. Nuclear medicine PET scan, whole body, on patient with known lung cancer. Findings from the study include a lesion in the left upper lobe of the lung, representing the patient's known lung carcinoma. No evidence of any metastases. Findings also significant for diverticulosis.

CPT code: _____

ICD-10-CM code: _____

References

Blausen.com staff. 2014. Blausen 0628 Mammogram.png. Digital image. Wikimedia Commons. https://commons.wikimedia.org/wiki/File:Blausen_0628_Mammogram.png.

Castellino, R. 2005 (August 23). Computer Aided Detection (CAD): An Overview. https://www.ncbi.nlm.nih.gov/pmc/articles/PMC1665219/.

Konijn, A. J. M., P. H. M. Egbers, and M. A. Kuiper. 2008. Pneumothorax Hemothorax Pneumomediastinum Contusion.JPG. Digital image. Journal of Medical Case Reports. https://jmedicalcasereports.biomedcentral.com/articles/10.1186/1752-1947-2-100.

National Cancer Institute (NCI). 1991. Mammogram Showing Small Lesion. Digital image. National Cancer Institute. https://visualsonline.cancer.gov/details.cfm?imageid=2553.

National Institute of Biomedical Imaging and Bioengineering (NIBIB). 2017. Ultrasounds. https://www.nibib.nih.gov/science-education/science-topics/ultrasound.

National Institute of Biomedical Imaging and Bioengineering (NIBIB). 2016. X-rays. https://www.nibib.nih.gov/science-education/science-topics/x-rays.

Rauscher, I., T. Maurer, W. P. Fendler, W. H. Sommer, M. Schwaiger, and M. Eiber. 2016. Gallium PSMA PET scan.png. Digital image. https://www.ncbi.nlm.nih.gov/pmc/articles/PMC4898465/.

Verhovshek, G. J. 2015 (November). Radiology Billing and Coding: Professional and Technical Components. http://www.radiologytoday.net/archive/rt1115p7.shtml.

Resources

American College of Radiology (ACR). 2017. What is a Radiologist? https://www.acr.org/Quality-Safety/Radiology-Safety/Patient-Resources/About-Radiology.

NYU Langone Health. 2017. Nuclear Medicine. https://med.nyu.edu/radiology/about-nyulmc-radiology/subspecialty-sections/nuclear-section.

CHAPTER

Laboratory and Pathology Services

Learning Objectives

- Understand the basics of billing and coding for independent laboratory and pathology services
- Examine procedural codes and guidelines for independent laboratory and pathology services
- Examine diagnosis coding and medical necessity for independent laboratory and pathology services
- Determine and apply ICD-10-CM, CPT, and HCPCS codes to independent laboratory and pathology services

Key Terms

Bacteriology
Cytopathology
Frozen block
Frozen section
Gross examination
Independent laboratory
Laboratory and pathology services
Methicillin-resistant *Staphylococcus aureus* (MRSA)

Microscopic examination
Mycology
Nonspecific test
Panel
Parasitology
Pass-through billing
Permanent block
Permanent section

Qualitative examination
Quantitative examination
Smear
Specific test
Specimen
Virology

Coding for laboratory and pathology services is a bit different than any other type of coding in the CPT code book. First, instead of performing procedures on the patient, **laboratory and pathology services** are diagnostic analyses of bodily tissue samples, such as urine, blood, or tissue. Often abbreviated as lab and path, laboratory and pathology services are designed to examine these specimens to determine a diagnosis, evaluate the quality of a specimen, or to assist in a surgical process. A **specimen** is a bodily tissue sample from the patient. Specimens come from all parts of the body—from blood, urine, and saliva to muscle tissues, stool, and even breath.

Coding for laboratory and pathology services requires an in-depth knowledge of the types of tests performed, the ways in which they are performed, and their many differences. It also requires a basic knowledge of the various practices that perform laboratory and pathology services, how these services are performed and billed, and the diagnosis codes that support the medical necessity for these services. This chapter discusses the basics of coding for laboratory and pathology services and covers the procedural and diagnostic guidelines for laboratory and pathology procedures.

Laboratory and Pathology Basics

Laboratory and pathology tests are a special type of service. While a handful of them may be performed in the healthcare office, such as Clinical Laboratory Improvement Amendments of 1988 (CLIA)-waived tests, many are performed in independent laboratories without the patient present. Billing and coding laboratory and pathology services require an understanding of the types of laboratory providers and how they bill and code for their services.

Key to Success

Rather than performing actual procedures on patients, laboratory and pathology services are only performing tests on specimens acquired from the patient. These codes are unique when compared to other CPT codes that identify procedures performed on patients. Indeed, the code structure and uses of the codes are the same, but the descriptions differ and identify only the test that was performed, not how it was obtained. It helps to keep this in mind when learning laboratory and pathology coding. Instead of performing surgical or medical procedures, evaluations, or managing patient conditions, laboratory and pathology services are only handling patient specimens—to perform a specific test on those specimens according to a doctor's request.

Laboratory and Pathology Settings and Billing for Services

In the United States, many healthcare offices have in-house CLIA-waived labs (discussed in chapter 8 [Primary Care Services]), which allow the clinical staff in the office to perform certain, low-complexity, low-risk laboratory tests and procedures. These include strep swabs, bacterial cultures, rapid influenza tests, mono spot cultures (for mononucleosis), blood counts, and simple urinalysis examinations. Additional CLIA-waived tests are **panels**, a group of specific tests (from the chemistry section) that are commonly performed together, such as a lipid or a comprehensive metabolic panel. When a healthcare office provides the lab test themselves, the code(s) for the lab(s) are billed along with the procedure codes for all other services provided at the encounter, such as E/M encounter and any other procedures.

When a more complex laboratory procedure is necessary, the patient (or a patient's sample specimen) is sent to an independent laboratory for analysis. An **independent laboratory** is a facility that is recognized and accredited to test and evaluate patient specimens as an independent entity free from a hospital or private practice. Accreditation of an independent laboratory is achieved by meeting a certain set of standards set by an accrediting body, such as Centers for Medicare and Medicaid Services (CMS) or other accrediting organization. An independent laboratory processes patient specimens according to orders given from healthcare providers, which identify the specimen to be examined and the purpose of the examination. When an independent laboratory provides the procedure, it can either bill for the lab directly, or send the ordering provider a bill for the services and the ordering provider bills the patient's insurance on the lab's behalf. This is a process called pass-through billing, discussed in more depth in the following section.

In the hospital setting, the hospital usually has an in-house lab that can process more complex laboratory and pathology procedures. When specimen testing is needed for a patient, the hospital staff or healthcare provider takes the patient sample and sends it directly to the in-house lab for processing and examination. If a diagnosis is determined, the lab sends the results to the ordering provider, who reads the results of the test and manages the patient accordingly. For example, a sample of wound exudate from a patient with a wound infection being treated in the hospital can be evaluated in the hospital's in-house laboratory to determine the infectious organism. Once the infectious organism is identified, then the treating provider can manage the patient's condition appropriately. Depending on the hospital, lab, and available equipment, some tests (such as a complex genetic sequencing test) may have to be sent to an outside independent lab with more specialized equipment to process the patient specimen for the exact test ordered. A common theme in healthcare, this all depends on the resources, availability, and need for the laboratory and pathology procedures. When a hospital performs the laboratory procedure in-house, the services performed are billed directly, together with other resources used during the patient's stay in the facility.

Laboratories are found in several healthcare settings, such as healthcare provider offices (which may only bill for CLIA-waived labs), inpatient and outpatient hospitals (including ASCs), and in the independent laboratory setting. The setting in which the laboratory service was provided depends on the needs of the patients and the resources available to the healthcare practice or facility. While this chapter focuses on coding for lab and path services in an independent lab, as a coder you will likely report lab or path services across a number of different settings.

Any type of laboratory or pathology procedure must be performed according to the orders of a healthcare provider. This provider has already examined or evaluated the patient and determined the need for the lab test. For example, a maternal fetal medicine specialist has performed an ultrasound on a patient and determined that there is a possibility that a chromosomal abnormality may be present. This doctor can do one of two things: either take a blood sample from the patient and send it to an independent lab, or send the patient to an independent lab to have them draw the blood sample. Either way, once the lab receives the blood sample with the orders to test the blood for the specific suspected chromosomal abnormality, the sample will be tested and results will be sent to the ordering doctor.

Sometimes laboratory procedures can be especially cost-prohibitive—very expensive—and may require special authorization from the patient's insurance before they may be performed. If the test is not paid for by the patient's insurance, then the patient will be responsible for payment. As a coder, prior authorization numbers may have to be reported on the claim (as discussed in chapter 2 [Healthcare Billing Basics]), together with the procedure codes for the authorized test and the diagnosis code that has been pre-approved to identify the medical necessity for the specific tests. Learning the basics for coding for laboratory and pathology services requires an understanding of pass-through billing and the technical versus professional components of laboratory services.

Pass-through Billing

Pass-through billing occurs when a laboratory performs an ordered lab test and sends the ordering provider a bill for the services (instead of billing the insurance company directly), and the ordering provider bills the patient's insurance on the lab's behalf. This is typically done when the ordering provider and the independent lab have some sort of agreement in place that identifies specific lab tests and costs for each procedure.

If an office engages in pass-through billing, the healthcare provider's office must bill for the lab test ordered, with all other procedures that were performed on the patient during the encounter. But to correctly identify that the laboratory test was not performed at the healthcare provider's office, three things must be done:

- Append modifier -90, Reference (outside) laboratory, to the laboratory procedure code. This indicates that the procedure was performed by an independent laboratory and that the healthcare office is billing for the services.
- Change the place of service code for the laboratory procedure to 81, Independent laboratory, rather than 11, Office. This indicates that the laboratory procedure was performed at an outside lab, and not in the healthcare provider's office.
- Identify the charges included in the pass-through billing in box 20 of the CMS-1500 claim form. This box further identifies that the laboratory procedures performed occurred at an outside lab and identifies the charge amount for the labs (see figure 14.1). Note that the charge amount included in this box must correspond to the actual charges billed for the lab services—the two amounts must match.

Figure 14.1. CMS-1500 box 20

20. OUTSIDE LAB?		$ CHARGES
[X] YES [ ] NO		159 00

Source: CMS 2019a.

Pass-through billing is not allowed by some insurance plans and it is more common to find that independent laboratories bill directly for the procedures performed. The labs are reimbursed according to a preset fee schedule that has been negotiated by the third-party payer and the lab. However, it is important to know how to code for these services when the situation arises.

Key to Success

When reporting pass-through billing for lab services, remember: append modifier -90, reference (outside) laboratory to the lab CPT code, change the place of service to 81, Independent laboratory, and add the charges in box 20 of the CMS-1500 form.

Technical versus Professional Components

Similar to radiological procedures, some laboratory and pathology procedures may be divided into technical versus professional components. The technical component of laboratory procedures consists of the testing of a sample using specialized equipment and highly trained clinical staff. The test may also require interpretation by a specially trained pathologist, who can decipher the complicated test results and provide a report of the findings—this is the professional component of the procedure.

> Just as in coding for either component of radiological procedures, modifier -TC, Technical component, or -26, Professional component, should be appended for either the technical or professional components of the procedure, respectively. When both the technical and professional components of the procedure are performed, do not append any modifier for the global service.

MOD

However, not all laboratory and pathology procedures may be broken into these two components. Some codes already identify only one component of the procedure, such as 85060, Blood smear, peripheral, interpretation by physician with written report. In this case, code 85060 already identifies the professional component and as such should not be appended with modifier -26. Furthermore, some insurance payers may choose to not recognize the two separate components for laboratory and pathology procedures, and instead pay only the global fee to the provider who performed the lab test. Again, being an effective coder requires an in-depth knowledge of the connection between coding and billing for the services performed in each specialty.

Laboratory and Pathology Testing Basics

Before discussing the codes for laboratory and pathology services, it is important to review the basic terminology and processes of laboratory tests. This includes the difference between specimen collection and specimen testing; definitions of specimens, blocks, and sections; and the difference between qualitative and quantitative examinations of specimens.

Specimen Collection versus Specimen Testing

Differentiation between the *collection* of a specimen, and the *testing* of a specimen is needed, as they are two very different procedures. To test any type of patient specimen, it must first be collected from the patient (see figure 14.2). This can be as simple as having the patient submit a urine sample in a specimen cup, or as complex as performing an invasive surgery to remove a tissue sample for a biopsy.

Reporting the code for the collection of the specimen depends on the provider who took the specimen. For example, if the doctor's office took a patient blood sample via venipuncture (code 36415, Collection of venous blood by venipuncture), and then performed a complete blood count (CBC) (85027, Blood count; complete (CBC), automated (Hgb, Hct, RBC, WBC, and platelet count) in the office, then this doctor's office should bill for both the venipuncture procedure and the CBC (36416 and 85025). Note that the venipuncture may be bundled into the CBC procedure depending on the insurance, as the insurance may determine that the blood draw is an inherent component of the CBC. Sometimes the collection of the specimen is included in the E/M encounter code for the service, such as having a patient urinate in a specimen

Figure 14.2. Specimen collection versus testing

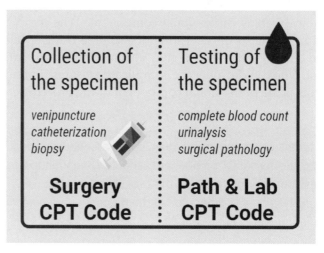

cup or taking a sample of wound exudate from an infected wound. In this case, the collection of the specimen is included in the work reported via the E/M code.

However, if the doctor's office drew the blood and then sent the sample to an independent lab, then the doctor's office would bill for the blood draw and the lab would bill for the testing of the blood. If the lab performed both the blood draw and the CBC, then it would bill for both procedures.

The collection procedure may be more invasive than a simple blood draw, as is often the case for biopsies and excision of organs or tissues examined for disease processes by a laboratory or pathologist. Remember to only report the procedure that was performed by the given office or facility. For example, if the coder is submitting codes for the independent laboratory, he or she should report only the codes that identify the services performed by the lab, and not by the doctor or surgeon who collected the specimen.

Specimens, Block, and Sections

All laboratory or pathology tests are performed on specimens, which can come from different sources. For example, a bacterial culture may be performed on a specimen obtained from wound exudate (pus from an infected wound). Or a specimen obtained from a breast lump may be examined for malignant cells (to check for breast cancer). Code selection for numerous laboratory and pathology codes depends on the type of the specimen tested in the procedure. For example, code 82565, Creatinine; blood, tests a blood sample for creatinine. Code 82570, Creatinine; other source, tests for the same substance (creatinine), but on a sample other than blood.

Once a specimen is obtained by the lab, it is prepared in several different ways, depending on the purpose of the test. Once the specimen is prepared, it is examined by the clinical laboratory and pathology staff. One type of examination is a **gross examination**—an examination of the physical characteristics of the specimen including the size, weight, consistency, and visual features such as discoloring. The laboratory technician may also place a label on the specimen to identify it, and note any additional tests performed on the specimen.

When a gross examination is not sufficient in determining the diagnosis, a microscopic examination is performed. A **microscopic examination** is the examination of the specimen at a minute level that allows the pathologist to see the cells of a specimen. These examinations are performed under a microscope on a slide that contains a small portion of the specimen and allows the individual cells to be seen. Obtaining a clear sample for the slide is done in various ways.

- Smear. If the specimen is a liquid or submerged in a fluid substance, it may be smeared onto the surface of a slide and then allowed to dry. It is then secured with a fixative agent, and then stained to allow for the visualization of certain cells. The process of applying the fixative agent or otherwise preparing the specimen for examination is included in the CPT code for the lab or path test and is not reported separately.

- Frozen section. For procedures that need a pathological examination quickly, the specimen may be frozen rapidly into a frozen block (a frozen piece of a specimen), which is cut into small slices of the tissue (a frozen section) and visualized under a microscope. This is a fast, yet impermanent method of preparing a specimen for pathological examination under a microscope. It is commonly used during surgical pathology services, in which a pathologist works together with a surgeon to evaluate tissue samples for malignancy during the surgical session.

- Permanent section. A permanent section procedure is similar to a frozen section, except that instead of freezing the block, it is placed in a fixative agent that immobilizes the cells so that they will not change. It is then placed in a small mold and surrounded with paraffin wax and cooled so the specimen is contained in a permanent block. This specimen block may be stored indefinitely for future evaluations. Once the block is formed, permanent sections may be cut from it and examined under a microscope by melting away the wax, adding water to the section, and staining it for microscopic examination.

Qualitative versus Quantitative Examinations

Laboratory and pathology procedures often differentiate between qualitative and quantitative examinations of specimens.

A **qualitative examination** is one that studies the *quality*, or characteristics and properties of a specimen. For example, is a drug or chemical present in the specimen? A qualitative examination answers the question with a yes or no answer. One example of a qualitative examinations is Presumptive Drug Class Screenings (80305–80307), which only identify whether a specific drug is identified in the specimen or not. The result of a qualitative examination is either a negative or a positive result, in that the substance being tested is either present or absent in the specimen.

A **quantitative examination** is one that identifies the *quantity*, or amount, of a specific substance found in a specimen. A quantitative examination answers the question: How much? For example, how much of a chemical is found in the specimen? An example of quantitative examinations is Therapeutic Drug Assays (80145–80299), which identify the amount of the specified drug in the specimen. In this case, the result of a quantitative examination is a number or measurement. See figure 14.3 for a visual representation of the differences between qualitative and quantitative examinations.

Whether the examination is qualitative or quantitative is identified in either the guidelines before the subsection of codes or in the code description itself. For example, 84119, Porphyrins urine; qualitative, is for a qualitative examination whereas code 84120, Porphyrins, urine; quantitation and fractionation, is for a quantitative examination. If the code description does not identify the examination as either qualitative or quantitative, refer to the guidelines at the beginning of the subsection of codes. For example, the guidelines for Therapeutic Drug Assays read: "Therapeutic Drug Assays are performed to monitor clinical response to a known, prescribed medication. The material for examination is whole blood, serum, plasma, or cerebrospinal fluid. *Examination is quantitative*. Coding is by parent drug; measured metabolites of the drug are included in the code, if performed" (AMA 2019). Therefore, all the procedures identified with these codes are quantitative examinations.

Figure 14.3. Qualitative versus quantitative

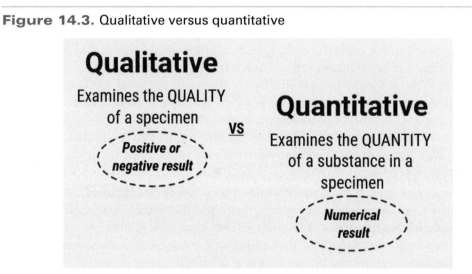

Some examinations can be both qualitative and quantitative, as described in either the code description or the guidelines before the codes in each subsection.

Complete the exercises in There's a Code for That 14.1 to practice identifying qualitative versus quantitative examinations.

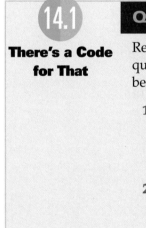

14.1

There's a Code for That

Qualitative versus quantitative

Refer to the following codes in the CPT code book and determine if the test is qualitative or quantitative. Tip: To find this information, read the guidelines at the beginning of each subsection of codes and code descriptions carefully.

1. Code 80150, Amikacin. This test is:
   a. Qualitative
   b. Quantitative
   c. Both qualitative and quantitative

2. Code 80202, Vancomycin. This test is:
   a. Qualitative
   b. Quantitative
   c. Both qualitative and quantitative

3. Code 83045, Hemoglobin; methemoglobin, qualitative. This test is:
   a. Qualitative
   b. Quantitative
   c. Both qualitative and quantitative

4. Code 84512, Troponin, qualitative. This test is:

a. Qualitative

b. Quantitative

c. Both qualitative and quantitative

5. Code 88741, Hemoglobin (Hgb), quantitative, transcutaneous, per day; methemoglobin. This test is:

a. Qualitative

b. Quantitative

c. Both qualitative and quantitative

Procedural Coding for Laboratory and Pathology Services

CPT procedure codes for laboratory and pathology services are all located in the Pathology and Laboratory Section of the CPT code book. They describe the test performed on the patient's specimen. Sometimes code descriptions are fairly detailed and identify the type of specimen or if the test was qualitative or quantitative; and other times code descriptions can be vague. Carefully read any subsection titles, guidelines, parenthetical notes, and any additional information included in this section to ensure complete understanding of the code descriptions. The modifiers used in reporting laboratory and pathology codes are also discussed.

Key to Success

Do not forget to use your resources when coding for lab and pathology services. A medical dictionary, CPT, ICD-10-CM, and HCPCS code books, as well as any other available resources can be helpful. Remember that coding for lab and pathology services is different than coding for medical procedures performed on the patient. The code descriptions only describe the type of test performed on the specimen. If you are not aware of what the test is used for and how it is performed, it may be helpful to research the procedure to ensure that you select the correct code. As you become more familiar with coding for laboratory and pathology services (or any specialty services), you will find that understanding the codes and procedures to report become easier with practice and experience.

Laboratory and Pathology Procedure Codes

The subsections of laboratory and pathology codes depend on the type of test performed on the specimen. When more than one test is performed on the same specimen, or if multiple specimens are tested, it may be necessary to code for more than one procedure. If multiple procedures are performed for the same patient on the same date of service, it is appropriate to report the services together.

The following sections discuss the different subsections of the Laboratory and Pathology section of the CPT code book.

Chemistry Tests and Organ or Disease-Oriented Panels

The Chemistry subsection of codes (82009–84999) is one of the largest sections of codes in the Pathology and Laboratory section. These codes describe tests for specific substances, such as potassium or lead. A **specific test** is one that evaluates a specimen for an identified substance. Some chemistry tests are qualitative and identify whether the specific substance is in the specimen or not, while others are quantitative and identify the exact amount of the specific substance in the specimen. For example, code 84106, Porphobilinogen, urine; *qualitative* is to determine whether porphobilinogen is present in the urine (qualitative), and code 84110, Porphobilinogen, urine; *quantitative* is to determine the amount of porphobilinogen in the urine (quantitative). If the word qualitative or quantitative is not included in the code description, then these qualities of the test do not impact code selection. If these qualities are described in the code description, then it is necessary to match the procedure performed with either the qualitative or quantitative code for the examination.

Note that the Chemistry section is organized in alphabetical order, according to the name of the chemical substance. To search for a chemistry code, look up the term *Pathology and Laboratory* in the Index of the CPT code book, and then refer to the subterm *Chemistry.* Then find the subterm for the specific substance for which the specimen is being tested.

Key to Success

The list of subterms under the Chemistry heading spans a number of pages. It helps to start at the beginning of the *Pathology and Laboratory* heading and search for the *Chemistry* subterm from there. If you do not start at the beginning, it is easy to get lost in the multiple subterms. It may also help to highlight or underline the first subterms for pathology and laboratory procedures in the Index to make them easier to find when searching through the CPT Index.

The Organ or Disease-Oriented Panels (80047–80081) subsection identifies groups of laboratory tests, called panels. A panel is a group of specific tests (from the chemistry section) that are commonly performed together. They are grouped together under one code description to make the reporting of the panel easier. For example, the code description for 80047 reads:

80047	Basic metabolic panel (Calcium, ionized)
	This panel must include the following:
	Calcium, ionized (82330)
	Carbon dioxide (bicarbonate) (82374)
	Chloride (82435)
	Creatinine (82565)
	Glucose (82947)
	Potassium (84132)
	Sodium (84295)
	Urea Nitrogen (BUN) (84520)

This means that the basic metabolic panel reported by code 80047 includes the following chemistry tests: Calcium ionized, Carbon dioxide (bicarbonate), Chloride, Creatinine, Glucose, Potassium, Sodium, and Urea nitrogen (BUN).

Note that the specific procedure code for each individual chemistry test is included after each of the components listed in the panel. For example, in the basic metabolic panel identified previously, each chemistry test included in the panel is listed in the

CPT book with the appropriate CPT code for just that chemistry test, such as Chloride (82435). This code identifies the chemistry test for that specific substance, if it was performed alone. This is a helpful reference for coders, because if not all components in the panel were performed, then the coder cannot report the panel code. The coder must report each of the components that were tested with their individual CPT codes. For example, if a provider ordered a basic metabolic panel (code 80047), but the Potassium and Sodium components of the test were not performed because they had been performed in an earlier lab test, for example, then the coder must *not* report the panel code. In this case, the coder can only report the codes for the procedures that were performed: 82330, Calcium; ionized, 82374, Carbon dioxide (bicarbonate), 82435, Chloride; blood, 82565, Creatinine; blood, 82947, Glucose; quantitative, blood (except reagent strip), and 84520, Urea nitrogen; quantitative.

Key to Success

A panel code can only be reported if *all* the components in the panel were performed. If not, then report the code for each individual test separately. In this way, panels are much like global packages of laboratory services. If all the components of the package were performed, then report the package code. If the entire package was not performed, report only the individual codes for the tests that *were* performed.

Complete the exercises in There's a Code for That 14.2 to practice assigning codes for panels and chemistry tests.

Panels and chemistry tests

14.2

There's a Code for That

Read the following documentation of the laboratory test and identify the correct chemistry or disease-oriented panel code(s).

1. Comprehensive metabolic panel.

   CPT code: _____

2. Hepatic function panel without bilirubin measurements.

   CPT codes: _____ , _____ , _____ ,

   _____ , _____

3. Tests completed: Lipid panel, comprehensive metabolic panel, and acute hepatitis panel.

   CPT codes: _____ , _____ , _____

4. Qualitative ketone test.

   CPT code: _____

5. Qualitative complete (40 acids) plasma amino acid analysis on a 40-year-old female with neuropsychiatric disorder.

   CPT code: _____

6. Direct measurement of HDL, VLDL, and LDL cholesterol.

   CPT codes: _____ , _____ , _____

Drug Assays

Drug assays, or procedures to test for drugs, are divided into three subsections: Drug Assay, Therapeutic Drug Assay, and Chemistry procedures. The selection of the code for the test depends on the purpose and desired result type (qualitative or quantitative).

Presumptive Drug Class Screenings and Definitive Drug Testing

The Drug Assays subsection is divided into Presumptive Drug Class Screening (80305–80307) and Definitive Drug Testing (80320–80377) codes. Presumptive drug class screening codes are used to report screening procedures performed to qualitatively determine if a drug is present in the specimen. These codes do not identify the drug being tested nor the purpose of the test, but rather the method in which the test was performed. There are three possible codes and only one code should be reported depending on the test type, per date of service, no matter how many drug classes are being assayed in the test.

- 80305, Drug test(s), presumptive, any number of drug classes, any number of devices or procedures; capable of being read by direct optical observation only (eg, utilizing immunoassay [eg, dipsticks, cups, cards, cartridges]) includes sample validation when performed, per date of service, identifies a drug test capable of being read by direct optical observation, such as dipsticks, cups, cards, or cartridges.

- 80306, Drug test(s), presumptive, any number of drug classes, any number of devices or procedures; read by instrument assisted direct optical observation (eg, utilizing immunoassay [eg, dipsticks, cups, card, cartridges]), includes sample validation when performed, per date of service, identifies a drug test capable of being read by instrument-assisted direct optical observation, such as if a cartridge is inserted into a device to aid in the optical reading of the test results.

- 80307, Drug test(s), presumptive, any number of drug classes, any number of devices or procedures, by instrument chemistry analyzers (eg, utilizing immunoassay [eg, EIA, ELISA, EMIT, FPIA, IA, KIMS, RIA]), chromatography (eg, GC, HPLC), and mass spectrometry either with or without chromatography (eg, DART, DESI, GC-MS, GC-MS/MS, LC-MS, LC-MS/MS, LDTD, MALD, TOF), includes sample validation when performed, per date of service, identifies a drug test capable of being read by any type of instrument chemical analyzers, including chromatography and mass spectrometry.

The results from any of these three tests are qualitative in nature, meaning that they only give a positive or negative result. These are nonspecific tests that only identify if a drug class is present, rather than test for the specific type of drug. A **nonspecific test** does not test for a specific chemical or substance, but rather tests for a quality, such as whether or not any type of drug from that drug class is present.

Definitive drug testing codes are used for both qualitative and quantitative analyses for drugs. These tests are specific and codes identify the exact substance that is being tested in the sample. Note that some code descriptions differ based on the number of specific substances tested. If the specific substance being tested is not listed within this code range, it is necessary to first search for the substance in the Therapeutic Drug Assays codes and Chemistry codes before assigning one of the unlisted drugs or substances codes (80375–80377).

Therapeutic Drug Assays

Therapeutic Drug Assays (80145–80299) codes are similar in nature to Drug Assay codes, except that the drugs tested in this subsection are therapeutic drugs taken upon the advice of a healthcare professional. These tests are run to monitor the clinical response to the prescribed drug. In this process, a patient takes a prescribed medication and the therapeutic drug assay test is performed to determine the amount of the drug in the patient's body after a specific amount of time. This is used to clinically determine the correct amount of time between doses for specific medications and to adjust dosing accordingly.

Chemistry

If the drug being tested is not listed in either the Drug Assays or Therapeutic Drug Assays sections previously noted, then it is necessary to check for a code for the test in the Chemistry section of codes (82009–84999) and report the test accordingly.

Complete the exercises in There's a Code for That 14.3 to practice assigning codes for drug testing.

Drug assays

14.3

There's a Code for That

Read the following documentation of the laboratory test and identify the correct drug assay code(s).

1. Presumptive drug test, five drug classes, via optically-read urine dipstick.

   CPT code: _____

2. DART mass spectrometry for three drug classes with sample validation.

   CPT code: _____

3. Patient with positive drug test results is tested for four classes of amphetamines.

   CPT code: _____

4. Alcohol breath test.

   CPT code: _____

5. Therapeutic drug assay for free phenytoin.

   CPT code: _____

6. Whole blood serum gabapentin assay.

   CPT code: _____

7. Drug assay for seven benzodiazepines.

   CPT code: _____

Evocative/Suppression Testing

Evocative/Suppression Testing (80400–80439) codes are used to report a test in which a substance in the body is measured both before and after the administration of another substance. For example, code 80422, Glucagon tolerance panel; for insulinoma, is an evocative/suppression evaluation that tests the patient for pancreatic tumor (insulinoma). The patient is tested for the two components in the test (as listed in the full code description): Glucose (82947) and Insulin (83525). After this initial test, a substance is administered, and after a specified amount of time the same two components are tested again (glucose and insulin). Then the results for both tests are compared. The result measure may be either evocative, meaning that the level of the first substance is stimulated, or suppressed. These tests are commonly performed to diagnose endocrine disorders, such as hypothyroidism, adrenal insufficiency, and Cushing's disease. The full code description for this laboratory procedure is 80422, Glucagon tolerance panel: for insulinoma. This panel must include the following: Glucose (82947 × 3), Insulin (83525 × 3).

Codes for evocative/suppression tests identify the type of test performed. Inherent in these tests is the administration of the agents administered to the patient during the test, which should be reported separately using codes from Hydration, Therapeutic, Prophylactic, Diagnostic Injections and Infusions, and Chemotherapy and Other Highly Complex Drug or Highly Complex Biologic Agent Administration (96365–96368, 96372, 96374–96376).

Consultations (Clinical Pathology)

A clinical pathology consultation should be reported when a pathologist must render a written interpretation and report of a test result that requires additional medical interpretation, as a response to a request from the ordering healthcare provider.

There are two code options in this section: a limited clinical consultation that does not require a review of the patient's healthcare history (80500), and a comprehensive clinical consultation, which requires a review of the patient's history and healthcare records (80502).

Urinalysis

Urinalysis (81000–81099) codes are for nonspecific tests on urine. They do not identify the quantitative evaluation of specific substances in the urine, but rather the quality of the urine itself. Code selection depends on the type of urinalysis performed and, in some cases, the purpose of the evaluation, such as 81025, Urine pregnancy test, by visual color comparison methods.

Gene Testing Procedures

There are a number of different genetic testing procedures included in the Pathology and Laboratory section of the CPT code book. These include Molecular Pathology procedures, Genomic Sequencing Procedures and Other Molecular Multianalyte Assays, and Multianalyte Assays with Algorithmic Analyses.

Molecular Pathology procedures (81105–81408, 81479) are highly specialized procedures performed on nucleic acid, such as DNA and RNA, to detect genetic variations and mutations. Code selection is based on the gene being analyzed.

Codes are listed in this section according to the gene name and organized in alphabetical order within their respective tiers. There are two divisions of molecular pathology codes, according to each tier: Tier 1 and Tier 2. Tier 1 tests are for a single analyte (component being tested for), and the code descriptions identify the specific analyte for which the pathology service is testing. For example, 81327, SEPT9 (Septin9) (eg, colorectal cancer) promoter methylation analysis, identifies the specific molecular pathology exam performed to test for the colorectal cancer gene. On the other hand, Tier 2 codes are less specific, as they test for less-common genetic attributes. Thus, Tier 2 code descriptions do not specify one analyte, but are more general in nature—for example, 81400, Molecular pathology procedure, Level 1 (eg, identification of single germline variant [eg, SNP] by techniques such as restriction enzyme digestion or melt curve analysis). Beneath this code description is a lengthy list of specific genes that may be tested with this procedure code. These lengthy code descriptions identify all of the many genes that may be tested for in the procedure, and result in this section of codes being multiple pages in length.

To assist coders in identifying the correct code for the gene being analyzed, the professional edition of the CPT code book includes a cross-reference section at the beginning of the Pathology and Laboratory section, which lists the genes by a claim designation, abbreviated gene name, full gene, name, and commonly associated proteins and diseases, also with the appropriate molecular pathology code for each specific gene. The CPT standard edition code book does not include this cross-reference.

Genomic Sequencing Procedures and Other Molecular Multianalyte Assays (81410–81471) are procedures that evaluate a selection of multiple genes or genetic regions relevant to a specific medical condition. Code selection depends on the type of genetic sequence being tested or the medical condition. Some genetic sequencing codes are similar to organ or disease-related panels, because they include a number of different molecular pathology procedures (for specific genes) into one panel of tests to evaluate for a range of genetic conditions.

Multianalyte Assays with Algorithmic Analyses (81490–81599) are complex procedures that identify specific biomarkers, genes, and proteins. Code selection depends on the disease type, material analyzed, number of markers included in the test, methodology of the test, number of functional domains (if indicated), specimen type, algorithm result type, and report produced from the test. For example, code 81503, Oncology (ovarian), biochemical assays of five proteins (CA-125, apolipoprotein A1, beta-2 microglobulin, transferrin, and pre-albumin), utilizing serum, algorithm reported as a risk score. Appendix O of the CPT code book includes a cross-reference of the proprietary lab that performs these tests, together with their descriptions and alpha-numeric lab requisition codes.

Hematology and Coagulation

Hematology and Coagulation (85002–85999) codes identify tests on blood and blood products. Code selection depends on the type of test performed, or which specific component is being tested in the blood (for example, 85007, Blood count; blood smear, microscopic examination with manual differential WBC count).

Immunology

Immunology (86000–86849) codes identify whether a specific immunological substance is present in the body. These procedures test for the presence of antibodies to specific infectious agents. Code selection depends on the identification of the specific antigen or antibody being tested, as well as other specifics of the procedure (for example, if it was qualitative or quantitative).

Transfusion Medicine

Transfusion Medicine (86850–86999) codes identify procedures performed on blood and blood products that are either collected from a blood donor or tested before storage and being given to a blood recipient. Code selection depends on the specific service performed on the blood or blood product.

Microbiology

Microbiology (87003–87999) codes identify procedures performed to identify specific microorganisms and infectious diseases, such as streptococcus or influenza. More specifically, the tests include **bacteriology**, the study of bacteria; **mycology**, the study of fungi; **parasitology**, the study of parasites; and **virology**, the study of viruses (see figure 14.4). Microbiology tests include swabs, smears, and cultures, all of which test a patient sample for a specific microbiological agent.

The same microorganism may be tested in several different ways, and it is possible that multiple tests may be conducted on the same date of service. For example, a lab may run streptococcal, influenza, and mononucleosis tests all on the same day, to rule out those three microorganisms as the cause of the patient's symptoms.

Coders should report each test conducted on the date of service. If the *same* test was performed on multiple sites (for example a bacterial culture from wound exudate on the buttock as well as one on the leg), append modifier -59, Distinct procedural service, to identify the procedures as distinct from each other. If the same test was run multiple times on the same date of service, append modifier -91, Repeat clinical laboratory diagnostic test.

Coding for microbiology tests relies on the identification of the specimen, the microorganism for which the study is testing, and the type of microbiology test. For example, with code 87086, Culture, bacterial; qualitative colony count, urine, the specimen is *urine*, the microorganism is *bacteria*, and the type of test is a *culture with qualitative colony count*. The microorganism in this code is only identified as bacteria,

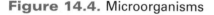

Figure 14.4. Microorganisms

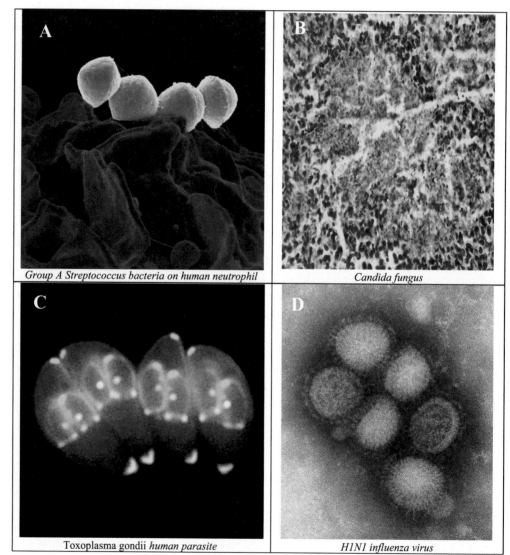

Group A Streptococcus bacteria on human neutrophil	*Candida fungus*
Toxoplasma gondii *human parasite*	*H1N1 influenza virus*

Sources: A) NIAID 2009; B) Rosen 2011; C) Hu et al. 2006; D) CDC 2010.

which means any type of bacteria. Some tests specify the exact bacteria for which the study is testing, but do not specify the type of specimen. For example, code 87880, Infectious agent antigen detection by immunoassay with direct optical observation; Streptococcus, group A, identifies the type of test, *immunoassay with direct optical observation*, and the specific bacteria, *group A streptococcus*, but does not specify the type of specimen.

Anatomic Pathology

Anatomic Pathology (88000–88099) codes identify services performed by a physician on a deceased patient for pathological examinations, such as an autopsy. These codes identify the type of examination, either gross or microscopic, and the components involved in the exam—for example, 88007, Necropsy (autopsy), gross examination only; with brain and spinal cord. Remember that a gross examination includes the physical components of the specimen, such as the size, weight, and visual characteristics, and that a microscopic examination is performed with a microscope.

Cytopathology

Cytopathology (88104–88199) codes identify **cytopathology** studies, which examine cells from a specimen to determine a cause or nature of a disease. The most common and widely used cytopathology study is the Pap smear, developed by George Nicolas Papanicolaou in 1928 (Tan 2015). A Pap smear is done by taking a sample of cells from the cervix that are then examined for cancerous cell changes. See figure 14.5, which displays a thin-prep cervical smear slide. Normal cervical cells are shown on the right, and HPV-infected cells appear on the left.

Codes in the cytopathology section identify the test technique and the source of the specimen. For example, code 88150, Cytopathology, slides, cervical or vaginal; manual screening under physician supervision, identifies the source of the specimen, *cervical or vaginal*, as well as the test technique, *slides...manual screening under physician supervision*.

Figure 14.5. Cells obtained from a Pap smear

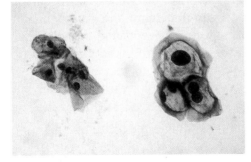

Source: Uthman 2006.

Cytogenic Studies

Cytogenic Studies (88230–88299), also known as cytogenetic studies, are performed on chromosomes to determine abnormalities. Code selection depends on the type and purpose of the test. For example, code 88248, Chromosome analysis for breakage syndromes; baseline breakage, score 50–100 cells, count 20 cells, 2 karyotypes (eg, for ataxia telangiectasia, Fanconi anemia, fragile X), identifies the type of test, *chromosome analysis*, and the purpose of the test, *breakage syndromes; baseline breakage, score 50–100 cells, count 20 cells, 2 karyotypes (eg, for ataxia telangiectasia, Fanconi anemia, fragile X).*

Complete the exercises in There's a Code for That 14.4 to practice assigning procedure codes for laboratory procedures.

14.4

There's a Code for That

Coding laboratory services

Read the following documentation of the laboratory test and identify the correct laboratory or pathology test code(s).

1. BRCA1 with BRCA2 gene analysis, full sequence analysis with detection of large gene rearrangements for patient with family history of breast cancer.

   CPT code: _____

2. Chorionic gonadotropin stimulation panel; estradiol response.

   CPT code: _____

3. Urine pregnancy test.

   CPT code: _____

4. Bacterial urine culture with quantitative colony count.

   CPT code: _____

5. Trichomonas vaginalis detection by DNA analysis, direct probe technique.

   CPT code: _____

Surgical Pathology

Surgical Pathology (88300–88399) codes identify the services performed by a surgical pathologist. Surgical pathology is the study of tissues removed during surgery that are examined intraoperatively by a surgical pathologist. During the pathological examination, the surgical pathologist examines the specimen (just removed from the patient) to distinguish between malignant and non-malignant cells, detect cancerous cell changes, and identify infectious agents and pathological diseases in tissues. This process involves both gross and microscopic examination of the tissue specimen (depending on the level of surgical pathology performed).

There are six levels of surgical pathology examinations, each of which is identified with a specific CPT code.

- 88300, Level I, Surgical pathology, gross examination only. Level I examinations should be used for any specimen that is accurately diagnosed without a microscopic examination.

- 88302, Level II, Surgical pathology, gross and microscopic examination. Level II examinations require both gross and microscopic examinations of the specimen to confirm the diagnosis, or the absence of a disease.

Levels III through VI examinations require both gross and microscopic examinations, with the higher levels of the service representing higher levels of physician work.

- 88304, Level III, Surgical pathology, gross and microscopic examination.
- 88305, Level IV, Surgical pathology, gross and microscopic examination.
- 88307, Level V, Surgical pathology, gross and microscopic examination.
- 88309, Level VI, Surgical pathology, gross and microscopic examination.

Each level of surgical pathology (except for Level I) has a list of tissue specimens after the code description. When coding for surgical pathology services, a coder must identify the tissue sample that is analyzed in the service, such as carpal tunnel tissue, and then locate that specific type of tissue in the list of a specific level of surgical pathology. For example, if the tissue examined was carpal tunnel tissue, find that specific tissue type in one of the levels for the surgical pathology service. In this case, code 88304, Level III, Surgical pathology, gross and microscopic examination, would be the correct code, because *Carpal tunnel tissue* is included in the list for that level of service.

The lists of tissue types are arranged in alphabetical order, according to the type of tissue, under each code heading for Levels II through Level VI surgical pathology services. Be careful, however, as sometimes the same tissue type appears in multiple different levels. For example, breast tissue is listed under Level IV, Level V, and Level VI. This requires careful reading to ensure the selection of the correct level of surgical pathology service: Level IV is for Breast, *biopsy, not requiring microscopic evaluation of surgical margins*; Level V is for Breast, *mastectomy-partial/simple* and Breast, *excision of lesion, requiring microscopic evaluation of surgical margins*; and Level VI is for Breast, *mastectomy-with regional lymph nodes*. Selection of the correct level depends on the correct identification of the type of tissue examined.

If the same tissue sample was examined in two different areas, report the appropriate code only once. If there were two separate tissue samples from the same body area that were examined, report one code for each sample examined.

Complete the exercises in There's a Code for That 14.5 to practice reporting procedure codes for surgical pathology services.

Surgical pathology coding

14.5

There's a Code for That

Read the following documentation of the surgical pathology service and identify the correct surgical pathology code(s).

1. Pathological examination of two skin tags.

   CPT code: _____ × _____

2. Labial biopsy examination, surgical pathology.

   CPT code: _____

3. Surgical pathology examinations of the following tissue samples: cervical conization, endometrial biopsy, and bladder biopsy.

   CPT code: _____ , _____ × _____

Other Procedures

Other procedures in the Pathology and Laboratory section include In Vivo (eg, Transcutaneous) Laboratory Procedures (88720–88749), Other Procedures (89049–89240), and Reproductive Medicine Procedures (89250–89398).

In vivo procedures are tests performed on living humans, rather than on a dead or partial specimen from a patient. These procedures are performed transcutaneously, or through an unbroken area of skin (such as a cardiac electrode being placed on an unbroken area of skin to read heart impulses). Code selection depends on the in vivo measurement performed. For example, code 88720, Bilirubin, total, transcutaneous, is the code reported for the in vivo examination of a patient's bilirubin level.

The Other Procedures subsection contains laboratory and pathology tests that are not classifiable into any other subsection, such as cell count of a body fluid other than blood (89050, Cell count, miscellaneous body fluids (eg, cerebrospinal fluid, joint fluid), except blood), or 89190, Nasal smear for eosinophils. Reproductive procedures are performed on both male and female reproductive products and the products of conception, such as oocytes, sperm, and embryos.

Proprietary Laboratory Analyses

Codes for proprietary laboratory analyses (PLA) identify laboratory tests that are commercially available for use of human specimens, and offered by a specific clinical laboratory or manufacturer. In other words, these are tests that are performed by a certain laboratory or manufacturer, and which no other laboratory can offer (they are proprietary). Note that these codes are also very different in format from other laboratory and pathology codes. All other codes in the Pathology and Laboratory section begin with the number 8 and are composed of five numbers. PLA test codes, on the other hand, all begin with a zero (0) and end with the letter *U*. For example, 0001U, Red blood cell antigen typing, DNA, human erythrocyte antigen gene analysis of 35 antigens from 11 blood groups, utilizing whole blood, common RBC alleles reported.

When reporting PLA codes, there are some important guidelines to ensure that the code is being reported correctly. If a PLA code is available to report a given laboratory procedure, then the coder should report the PLA code. Appendix O also lists all PLA codes, along with the procedure's proprietary name, to help with code selection. Furthermore, it is important to note the "Duplicate PLA test" symbol next to some of the codes, which identifies codes with identical code descriptors. For codes with identical descriptions, it is necessary to pay attention to parenthetical notes in the CPT code book, and refer to Appendix O, to ensure accurate code selection.

Handling of Drug Specimen

In some cases, patients may leave a specimen—such as a urine or stool sample—at their healthcare provider's office. If the needed test is not CLIA-waived, or otherwise cannot be performed at the healthcare provider's office, then the provider's office will have to send this specimen to an independent laboratory. Many independent labs collect specimens from their local area and use couriers to drive to nearby healthcare offices to pick up these samples.

Code 99000, Handling and/or conveyance of specimen for transfer from the office to a laboratory, is reported when a specimen collected in the outpatient office is packed and taken to the laboratory by someone other than the patient. For example, if an outpatient office took a blood or urine sample from a patient, and this sample was picked up by a lab courier service and then delivered to an independent lab, the office would bill code 99000 to identify that the sample was taken at the office, prepared and packed by the office, and then transported to the laboratory.

If a patient dropped off the specimen directly to the lab, or of the lab drew the specimen (such as a blood draw), then code 99000 would *not* be reported, as the specimen was not transferred from one office to another.

Modifiers for Laboratory and Pathology Services

There are three CPT modifiers that are specifically designed for use with pathology and laboratory codes.

- Modifier -90, Reference (outside) laboratory. This modifier should be used when the healthcare office practices pass-through billing and bills for the laboratory service directly, rather than the laboratory billing for the test. This is only done when the two parties have a prior agreement to bill for services in this manner.

- Modifier -91, Repeat clinical diagnostic laboratory test. This modifier should be used when the exact same laboratory test is re-run on the same date of service for the same patient. However, it may *not* be used if the test was re-run either to confirm the previous result or if the previous test was faulty or questionable. For example:

    > A patient received a CBC in the outpatient office and it was determined that the patient was fighting off a severe infection. The healthcare provider, suspecting that it was bacterial, administered an antibiotic injection in the office to immediately control the infection. The CBC was repeated after two hours to verify the effect on the patient's system.

    In this case, the test was repeated for the same patient on the same date of service, but was conducted to determine separate results. In this example, the second CBC wound be appended with modifier -91.

Note that modifier -51, Multiple procedures, may not be appended to laboratory and pathology procedures. This is because modifier -91, Repeat clinical diagnostic laboratory test, is more appropriate. If the same test was run multiple times, it may only be billed for in the circumstances described previously. If it was re-run because the initial test was faulty or questionable, or if the test was re-run to confirm the initial results, only one test can be reported for the date of service. If multiple different tests were performed on the same date of service, none of which were repeated on that day, then no modifiers are necessary.

- Modifier -92, Alternative laboratory platform testing. This modifier should be appended when a laboratory test is performed using a kit or a transportable device that consists of a single-time use, disposable analytic chamber. For example, HIV tests may be performed using single, one-time use analytic chambers, so if the HIV test was performed in a mobile unit, then the code for the HIV test (86701, HIV-1) would be appended with modifier -92, Alternative laboratory platform testing (86701-92).

Other modifiers that may be appropriate for laboratory services include modifier -QW, CLIA-waived test, for specifically identified CLIA-waived tests, modifier -XS, Separate structure, and modifier -XU, Unusual non-overlapping service. Both -XS and -XU should be used in lieu of modifier -59, Distinct procedural service, when the same laboratory test is conducted more than once on different specimens on the same day, to better describe the circumstances of the encounter.

Diagnostic Coding for Laboratory and Pathology Services

Diagnosis coding for pathology and laboratory services requires an in-depth knowledge of Chapter 1 (Certain Infectious and Parasitic Diseases in the ICD-10-CM) code book. This chapter includes codes that identify certain infectious and parasitic diseases, as well as those certain infectious and parasitic diseases as the cause of conditions coded elsewhere. It contains important guidelines for coding HIV and AIDS, sepsis (discussed in chapter 10 [Urgent Care and Emergency Department Services]), and methicillin-resistant *Staphylococcus aureus* (MRSA).

Infectious Diseases and Infectious Diseases as the Cause of Conditions Coded Elsewhere

There are two divisions of codes in the infectious diseases chapter in the ICD-10-CM code book: codes for specific infectious diseases, including specified bacteria, viruses, fungi, and other pathogens; and codes for these infectious diseases as the cause of a condition classified elsewhere.

Codes for the infectious diseases themselves should be used when that specific infectious organism has not been confirmed as causing any specific medical condition. For example, if a lab sample runs a test on a specimen and determines that the sample is contaminated with Enterotoxigenic E. coli, then the coder should report the procedure code for the lab test along with the code for the infectious organism, in this case A04.1, Enterotoxigenic Escherichia coli infection.

However, if a healthcare office sent a urine sample to the lab to determine the infectious agent for a patient with a urinary tract infection, and it was determined that the infectious agent was E. coli, then the code selected to identify the E. coli would be B96.20, Unspecified Escherichia coli [E. coli] as the cause of diseases classified elsewhere. An additional code would also be assigned to identify the manifestation of the E. coli infection, in this case a urinary tract infection, N39.0, Urinary tract infection, site not specified. Refer to chapter 4 (Learning the ICD-10-CM Code Book) for a refresher of etiology and manifestation coding.

Note that in the first example, the lab is testing the specimen, identifying the infectious agent, and assigning a code to identify the organism. In the second example, the provider's office received the information from the lab and assigns a code from category B95 to B97, Bacterial and viral infectious agents (as the cause of disease classified elsewhere). The codes in these categories identify that the infectious agent has caused a specific manifestation, condition, or disease.

Figure 14.6. OGCR I.C.1.b

---

b. Infectious agents as the cause of diseases classified to other chapters

Certain infections are classified in chapters other than Chapter 1 and no organism is identified as part of the infection code. In these instances, it is necessary to use an additional code from Chapter 1 to identify the organism. A code from category B95, Streptococcus, Staphylococcus, and Enterococcus as the cause of diseases classified to other chapters, B96, Other bacterial agents as the cause of diseases classified to other chapters, or B97, Viral agents as the cause of diseases classified to other chapters, is to be used as an additional code to identify the organism. An instructional note will be found at the infection code advising that an additional organism code is required.

Source: CMS 2019b.

Because labs identify the infectious organism, when present, they are more likely to use the infectious and parasitic agent codes. On the other hand, because healthcare providers diagnose and treat known healthcare conditions, they are more likely to report codes for bacterial and viral infectious agents as the cause of a disease classified elsewhere. Remember that according to coding guidelines, if the infectious organism is known, then it should be identified with the appropriate ICD-10-CM code. See figure 14.6 for the OGCR related to infectious agents as the cause of diseases classified elsewhere.

Coding for HIV and AIDS

Coding for HIV and AIDS must be done with the utmost caution, as this condition is closely tracked by public health agencies, health insurance providers, and third-party payers. There are also several ICD-10-CM guidelines that specify which and how HIV codes should be used.

When a patient presents for HIV testing, report code Z11.4, Encounter for screening for human immunodeficiency virus [HIV]. If HIV counseling is performed at this visit, then report the additional code Z71.7, Human immunodeficiency virus [HIV] counseling. If the patient engages in high-risk sexual behavior, then the appropriate code from category Z72.5-, High-risk sexual behavior, should also be reported. For example, a patient with multiple heterosexual partners presents because he is worried about contracting HIV. An HIV test is performed after the provider counsels the patient on HIV risks and testing. The codes for this encounter would be as follows:

- Z11.4, Encounter for screening for human immunodeficiency virus [HIV]
- Z71.7, Human immunodeficiency virus [HIV] counseling
- Z72.51, High-risk heterosexual behavior

Furthermore, if the patient has been exposed to HIV, report code Z20.6, Contact with and (suspected) exposure to human immunodeficiency virus [HIV]. The exposure to HIV code should not be reported with codes for HIV positive status.

There are three possible outcomes from an HIV test:

- *The results are inconclusive.* If the results from this HIV test are inconclusive, then report code R75, Inconclusive laboratory evidence of human immunodeficiency virus [HIV].
- *The result is negative.* If the results are negative and the patient returns to discuss the findings, then report code Z71.7, Human immunodeficiency virus [HIV] counseling.
- *The result is positive.*
  - If the result is positive, and the patient is not experiencing any HIV-related symptoms, then report code Z21, Asymptomatic human immunodeficiency virus [HIV] infection status.
  - If the result is positive, and the patient is experiencing HIV-related symptoms, report code B20, Human immunodeficiency virus [HIV] disease. This code should be reported for all HIV or AIDS patients that have a positive HIV test and any HIV-related symptoms, ranging all the way to AIDS. Sequence B20 first, followed by any additional codes for HIV-related conditions. Note that even if the patient is not currently exhibiting any symptoms, it is still necessary to assign code B20, if he or she has ever exhibited HIV-related symptoms. Once a patient has been assigned code B20, he or she can never go back to asymptomatic status.

○ If the result is positive and the patient is pregnant, report a code from category O98.7-, Human immunodeficiency virus [HIV] disease complicating pregnancy, childbirth and the puerperium, as well as code B20, followed by any additional code to identify HIV-related conditions, or Z21.7, for asymptomatic HIV status. For example, an asymptomatic HIV-positive patient that is currently in the third trimester of pregnancy would be coded as follows: O98.713, Human immunodeficiency virus [HIV] disease complicating pregnancy, third trimester, and Z21, Asymptomatic human immunodeficiency virus [HIV] infection status.

See figure 14.7 for a graphic illustrating the coding process for HIV cases.

Figure 14.7. HIV coding

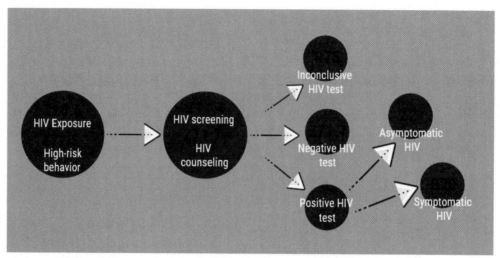

Once a patient receives an HIV-related diagnosis (either Z21 or B20), then either of these codes must be reported for *every* encounter with the patient, as this is a lifelong condition that is not currently curable.

Sequencing of the HIV positive codes is also important (see figure 14.8 for the OGCR related to HIV coding).

- When a patient presents for an HIV-related condition, sequence B20 first, followed by any HIV-related condition(s). For example, an HIV positive patient presents for management of her pneumocystis carinii, which is related to her HIV status, the following codes would be reported in this order:
  ○ B20, Human immunodeficiency virus [HIV] disease
  ○ B59, Pneumocystosis

- When a patient presents for a condition that is *not* related to HIV, sequence the unrelated condition first, followed by B20 and any codes for HIV-related condition(s). For example, if the HIV positive patient with pneumocystis carinii presented for a fracture of the right wrist, then the following codes would be reported in this order:
  ○ S62.101A, Fracture of unspecified carpal bone, right wrist, initial encounter for closed fracture
  ○ B20, Human immunodeficiency virus [HIV] disease
  ○ B59, Pneumocystosis

Figure 14.8. OGCR I.C.1.a

---

1. **Chapter 1: Certain Infectious and Parasitic Diseases (A00-B99)**

    a. **Human Immunodeficiency Virus (HIV) Infections**

        1) **Code only confirmed cases**

            Code only confirmed cases of HIV infection/illness. This is an exception to the hospital inpatient guideline Section II, H.

            In this context, "confirmation" does not require documentation of positive serology or culture for HIV; the provider's diagnostic statement that the patient is HIV positive, or has an HIV-related illness is sufficient.

        2) **Selection and sequencing of HIV codes**

            (a) **Patient admitted for HIV-related condition**

                If a patient is admitted for an HIV-related condition, the principal diagnosis should be B20, Human immunodeficiency virus [HIV] disease followed by additional diagnosis codes for all reported HIV-related conditions.

            (b) **Patient with HIV disease admitted for unrelated condition**

                If a patient with HIV disease is admitted for an unrelated condition (such as a traumatic injury), the code for the unrelated condition (e.g., the nature of injury code) should be the principal diagnosis. Other diagnoses would be B20 followed by additional diagnosis codes for all reported HIV-related conditions.

            (c) **Whether the patient is newly diagnosed**

                Whether the patient is newly diagnosed or has had previous admissions/encounters for HIV conditions is irrelevant to the sequencing decision.

            (d) **Asymptomatic human immunodeficiency virus**

                Z21, Asymptomatic human immunodeficiency virus [HIV] infection status, is to be applied when the patient without any documentation of symptoms is listed as being "HIV positive," "known HIV," "HIV test positive," or similar terminology. Do not use this code if the term "AIDS" is used or if the patient is treated for any HIV-related illness or is described as having any condition(s) resulting from his/her HIV positive status; use B20 in these cases.

            (e) **Patients with inconclusive HIV serology**

                Patients with inconclusive HIV serology, but no definitive diagnosis or manifestations of the illness, may be assigned code R75, Inconclusive laboratory evidence of human immunodeficiency virus [HIV].

            (f) **Previously diagnosed HIV-related illness**

                Patients with any known prior diagnosis of an HIV-related illness should be coded to B20. Once a patient has developed an HIV-related illness, the patient should always be assigned code B20 on every subsequent admission/encounter. Patients previously diagnosed with any HIV illness (B20) should never be assigned to R75 or Z21, Asymptomatic human immunodeficiency virus [HIV] infection status.

            (g) **HIV Infection in Pregnancy, Childbirth and the Puerperium**

                During pregnancy, childbirth or the puerperium, a patient admitted (or presenting for a health care encounter) because of an HIV-related illness should receive a principal diagnosis code of O98.7-, Human immunodeficiency [HIV] disease complicating pregnancy, childbirth and the puerperium, followed by B20 and the code(s) for the HIV-related illness(es). Codes from Chapter 15 always take sequencing priority. Patients with asymptomatic HIV infection status admitted (or presenting for a health care encounter) during pregnancy, childbirth, or the puerperium should receive codes of O98.7- and Z21.

            (h) **Encounters for testing for HIV**

                If a patient is being seen to determine his/her HIV status, use code Z11.4, Encounter for screening for human immunodeficiency virus [HIV]. Use additional codes for any associated high risk behavior.

                If a patient with signs or symptoms is being seen for HIV testing, code the signs and symptoms. An additional counseling code Z71.7, Human immunodeficiency virus [HIV] counseling, may be used if counseling is provided during the encounter for the test.

                When a patient returns to be informed of his/her HIV test results and the test result is negative, use code Z71.7, Human immunodeficiency virus [HIV] counseling.

                If the results are positive, see previous guidelines and assign codes as appropriate.

Source: CMS 2019b.

Note also that both codes for HIV infection are HCC codes, so special attention should be paid to the accurate and complete documentation of these conditions.

Coding for MRSA

Methicillin-resistant *Staphylococcus aureus* (MRSA) is a bacterium that can cause infections throughout the human body. It is resistant to certain antibiotics, making it especially hard to treat and cure. There are a handful of MRSA guidelines that are important to know when coding for this condition. See figure 14.9 for the official OGCR related to MRSA conditions.

Figure 14.9. OGCR I.C.1.e

---

e. Methicillin Resistant Staphylococcus aureus (MRSA) Conditions

1) Selection and sequencing of MRSA codes

(a) Combination codes for MRSA infection

When a patient is diagnosed with an infection that is due to methicillin resistant Staphylococcus aureus (MRSA), and that infection has a combination code that includes the causal organism (e.g., sepsis, pneumonia) assign the appropriate combination code for the condition (e.g., code A41.02, Sepsis due to Methicillin resistant Staphylococcus aureus or code J15.212, Pneumonia due to Methicillin resistant Staphylococcus aureus). Do not assign code B95.62, Methicillin resistant Staphylococcus aureus infection as the cause of diseases classified elsewhere, as an additional code because the combination code includes the type of infection and the MRSA organism. Do not assign a code from subcategory Z16.11, Resistance to penicillins, as an additional diagnosis.

See Section C.1. for instructions on coding and sequencing of sepsis and severe sepsis.

(b) Other codes for MRSA infection

When there is documentation of a current infection (e.g., wound infection, stitch abscess, urinary tract infection) due to MRSA, and that infection does not have a combination code that includes the causal organism, assign the appropriate code to identify the condition along with code B95.62, Methicillin resistant Staphylococcus aureus infection as the cause of diseases classified elsewhere for the MRSA infection. Do not assign a code from subcategory Z16.11, Resistance to penicillins.

(c) Methicillin susceptible Staphylococcus aureus (MSSA) and MRSA colonization

The condition or state of being colonized or carrying MSSA or MRSA is called colonization or carriage, while an individual person is described as being colonized or being a carrier. Colonization means that MSSA or MSRA is present on or in the body without necessarily causing illness. A positive MRSA colonization test might be documented by the provider as "MRSA screen positive" or "MRSA nasal swab positive".

Assign code Z22.322, Carrier or suspected carrier of Methicillin resistant Staphylococcus aureus, for patients documented as having MRSA colonization. Assign code Z22.321, Carrier or suspected carrier of Methicillin susceptible Staphylococcus aureus, for patient documented as having MSSA colonization. Colonization is not necessarily indicative of a disease process or as the cause of a specific condition the patient may have unless documented as such by the provider.

(d) MRSA colonization and infection

If a patient is documented as having both MRSA colonization and infection during a hospital admission, code Z22.322, Carrier or suspected carrier of Methicillin resistant Staphylococcus aureus, and a code for the MRSA infection may both be assigned.

Source: CMS 2019b.

- If the manifestation of the MRSA infection is not known or specified, code only for the organism with code A49.02, Methicillin-resistant *Staphylococcus aureus* infection, unspecified site. If the MRSA is the infectious agent causing sepsis, report code A41.02, Sepsis due to Methicillin-resistant *Staphylococcus aureus*.

- Use a combination code when available. There are several combination codes for MRSA as the infectious agent and the healthcare condition (the etiology and manifestation). When a combination code is present, it is only necessary to report the combination code. Do not report the combination code and the code for the infectious organism. One example of a MRSA combination code is J15.212, Pneumonia due to Methicillin-resistant *Staphylococcus aureus*. This code combines the etiology (MRSA) with the manifestation (pneumonia) into one code.

- When a combination code is not available, code for the condition and MRSA as the cause of the condition. When a combination code is available, report one for the manifestation of the disease, along with B95.62, Methicillin-resistant *Staphylococcus aureus* infection as the cause of diseases classified elsewhere.

- If the patient is documented as an MRSA carrier or that he or she has an MRSA colonization, report code Z22.322, Carrier or suspected carrier of Methicillin-resistant *Staphylococcus aureus*. This code may be reported with the code for MRSA infection, if the patient has both conditions at the same time.

Key to Success

When reporting codes for MRSA, read the code descriptions carefully, as they are similar and in close proximity to MSSA codes. Methicillin-susceptible *Staphylococcus aureus* (MSSA) is a strain of the same bacteria that is susceptible to antibiotics, rather than resistant to them like MRSA. MSSA codes and MRSA codes read almost exactly alike, and only differ by one word, so they are easy to mistake for each other. For example, compare codes Z22.321, Carrier or suspected carrier of Methicillin-susceptible *Staphylococcus aureus*, and Z22.322, Carrier or suspected carrier of Methicillin-resistant *Staphylococcus aureus*.

HCC Coding Corner

HCC codes are scattered throughout chapter 1 (Certain Infectious and Parasitic Diseases) of the ICD-10-CM code book. Most conditions that qualify as HCCs have a long-term impact on the patient's health. Additional categories of codes that all qualify as HCC codes include: Streptococcal sepsis (A40.-), Viral infections of the central nervous system (A81.-), Chronic viral hepatitis (B18.-), Human immunodeficiency virus disease (B20), Cytomegaloviral diseases (B25.-), Aspergillosis (B44.-), Cryptococcosus (B45.-), and Zygomycosis (B46.-). Codes that fit into an HCC should be documented carefully with all required components of HCC documentation.

Complete the exercises in There's a Code for That 14.6 to practice assigning diagnostic codes for laboratory procedures.

14.6 Diagnostic coding for laboratory procedures

Read the following documentation of the laboratory or pathology service and identify the correct diagnosis code(s).

1. A 23-year-old female with high-risk heterosexual behavior and exposure to HIV presents for HIV counseling and screening.

    ICD-10-CM codes: _____ , _____ ,

    _____ , _____

2. Lab culture positive for MRSA.

    ICD-10-CM code: _____

3. Group A streptococcal septicemia.

    ICD-10-CM code: _____

4. HIV positive patient is seen for management of AIDS-related Kaposi's sarcoma of the right lung.

    ICD-10-CM codes: _____ , _____

5. Influenza due to novel influenza A/H5N1 virus.

    ICD-10-CM code: _____

6. Chlamydial epididymitis.

    ICD-10-CM code: _____

7. Salmonella gastroenteritis.

    ICD-10-CM code: _____

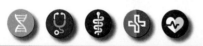

Putting It All Together: Coding for Laboratory and Pathology Services

Coding correctly for laboratory and pathology services requires an understanding of the various types of laboratory and pathology tests and the components of each test, as listed in the code descriptions.

Determination of the correct codes relies on the answers to the following questions.

- What type of laboratory or pathology procedure was performed?
    - For specific tests, what substance was tested?
    - For nonspecific tests, what type of specimen was tested?
    - What technique was used for the test?

- Was it qualitative or quantitative?

- How many tests were performed, and how many specimens were tested?

- How was the specimen collected?
    - Which facility collected the specimen? If it was the coder's facility, code for the collection technique (for example, venipuncture).

- - Did your facility test the specimen? If so, code for the laboratory procedure (for example, CBC).
  - - Did your facility both collect and test the specimen? If so, code for both the collection and the testing.
- Is there an infectious organism present in the specimen?
  - - If so, assign a diagnosis code to identify the infectious agent.
    - ◻ If the manifestation of the infection is known, use either a combination code to identify both the manifestation and etiology of the infection, or separate codes to identify each.
  - - If no, then code for the signs, symptoms, or abnormal finding code.

The following vignette demonstrates how to select the appropriate diagnosis and procedure codes. After reviewing the vignette, complete the following exercises in There's a Code for That 14.7 to practice coding for laboratory and pathology services.

Jessie has been working in healthcare billing and coding for a few years and most of her experience has been in primary care billing. She just moved to a new city and found a job as a coder for an independent laboratory clinic. The lab is large and employs numerous clinical and surgical pathologists, as well as several labs throughout the state that perform a wide range of tests. Jessie is studying some reference materials she bought in order to prepare for her new job at the independent lab. She is currently coding from the following surgical pathology report.

SURGICAL PATHOLOGY
Specimen: 0.5 cm polyp of the ascending colon 0.2 cm polyp in the sigmoid colon
Clinical History: Patient presents for a screening colonoscopy. Family history significant for maternal history of adenocarcinoma of colon.

Gross Examination:
A. Cassette A labeled "ascending colon" contains a polypoid piece of tan mucosal tissue measuring 0.5 cm.
B. Cassette B labeled "sigmoid colon" contains one piece of light tan mucosal tissue 0.2.

Microscopic Examination:
Supportive of sessile serrated adenomatous polyp with low-grade adenomatous dysplasia in the ascending colon and tubular adenoma of the sigmoid colon.

Jessie knows from the report that the service performed was a surgical pathology test. She asks herself: What did the doctor do? In this case, the pathologist examined two polyps that were located in the colon. These were two separate tissue samples, so there should be one code assigned for each pathological examination. She searches the lists of tissues within each surgical pathology code, and locates Polyp, colorectal, *in the list of tissues for Level IV Surgical pathology. She assigns the following code:*

- *88305, Level IV Surgical pathology, gross and microscopic*

Now that Jessie has her procedure code, she asks herself: Why did the doctor do it? She notes that the patient has a family history of colon cancer, which should be reported with the appropriate family history code (chapter 8). Also, in the microscopic examination section of the report, she notes that the doctor wrote that the findings were "supportive of sessile serrated adenomatous polyp with low-grade adenomatous dysplasia in the ascending colon and tubular adenoma of the sigmoid colon."

She searches for the term Polyp *in the ICD-10-CM Index, and the subterm* Adenomatous, *which refers her to see also Neoplasm, benign, by site. She then refers to the Neoplasm Table, and locates the* colon *entry, with the cross-reference to see also*

Neoplasm, intestine, large. *She refers to the entry* Intestine, intestinal, *and then the subterm* large *in the Table of Neoplasms. Here she finds multiple locations in the colon. The first polyp examined in the procedure was located in the ascending colon and was determined to be a sessile serrated adenomatous polyp (benign neoplasm of the ascending colon). She selects code D12.2. Now she locates the code for the second polyp, determined to be a tubular adenoma of the sigmoid colon (benign neoplasm of the sigmoid colon), so she selects code D12.5. She verifies each code in the Tabular List and reports the following diagnosis codes:*

- *D12.2, Benign neoplasm of the ascending colon*
- *D12.5, Benign neoplasm of the sigmoid colon*
- *Z80.0, Family history of malignant neoplasm of digestive organs*

She then rechecks the documentation to make sure she has coded everything for the encounter and reports the chosen codes.

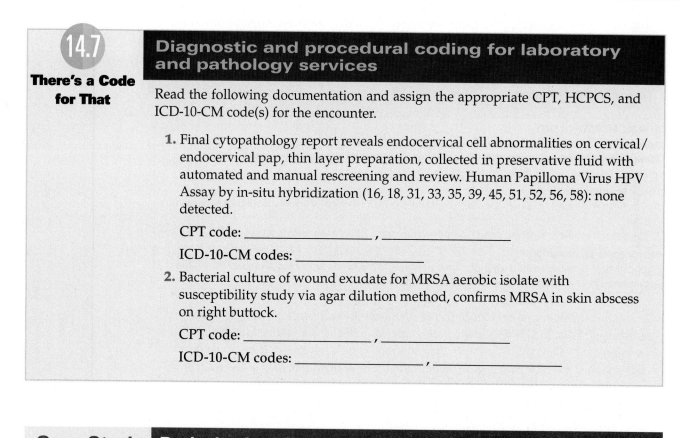

14.7 Diagnostic and procedural coding for laboratory and pathology services

There's a Code for That

Read the following documentation and assign the appropriate CPT, HCPCS, and ICD-10-CM code(s) for the encounter.

1. Final cytopathology report reveals endocervical cell abnormalities on cervical/endocervical pap, thin layer preparation, collected in preservative fluid with automated and manual rescreening and review. Human Papilloma Virus HPV Assay by in-situ hybridization (16, 18, 31, 33, 35, 39, 45, 51, 52, 56, 58): none detected.

   CPT code: _____ , _____

   ICD-10-CM codes: _____

2. Bacterial culture of wound exudate for MRSA aerobic isolate with susceptibility study via agar dilution method, confirms MRSA in skin abscess on right buttock.

   CPT code: _____ , _____

   ICD-10-CM codes: _____ , _____

Case Study Pathological Examination of Moles

PATIENT: Jacqueline K. Mossman

ORDERING PROVIDER: Susan Alameda, DO

SURGICAL PATHOLOGY: TISSUE BIOPSIES

Material submitted:
PART A: ANTERIOR LEFT ABDOMEN (Raised regular brown speckled lesion). Gross description: Received is a 0.8 x 0.7 x 0.4 cm gray-tan unoriented skin shave. The surgical margins are inked. It is trisected and submitted in one cassette.
PART B: LOWER RIGHT LUMBAR (Pedunculated flesh tone lesion). Gross description: Received is a 0.6 x 0.5 x 0.3 cm gray-tan unoriented popular skin shave. The surgical margins are inked. It is bisected and submitted in one cassette.
PART C: RIGHT CHEST (7 mm raised irregular border lesion). Gross description: Received is a 0.8 x 0.7 x 0.3 cm gray-tan unoriented segment of skin. The surgical margins are inked. It is trisected and submitted on one cassette.
PART D: LEFT UPPER BACK/SHOULDER (7 mm raised regular dark brown lesion). Gross description: Received is a 0.7 x 0.7 x 0.4 cm gray-tan unoriented popular segment of skin. The surgical margins are inked. It is trisected and submitted on one cassette.

Diagnosis: Microscopic examination of sample reveals the following:
PART A: ANTERIOR LEFT ABDOMEN
Intradermal melanocytic nevus, incompletely excised
PART B: LOWER RIGHT LUMBAR
Intradermal melanocytic nevus, incompletely excised
PART C: RIGHT CHEST
Intradermal melanocytic nevus, incompletely excised
PART D: LEFT UPPER BACK/SHOULDER
Intradermal melanocytic nevus, incompletely excised

SIGNED: Dr. Melissa Huffy, DO

Use the following steps to select the appropriate code(s) for the case study.

1. Read through the case study and answer the question: *What did the doctor do?* In the case study, identify the name of the laboratory procedure:

_____

_____

2. Now that you have identified the procedure, locate the code for the procedure in the CPT code book.

a. Search the Index for the procedure and search through the options.

b. In the listing of codes, check for any guidelines, important definitions, or parenthetical notes. Select the appropriate code and list it here.

_____

_____

c. Are there any modifiers that need to be added to identify any special circumstance surrounding the procedure(s)? If yes, refer to Appendix A of the CPT code book to assign all appropriate modifiers.

_____

_____

3. Now that the procedure(s) and modifier(s) have been identified, review the case study and answer the following question: *Why did the doctor do it?*

_____

_____

4. Now that you have identified the patient's diagnoses, search the ICD-10-CM code book for the correct codes for these conditions. Follow these steps for each of the diagnoses identified:

a. Search the Main Index for the name of each condition and search through any applicable subterms and cross-references to locate the appropriate code.

_____

_____

b. Verify the code in the Tabular List. Locate the code identified previously in the Tabular Listing of codes and refer to any applicable guidelines, notes, and symbols. Does the code selected correctly identify the patient's condition? If yes, list the code.

i. _____

_____

ii. _____

_____

5. Now that the procedure and diagnosis codes have been identified, list them on the CMS-1500 form.

21. DIAGNOSIS OR NATURE OF ILLNESS OR INJURY Relate A-L to service line below (24E)	ICD Ind.		
A.	B.	C.	D.
E.	F.	G.	H.
I.	J.	K.	L.

24. A. DATE(S) OF SERVICE From / To	B. PLACE OF	C.	D. PROCEDURES, SERVICES, OR SUPPLIES (Explain Unusual Circumstances)	E.
MM DD YY MM DD YY	SERVICE	EMG	CPT/HCPCS MODIFIER	DIAGNOSIS POINTER
1				
2				
3				
4				

End-of-Chapter Content

Instructions: Indicate whether the following statements are true or false (T or F). For false statements, rewrite the statement on the line below to make the statement true.

1. The patient must be present in order to run a laboratory test.

_____

_____

2. An independent laboratory is accredited to test and evaluate patient specimens free from a hospital or private practice.

_____

_____

3. Modifier -90 should be used when practicing pass-through billing.

_____

_____

4. Outside lab charges should be placed in box 24.B of the CMS-1500 claim form.

_____

_____

5. In laboratory coding, the modifier for the professional component is -PC.

_____

_____

6. Laboratories are prohibited from billing for the collection of lab samples via venipuncture.

_____

_____

7. Code selection for many laboratory and pathology codes depends on the type of the specimen tested.

_____

_____

(Continued on next page)

(Continued)

8. A permanent block is embedded in ice so that it can be stored indefinitely.

_____

_____

9. The result of a quantitative examination is numerical.

_____

_____

10. A disease-oriented panel code may only be reported if more than half of the tests were performed.

_____

_____

Instructions: Choose the best answer.

1. What is the name of the billing practice in which a private practice bills for the laboratory service performed by an independent lab, and the lab bills the provider directly for the service?
   a. Fee for service billing
   b. Capitation
   c. Independent laboratory billing
   d. Pass-through billing

2. Which place of service code should be reported for services that were performed at an independent laboratory?
   a. 11
   b. 81
   c. 23
   d. 42

3. The professional component of a laboratory procedure is performed by which of the following?
   a. A pathologist
   b. A primary care provider
   c. A registered nurse
   d. An anesthesiologist

4. A doctor's office collected a patient blood sample and sent it to a lab for analysis. For what will the lab bill?
   a. The collection of the blood sample
   b. The testing of the blood
   c. Both the collection and the testing of the blood
   d. The lab handling fee only

5. A doctor's office collected a patient blood sample and sent it to a lab for analysis. For what will the doctor's office bill?
   a. The collection of the blood sample
   b. The testing of the blood
   c. Both the collection and the testing of the blood
   d. The lab handling fee only

6. A lab collected a blood sample from a patient and then tested the blood. For what will the lab bill?
   a. The collection and testing of the blood sample
   b. The preparation and testing of the blood
   c. The collection and preparation of the blood sample
   d. The lab handling fee only

7. An examination of the physical characteristics of a specimen is known as which of the following?

a. Gross examination
b. Microscopic examination
c. Smear
d. This type of exam is not included in lab services

8. The result from a specific test determined that it was contaminated with a substance. Which kind of test was it?

a. Qualitative
b. Quantitative
c. A drug assay
d. A chemistry study

9. Which type of laboratory procedure evaluates chromosomes for abnormalities?

a. Cytogenetic studies
b. Cytopathology
c. Genomic sequencing procedures
d. Multianalyte assays

10. Which code should be reported for a qualitative drug test read by instrument-assisted optical observation?

a. 80305
b. 80306
c. 80307
d. 80375

11. Which of the following codes is a nonspecific test?

a. 81005
b. 80047
c. 82085
d. 82017

12. Which code should be reported for a gross and microscopic full body autopsy, including the brain and spinal cord?

a. 88007
b. 88028
c. 88027
d. 88005

Instructions: Answer the following questions with the appropriate code(s) and modifier(s).

1. Therapeutic drug monitoring for quinidine in patient with atrial fibrillation.

CPT code: _____

ICD-10-CM code: _____

2. Hematocrit blood count for patient with polycythemia vera.

CPT code: _____

ICD-10-CM code: _____

3. Diphtheria immunoassay performed on patient recently returned from traveling abroad in Russia confirms presence of diphtheria.

CPT code: _____

ICD-10-CM code: _____

References

American Medical Association (AMA). 2019. *CPT 2020 Professional Edition.* Chicago: AMA.

Centers for Disease Control and Prevention (CDC). 2010 (March). "H1N1 influenza virus.jpg." Digital Image. Wikimedia Commons. https://commons.wikimedia .org/wiki/File:H1N1_influenza_virus.jpg.

Centers for Medicare and Medicaid Services (CMS). 2019a. CMS 1500. https://www.cms.gov/Medicare/CMS -Forms/CMS-Forms/CMS-Forms-Items/CMS1188854 .html.

Centers for Medicare and Medicaid Services (CMS). 2019b. ICD-10-CM Official Guidelines for Coding and Reporting FY 2020. https://www.cms.gov/Medicare /Coding/ICD10/Downloads/2020-Coding-Guidelines .pdf.

Hu, K., J. Johnson, L. Florens, M. Fraunholz, S. Suravajjala, C. DiLullo, J. Yates, D.S. Roos, and J.M. Murray. 2006 (February). "Toxoplasma gondii.jpg." Digital Image. Wikimedia Commons. https://commons.wikimedia .org/wiki/File:Toxoplasma_gondii.jpg.

National Institute of Allergy and Infectious Diseases (NIAID). 2009 (November). "Group A Streptococcus Bacteria on Human Neutrophil (8517040030).jpg." Digital Image. Wikimedia Commons. https://commons .wikimedia.org/wiki/File:Group_A_Streptococcus _Bacteria_on_Human_Neutrophil_(8517040030).jpg.

Rosen, Y. 2011 (January). "Candidiasis (5494228342).jpg." Digital Image. Wikimedia Commons. https://commons .wikimedia.org/wiki/File:Candidiasis_(5494228352).jpg.

Tan, S. Y. and Y. Tatsumara. 2015 (October). George Papanicolaou (1883–1962): Discoverer of the Pap smear. *Singapore Med J* 56(10): 586–587. https://www.ncbi.nlm.nih.gov/pmc/articles/PMC4613936/.

Uthman, E. 2006 (July). "ThinprepHPV.jpg." Digital Image. Wikimedia Commons. https://commons.wikimedia.org/wiki/File:ThinPrep_Pap_smear_HPV.jpeg.

Resources

American Society of Cytopathology (ASC). n.d. About Us. https://cytopathology.org/page/AboutUs.

Cancer.Net. 2018 (March). After a Biopsy: Making the Diagnosis. http://www.cancer.net/navigating-cancer-care/diagnosing-cancer/reports-and-results/after-biopsy-making-diagnosis.

Centers for Medicare and Medicaid Services (CMS). 2018 (October). CLIA Program and Medicare Laboratory Services. https://www.cms.gov/Outreach-and-Education/Medicare-Learning-Network-MLN/MLNProducts/downloads/CLIABrochure.pdf.

Johns Hopkins Medicine. 2019. Surgical Pathology. https://www.hopkinsmedicine.org/health/treatment-tests-and-therapies/surgical-pathology.

Rolls, G. 2019. An Introduction to Specimen Preparation. https://www.leicabiosystems.com/knowledge-pathway/an-introduction-to-specimen-preparation/.

CHAPTER

Orthopedic Services

Learning Objectives

- Understand the basics of billing and coding for orthopedic services
- Examine procedural codes and guidelines for orthopedic services
- Examine diagnosis coding and medical necessity for orthopedic services
- Determine and apply ICD-10-CM, CPT, and HCPCS codes to orthopedic services

Key Terms

Amputation
Arthritis
Arthrocentesis
Arthrodesis
Arthropathy
Arthroplasty
Arthroscopy
Bursa
Chiropractor
Closed fracture
Closed treatment
Comminuted fracture
Compound fracture
Compression fracture
Displaced fracture
Fascia
Gout
Greenstick fracture
Gustilo-Anderson classification

Impacted fracture
Internal fixation device
Interspace
Kyphosis
Malunion
Manipulation
Monoarthritis
Musculoskeletal system
Non-displaced fracture
Nonunion
Oblique fracture
Open fracture
Open treatment
Orthopedic services
Orthopedist
Osteoarthritis
Osteopathic manipulative treatment (OMT)
Pathological fracture

Percutaneous
Percutaneous skeletal fixation
Physeal fracture
Polyarthritis
Salter-Harris classification
Scoliosis
Segment
Segmental fracture
Skeletal traction
Skin traction
Spiral fracture
Sprain
Strain
Tophus
Torus fracture
Traction
Transverse fracture
Traumatic fracture

Orthopedic services focus on the management and treatment of conditions affecting the musculoskeletal system—such as fractures, arthritis, joint sprains and strains, and osteoporosis. Orthopedics services may be performed in the outpatient office, inpatient hospital, or outpatient hospital setting, depending on the type of service and the needs of the patient. This chapter discusses the various orthopedic service procedure codes, as well as the diagnosis codes that identify the medical necessity for orthopedic services.

Orthopedics Basics

The **musculoskeletal system** is the body system comprised of all the bones, joints, muscles, cartilage, tendons, and ligaments in the human body. Comprehensively, the musculoskeletal system works to provide movement, stability, and form to the human body. Due to the wide range of elements (like muscles, bones, or joints) in the musculoskeletal system, and the various medical conditions that can affect these elements, there are numerous subspecialties within the field of orthopedics. Orthopedic specialists focus on certain types of injuries, medical conditions, or treatment strategies.

Figure 15.1. Human skeleton

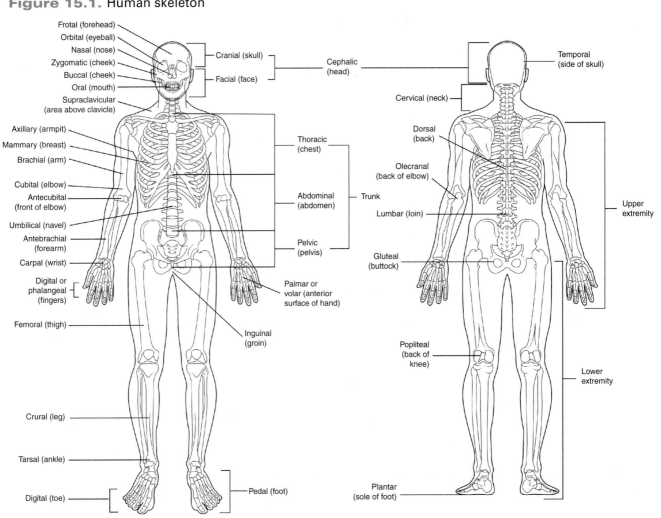

Source: ©AHIMA.

At the fundamental level, an **orthopedist** is a medical doctor who specializes in correcting congenital or acquired abnormalities of the bones and musculoskeletal system through the use of casting, bracing, and surgical techniques. Orthopedic specialists (also spelled orthopaedic specialists) may also treat and manage musculoskeletal conditions with physical therapy or medication. They may be referred to as "orthopods," or the specialty referred to as "ortho."

Additional orthopedic specialties include surgical specialties that focus solely on performing invasive surgeries on the orthopedic system, much like general surgeons focus on performing surgeries on the organ systems of the human body. Orthopedic surgeons are further subspecialized in specific musculoskeletal areas on which they focus, including the hand, knee, foot and ankle, hip, shoulder, and spine. Sports medicine is another type of orthopedic specialty that focuses on sports injuries and the treatment (both surgical and nonsurgical) and management of injuries sustained in sports, with the goal of returning the patient to his or her pre-injury health.

Billing and coding of orthopedic services is similar to any other type of outpatient coding and uses procedure codes from across several different sections of the Current Procedural Terminology (CPT) code book, including evaluation and management (E/M) codes and codes from the Surgery and Radiology sections. Diagnosis codes used for orthopedic coding are found throughout the ICD-10-CM code book but are mainly located in chapter 13 (Diseases of the Musculoskeletal System and Connective Tissue) and chapter 19 (Injury, Poisoning, and Certain Other Consequences of External Causes).

Being an effective orthopedic coder requires strict attention to detail and a solid knowledge of the musculoskeletal system including muscles, bones, tendons, and ligaments that hold the body together. See figure 15.1 for the front and back view of the human skeleton.

Procedural Coding for Orthopedic Services

Without a doubt, the most important subsection of procedure codes for orthopedics is the Musculoskeletal System subsection of the Surgery section. This subsection includes codes for fracture repair and manipulation, application of casts and strapping, joint injections, excision of both soft tissue and bone tumors, amputations, and arthrodesis. These procedures are stretched across the entirety of the Musculoskeletal System subsection, so coders will find themselves going back and forth in it. Therefore, it is important to review the table of contents at the beginning of the Musculoskeletal subsection closely before coding for these procedures.

The following sections of this chapter discuss the format of the Musculoskeletal System subsection of the CPT code book, followed by specific procedures that include excision of bone and soft tissue tumors, arthrocentesis and joint injections, fracture repairs, application of casts and strapping, hip and knee replacements, arthrodesis and spinal instrumentation, amputations, and arthroscopies.

Format of the Musculoskeletal System Subsection

The Musculoskeletal System subsection is one of the most extensive subsections in the CPT code book because it contains codes for procedures for the largest list of body elements—including all of the bones, muscles, ligaments, and tendons in the human body. Because of its complexity, coders should first review and understand the format of the subsection and how codes are organized in it.

Figure 15.2. Organization of the Musculoskeletal System subsection

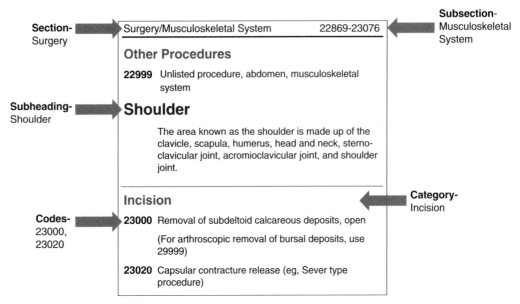

Source: AMA 2019, 145.

This subsection is organized by body area first, with categories for specific types of procedures in each subheading (see figure 15.2). The only exceptions to this are the subheadings General, Application of Casts and Strapping, and Endoscopy/ Arthroscopy. These subheadings are organized according to the type of procedure performed rather than by body area.

Within each subheading are the categories of procedures for that body area: Incision; Excision; Manipulation; Introduction or Removal; Repair, Revision, and/ or Reconstruction; Fracture and/or Dislocation; Arthrodesis; Amputation; and Other Procedures. These categories are located throughout the Surgery section of the CPT code book, as discussed in chapter 11 (Surgical Services). However, several categories of procedure are specific to the Musculoskeletal System subsection, all of which are discussed in this chapter, including:

- *Fracture and/or Dislocation.* This category of codes identifies services performed specifically to treat fractures and dislocations.
- *Arthrodesis.* This category of codes includes all arthrodesis procedures only, performed to surgically fix a joint (that is, immobilize the joint by fusing the bones together).
- *Amputation.* This category identifies procedures performed to amputate parts of the body.

The categories of codes listed beneath each subheading are specific to the procedures that can be performed on that particular body area. It is important to pay attention to these headings to ensure you are in the correct section of codes for the procedure being reported.

Musculoskeletal system coding requires an understanding of the basic components of these procedure categories, and the ability to apply this understanding to codes across all body areas. For example, once a coder knows the basics of coding for arthrodesis procedure, he or she can apply that knowledge to code for arthrodesis of the shoulder, humerus, or forearm or wrist.

Because the Musculoskeletal System subsection is so extensive, it is easy to get lost while searching for the correct code. Refer to the table of contents at the beginning of the subsection to find your bearings and get back on track. First, find the body area on which the procedure was performed, and then locate the category for the type of procedure performed. Go to this section of codes and search through the code descriptions until you find a code that looks correct. Then refer to the Index of the CPT code book to see if the code you chose in the Tabular List matches the one in the Index. If they match, you have the right code. If not, find where you went wrong by referring to the Index and starting the process over again.

Key to Success

Learning how to maneuver through the CPT code book takes time, and every time you get lost, you learn something new—so do not get frustrated! It is all part of the learning process.

Remember that the Musculoskeletal System subsection is part of the Surgery section, so surgical guidelines and terminology are used in these codes. For a refresher on surgery basics, refer to chapter 11. Common procedural terminology in this section include the following:

- *-ectomy*, which means surgical removal; as in ostectomy, the removal of bone
- *-desis*, which means surgical fixation; as in arthrodesis, the surgical fixation of a joint
- *-tomy*, which means surgical incision; as in arthrotomy, the surgical incision of a joint
- *-plasty*, which means surgical repair; as in arthroplasty, the surgical repair of a joint
- *-centesis*, which means surgical puncture (often used to remove fluid); as in arthrocentesis, the removal of fluid from a joint
- *-scopy*, which means an examination or procedure performed with a scope; as in arthroscopy, an endoscopic-assisted procedure of the joint

Key to Success

Notice how the subheadings of the Musculoskeletal System subsection are generally organized from the head to the toes. This is common across the various subsections in the Surgery section of the CPT code book, as the subheadings are organized from one area of the body to another. As you become more accustomed to the ways in which the Surgery subsections are organized, you may find that locating codes is easier by accessing the specific body area or organ system, and then the type of procedure in each body area or organ system.

Excision of Bone and Soft Tissue Tumors

The Musculoskeletal System subsection of the CPT code book contains a number of codes for excision of both soft tissue and bone tumors, which may be either benign or malignant. It is highly probable that some of these excisions would be performed by a specialist other than an orthopedic surgeon, such as a general surgeon. However, they are discussed here in full as they are best understood in relation to each other.

Codes for the excision of tumors are based on the depth of the excision. Excisions of the skin, such as excisions of benign or malignant lesions, are identified with codes from the Integumentary System subsection. The excision codes found in the Musculoskeletal System subsection are for excisions of deeper structures, such as the subcutaneous tissues, fascial and subfascial tissues, connective tissues within the subcutaneous and subfascial layers, and bone. Fascia is a sheet of connective tissue that encloses the structures of the muscles and other internal organs, and subfascial tissues are underneath the fascial layers, such as muscles. Procedures that are not performed on these deep structures are listed in the Integumentary System subsection of the CPT code book.

The tissue excised within any layer is only identified by the area from which it was excised and does not depend on the type of tissue excised (that is, benign, malignant, or metastatic). Code selection is usually based on the location and size of the tumor, with the exception of bone tumors. All of the following procedures listed are found in the Musculoskeletal System subsection of codes.

- *Excision of subcutaneous soft tissue tumors.* These tumors are below the skin but above the deep fascia. Code selection depends on the location and size of the tumor, which is based on the greatest diameter of the tumor plus the excisional margins (similar to the margins included in the excision of skin lesions). For example, code 22902, Excision, tumor, soft tissue of abdominal wall, subcutaneous; less than 3 cm.

- *Excision of fascial or subfascial soft tissue tumors.* These tumors are located in or below the deep fascia but do not involve the bone. Code selection depends on the location and the size of the tumor, including excisional margins. For example, code 23076, Excision, tumor, soft tissue of shoulder area, subfascial (eg, intramuscular); less than 5 cm.

- *Radical resection of soft connective tissue tumors.* These tumors have wide margins, and removal may involve excision of more than one layer of tissue. Code selection is based on the location and size of the tumor, including excisional margins. For example, 21557, Radical resection of tumor (eg, sarcoma), soft tissue of neck or anterior thorax; less than 5 cm.

- *Excision of bone tumors.* These tumors are in the bone and are typically very aggressive benign or malignant tumors. Code selection is based on the location of the tumor, and not on the size or type of tumor removed. For example, code 27360, Partial excision (craterization, saucerization, or diaphysectomy) bone, femur, proximal tibia and/or fibula (eg, osteomyelitis or bone abscess).

To search for codes for the excision of tumors, look up the term *Excision* in the CPT Index, and refer to the subterm *Tumor*. There is a large section of subterms identifying codes for the removal of tumors. Many of these are within the code range 20100 through 29999, so they are musculoskeletal system procedure codes.

An alternate method of locating the code for the tumor is to search for the subterm for the body area, organ, or bone under the Excision heading. For example, to find the code for the excision of a tumor in the humerus, search for the subterm *Humerus* under *Excision,* and note the subterm for *Tumor* and the possible codes: 23150, 23155, 23156, 24110, 24115, 24116.

Complete the exercises in There's a Code for That 15.1 to practice assigning codes for excisions of bone and soft tissue.

Excisions of bone and soft tissue

15.1

There's a Code for That

Read the following documentation of the procedure test and identify the correct excision of bone or soft tissue procedure code(s).

1. Excision of osteoid osteoma on right femur, with allograft and placement of internal fixation device.

   CPT code: _____ , _____

2. Excision of 7 cm subfascial tumor of the left upper arm.

   CPT code: _____

3. Radical resection of squamous cell carcinoma of the mandible, with bone graft.

   CPT code: _____ , _____

4. Excision of 2 cm benign soft tissue tumor in right foot.

   CPT code: _____

Arthrocentesis and Joint Injections

Arthrocentesis is the aspiration of a joint, a process that involves inserting a hollow needle into a joint or bursa to allow for the removal of fluid. **Bursae** are fluid-filled sacs beneath the skin that lie between tendons, ligaments, and bones, and assist in lubricating the joints. Inflammation of the bursa creates a condition called bursitis, which causes swelling and pain, and requires aspiration. Joint aspirations are performed for either diagnostic purposes—to obtain a sample of fluid from the joint and test it, or for therapeutic purposes by removing inflammation of effusive fluid from a joint, thereby relieving pressure and pain.

CPT codes for arthrocentesis (20600–20611) are based on the joint or bursa being aspirated, and whether or not imaging guidance is used during the procedure. For example, code 20610, Arthrocentesis, aspiration, and/or injection, major joint or bursa (eg, shoulder, hip, knee, subacromial bursa); without ultrasound guidance, identifies the joint involved (*major joint or bursa*) and if imaging guidance was used (*without ultrasound guidance*). The parenthetical guidance below the codes identifies which codes should be used when imaging guidance is performed with the arthrocentesis. See figure 15.3 for an illustration of the bursae located at the knee joint.

Codes 20600 through 20611 include both the aspiration of fluid from a joint (arthrocentesis) and injection of a joint. As discussed in chapter 12 (Anesthesia and Pain Management), joint injections are performed for treatment of pain, to reduce inflammation, and to help lubricate the joint. Depending on the orthopedic specialty and the resources available to the provider, some orthopedic providers may choose to perform anesthetic joint injections for pain management. This procedure may also sometimes be performed by the patient's primary care physician. Refer to figure 15.4 for an illustration of arthrocentesis techniques.

Key to Success

Do not confuse arthro*centesis* with arthro*desis*. Arthro*centesis* is the aspiration of a joint, while arthro*desis* is the surgical fixation of a joint—two completely different procedures. Arthrodesis procedures are discussed in depth later in this chapter.

Figure 15.3. Bursae of the knee joint

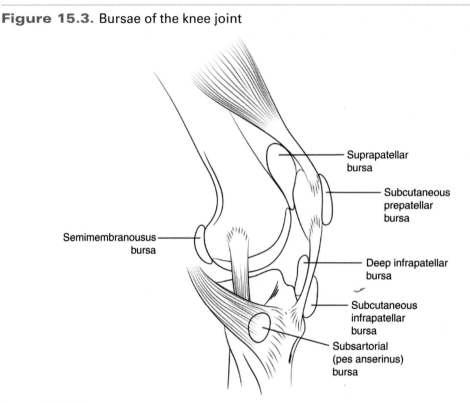

Source: © AHIMA.

Complete the exercises in There's a Code for That 15.2 to practice reporting arthrocentesis procedures.

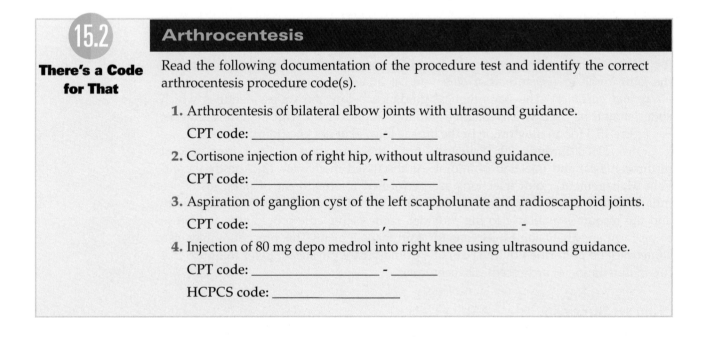

15.2

There's a Code for That

Arthrocentesis

Read the following documentation of the procedure test and identify the correct arthrocentesis procedure code(s).

1. Arthrocentesis of bilateral elbow joints with ultrasound guidance.

   CPT code: _____ - _____

2. Cortisone injection of right hip, without ultrasound guidance.

   CPT code: _____ - _____

3. Aspiration of ganglion cyst of the left scapholunate and radioscaphoid joints.

   CPT code: _____ , _____ - _____

4. Injection of 80 mg depo medrol into right knee using ultrasound guidance.

   CPT code: _____ - _____

   HCPCS code: _____

Fracture Repair

Fracture repair and treatment is a large part of the job of an orthopedist. Coding correctly for fracture repair requires knowing the types of fractures as well as the various

Figure 15.4. Arthrocentesis techniques

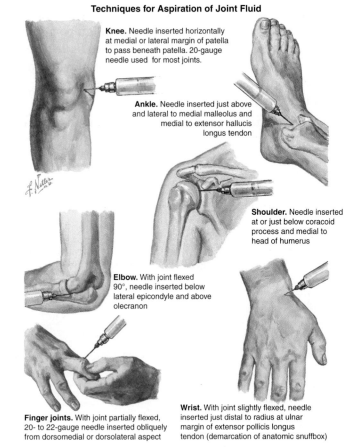

Techniques for Aspiration of Joint Fluid

Knee. Needle inserted horizontally at medial or lateral margin of patella to pass beneath patella. 20-gauge needle used for most joints.

Ankle. Needle inserted just above and lateral to medial malleolus and medial to extensor hallucis longus tendon

Shoulder. Needle inserted at or just below coracoid process and medial to head of humerus

Elbow. With joint flexed 90°, needle inserted below lateral epicondyle and above olecranon

Finger joints. With joint partially flexed, 20- to 22-gauge needle inserted obliquely from dorsomedial or dorsolateral aspect

Wrist. With joint slightly flexed, needle inserted just distal to radius at ulnar margin of extensor pollicis longus tendon (demarcation of anatomic snuffbox)

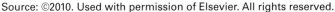

treatment techniques; this includes the differences in closed, open, and percutaneous skeletal fixation treatments for fractures.

Closed Treatment of Fractures

Closed treatment of a fracture means that the site of the fracture is not surgically opened to perform the repair. Closed treatment of a fracture is performed via four different methods.

- *With manipulation.* **Manipulation** is the attempt to return a fractured bone to its original location with manually applied forces. In other words, manipulation is the orthopedist applying forces by hand to put the bones back in place—pushing, pulling, or twisting the bone until it is in the original location (see figure 15.5).

- *Without manipulation.* Some fractures are not displaced and do not require manipulation in order to return the bone into its original location. If the fracture care did not include manipulation of the bone(s) back into place, select the "without manipulation" option, if available.

- *With traction.* **Traction** is the use of mechanical devices and mechanisms to straighten bones or relieve pressure. This is different than manipulation, which is done with hands. Traction employs the use of straps and sometimes mechanical devices such as pins or screws. There are two types of traction—skin traction and skeletal traction.

- **Skin traction** uses straps, ropes, pulleys, and weights that are applied externally to the skin to slowly stretch and realign bones into place until they can be set and casted until fully healed (see figure 15.6).
- **Skeletal traction** is an invasive form of traction in which a screw, pin, or wire is inserted into the bone, after which weights, ropes, and pulleys are used to pull the bone into the correct position.

- *Without traction.* Some fractures do not require traction in order to set the bone(s) back into place. If traction was not used, select the "without traction" option, if available.

Figure 15.5. Closed treatment of Colles' fracture with manipulation

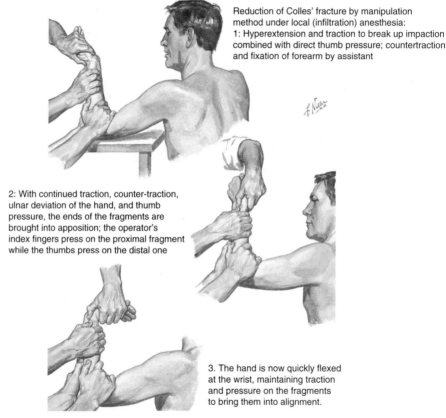

Reduction of Colles' fracture by manipulation method under local (infiltration) anesthesia:
1: Hyperextension and traction to break up impaction combined with direct thumb pressure; countertraction and fixation of forearm by assistant

2: With continued traction, counter-traction, ulnar deviation of the hand, and thumb pressure, the ends of the fragments are brought into apposition; the operator's index fingers press on the proximal fragment while the thumbs press on the distal one

3. The hand is now quickly flexed at the wrist, maintaining traction and pressure on the fragments to bring them into alignment.

A Colles' fracture is a common fracture of the distal radius, which often occurs as a result of a fall onto an outstretched hand.
Source: ©2017. Used with permission of Elsevier. All rights reserved.

Open Treatment of Fractures

Open treatment of a fracture means that the fracture site has been surgically opened to see the fracture area or apply internal fixation devices. An **internal fixation device** is a device inserted into or across a bone or set of bones to fix it into place. Internal fixation devices are typically made from stainless steel or titanium and include plates, screws, nails, rods, wires, or pins (see figure 15.7).

Figure 15.6. Closed treatment of Colles' fracture with skin traction

Closed Reduction and Plaster Cast Immobilization of Colles Fracture

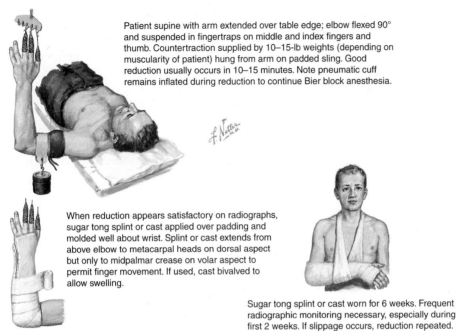

Patient supine with arm extended over table edge; elbow flexed 90° and suspended in fingertraps on middle and index fingers and thumb. Countertraction supplied by 10–15-lb weights (depending on muscularity of patient) hung from arm on padded sling. Good reduction usually occurs in 10–15 minutes. Note pneumatic cuff remains inflated during reduction to continue Bier block anesthesia.

When reduction appears satisfactory on radiographs, sugar tong splint or cast applied over padding and molded well about wrist. Splint or cast extends from above elbow to metacarpal heads on dorsal aspect but only to midpalmar crease on volar aspect to permit finger movement. If used, cast bivalved to allow swelling.

Sugar tong splint or cast worn for 6 weeks. Frequent radiographic monitoring necessary, especially during first 2 weeks. If slippage occurs, reduction repeated.

Figure 15.7. Internal fixation device of the humerus

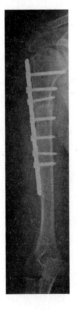

Source: Dilmen 2011.

Key to Success

Do not confuse open and closed *treatment* of fractures with open and closed *fractures*. Open and closed treatments refer to the way in which a fracture is treated.

> Open and closed fractures refer to the clinical presentation of the fracture (fracture types are discussed later in the chapter).

Percutaneous Skeletal Fixation

Percutaneous skeletal fixation is a type of fracture treatment in which fixation devices are placed across the fracture site, usually under x-ray imaging guidance. This procedure is neither closed (because it does break the skin), nor open (as the fracture site or bone is not surgically opened for visualization), but rather percutaneous. **Percutaneous** means through the skin, which is achieved by creating a small puncture in the skin and then inserting the medical instrument into the body through this opening. Percutaneous fixation is a process in which the fixation device(s) are placed through the skin and into the bone (see figure 15.8).

Figure 15.8. Percutaneous skeletal fixation of the tibia

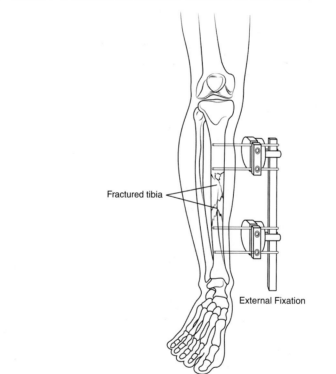

Fractured tibia

External Fixation

Source: ©AHIMA.

Coding for Fracture Repair

Codes for fracture repair depend on the bone and the type of fracture treatment, including the elements discussed previously—with or without manipulation, open versus closed treatment, with or without traction (identify the type of traction, such as skin traction or skeletal traction), or with percutaneous skeletal fixation. To find the code for the fracture repair, search for the term *Fracture* in the CPT Index, followed by the subterm for the fracture site, and then the treatment type. If percutaneous skeletal fixation is provided along with fracture repair, report one code for each repair performed. For example, code 27517, Closed treatment of distal femoral epiphyseal separation; with manipulation, with or without skin or skeletal traction, identifies whether it was open or closed (*closed*), the manipulation (*with manipulation*), and traction (*with or without skin or skeletal traction*). Note that skeletal fixation is not described in this code, which means that it was not an element in this fracture repair. See figure 15.9 for the elements of fracture repair coding. When coding for fracture repair procedures, it is important to keep these questions in mind to ensure that you capture all of the components of the repair procedure.

Fracture repair codes carry a global period, typically 90 days, which includes all services related to treating the fracture until it is healed. This includes removal of any traction or percutaneous skeletal fixation devices, routine follow-up care, and casting and strapping for immobilization of the bones at the fracture site. When a patient presents to the orthopedist for typical routine fracture follow-up care within the global period, the orthopedist reports code 99024, Postoperative follow-up visit, normally included in the surgical package, to indicate that an evaluation and management service was performed during a postoperative period for a reason(s) related to the original procedure, to identify that the patient received care within the postoperative period.

Figure 15.9. Fracture repair coding

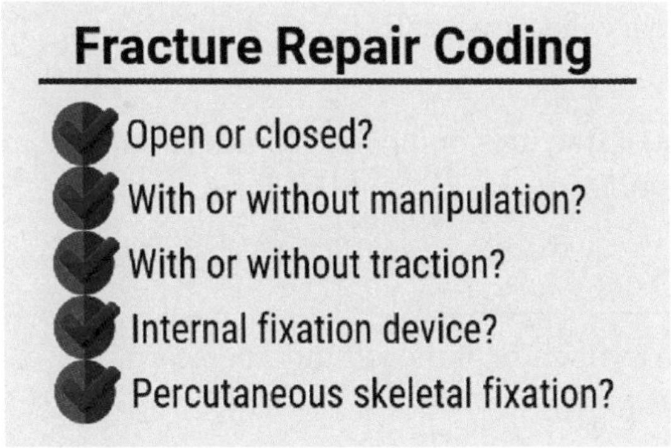

Application of Casts and Strapping

Typically, after a fracture is repaired or set, a cast or strapping is applied to the body to immobilize the fracture site during the healing process. This initial application of casts or strapping is included in the global service for the fracture repair procedure and is not billed separately.

Codes for the application of casts or strapping (29000–29799) should be reported only in the following instances:

- When the cast or application procedure is a replacement procedure performed during or after the period of follow-up care (either within the global period or after the global period has ended). For example, if the initial cast was removed to gain access to the fracture site or due to damage, the reapplication of the cast or strapping may be coded.

- When the application of cast or strapping is an initial service performed on a fracture, dislocation, or other injury that requires stabilization. For example, if the initial fracture did not require manipulation, fixation, or surgical repair, and only a cast was applied for mobilization, then only the cast or strapping code would be reported, not the fracture repair code. (AMA 2019)

Codes for the application of casts and strapping include removal of the cast or strapping, so when a patient presents for the removal of a cast it is not billable as a separate service.

Code selection depends on the site of the application of cast or strapping, and the type of cast or strapping used. When a separate brace, splint, or other permanent supply item is used, report the supply with the appropriate HCPCS code (as discussed in chapter 6 [Supplies and Services]), such as HCPCS code A4580, Cast supplies (e.g., plaster), or A4590, Special casting material (e.g., fiberglass).

Complete the exercises in There's a Code for That 15.3 to practice reporting procedure codes for fracture repair, casts, and strapping procedures.

15.3

There's a Code for That

Fracture repair, casts, and strapping

Read the following documentation of the procedure test and identify the correct fracture repair, cast, and/or strapping procedure code(s).

1. Closed repair of right humeral fracture with manipulation and skeletal traction.

   CPT code: _____ - _____

2. Open treatment of fracture of displaced intraarticular calcaneous with internal fixation and primary iliac autograft.

   CPT code: _____

3. Closed treatment of fractures of the first, second, and third metacarpal bones, with manipulation.

   CPT code: _____ , _____ - _____ ,

   _____ - _____

4. Closed reduction of fracture of the left fifth metacarpal base, with manipulation and percutaneous pinning.

   CPT code: _____ , _____

5. Established patient with distal fracture of the left radius and ulna present for x-ray and evaluation of healing. She is one-month status post initial treatment, which involved a closed treatment of the fracture with skin traction and manipulation, and the insertion of pins. Complete x-ray of the left wrist completed today reveals a normally healing bone. Pins are stable and in original location. Fracture is re-casted with short-arm cast for immobility and patient is advised to return to office in two weeks for follow-up x-ray and evaluation.

   CPT code: _____ , _____

Hip and Knee Replacements

Hip and knee replacements are commonly performed by orthopedic hip or knee surgeons. Known as **arthroplasty** procedures (surgical repair of a joint), they replace the joint with a prosthetic device, with the goal of returning the joint to its previous functionality.

Coding for hip replacements depends on whether the replacement was a hemiarthroplasty (partial replacement), coded with 27125, Hemiarthroplasty, hip, partial (eg, femoral stem prosthesis, bipolar arthroplasty), or if the procedure was a total hip replacement. A total hip replacement is coded with 27130, Arthroplasty, acetabular and proximal femoral prosthetic replacement (total hip arthroplasty), with or without autograft or allograft. Additional codes (27132–27138) identify revision of previous hip replacement components and conversion from hip surgery to total hip arthroplasty. Hip prosthesis revisions are commonly performed to repair a hip prosthesis that has become damaged due to infection or due to regular wear and tear of the joint. See figure 15.10 for basic anatomy of the hip joint.

Codes for knee replacements, such as 27445, Arthroplasty, knee, hinge prosthesis (eg, Walldius type), and knee prosthesis revisions, such as 27486, Revision of total knee arthroplasty, with or without allograft; 1 component, are dependent on the components included in the procedure. For example: 27446, Arthroplasty, knee, condyle and plateau; *medial OR lateral compartment*, and 27447, Arthroplasty, knee, condyle and plateau; *medial AND lateral compartments with or without patella resurfacing (total knee arthroplasty)*, both describe different components included in the knee arthroplasty procedure. See figure 15.11 for an illustration of a total knee arthroplasty.

Figure 15.10. Basic anatomy of the hip joint

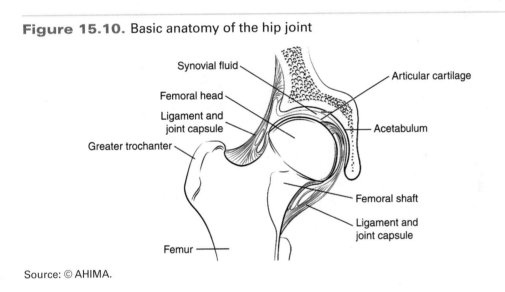

Source: © AHIMA.

Figure 15.11. Total knee arthroplasty

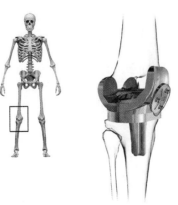

Source: BruceBlaus 2015.

Arthrodesis, Spinal Instrumentation, and Additional Spinal Procedures

Arthrodesis is the surgical fixation of a joint, performed to treat deformities of the bones and pain and may be performed throughout the body (see figure 15.12 for an image of arthrodesis of the spine). Codes for arthrodesis are based on the joint(s) involved, extent of the procedure, type of internal fixation (if applicable), and whether or not any grafts were used during the procedure. For example, an arthrodesis of the wrist could be reported with code 25820, Arthrodesis, wrist; limited, without bone graft (eg, intercarpal or radiocarpal).

Arthrodesis of the spine is by far the most complex area for coding arthrodesis procedures. Arthrodesis of the spine codes first rely in the approach: lateral extracavitary (22532–22534); anterior or anterolateral (22548–22586); or posterior, posterolateral, or lateral transverse process (22590–22634); or by spinal deformity, such as scoliosis or kyphosis (22800–22819). For example, 22800, Arthrodesis, posterior, for spinal deformity, with or without cast; up to 6 vertebral segments.

Figure 15.12. Arthrodesis of the spine

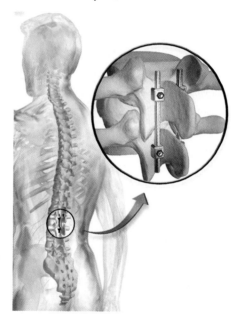

Source: BruceBlaus 2013.

The approach technique, such as anterior or posterior, should be listed in the procedural description, and the coder should be able to discern this information to select the correct code. After the approach technique or medical condition is identified, codes depend on the site of the fusion, and may identify either the general vertebral area (cervical, thoracic, lumbar), or specific vertebrae involved in the procedure. Types of fusion procedures include:

- Anterior Lumbar Interbody Fusion (ALIF)
- Posterior Lumber Interbody Fusion (PLIF)
- Transforaminal Lumbar Interbody Fusion (TLIF)
- Direct Lateral Interbody Fusion (DLIF)
- Anterior Cervical Discectomy with Interbody Fusion (ACDF) (Medtronic 2017)

Because a vertebra cannot be fused to itself, it must be fused to another vertebra, either above or below it. The space between the two vertebrae is referred to as an **interspace** and the two vertebrae with the space between it is referred to as a **segment**. The CPT code book uses these two terms interchangeably when reporting the codes for the spaces between vertebrae. Some codes for arthrodesis procedures refer to the spaces between as segments, such as code 22802, Arthrodesis, posterior, for spinal deformity, with or without cast; 7 to 12 vertebral segments, while others refer to the spaces between as interspaces, such as 22585, Arthrodesis, anterior interbody technique, including minimal discectomy to prepare interspace (other than for decompression); each additional interspace.

When reporting arthrodesis for more interspaces than listed in the primary code, the coder should report the add-on code according to the additional number of interspaces. For example, if a surgeon performed an arthrodesis of the thoracic vertebra T1 through T3, then this wound counts as two interspaces (or segments) (the space between T1 and T2, and T2 and T3), and would be coded as follows (count the spaces between the two vertebrae to total the correct number of procedures):

> 22532, Arthrodesis lateral extracavitary technique, including minimal discectomy to prepare interspace (other than for decompression); *thoracic*
>
> 22534, Arthrodesis lateral extracavitary technique, including minimal discectomy to prepare interspace (other than for decompression); thoracic or lumbar, *each additional vertebral segment*

Code 22532 identifies the surgical fixation of the first space (between T1 and T2), and code 22534 identifies the surgical fixation of the second space (between T2 and T3). 22534 is an add-on code, which is used to identify each additional vertebral segment involved in the procedure, and should be reported as many times as necessary to identify each segment. Count the spaces between the two vertebrae to count the correct number of procedures.

Note that the previous examples describe more than just arthrodesis. In this case, they include a minimal discectomy to prepare the interspace. This means that the surgeon removed a small amount of the intervertebral disc in-between the vertebrae in addition to the arthrodesis procedure. Pay careful attention to these code descriptions, as many include additional spinal procedures. On the other hand, add-on codes may be necessary to identify all of the components that were included within the procedure.

If spinal instrumentation was used, an appropriate add-on code may be necessary to identify the placement of the instrumentation. In the previous example, if a non-segmental posterior instrumentation was placed in order to complete the arthrodesis procedure, then an add on code should be used to identify this instrumentation: 22840, Posterior non-segmental instrumentation (eg, Harrington rod technique, pedicle fixation across 1 interspace, atlantoaxial transarticular screw fixation, sublaminar wiring at C1, facet screw fixation) (List separately in addition to code for primary procedure).

If a graft was used, report the necessary add-on code to identify the type of graft, such as allograft or autograft, and whether the graft was morselized (small pieces of the graft material) or structural (a larger or structural piece of the graft material). For example, if the arthrodesis listed in the previous example (22532, 22534) was performed with a morselized autograft, then the following add-on code would be used to identify the graft: 20930, Allograft, morselized, or placement of osteopromotive material, for spine surgery only (List separately in addition to code for primary procedure).

Key to Success

Note that there are many CPT guidelines and parenthetical notes in the codes for spinal surgeries. Pay close attention to this guidance, as it will help you select the correct code(s) as well as to tell you when an additional code may be necessary to fully report all components of the procedure.

Additional spinal procedures may be performed to treat vertebral conditions such as herniated or compressed discs, or fractured, compressed, or weakened vertebra. These additional procedures include corpectomy to remove the vertebral body, laminectomy to remove the lamina of the vertebra, facetectomy to remove a facet joint from a vertebra, foraminotomy to remove pressure on compressed nerves within the spinal column, and kyphoplasty and vertebroplasty to treat a spinal compression fracture. See figure 15.13 for a diagram of vertebral anatomy

Figure 15.13. Vertebral anatomy

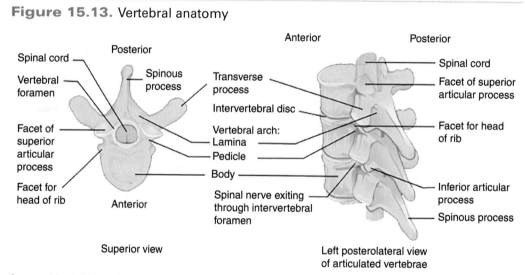

Source: March i Nogué 2015.

Amputation

An **amputation** is the complete removal of a body part, performed to remove dead, diseased, or damaged tissue, leaving only healthy and functional tissue behind. Depending on the site and cause of the amputation, it may be necessary to perform multiple amputations at the same site in staged procedures, moving from distal toward more proximal areas. Codes for amputations are based on the site of the amputation, any additional procedures, and whether the procedure is an initial (first) or a re-amputation (a subsequent amputation at the same body site, at a higher—more proximal—level).

To find the code for an amputation, search for the term *Amputation* in the CPT Index, and then the subterm for the area that was amputated. For example, the code for a single toe amputation would be 28810, Amputation, metatarsal, with toe, single.

Arthroscopy

An **arthroscopy** is an endoscopically assisted procedure of a joint. Arthroscopies are less invasive than open surgeries and are used to perform repairs of a joint without open surgery (see figure 15.14). Codes for arthroscopies are initially based on the joint involved, and then whether the procedure was diagnostic (with or without biopsy) or surgical. Codes for surgical arthroscopies are based on the type of surgery performed during the procedure. For example, see code 29866, Arthroscopy, knee surgical; osteochondral autograft(s) (eg, mosaicplasty) (includes harvesting of the autograft[s]).

Figure 15.14. Arthroscopic surgery of the patella

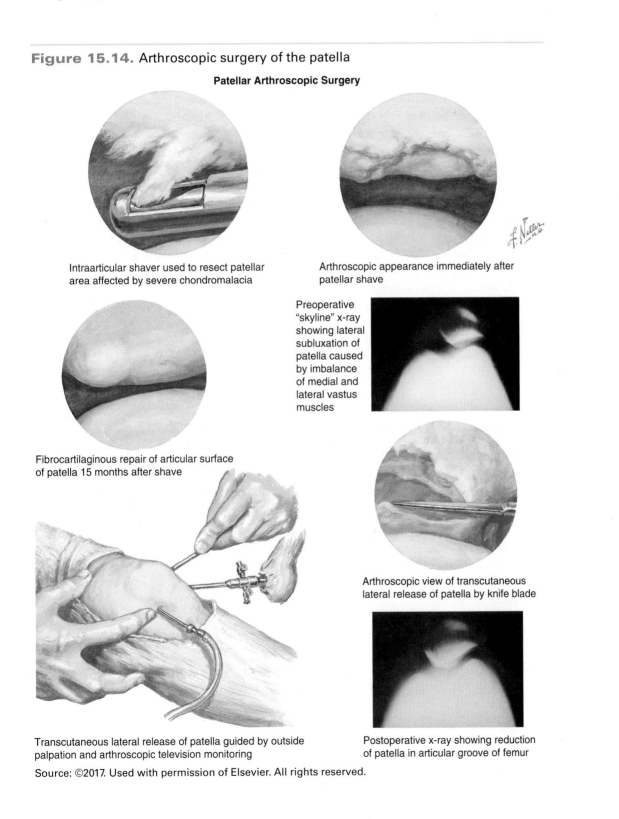

Patellar Arthroscopic Surgery

Intraarticular shaver used to resect patellar area affected by severe chondromalacia

Arthroscopic appearance immediately after patellar shave

Fibrocartilaginous repair of articular surface of patella 15 months after shave

Preoperative "skyline" x-ray showing lateral subluxation of patella caused by imbalance of medial and lateral vastus muscles

Arthroscopic view of transcutaneous lateral release of patella by knife blade

Transcutaneous lateral release of patella guided by outside palpation and arthroscopic television monitoring

Postoperative x-ray showing reduction of patella in articular groove of femur

Chiropractic and Osteopathic Procedures

Outside of the strict realm of orthopedics is a related specialty, chiropractics. A **chiropractor** is a practitioner of manual spinal manipulation therapy through spinal subluxation techniques. Spinal manipulation involves placing pressure on the vertebrae and applying stretching and twisting to realign the vertebrae. A chiropractor is not a medical doctor but holds a special license as required by state law to practice chiropractics. Codes for Chiropractic Manipulative Treatment are found in the CPT code book under code range 98940 to 98943 and depend the area being manipulated and how many spinal regions were involved, if necessary. For example, spinal manipulation of two spinal regions would be reported with code 98940, Chiropractic manipulative treatment (CMT); spinal, 1-2 regions.

Osteopathic procedures are similar to chiropractic procedures, although they are aimed at all areas of the body, including the muscles, underlying fascia, and joints. **Osteopathic manipulative treatments (OMT)** involve the application of pressure, stretching, and resistance to body structures to relieve pain and improve range of motion. OMT is performed by a Doctor of Osteopathy (DO), who is a trained as a medical doctor but receives extra training in osteopathy. Codes for Osteopathic Manipulative Treatments are found in the CPT code book in code range 98925 through 98929. Code selection depends on the amount of body areas involved in the treatment. For example, OMT of the skull for migraines would be reported with code 98925, Osteopathic manipulative treatment (OMT); 1-2 body regions involved.

Although codes exist for both of these therapies, a patient's insurance coverage may or may not actually cover the services included in these codes. Chiropractic medicine may be considered an alternative medical treatment, and as such may be excluded from coverage.

Complete the exercises in There's a Code for That 15.4 to practice reporting codes for orthopedic procedures.

15.4

There's a Code for That

Orthopedic procedures

Read the following documentation of the procedure test and identify the procedure code(s).

1. Arthrodesis of T9 through T12, posterior approach.

   CPT code: _____ , _____ × _____

2. Arthroscopic rotator cuff repair with partial acromioplasty, distal clavicle resection, and biceps tenodesis. (Hint: All these procedures were performed arthroscopically.)

   CPT code: _____ , _____ - _____ ,

   _____ - _____ , _____

3. OMT provided to patient with fibromyositis in the following areas: cranial manipulation, right and left shoulders, and acromioclavicular joints bilaterally (three body regions total).

   CPT code: _____

   ICD-10-CM code: _____

4. ALIF with anterior instrumentation, L1 through L3. Synthetic cage with anterior instrumentation placed at each interspace with structural allograft used for L1-L2 interspace.

   CPT codes: _____ , _____ , _____ ,

   _____

5. Total bilateral hip arthroplasty for patient with bilateral osteoarthritis of the hips.

   CPT code: _____ - _____

   ICD-10-CM code: _____

Diagnostic Coding for Orthopedic Services

Diagnosis coding for orthopedic services requires an in-depth knowledge of two chapters in the ICD-10-CM code book—chapter 13 (Diseases of the Musculoskeletal System and Connective Tissue) and chapter 19 (Injury, Poisoning, and Certain Other Consequences of External Causes). Chapter 13 includes the myriad medical conditions that affect the musculoskeletal system, such as arthritis and osteoarthritis, gout, acquired joint disorders, joint pain and effusion, connective tissue disorders, spinal and vertebral conditions, and soft tissue disorders. Chapter 19 includes the numerous injuries to the musculoskeletal system, like fractures, sprains, and strains. Additional codes used by orthopedists may include those for congenital anomalies, nervous system disorders, and codes to identify underlying and comorbid conditions.

Coding for orthopedic diagnoses requires strict attention to detail, especially when it comes to fracture coding because fracture diagnosis codes are by far the most extensive set of diagnosis codes in the ICD-10-CM code book. Many codes require the following:

- *The specific identification of the site involved, including laterality.* Remember that if a condition presents bilaterally but no bilateral code exists, assign one code for each side (right and left).
- *Type of encounter.* The type of encounter is especially complicated for fracture codes, which can have up to 16 different encounter types.
- *External causes of injury.* If the patient has suffered any type of injury, the external cause codes for the injury need to be reported in addition to the primary code for the injury. (Refer to chapter 4 for instructions on how to use the Index to External Causes and chapter 10 for discussion of coding for external causes).

The following sections discuss diagnostic coding for fractures, arthropathies, spinal and vertebral conditions, sprains and strains, congenital and acquired deformities, and amputations.

Coding for Fractures

Fracture coding is detailed and includes many different components of the condition. When a patient has multiple fractures, sequence the worst or most severe fracture first. Code selection for fractures depends on the fracture type, fracture pattern, displacement of the bone, location of the fracture, the episode of care and healing status, and the external causes of the injury.

Key to Success

Remember, "worst comes first" when sequencing any injuries. This includes fractures. When multiple fractures are present, sequence the most severe fracture before less severe fractures.

Fracture Type

There are two main divisions in fracture coding—traumatic or pathological fractures. Pathological fractures are reported with codes from chapter 13 of the ICD-10-CM code book (the musculoskeletal system chapter), whereas traumatic fractures are reported with codes from chapter 19 of the ICD-10-CM code book (the injury chapter). See figure 15.15 for the OGCR related to coding for pathological fractures.

- A **pathological fracture** is one that occurs in a diseased bone, such as osteoporosis or neoplastic disease (bone cancer). These conditions are reported with codes from category M84, Disorder of continuity of bone. Pathological fractures that occur with osteoporosis are reported with the appropriate code from category M80, Osteoporosis with current pathological fracture. Stress or fatigue fractures are also classified within category M84.
- A **traumatic fracture** is one that occurs as a result of some sort of traumatic injury. These conditions are reported with codes from chapter 19, to report the injury (fracture). Traumatic fractures can be either open or closed.
    - A **closed fracture** is one in which the broken bone does not penetrate the skin. If a fracture is not documented as either open or closed, report the code for the closed fracture (closed fracture is the default code).
    - An **open fracture**, also known as a **compound fracture**, is one in which the bone penetrates the skin. Open fractures can range from minor to complex, with vascular involvement. To classify the severity of an open fracture, the ICD-10-CM code book employs the Gustilo-Anderson classification system, discussed as follows.

Key to Success

If the documentation of the fracture does not specify if the fracture is open or closed, report the code for a closed fracture. If the fracture is not specified as open, report the closed fracture code.

Key to Success

When coding for fractures, it is important to distinguish between traumatic and non-traumatic fractures first, as each will lead you in two completely different directions. When searching for fractures in the Index of the ICD-10-CM code book, look up the term *Fracture*. (This is a large section.) The very first section of fracture entries is *Fracture, nontraumatic*, and then *Fracture, pathological*. All subsequent subterms are for pathological or non-traumatic fractures. Next, scan for the next fracture heading for *Fracture, traumatic*; all of these subterms are for traumatic fractures. If necessary, draw a line in the Index of your ICD-10-CM code book to make this difference more obvious.

Figure 15.15. OGCR I.C.13.c and d

> **13. Chapter 13: Diseases of the Musculoskeletal System and Connective Tissue (M00-M99)**
>
> **c. Coding of Pathologic Fractures**
>
> 7th character A is for use as long as the patient is receiving active treatment for the fracture. While the patient may be seen by a new or different provider over the course of treatment for a pathological fracture, assignment of the 7th character is based on whether the patient is undergoing active treatment and not whether the provider is seeing the patient for the first time.
>
> 7th character, D is to be used for encounters after the patient has completed active treatment for the fracture and is receiving routine care for the fracture during the healing or recovery phase. The other 7th characters, listed under each subcategory in the Tabular List, are to be used for subsequent encounters for routine care of fractures during the healing and recovery phase as well as treatment of problems associated with the healing, such as malunions, nonunions, and sequelae.
>
> Care for complications of surgical treatment for fracture repairs during the healing or recovery phase should be coded with the appropriate complication codes.
>
> *See Section I.C.19. Coding of traumatic fractures.*
>
> **d. Osteoporosis**
>
> Osteoporosis is a systemic condition, meaning that all bones of the musculoskeletal system are affected. Therefore, site is not a component of the codes under category M81, Osteoporosis without current pathological fracture. The site codes under category M80, Osteoporosis with current pathological fracture, identify the site of the fracture, not the osteoporosis.
>
> **1) Osteoporosis without pathological fracture**
>
> Category M81, Osteoporosis without current pathological fracture, is for use for patients with osteoporosis who do not currently have a pathologic fracture due to the osteoporosis, even if they have had a fracture in the past. For patients with a history of osteoporosis fractures, status code Z87.310, Personal history of (healed) osteoporosis fracture, should follow the code from M81.
>
> **2) Osteoporosis with current pathological fracture**
>
> Category M80, Osteoporosis with current pathological fracture, is for patients who have a current pathologic fracture at the time of an encounter. The codes under M80 identify the site of the fracture. A code from category M80, not a traumatic fracture code, should be used for any patient with known osteoporosis who suffers a fracture, even if the patient had a minor fall or trauma, if that fall or trauma would not usually break a normal, healthy bone.

Source: CMS 2019.

- ▫ *Gustilo-Anderson classification* is used to identify the type of open fracture, which is included as part of the code description for open fractures. The classification system is as follows (see figure 15.16):
  - ○ Type I. This is an open fracture with a clean wound less than 1 cm long.
  - ○ Type II. This is an open fracture with an open wound greater than 1 cm long, which does not have extensive soft tissue damage, flaps, or avulsions of tissue.
  - ○ Type IIIA. This is an open fracture with soft tissue coverage of the wound measuring more than 10 cm, with extensive soft tissue lacerations or flaps, or one due to high-energy trauma.
  - ○ Type IIIB. This is an open fracture with extensive soft tissue injury and bone exposure, usually highly contaminated with foreign material.
  - ○ Type IIIC. This is an open fracture that involves a large wound with arterial injury. (Kim 2012)

Figure 15.16. Gustilo-Anderson classification

Gustilo and Anderson classification of open fracture

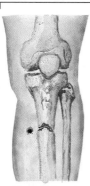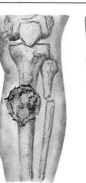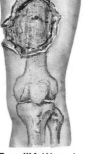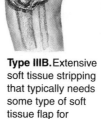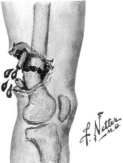

Type I. Wound <1 cm long

Type II. Wound 1 to 10 cm long but without significant soft tissue stripping, gross contamination, or high-energy fracture patterns

Type IIIA. Wound >10 cm long or lesser skin lesions with gross contamination and/or high-energy fracture patterns. Bone coverage adequate

Type IIIB. Extensive soft tissue stripping that typically needs some type of soft tissue flap for coverage

Type IIIC. Large wound with major arterial injury

Key to Success

Don't worry about being able to diagnose a specific type of open fracture according to the Gustilo classification type! This is something that the clinician must determine, not the coder. If the documentation of an open fracture is unclear or incomplete, query the physician to determine the type of fracture. This includes Gustilo classification as well as the type or site of fracture, as discussed in the following sections.

Fracture Pattern

The pattern of the fracture identifies the way in which the bone broke, which is an important consideration in the way the fracture is treated. The treatment performed for each of these fractures depends on the severity and location of the fracture. For example, a mild transverse fracture may be treated without manipulation and a simple cast, whereas a severe transverse fracture of a long bone of the upper extremity may require open treatment or skeletal fixation. The following fracture types impact code selection for certain bones, when applicable (see figure 15.17):

- **Greenstick fractures** occur when a bone bends and cracks on one side (similar to a green branch, which may bend and only break one side). This fracture type occurs most often in children, as their bones are less brittle and more flexible, which results in incomplete fractures.

- **Transverse fractures** travel horizontally across the bone.

- **Spiral fractures** spiral around and extend down the length of the bone.

- **Oblique fractures** travel diagonally across the bone.

- **Comminuted fractures** have more than two parts, usually with multiple broken pieces.

- **Segmental fractures** are made up of at least two fracture lines, which isolate a larger section of bone.

- **Torus fractures** occur in children, when only one part of the bone buckles. This is also referred to as an incomplete fracture.
- **Impacted fracture** are ones in which the ends of a bone are pushed into each other. This is also referred to as a buckle fracture.
- **Compression fractures** are found in the spine, and occur when one or more vertebrae collapse under their own pressure.

Displacement

Fractures are identified as either displaced or non-displaced. A **displaced fracture** is one in which the bone moves so the two ends of the bones are misaligned (see figure 15.18). A **non-displaced fracture** is one in which the bone itself is fractured, but the bone has not moved and is still properly aligned. If a fracture is not documented as

Figure 15.17. Fracture patterns

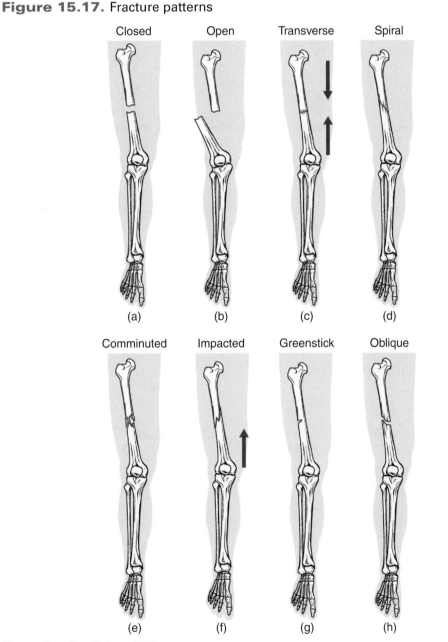

Source: OpenStax College 2013.

either displaced or non-displaced, report the code for the displaced fracture (displaced fracture is the default code).

Location

Fracture codes often identify the exact location of the fracture—both the involved in the fracture and the precise site of the fracture, such as the shaft, head, neck, distal, proximal, styloid process, epiphysis, and such. The laterality is also indicated as left or right. There are no bilateral fracture codes; if the condition presents bilaterally, assign one code for each side. **Physeal fractures**, fractures of the growth plate in long bones in

Figure 15.18. Types of fracture displacement

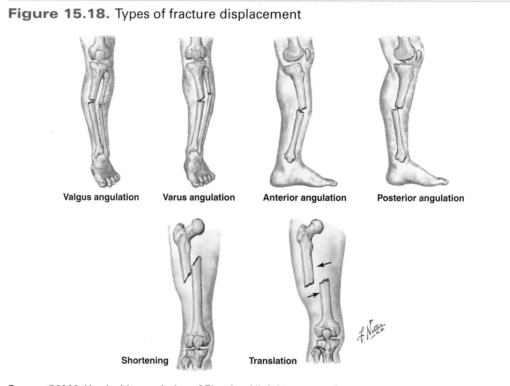

Valgus angulation   Varus angulation   Anterior angulation   Posterior angulation

Shortening   Translation

Figure 15.19. Salter-Harris classification

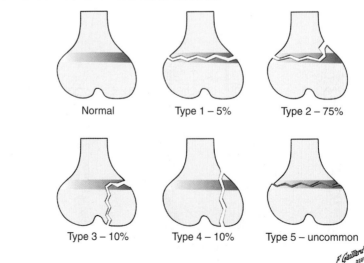

Normal   Type 1 – 5%   Type 2 – 75%

Type 3 – 10%   Type 4 – 10%   Type 5 – uncommon

Source: Gaillard 2012.

children, are identified using the **Salter-Harris classification** system (see figure 15.19). This classification identifies the type of physeal fracture, according to the following:

- Type I fractures pass all the way through the growth plate, completely missing the bone.
- Type II fractures pass through most of the growth plate and upward through the metaphysis of the bone.
- Type III fractures pass through the growth plate and down through the epiphysis.
- Type IV fractures pass through the entire growth plate, including the metaphysis and the epiphysis.
- Type V are a crushing type injury, which do not displace the growth plate but cause direct damage to it (Cepela 2016).

Figure 15.20 lists additional OGCR related to coding for traumatic fractures.

Figure 15.20. OGCR I.C.19.c.

---

c. Coding of Traumatic Fractures

The principles of multiple coding of injuries should be followed in coding fractures. Fractures of specified sites are coded individually by site in accordance with both the provisions within categories S02, S12, S22, S32, S42, S49, S52, S59, S62, S72, S79, S82, S89, S92 and the level of detail furnished by medical record content.

A fracture not indicated as open or closed should be coded to closed. A fracture not indicated whether displaced or not displaced should be coded to displaced.

More specific guidelines are as follows:

1) Initial vs. Subsequent Encounter for Fractures

Traumatic fractures are coded using the appropriate 7th character for initial encounter (A, B, C) for each encounter where the patient is receiving active treatment for the fracture. The appropriate 7th character for initial encounter should also be assigned for a patient who delayed seeking treatment for the fracture or nonunion.

Fractures are coded using the appropriate 7th character for subsequent care for encounters after the patient has completed active treatment of the fracture and is receiving routine care for the fracture during the healing or recovery phase.

Care for complications of surgical treatment for fracture repairs during the healing or recovery phase should be coded with the appropriate complication codes.

Care of complications of fractures, such as malunion and nonunion, should be reported with the appropriate 7th character for subsequent care with nonunion (K, M, N,) or subsequent care with malunion (P, Q, R).

Malunion/nonunion: The appropriate 7th character for initial encounter should also be assigned for a patient who delayed seeking treatment for the fracture or nonunion.

The open fracture designations in the assignment of the 7th character for fractures of the forearm, femur and lower leg, including ankle are based on the Gustilo open fracture classification. When the Gustilo classification type is not specified for an open fracture, the 7th character for open fracture type I or II should be assigned (B, E, H, M, Q).

A code from category M80, not a traumatic fracture code, should be used for any patient with known osteoporosis who suffers a fracture, even if the patient had a minor fall or trauma, if that fall or trauma would not usually break a normal, healthy bone.

See Section I.C.13. Osteoporosis.

The aftercare Z codes should not be used for aftercare for traumatic fractures. For aftercare of a traumatic fracture, assign the acute fracture code with the appropriate 7th character.

2) Multiple fractures sequencing

Multiple fractures are sequenced in accordance with the severity of the fracture.

3) Physeal fractures

For physeal fractures, assign only the code identifying the type of physeal fracture. Do not assign a separate code to identify the specific bone that is fractured.

Source: CMS 2019.

Episode of Care and Healing Status

Identifying the episode of care for fracture codes is complex, and for some fracture types there are as many as 16 different classifications (see figure 15.21 for a list of the 16 seventh-character encounter types). Follow these steps to identify the correct encounter of care:

- The episode of care should be identified as either initial, subsequent, or sequela.
- For open fracture, identify the Gustilo classification for the fracture, in terms of type I or II, or type IIIA, IIIB, or IIIC.
- For subsequent encounters, identify the healing status of the fracture, in terms of:
  - Routine healing
  - Delayed healing
  - **Nonunion** of fracture (when the bones have not fused back together)
  - **Malunion** of fracture (when the bones have fused back together in the wrong position)

Figure 15.21. Encounters of care for fracture codes*

The appropriate seventh character is to be added to all codes form category S52	
A	initial encounter for closed fracture
B	initial encounter for open fracture type I or II initial encounter for open fracture NOS
C	initial encounter for open fracture type IIIA, IIIB, or IIIC
D	subsequent encounter for closed fracture with routine healing
E	subsequent encounter for open fracture type I or II with routine healing
F	subsequent encounter for open fracture type IIIA, IIIB, or IIIC with routine healing
G	subsequent encounter for closed fracture with delayed healing
H	subsequent encounter for open fracture type I or II with delayed healing
J	subsequent encounter for open fracture type IIIA, IIIB, or IIIC with delayed healing
K	subsequent encounter for closed fracture with nonunion
M	subsequent encounter for open fracture type I or II with nonunion
N	subsequent encounter for open fracture type IIIA, IIIB, or IIIC with nonunion
P	subsequent encounter for closed fracture with malunion
Q	subsequent encounter for open fracture type I or II with malunion
R	subsequent encounter for open fracture type IIIA, IIIB, or IIIC with malunion
S	sequela

⇧ Encounter   ⇧ Open or closed fracture   ⇧ Gustilo classification   ⇧ Healing status

*Not all 16 episodes of care are options for all fracture codes.

External Causes of the Injury

Codes for the external cause of the injury identify the injury mechanism (how the patient was injured), place of occurrence when the injury happened, activity in which the patient was engaged when the injury occurred, and patient status at the time of injury.

Review figures 15.22 and 15.23, which illustrate the components of fracture codes and a decision process for fracture coding, then complete the exercises in There's a Code for That 15.5 to practice reporting fracture diagnosis codes.

Figure 15.22. Fracture code components

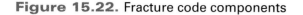

> **S52.342M, Displaced spiral fracture of shaft of radius, left arm, subsequent encounter for open fracture type I or II with nonunion**
>
> **Fracture type:** open
> **Gustilo classification:** type I or II
> **Pattern:** spiral
> **Displacement:** displaced
> **Location:** shaft of radius
> **Laterality:** left
> **Encounter:** subsequent
> **Healing status:** nonunion

Figure 15.23. Fracture coding

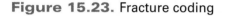

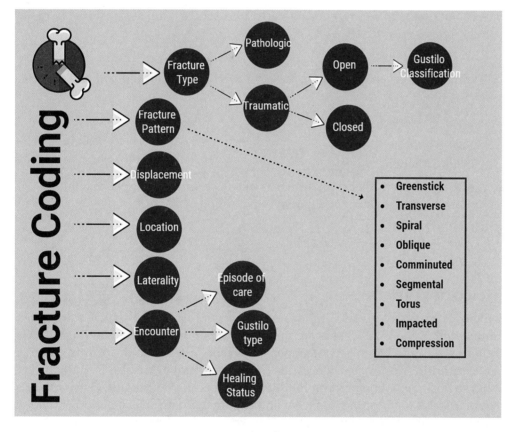

Fracture coding

15.5

Read the following documentation and assign the appropriate diagnosis code(s) for the fracture and any additional conditions.

There's a Code for That

1. A 27-year-old male presents for initial treatment of his closed trimalleolar fracture of the left ankle.

   ICD-10-CM code: _____

(Continued on next page)

15.5

Continued

2. A 27-year-old male presents for removal of cast and subsequent x-ray of his trimalleolar fracture of the left ankle. X-ray reveals nonunion of the fracture.

   ICD-10-CM code: _____

3. X-ray results reveal an open, type II, displaced compound comminuted fracture of the right radial shaft.

   ICD-10-CM code: _____

4. Frontal skull fracture with subsequent subdural hemorrhage.

   ICD-10-CM codes: _____ , _____

5. Sports-related injuries resulting in fractures of three right ribs, fractured right wrist, and contusion of right chest over rib fractures.

   ICD-10-CM codes: _____ , _____

6. A 60-year-old female presents with arthritis of the left hip as a residual of hip fracture five years ago.

   ICD-10-CM codes: _____ , _____

7. Traumatic lateral epicondyle fracture of the left elbow, subsequent encounter with routine healing.

   ICD-10-CM codes: _____

8. Stress fracture of right foot, subsequent encounter with delayed healing.

   ICD-10-CM codes: _____

9. Pathological fracture of right humerus due to secondary neoplasm of bone. Secondary encounter for evaluation of nonunion of fracture.

   ICD-10-CM codes: _____ , _____

HCC Arthropathies

An **arthropathy** is any disease of the joints, the most common of which is **arthritis**, an inflammation of the joints. There are numerous types of arthritis including infectious arthritis (as a response to an infectious organism), rheumatoid arthritis (RA), and juvenile arthritis. Most forms of arthritis (not osteoarthritis) are also included in HCC coding, so documentation of these conditions is especially important. **Osteoarthritis** is a type of arthritis that results from wear and tear on the joints over a period of time, and often occurs in the hips and knees.

Coding for arthritis thus requires identification of the type of arthritis. It further requires identification of the location and the specific joint(s) involved. Arthritis that occurs in many different areas is referred to as **polyarthritis** or polyosteoarthritis, while arthritis in a localized joint is referred to as **monoarthritis**. It is also important to identify any underlying or comorbid conditions. For example, M08.261, Juvenile rheumatoid arthritis with systemic onset, right knee, identifies the type of arthritis (*juvenile RA with systemic onset*), the location, and joint involved (*right knee*).

Spinal and Vertebral Conditions

Many of the spinal and vertebral conditions discussed in chapter 12 (Anesthesia and Pain Management) may also be treated by orthopedic spinal surgeons for definitive repair and treatment. These conditions include intervertebral disc disorders, spinal stenosis, neck and back pain, and radiculopathy. Remember that most of these conditions require specific identification on where exactly the condition occurs: occipito-atlanto-axial, cervical, cervicothoracic, thoracic, thoracolumbar, lumbar, lumbosacral, sacral, and sacrococcygeal sites.

Sprains and Strains

Sprains and strains are common joint injuries, especially for patients involved in sports, and are usually managed by sports medicine providers. Though sprain and strain sound alike, do not get them confused—they are two separate conditions and are coded separately. A **sprain** is the stretching or tearing of a ligament (see figure 15.24). A **strain** is an injury to a muscle or tendon, which ranges from a simple stretching of the muscle or tendon to complete tear of the muscle and tendon (see figure 15.25).

Figure 15.24. Sprain

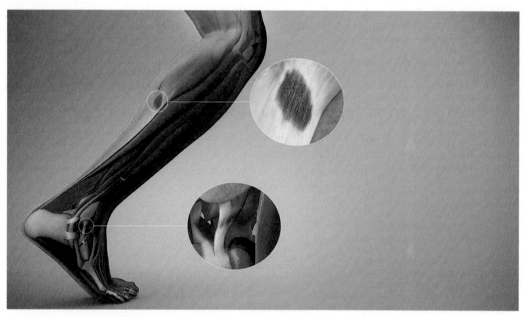

A sprain stretches the ligaments in the ankle and lower leg.
Source: Scientificanimations.com 2016.

Codes for sprains and strains identify the specific joint involved and the ligament, tendon, or muscle, if known. Furthermore, since these are all classified as injury codes, they all require the identification of the episode of care for the encounter. To look up the code for a sprain, search for the main term *Sprain* in the ICD-10-CM Index, and then search for the specific area of sprain. For example: S93.411A, Sprain of calcaneofibular ligament of right ankle, initial encounter. To search for a strain in the Index of the ICD-10-CM code book, search for either the main term *Strain*, or if the strain is of a muscle, search for the main term *Injury*, followed by *muscle*, then search for the specific muscle strained. For example: S76.311A, Strain of muscle, fascia and tendon of the posterior muscle group at thigh level, right thigh, initial encounter.

Figure 15.25. Strain

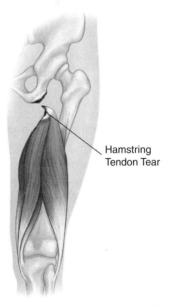

Hamstring
Tendon Tear

A severe hamstring strain in which the tendon has been torn from the bone.
Source: Reproduced with permission from *OrthoInfo*.© American Academy of Orthopaedic Surgeons (AAOS) 2015. http://orthoinfo.aaos.org.

Congenital and Acquired Deformities

Both congenital and acquired deformities are treated by orthopedists and orthopedic surgeons to correct and return the body area to its original function, improve function, or to reduce pain. Congenital deformities are ones present at birth, whereas acquired conditions develop over a period of time or later in life because of a traumatic event or disease state.

Scoliosis, a condition in which the spine curves sideways (see figure 15.26), and **kyphosis**, a condition in which the back rounds forward, are two examples of musculoskeletal deformities that can be either congenital or acquired. When looking up a code for a musculoskeletal deformity, search for the specific term for the type of deformity, such as *Scoliosis*, and then either *acquired, congenital,* or the specified type of the deformity. Congenital disorders are all coded from chapter 17 (Congenital Malformations, Deformations and Chromosomal Abnormalities) of the ICD-10-CM code book.

Amputation

When coding for an amputation, search for the term *Amputation* in the ICD-10-CM Index, and then locate the code for the site of the amputation. Codes for amputations of the extremities may also identify the level of amputation, such as amputation of the lower leg (S88), which can be reported as at the knee level (S88.0-) or at level between knee and ankle (S88.1-). They further identify the amputation as either complete, in that the entire extremity has been amputated, or if the patient has suffered only a partial amputation of the extremity (in which some of the soft tissue, vascular structures, or bone remains).

Figure 15.26. Scoliosis

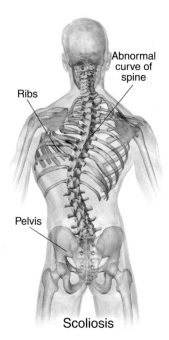

Scoliosis

Source: Blausen.com staff 2013.

If the documentation does not identify the amputation as either partial or complete, code it as a complete amputation. Because an amputation is a life-long medical condition that may require healthcare services for the rest of the patient's life, diagnosis codes for amputations do impact HCC coding and thus require complete documentation and careful code selection.

Orthopedic Aftercare

Aftercare is the healthcare provided to patients after the healing phase of an injury or illness has completed. Orthopedic aftercare is the care provided to patients that have sustained fractures, joint replacements, or other orthopedic services. These aftercare encounters are reported with E/M codes to identify the encounter with the patient; and medical necessity for the services is identified with the appropriate code from category Z47, Orthopedic aftercare. These aftercare services include:

- Z47.1, Aftercare following joint replacement surgery
- Z47.2, Encounter for removal of internal fixation device
- Z47.31, Aftercare following explantation of shoulder joint prosthesis
- Z47.32, Aftercare following explantation of hip joint prosthesis
- Z47.33, Aftercare following explantation of knee joint prosthesis
- Z47.81, Encounter for orthopedic aftercare following surgical amputation
- Z47.82, Encounter for orthopedic aftercare following scoliosis surgery
- Z47.89, Encounter for other orthopedic aftercare

These aftercare codes should not be used to identify care for an acute injury, but they may be used with additional codes to describe the patient's condition. For example, if a patient received a right hip joint prosthesis two months ago, and presents to his or her orthopod's office for an aftercare appointment and complains of difficulty walking, then the coder would assign the Z code for the aftercare (Z47.1, Aftercare following joint replacement surgery), and the code for difficulty walking (R26.2, Difficulty in walking, not elsewhere classified). If a problem was found with the prosthesis itself, then a code would be assigned to identify the specific mechanical problem with the device. For example, if the pain was found to be due to an inflammatory reaction to the hip joint prosthesis, then the coder should assign code T84.51XA, Infection and inflammatory reaction due to internal right hip prosthesis, initial encounter. See figure

Figure 15.27. OGCR I.C.21.c.7 Aftercare

7. Aftercare

Aftercare visit codes cover situations when the initial treatment of a disease has been performed and the patient requires continued care during the healing or recovery phase, or for the long-term consequences of the disease. The aftercare Z code should not be used if treatment is directed at a current, acute disease. The diagnosis code is to be used in these cases. Exceptions to this rule are codes Z51.0, Encounter for antineoplastic radiation therapy, and codes from subcategory Z51.1, Encounter for antineoplastic chemotherapy and immunotherapy. These codes are to be first-listed, followed by the diagnosis code when a patient's encounter is solely to receive radiation therapy, chemotherapy, or immunotherapy for the treatment of a neoplasm. If the reason for the encounter is more than one type of antineoplastic therapy, code Z51.0 and a code from subcategory Z51.1 may be assigned together, in which case one of these codes would be reported as a secondary diagnosis.

The aftercare Z codes should also not be used for aftercare for injuries. For aftercare of an injury, assign the acute injury code with the appropriate 7th character (for subsequent encounter).

The aftercare codes are generally first-listed to explain the specific reason for the encounter. An aftercare code may be used as an additional code when some type of aftercare is provided in addition to the reason for admission and no diagnosis code is applicable. An example of this would be the closure of a colostomy during an encounter for treatment of another condition.

Aftercare codes should be used in conjunction with other aftercare codes or diagnosis codes to provide better detail on the specifics of an aftercare encounter visit, unless otherwise directed by the classification. Should a patient receive multiple types of antineoplastic therapy during the same encounter, code Z51.0, Encounter for antineoplastic radiation therapy, and codes from subcategory Z51.1, Encounter for antineoplastic chemotherapy and immunotherapy, may be used together on a record. The sequencing of multiple aftercare codes depends on the circumstances of the encounter.

Certain aftercare Z code categories need a secondary diagnosis code to describe the resolving condition or sequelae. For others, the condition is included in the code title.

Additional Z code aftercare category terms include fitting and adjustment, and attention to artificial openings.

Status Z codes may be used with aftercare Z codes to indicate the nature of the aftercare. For example code Z95.1, Presence of aortocoronary bypass graft, may be used with code Z48.812, Encounter for surgical aftercare following surgery on the circulatory system, to indicate the surgery for which the aftercare is being performed. A status code should not be used when the aftercare code indicates the type of status, such as using Z43.0, Encounter for attention to tracheostomy, with Z93.0, Tracheostomy status.

The aftercare Z category/codes:

Z42	Encounter for plastic and reconstructive surgery following medical procedure or healed injury
Z43	Encounter for attention to artificial openings
Z44	Encounter for fitting and adjustment of external prosthetic device
Z45	Encounter for adjustment and management of implanted device
Z46	Encounter for fitting and adjustment of other devices
Z47	Orthopedic aftercare
Z48	Encounter for other postprocedural aftercare
Z49	Encounter for care involving renal dialysis
Z51	Encounter for other aftercare and medical care

15.27 for additional ICD-10-CM OGCR related to aftercare codes in general and figure 15.28 for OGCR related to complications of medical devices.

Figure 15.28. OGCR I.C.19.g.2 Pain due to medical devices

> **2. Pain due to medical devices**
>
> Pain associated with devices, implants or grafts left in a surgical site (for example painful hip prosthesis) is assigned to the appropriate code(s) found in Chapter 19, Injury, poisoning, and certain other consequences of external causes. Specific codes for pain due to medical devices are found in the T code section of the ICD-10-CM. Use additional code(s) from category G89 to identify acute or chronic pain due to presence of the device, implant or graft (G89.18 or G89.28).

Pay close attention to the instructions in Tabular List for this range of codes to ensure that all codes are reported. For example, under code Z47.81, Encounter for orthopedic aftercare following surgical amputation, there is a note to use an additional code to identify the limb that was amputated.

Gout

Gout, a type of arthritis, is a painful condition that results from a buildup of uric acid in the bloodstream, which forms needle-like crystals, causing swelling, redness, heat, and stiffness in the joints. Often gout first attacks the big toe, but may eventually travel to other joints in the body, including the fingers, wrists, elbows, knees, ankles, and heels (Medline Plus 2019).

Many of the ICD-10-CM codes for gout require six to seven characters, and identify the acuity of the condition, underlying disease or causative agent, specific joint involved, laterality of the condition, and whether the condition presents with or without tophus, or tophi (plural). A tophus is a lump or nodule under the skin that is composed of the uric acid buildup. For example, code M1A.10X1, Lead-induced chronic gout, unspecified site, with tophus (tophi), identifies the gout acuity (*chronic*), the underlying cause (*lead-induced*), the site (*unspecified*), and with or without tophus (*with tophus*).

Complete the exercises in There's a Code for That 15.6. to practice reporting diagnosis codes for orthopedic conditions.

Orthopedic diagnosis coding

15.6

There's a Code for That

Read the following documentation and assign the appropriate diagnosis code(s) for the patient's condition(s).

1. A 54-year-old male presents with instability of the right knee due to old complex tear of lateral meniscus of the right side.

   ICD-10-CM code: _____ , _____

2. A 25-year-old athlete presents with peripheral tear of the medial meniscus of the left knee. She was seen at urgent care last night after sustaining the injury.

   ICD-10-CM code: _____

3. Strain of right Achilles tendon, initial encounter.

   ICD-10-CM code: _____

(Continued on next page)

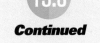

Continued

4. Left ACL sprain, initial encounter.

   ICD-10-CM code: _____

5. Chronic gout due to renal impairment, right hand, without tophus (tophi).

   ICD-10-CM code: _____

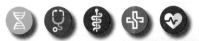

Putting It All Together: Coding for Orthopedic Services

Coding correctly for orthopedic services requires an in-depth understanding of the Musculoskeletal System subsection of the CPT code book, as well as the ability to code for E/M and Radiology procedures, when necessary.

Determination of the correct codes relies on the answers to the following questions.

- What type of orthopedic procedure was performed?
  - Fracture repair, excision of tumor, arthrodesis, arthrocentesis, and so forth.
  - What technique was used for the procedure? What components were included? Were any additional procedures performed? Check for all applicable add-on codes to fully report all components of the procedure, if necessary.

- Are there any applicable modifiers for the procedure?
  - Remember to add modifiers for bilateral procedures, distinct procedural services, repeat services, and multiple procedures.

- Is there a definitive diagnosis for the procedure? If so, then code for the definitive diagnosis. If not, then code for the signs and symptoms, such as joint pain.

The following vignette demonstrates how to select the appropriate diagnosis and procedure codes. After reviewing the vignette, complete the exercises in There's a Code for That 15.7 to practice coding for orthopedic services.

It is Towana's first day on the job in the orthopedics office, and her office manager has given her a handful of easy coding cases to work on while she is still in training. She is coding the following: Two-view x-ray of the fingers of the left hand reveal closed displaced fracture of medial phalanx of left middle finger. Closed reduction with manipulation of the phalangeal shaft of the middle phalanx with application of static finger splint.

She asks herself: What did the doctor do? In this case, the doctor performed an x-ray of the fingers, then reduced the fracture with manipulation, and applied a static finger splint. Since her office owns the radiology equipment and employs the orthopedist, she knows that she will bill the global fee for the x-ray. She will also need to bill for the fracture treatment as well as the cast. Because the application of the cast is included in the initial fracture treatment service, she only needs to code for the cast supply, and not the application of the cast. She selects the following codes:

- *26720, Closed treatment of phalangeal shaft fracture, proximal or middle phalanx, finger or thumb; without manipulation, each*
- *73140, Radiologic examination, finger(s), minimum of 2 views*
- *Q4049, Finger splint, static*

Now that Towana has her procedure codes, she asks herself: Why did the doctor do it? The patient was diagnosed with a closed displaced fracture of medial phalanx of left middle finger. This was an initial encounter for the fracture because this the first time the patient has been seen for this injury, which just occurred. She searched the ICD-10-CM Index for Fracture, traumatic, selects the location, laterality, and type of fracture, and adds the seventh character extension to the end of the code for initial encounter for closed fracture. She reports the following diagnosis code:

- *S62.623A, Displaced fracture of medial phalanx of left middle finger, initial encounter for closed fracture*

She then rechecks the documentation to make sure she has coded everything for the encounter and reports the chosen codes.

Diagnostic and procedural coding for orthopedic services

15.7

There's a Code for That

Read the following documentation and assign the appropriate CPT, HCPCS, and ICD-10-CM code(s) for the encounter.

1. A 40-year-old morbidly obese (due to excess calories) male with fever and chills presents with swelling, pain, and redness of his right knee, which has progressed over the last two days. He is a type 2 diabetic and currently dependent on chewing tobacco. Three-view x-ray of right knee are negative for fracture but are indicative of effusion. Joint aspirated of effusive fluid in office. Impression: infective tenosynovitis of the right knee.

   CPT code: _____ -_____ , _____ -_____

   ICD-10-CM codes: _____ , _____ , _____ ,

   _____

2. An 82-year-old otherwise healthy female slipped in the kitchen of her single-family home and fell on her left hip. AP x-ray performed in the hospital facility ED revealed displaced oblique fracture of the center of the femoral neck. Midcervical fracture of the right femur treated via open treatment of femoral fracture with placement of internal fixation device. (Tip: In this case, do not code for the x-ray, as it is performed in the emergency department setting of a hospital facility.)

   CPT code: _____ -_____

   ICD-10-CM codes: _____ , _____ , _____

Case Study | Carpal Tunnel Release

PATIENT: Benjamin Manson

PREOPERATIVE DIAGNOSIS: Bilateral carpal tunnel syndrome

POSTOPERATIVE DIAGNOSIS: Bilateral carpal tunnel syndrome

PROCEDURE: Bilateral carpal tunnel release (open)

ANESTHESIA: Local with MAC

INDICATIONS: Mr. Manson is a 61-year-old male with a history of bilateral carpal tunnel syndrome with electromyography (EMG) confirmation. He failed a conservative treatment program of activity restriction, nighttime splinting, and oral medications. He was thus indicated for above-mentioned procedures.

PROCEDURE IN DETAIL: The patient was properly identified and brought to the OR. Patient was given IV sedation and perioperative antibiotics. Both upper extremities were prepped and draped in the usual sterile fashion, a time out was called, and we proceeded with the case.

Starting with the right upper extremity, Esmarch bandage was used to exsanguinate the upper extremity. Curvilinear incision was made in the proximal part of the palmar crease. Skin and subcutaneous structures were divided sharply with the knife. Dissection continued down to the superficial palmar fascia, which was divided sharply with the knife. Retractors were placed deeper and the transverse carpal ligament divided carefully until the median nerve was visualized. Groove director was directed distally and full release of the median transverse carpal ligament was performed until deep palmar fat was visualized. The groove director was then redirected proximally and the rest of the ligament and the dissection of the flexor retinaculum was divided fully releasing the median nerve. Irrigation was performed followed by a release of the Esmarch bandage. Hemostasis was achieved and wound was closed in single layers of interrupted 4-0 nylon sutures. Sterile dressing was placed. We then moved to the left upper extremity. Procedure was performed identically to that performed on the right upper extremity.

Patient's postoperative plan will be for immobilization with early home range of motion exercises for tendon gliding. We will plan to see him back in the clinic in 7 to 10 days for wound check and suture removal.

SIGNED: Dr. Kameron L. Snill, MD

Use the following steps to select the appropriate codes for the case study.

1. Read through the case study and answer the question: *What did the doctor do?* In this case study, identify the name of the procedure.

_____

_____

2. Now that you have identified the procedure, locate the code for the procedure in the CPT code book.

    a. Search the Index for the procedure and search through the options. If there are multiple options, identify the most appropriate code option and refer to the code listed in the Tabular section.

_____

_____

    b. In the listing of codes, check for any guidelines, important definitions, or parenthetical notes. Select the code that correctly identifies all of the components of the procedure and list it.

_____

_____

    c. Are there any additional procedures that need to be added to identify all of the procedures performed? If yes, follow the previous steps to identify the codes for the additional procedures.

_____

_____

    d. Are there any modifiers that need to be added to identify any special circumstance surrounding the procedure(s)? If yes, refer to Appendix A of the CPT code book to assign all appropriate modifiers.

_____

_____

3. Now that the procedure(s) and modifier(s) have been identified, refer to the case study and answer the following question: *Why did the doctor do it?* In this case study, identify the patient's diagnosis (note that there may be multiple diagnoses).

_____

_____

4. Now that you have identified the patient's diagnoses, search the ICD-10-CM code book for the correct code for this condition.

    a. Search the Main Index for the name of the condition and search through any applicable subterms and cross-references to locate the appropriate code.

_____

_____

    b. Verify the codes in the Tabular List. Locate the code identified previously in the Tabular Listing of codes and refer to any applicable guidelines, notes, and symbols. Does the code selected correctly identify the patient's condition? If yes, list the code:

_____

_____

5. Now that the procedure and diagnosis codes have been identified, list them on the CMS-1500 form. Be sure to correctly link the procedure and diagnosis codes.

21. DIAGNOSIS OR NATURE OF ILLNESS OR INJURY Relate A-L to service line below (24E)			ICD Ind.	
A. _____	B. _____	C. _____	D. _____	
E. _____	F. _____	G. _____	H. _____	
I. _____	J. _____	K. _____	L. _____	

24. A. DATE(S) OF SERVICE						B. PLACE OF SERVICE	C. EMG	D. PROCEDURES, SERVICES, OR SUPPLIES (Explain Unusual Circumstances)		E. DIAGNOSIS POINTER
From			To					CPT/HCPCS MODIFIER		
MM	DD	YY	MM	DD	YY					

End-of-Chapter Content

Instructions: Indicate whether the following statements are true or false (T or F). For false statements, rewrite the statement on the line below to make the statement true.

1. An orthopedic surgeon is an orthopedic doctor who specializes in surgeries of the musculoskeletal system.

_____

_____

2. Orthopedic services may only be performed in the surgical suite of an outpatient hospital.

_____

_____

3. Arthrodesis procedures aspirate fluid from a joint.

_____

_____

4. The Musculoskeletal System subsection in the CPT code book is organized by body area first.

_____

_____

5. To search for the code for an excision of a soft tissue tumor in the CPT Index, first look up the term *soft tissue.*

_____

_____

6. When coding for arthrodesis, vertebral segments and interspaces are measured in the same manner.

_____

_____

7. Manipulation of a fracture is the attempt to return the bone to its original location.

_____

_____

8. There are three types of traction for fracture treatments.

_____

_____

9. The application of a cast or strapping is included in the initial fracture repair code.

_____

_____

10. Codes for the excision of a soft tissue tumor rely on the location of the tumor, but not the size.

_____

_____

Instructions: Choose the best answer.

1. Which type of orthopedic specialist would perform a surgery of the metacarpals?
   a. Orthopedic spine surgeon
   b. Orthopedic hand surgeon
   c. Orthopedic foot and ankle surgeon
   d. Orthopedic shoulder surgeon

2. Which chapter of the ICD-10-CM code book includes the codes for fractures?
   a. Diseases of the Musculoskeletal System
   b. Injury, Poisoning, and Certain Other Consequences of External Causes
   c. External Causes of Morbidity
   d. Congenital Malformations, Deformations, and Chromosomal Abnormalities

3. Which of the following suffixes means surgical incision?
   a. *-desis*
   b. *-centesis*
   c. *-ectomy*
   d. *-tomy*

4. Which type of tumor excision includes the removal of a tumor below the skin but above the deep fascia?
   a. Excision of subcutaneous soft tissue tumors
   b. Excision of fascial or subfascial soft tissue tumors
   c. Excision of soft connective tissue tumors
   d. Excision of bone tumors

5. Which of the following arthrocentesis codes would be assigned for the finger joint?

   a. 20600
   b. 20605
   c. 20610
   d. 20612

6. Which type of fracture treatment employs the use of straps, ropes, pulleys, and weights applied externally to the body?

   a. Skin traction
   b. Skeletal traction
   c. Percutaneous skeletal fixation
   d. Internal fixation

7. Which type of fracture repair surgically opens the body to visualize the fracture site?

   a. Open
   b. Closed
   c. Internal fixation
   d. Percutaneous skeletal fixation

8. Which of the following codes would be reported for a total hip arthroplasty?

   a. 27438
   b. 27138
   c. 27130
   d. 27447

9. Which of the following ICD-10 categories would be used for a pathological fracture in osteoporosis?

   a. S52
   b. M80
   c. M84
   d. M85

10. An open fracture is also known as which of the following?

    a. Closed
    b. Comminuted
    c. Gustilo
    d. Compound

11. Which classification system is used to classify physeal fractures?

    a. Gustilo-Anderson
    b. Salter-Harris
    c. ICD-10-CM codes
    d. Rule of Nines

12. Which of the following types of fractures results in two or more fracture lines that isolate a large section of bone?

    a. Comminuted
    b. Compound
    c. Torus
    d. Segmental

13. Which of the following injuries identifies a strain?

    a. The stretching of ligaments in the ankle
    b. The stretching of ligaments in the shoulder
    c. The tearing of muscle in the groin
    d. The tearing of a ligament in the groin

Instructions: Answer the following questions with the appropriate code(s) and modifier(s).

1. Fracture of shaft of right femur, subsequent encounter for open type IIIA fracture with delayed healing. AP x-ray performed in office confirms slow healing. Long-leg cast reapplied in office and patient will follow up in three weeks.

   CPT codes: _____-_____ ,

   _____-_____

   ICD-10-CM code: _____

2. A 30-year-old male was playing basketball when he felt a snap in his left ankle and intense calf pain. This is a healthy man with unremarkable medical history. Does not smoke or drink. Physical examination revealed passive range of motion and inability to plantarflex the left foot. Two-view radiography of the left ankle is negative for fracture. Clinical impression: spontaneous rupture of Achilles tendon. Definitive procedure performed was a surgical repair and reattachment of Achilles tendon, without graft.

   CPT codes: _____-_____ ,

   _____-_____

   ICD-10-CM code: _____ , _____

3. Trigger finger of the left index, middle, and ring fingers.

   ICD-10-CM code: _____ , _____ ,

   _____

4. Radial styloid tenosynovitis.

   ICD-10-CM code: _____

5. Ganglion cyst of left wrist and right hip.

   ICD-10-CM code: _____

6. Complete tear of the rotator cuff of the right shoulder.

   ICD-10-CM code: _____

7. A 43-year-old male presents with pain in the right leg and knee joint. He plays tag football on the weekend and reports falling on his knee this past weekend. X-rays negative for fracture.

   ICD-10-CM code: _____

References

American Academy of Orthopaedic Surgeons (AAOS). 2015. Hamstring Tendon Tear. Digital Image. American Academy of Orthopedic Surgeons. https://orthoinfo.aaos.org/en/diseases-conditions/sprains-strains-and-other-soft-tissue-injuries.

American Medical Association (AMA). 2019. *CPT 2020 Professional Edition*. Chicago: AMA.

Blausen.com staff. 2013. Blausen 0785 Scoliosis 01.png. Digital image. Wikimedia Commons. https://en.wikipedia.org/wiki/Scoliosis#/media/File:Blausen_0785_Scoliosis_01.png.

BruceBlaus. 2015. Knee Replacement.png. Digital image. Wikimedia Commons. https://commons.wikimedia.org/wiki/File:Knee_Replacement.png.

BruceBlaus. 2013. Blausen 0446 HarringtonRods.png. Digital image. Wikimedia Commons. https://commons.wikimedia.org/wiki/File:Blausen_0446_HarringtonRods.png.

Centers for Medicare and Medicaid Services (CMS). 2019. ICD-10-CM Official Guidelines for Coding and Reporting FY 2020. https://www.cms.gov/Medicare/Coding/ICD10/Downloads/2020-Coding-Guidelines.pdf.

Cepela, D. J., Tartaglione, J. P., and T. P. Dooley. 2016 (November). Classifications in Brief: Salter-Harris Classification of Pediatric Physeal Fractures. https://doi.org/10.1007/s11999-016-4891-3.

Dilmen, N. 2011. Medical X-Ray imaging LHH05 nevit.jpg. Digital image. Wikimedia Commons. https://commons.wikimedia.org/wiki/Category:X-rays_of_internal_fixation#/media/File:Medical_X-Ray_imaging_LHH05_nevit.jpg.

Gaillard, F. 2012. SalterHarris.svg. Digital image. Wikimedia Commons. https://commons.wikimedia.org/wiki/File:SalterHarris.svg.

Kim, P. H. and S. S. Leopold. 2012 (May 9). Gustilo-Anderson Classification. *Clin Orthop Relat Res* (11): 3270–3274. https://www.ncbi.nlm.nih.gov/pmc/articles/PMC3462875/#CR17.

March i Nogué, J. 2015 (December). "Vertebra-en.svg." Digital image. Wikimedia Commons. https://commons.wikimedia.org/wiki/File:718_Vertebra-en.svg.

Medline Plus. 2019. Gout. https://medlineplus.gov/gout.html.

Medtronic. 2017. CPT Coding Examples. https://www.medtronic.com/content/dam/medtronic-com/products/spinal-orthopaedic/reimbursement/documents/PMD004287-10-0-2017-cpt-coding-examples.pdf.

OpenStax College. 2013. 612 Types of Fractures.jpg. Digital Image. Wikimedia Commons. https://en.wikipedia.org/wiki/Bone_fracture#/media/File:612_Types_of_Fractures.jpg.

Scientificanimations.com. 2016. Sprain SAG.jpg. Digital image. Wikimedia Commons. https://commons.wikimedia.org/wiki/File:Sprain_SAG.jpg.

Resources

American Academy of Orthopaedic Surgeons (AAOS). 2017. Sprains, Strains and Other Soft-Tissue Injuries. http://orthoinfo.aaos.org/topic.cfm?topic=a00111.

American Medical Association (AMA). 2013. *Advanced Anatomy and Physiology for ICD-10-CM/PCS*. Salt Lake City, UT: Contexo Media.

Beach, W., and J. B. Samora. 2017. Coding and Billing: A Global Perspective. http://www.aaos.org/CustomTemplates/Content.aspx?id=22436.

Centers for Medicare and Medicaid Services (CMS). 2015 (October 1). ICD-10 Clinical Concepts for Orthopedics. https://www.cms.gov/medicare/coding/icd10/downloads/icd10clinicalconceptsorthopedics1.pdf.

Haralson III, R. H. and M.S. Vaught. 2004 (August). Coding Spinal Procedures Avoid Confusion by Following These Tips. http://www2.aaos.org/bulletin/aug04/code.htm.

Jones, L. n.d. Lesion / Tumor Excision & Would Repair CPT Guidelines. https://newsletters.ahima.org/Newsletters/Code_Write/2016/November/CW1116_LesiontumorTool.pdf.

Lohr, K. M., A. Gonsalves, L. Root, and J. K. Talbot-Stern. 2016 (September 26). Bursitis. http://emedicine.medscape.com/article/2145588-overview.

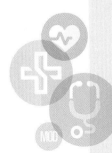

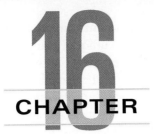

CHAPTER 16

Physical, Occupational, and Speech Therapy Services

Learning Objectives

- Understand the basics of billing and coding for physical, occupational, and speech therapy services
- Examine procedural codes and guidelines for physical, speech, and occupational therapy services
- Examine diagnosis coding and medical necessity for physical, speech, and occupational therapy services
- Determine and apply ICD-10-CM, CPT, and HCPCS codes to physical, speech, and occupational therapy services

Key Terms

8-minute rule

Amputation

Amputee

Amyotrophic lateral sclerosis (ALS)

Aphonia

Augmentative and alternative communication (AAC)

Cognitive communication disorder

Constant attendance code

Dominant side

Dyslexia

Dysphagia

Electrical stimulation

Habilitative services

Hubbard tank

Hypernasality

Iontophoresis

Language disorder

Multiple sclerosis (MS)

Occupational therapist (OT)

Occupational therapy services

Physical therapist (PT)

Physical therapy services

Rehabilitative services

Service-based code

Social communication disorder

Speech-language pathologist (SLP)

Speech therapy services

Therapy services

Time-based code

Traumatic brain injury (TBI)

Treatment modality

Vasopneumatic device

Therapy services are treatments aimed at rehabilitating the patient to optimal bodily function. These services are uniquely tailored to the needs of individual patients so that patients can receive the best possible rehabilitation or functional training to live their lives without outside support. Discussed in this chapter are physical, occupational, and speech therapy services, all of which are designed to help patients reduce pain, improve function, and live as independently as possible.

Physical therapy services are noninvasive procedures and treatments that alleviate pain and improve and restore mobility to limbs and areas of the body. **Occupational therapy services** are noninvasive procedures aimed at improving fine motor skills and functions (such as brushing teeth or writing with a pencil). **Speech therapy services**, also referred to as speech language pathology, help adults and children improve their speech, advance social and cognitive communication skills, and treat swallowing disorders. Some speech therapy services may also be performed by otorhinolaryngologists, otherwise known as ear, nose, and throat doctors (ENTs), who may treat or study the medical causes of speech and swallowing disorders.

Procedural codes for therapy services make up a small slice of CPT codes, so coding for physical, occupational, or speech therapy services is not as complicated as some other specialties. This chapter discusses the basics of coding for therapy services, as well as procedural coding for therapy services and common therapy diagnosis codes.

Therapy Basics

Physical, speech, and occupational therapy services are often combined so that several providers of multiple therapy types can work together to help patients with multiple needs, such as a patient who might need physical and occupational training after receiving a lower arm prosthesis. Individual therapists may also work with healthcare specialists to help improve patient function and outcomes. For example, a physical therapist may work with an orthopedist or sports medicine doctor to help patients recover from sports injuries. Physical, speech, and occupational therapists must be licensed to practice in their state and may not determine patient medical diagnoses. All of the services they perform must be requested by an authorized provider who has determined the patient's diagnosis and the need for therapy services.

When coding for therapy services, coding professionals focus on the relatively small selection of therapy codes for physical, occupational, and speech therapy services located in the Medicine section of the CPT code book, and base diagnosis code selection on the documentation provided by the patient's requesting provider. The healthcare provider diagnoses the patient and then requests a specific therapy service from either a physical, occupational, or speech therapist to help treat a deficit (discussed in full later in this chapter). Coders must also keep in mind the basics of billing for all three types of therapy services.

Speech, physical, and occupational therapists also develop a plan of care that is individualized for each patient, which includes an evaluation of the patient and his or her speech, physical, or occupational functioning, as well as a plan of interventions to help the patient reach his or her goals.

This chapter discusses three types of therapy—physical, occupational, and speech—and their providers and services performed. It also identifies the settings in which services are provided, the basics of billing and coding for therapy services, and also physician orders, authorizations for therapy services, and advance beneficiary notices (ABNs).

Physical Therapy

A **physical therapist (PT)** is a licensed healthcare professional who focuses on noninvasive procedures that alleviate pain and improve and restore mobility. Unlike surgeons, who perform invasive restorative procedures, physical therapists perform an in-depth functional evaluation of each individual patient (upon physician orders) to develop a plan of care that includes multiple methods or procedures (modalities) to help improve movement, reduce pain, restore body functionality, and prevent patient disability. These services are typically provided in one or more individual treatment periods, or rehabilitative sessions, in which the therapist focuses on gross motor skills, range of motion for large joints, and body movement. PTs teach patients how to manage their own condition to achieve long-term health benefits and bodily function, often without the use of prescription medications.

PT services are usually performed immediately after an injury, surgery, or onset of another medical condition, which may result in loss of function or disability. For example, a patient who has just received a total hip arthroplasty may receive physical therapy services after surgery to retrain the body to use the new hip joint and ensure total functionality of the hip prosthesis. This would include training in coordination, endurance, muscle function, and range of motion. PT services in this case not only help restore function but also help to regain strength, balance, prevent patient falls, and decrease pain.

Physical therapists may perform their services in various settings, including inpatient and outpatient hospitals, private practices, home healthcare agencies, nursing homes, schools, and sports and fitness facilities. For example, they may see patients in a sports facility on the weekends, at a private practice during the week, and in the outpatient hospital setting on occasion. Therefore, when coding for PT services it is important to verify the place of service (POS) code for each service performed.

Occupational Therapy

An **occupational therapist (OT)** is a healthcare professional who uses constructive activities to help restore a patient's ability to perform essential activities of daily living (occupations) and improve or maintain functional ability. Unlike physical therapists, occupational therapists focus more on fine motor skills that allow individuals to perform activities of daily living, such as brushing teeth, eating with a fork, or holding a pencil.

Occupational therapy interventions include helping children and adults with disabilities to participate in school and social settings, assisting patients with recovery from illness or injury, and restoring full function of abilities to adult patients who have suffered physical or cognitive problems, such as a stroke.

Just as physical therapists may perform their services in a number of different settings, occupational therapists also provide services across settings such as hospitals, private practices, nursing homes, and schools. Again, always select the appropriate POS code that corresponds to the location in which services were rendered. For a reminder of the different types of settings, please refer to chapter 1 (Your Coding Career).

Speech Therapy

A healthcare professional who provides speech therapy services is referred to as a **speech-language pathologist (SLP)**. SLPs perform a number of different procedures in the form of therapeutic services that help adults and children improve speech and social and cognitive communication skills; they also treat swallowing disorders. Speech therapy may include treatment of speaking problems (such as fluency), problems with voice resonance, and difficulties with pronunciation.

SLPs provide a wide range of services depending on the needs of the patient and include rehabilitation for patients with hearing problems, development of communication systems for patients with expressive or language comprehension problems, strengthening of oral muscle function for patients with swallowing disorders, and even treatment of cognitive status such as orientation, memory, and reasoning skills.

Note that SLPs, just like PTs and OTs, may perform services across a wide range of settings including inpatient and outpatient hospitals, private practices, home healthcare agencies, nursing homes, and schools. Thus, the POS for SLP services should always be verified when reporting codes.

Physician Orders, Authorizations, and Advance Beneficiary Notices

When a PT, OT, or SLP provides services to a patient, is it upon the order of a healthcare provider or primary care physician (PCP) who has either diagnosed the patient with the medical condition, disorder, or disability, or the surgeon who performed the surgery. In either case, the healthcare professional has identified that the patient needs a certain therapeutic service (PT, OT, or SLP) and referred the patient to the therapist for services. The patient's diagnosis (or signs and symptoms) are usually included on the orders for the therapy service. Because they are not medical doctors, PTs, OTs, and SLPs are not authorized to diagnose patients—they must rely on the diagnosis code(s) included on the orders for services.

Understanding the billing process for therapy claims is essential, as it may impact the way in which the claim for therapy services is coded and the amount or frequency of therapy services the patient is allowed to receive. For example, if the insurance requires that a referral is on file before the therapy services are provided, then it will not pay for any services rendered until the referral is authorized and on file.

Certain insurance companies may have a specific dollar amount capped annually for therapy services; for example, Medicare only permits a specific dollar amount for therapy services per year (CMS 2018a). Anything over this amount must be specifically documented as reasonable and medically necessary or it will not be paid. Determination that a therapy service is medically necessary is dependent on more than just assigning an ICD-10-CM code and may require statements from the healthcare provider or therapist explaining why services are still required. This documentation could include progress reports or range of motion measurements, for example. The determination is made by the therapy provider, patient, and the patient's requesting healthcare provider. Ultimately, the patient's insurance can decide to approve or deny additional services (unless the patient chooses to pay for the services out-of-pocket).

If a service is provided to a Medicare patient and it is expected that Medicare will not reimburse for the service (and the patient will be responsible for payment), the patient must be given an advance beneficiary notice of non-coverage (ABN), as discussed in chapter 2 (Healthcare Billing Basics). This document notifies the patient that Medicare may not pay for the service, and that the patient may have to assume full financial responsibility for the services provided (CMS 2018a).

When an ABN is given to the patient, the coder must append a modifier to the procedure code indicating to Medicare that the ABN was provided. These include the following:

- GA, Waiver of liability statement issued as required by payer policy, individual case. This modifier indicates that the ABN was signed and is on file at the provider's office, which allows the provider to bill the patient for the service if the service is denied by Medicare.

- GX, Notice of liability issued, voluntary under payer policy. This modifier is used to indicate that an ABN was signed for a noncovered service that will not be paid by Medicare. This service will be billed to the patient.

- GY, Item or service statutorily excluded, does not meet the definition of any Medicare benefit or, for non-Medicare insurers, is not a contract benefit. This modifier is used to notify Medicare that the provider understands that this is a noncovered service and will not be reimbursed.

- GZ, Item or service expected to be denied as not reasonable or necessary. This modifier is used to identify instances in which an ABN may have been required but was not obtained from the patient. (CMS 2018b)

Other insurance payers may set a limit of services rather than a dollar amount. For example, a commercial insurance company may authorize five rehabilitation sessions for a physical therapy patient. If additional services are needed after those five services have been provided, then the insurance company must approve a new request. If it is not approved, then the patient will be responsible to pay for the additional services.

The services provided by each individual therapy provider are distinct and intended to treat a specific functionality or disability with a particular modality. Procedure codes for PT, OT, and SLP services are found in the Medicine section of the CPT code book.

Key to Success

Therapy providers are not typically classified as healthcare professionals according to CMS or CPT guidelines, and are therefore unable to provide any type of healthcare service other than the therapy services they are qualified to perform. In other words, PTs, OTs, and SLPs are not qualified to provide evaluation and management (E/M) encounters, surgical procedures, or medical procedures other than their approved therapy services. Qualification for therapy providers depends on state licensing regulations and insurance regulations, so the exact services allowed may differ from state to state or by insurance company.

Procedural Coding for Therapy Services

Procedure codes for physical and occupational therapy, and speech language pathology services are all included in the Medicine section of the CPT code book. Physical and occupational therapy use similar modalities, whereas speech language services use a different set of modalities and procedures. A small selection of HCPCS codes are employed for both in addition to CPT codes. There are also two CPT modifiers that apply specifically to therapy procedures.

Physical and Occupational Therapy Procedures

Physical and occupational therapy codes are found in the Medicine section of the CPT code book, in the Physical Medicine and Rehabilitation subsection (97010–97799).

Codes in this section identify physical and occupational therapy evaluation and re-evaluations, treatment modalities, therapeutic procedures, tests and measurements, and orthotic and prosthetic management. The services identified in this section may be reported for some physical or occupational therapists but may not be reported for others; this depends on the types of services for which each individual therapy provider is qualified, trained, and has the resources to perform. For example, a physical therapist with the necessary equipment to perform Hubbard tank treatments may do so, and report the service with the code 97036, Application of a modality to 1 or more areas; Hubbard tank, each 15 minutes.

Physical and Occupational Therapy Evaluations

Both physical and occupational therapy services are initiated with an evaluation service, which includes a patient history, examination or assessment, and the development of a plan of treatment used to deliver the physical or occupational therapy services to the patient.

Physical therapy evaluations (97161–97164) include a patient history and examination, and the development of a plan of care. They are similar in nature to E/M codes, as they include the three key components of history, examination, and clinical decision-making in addition to the development of a plan of care (see figure 16.1). There are three levels of physical therapy evaluations—low complexity, moderate complexity, and high complexity, which depend on the level of difficulty for each of the key components in the code description. Note that the levels of complexity listed in these codes are not the same as the levels of complexity for E/M codes. The exact components within each level of complexity are included in the full code description for each respective therapy evaluation service. For example, codes 97161, Physical therapy evaluation: low complexity through 97163, Physical therapy evaluation: high complexity, identify the *initial* evaluation service, whereas code 97164, Re-evaluation of physical therapy established plan of care is reported for a *re-evaluation* of the established physical therapy plan of care.

Occupational therapy evaluations (97165–97168) are also similar to E/M codes, except the key component of the codes differ slightly from physical therapy evaluation codes. The key components for occupational therapy evaluations include an occupational profile and client medical and therapy history, an assessment of occupational performance, clinical decision-making, and the development of a plan of care. There are three levels of codes for occupational therapy evaluations—low complexity, moderate complexity, and high complexity—that depend on the levels of the four key components. Codes 97165, Occupational therapy evaluation, low complexity through 97167, Occupational therapy evaluation, high complexity, identify *initial* evaluations, whereas code 97168, Re-evaluation of occupational therapy established plan of care, is reported for a *re-evaluation* of an established occupational therapy plan of care. See figure 16.1 for the key components of physical and occupational therapy evaluations.

Evaluations for either physical or occupational therapy are performed as an initial service, and the plan of care is developed for the remaining therapy services that will be provided to the patient. A re-evaluation is used to perform an additional assessment of the patient and make any necessary changes to the plan of care. Neither of these services are performed at every visit. Rather, once the evaluation is completed and the plan of care is developed, only the specific therapeutic modalities or procedures will be performed. The only exception to this is if the patient needs a re-evaluation, in which case a new plan of care will determine the services the patient will receive. For example, after an initial evaluation, a physical therapist may create a plan of care including the gross motor function of a lower-limb amputee and include 10 treatments over the course of three months. After the three-month period, the physical therapist notes that the patient has not made as much progress as anticipated by the original plan of care, and performs a re-evaluation and the development of a new plan of care that includes additional treatments (Jannenga 2014).

Figure 16.1. Key components of therapy evaluations

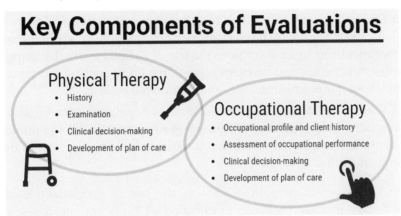

Physical and Occupational Therapy Modalities and Procedures

Physical and occupational treatment services employ a range of treatment modalities—methods of therapeutic treatment designed to treat or rehabilitate a specific patient condition. Codes for therapy services identify the specific modality employed during the service, which is either service-based or time-based.

Treatment Modalities

Treatment modalities for physical therapy services help to strengthen, relax, or heal a specific muscle or group of muscles. Modalities for occupational therapy services help to improve circulation, decrease pain, improve elasticity of muscles and body movement, improve joint mobility, and reduce inflammation and swelling. The codes for the specific modality do not change depending on if they were employed for occupational or therapeutic services. Coders should select the appropriate code according to the modality used, without regard to the type of healthcare provider who performed the service.

Some of the more common modalities used by physical therapists involve the use of manual techniques and therapeutic activities. These therapy services are reported with the following codes (along with others):

- 97110, Therapeutic procedure, 1 or more areas, each 15 minutes; therapeutic exercises to develop strength and endurance, range of motion and flexibility. In this therapeutic service, the therapist may employ the use of various methods to increase endurance, range of motion, and flexibility as well as various stretching and strengthening exercises, such as a treadmill or gymnastic ball.

- 97112, Therapeutic procedure, 1 or more areas, each 15 minutes; neuromuscular reeducation of movement, balance, coordination, kinesthetic sense, posture, and/or proprioception for sitting and/or standing exercises. In this service, the therapist may employ various neuromuscular techniques, such as the use of desensitization techniques or the use of a biomechanical ankle platform system (BAPS) board, to help recondition the patient's lower limb joints.

- 97113, Therapeutic procedure, 1 or more areas, each 15 minutes; aquatic therapy with therapeutic exercises. In this exercise, the therapist employs the use of aquatic therapy, such as swimming exercises.

- 97116, Therapeutic procedure, 1 or more areas, each 15 minutes; massage, including effleurage, petrissage and/or tapotement (stroking, compression, percussion).

- 97140, Manual therapy techniques (eg, mobilization/manipulation, manual lymphatic drainage, manual traction), 1 or more regions, each 15 minutes. This therapeutic technique employs the use of various manual manipulative therapies directed toward problem areas of the body, such as soft tissue or joint mobilization, lymphatic drainage, and myofascial release.

- 97530, Therapeutic activities, direct (one-on-one) patient contact (use of dynamic activities to improve functional performance), each 15 minutes. These therapeutic activities involve the use of various movements, such as throwing, catching, or lifting.

Additional therapeutic modalities include the use of specialized equipment or devices, and may include massage, application of tape, and exercises. Additional therapeutic modalities are as follows:

- *Hot and/or cold packs.* Coded with 97010, Application of a modality to 1 or more areas; hot or cold packs, hot packs are used to help relax tight muscles and decrease pain and muscle spasms and are typically applied before a treatment session. Cold packs are used after a treatment session to reduce pain and inflammation.

- *Electrical stimulation.* **Electrical stimulation** causes one muscle or a group of muscles to contract, helping to increase muscle strength and blood supply to the muscle and decrease pain. Codes for electrical stimulation identify the type of stimulation performed and differ depending on whether the code selected is service based or time based (discussed later in this chapter). Code 97014, Application of modality to 1 or more areas; *electrical stimulation (unattended),* should be reported for electrical stimulation treatment for a patient when the therapist is not in constant physical attendance. Alternatively, code 97032, Application of modality to 1 or more areas; *electrical stimulation (manual), each 15 minutes,* should be reported when the therapist is in constant physical attendance. **Iontophoresis** (97033) is a form of electrical stimulation used to push medication through the skin to the affected body area, muscle, tendon, or ligament (see figure 16.2). Note that the medication administered during the iontophoresis must be prescribed by the patient's healthcare provider.

- *Ultrasound.* The high or low frequency sound waves from an ultrasound machine are used by therapists to penetrate muscle tissues to warm them and help in relaxation techniques, as well as increase circulation and reduce inflammation. This is coded with 97035, Application of a modality to 1 or more areas; *ultrasound, each 15 minutes.*

- *Paraffin bath.* Paraffin is a wax heated together with mineral oil and used as a treatment for patients with arthritis or joint conditions. The procedure is performed by coating the hand with multiple coats of the wax mixture, letting

Figure 16.2. Iontophoresis

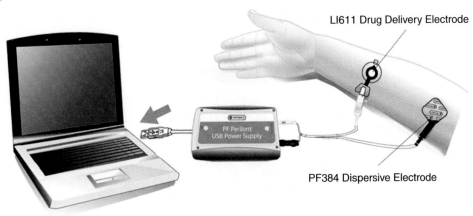

LI611 Drug Delivery Electrode

PF384 Dispersive Electrode

Source: ©2017. Image courtesy of Perimed.

it to dry between coats, and allowing it to heat the hand for a small amount of time. It is reported with code 97018, Application of a modality to 1 or more areas; *paraffin bath*.

- *Ultraviolet therapy.* This procedure is used to help improve circulation and bring oxygen to body tissues by employing ultraviolet rays. It is coded with 97028, Application of a modality to 1 or more areas; *ultraviolet*.

- *Diathermy and infrared therapy.* These two therapeutic procedures produce a warming sensation directed at a specific body area or muscle. They are reported with 97024, Application of a modality to 1 or more areas; diathermy (eg, microwave), and 97026, Application of a modality to 1 or more areas; infrared.

- *Whirlpool and immersion.* A whirlpool is a large tank or tub filled with warm water that uses water jets and bubbles to help clean wounds or improve flexibility of muscles. Whirlpool treatments are reported with code 97022, Application of a modality to 1 or more areas; whirlpool. A **Hubbard tank** (reported with code 97036, Application of a modality to 1 or more areas; Hubbard tank, each 15 minutes), is a large tub in which the patient can be fully immersed, allowing patients to perform exercises while in the water.

- *Vasopneumatic device.* A **vasopneumatic device** is used on the external extremities, like the arms and legs, applying external pressure to the soft tissues and decreasing swelling. Use of a vasopneumatic device is reported with code 97016, Application of a modality to 1 or more areas; vasopneumatic devices.

Figure 16.3 illustrates a physical therapist providing care to a patient.

Medicare may require the submission of HCPCS codes for certain services, when HCPCS codes are available. HCPCS codes for therapy services can be found in the HCPCS code book by searching under the term *Therapy* and then selecting the subterm for the specific type of therapy service provided, or by searching the Index for the specific type of therapy service provided. Most, but not all, therapy services in the HCPCS code book are found in Temporary Procedures/Professional Services (G0000–G9999). For example, code G0129, Occupational therapy services requiring the skills of a qualified occupational therapist, furnished as a component of a partial hospitalization treatment program, per session (45 minutes or more).

Figure 16.3. Physical therapy

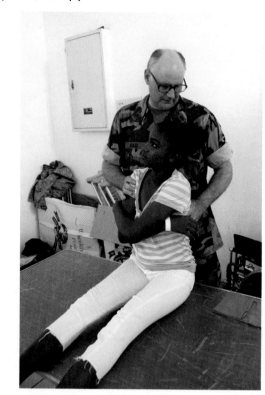

Source: Airman First Class Danielle Grannan 2009.

MOD *Modifiers Used in Therapy Services*

There are two CPT modifiers designed specifically for therapy services such as those provided by physical, occupational, and speech therapists.

- Modifier -96, Habilitative Services. This modifier should be appended to codes for **habilitative services** that help a patient keep, learn, or improve skills and functions of daily living. For example, an occupational therapy service provided to a pediatric patient with a physical disability that helps the patient learn activities of daily living would be appended with this modifier.

- Modifier -97, Rehabilitative Services. This modifier should be appended to codes for **rehabilitative services** that help a patient keep, recover, or improve skills, functions, and activities of daily living after they have been lost or impaired due to illness, injury, or disability. For example, a physical therapy service provided to an older adult to help him re-learn how to walk after an injury would be classified as a rehabilitative service and would thus be appended with this modifier.

Service-Based and Time-Based Codes

Physical and occupational therapy services are divided into two types of codes: service based and time based. A **service-based code** is one that describes a full service, such as a physical therapy evaluation (97161–97163), application of hot or cold packs (97010), or the performance of electrical stimulation (97014). Service-based codes are *untimed,* and one code should be reported no matter how long the provider spent performing the service.

Time-based codes, also known as **constant attendance codes**, are reported according to the length of time the provider spent performing the service. These are easily distinguished from service-based codes, as the code description identifies the amount of time per code. For example, code 97110, Therapeutic procedure, 1 or more areas, each 15 minutes; therapeutic exercises to develop strength and endurance, range of motion and flexibility, describes the amount of time during which the provider must be in constant attendance in order to report the code (15 minutes). In this case, the therapy provider must be face-to-face with the patient, constantly attending the patient's side, for the amount of time described in the code.

Reporting time-based codes becomes a bit more complicated when the healthcare practitioner does not provide the full 15 minutes of the therapy service, as identified in the code. In order to bill for the full code, the provider must perform at least 8 minutes of the service. For example, if the provider was in constant attendance for 10 minutes, then he or she would be able to bill for the service, with one unit. For any time *over* 15 minutes, the additional time must be at least 8 minutes over the 15-minute unit to report an additional unit of the service. This is known as the **8-minute rule**. For example, if a provider performed 23 minutes of electrical stimulation to a patient with atrophy of leg muscles, the code for the service would be 97032, Application of a modality to 1 or more areas; electrical stimulation (manual), each 15 minutes, reported with two units: 97032 × 2 (the first unit would account for the initial 15 minutes of the service, and the second unit would account for the additional 8 minutes of the service). Each additional 8 minutes over the last 15-minute mark equals one additional unit. If less than 8 additional minutes are spent (over the last 15-minute mark), do not report an additional unit (see figure 16.4).

Figure 16.4. The 8-minute rule

97032	15 (1 unit)
97032	8 (1 unit)
Code(s) reported: **97032 × 2**	**Total time spent:** **23 minutes**

97032	15 (1 unit)
97032	15 (1 unit)
97032	5 (not reported)
Code(s) reported: **97032 × 2**	**Total time spent:** **35 minutes**

It is important to note that Medicare follows the 8-minute rule, but not all third-party payers follow suit. When reporting time-based codes for insurance plans other than Medicare, be sure to follow the specific guidelines for each insurance for reporting time-based services.

Complete the exercises in There's a Code for That 16.1 to practice reporting physical and occupational therapy procedures.

16.1 Physical and occupational therapy procedures

There's a Code for That

Read the following documentation of the service and identify the procedure code(s).

1. Application of hot packs to right ankle and knee joints.

   CPT code: _____

2. Patient received paraffin bath treatment on both hands.

   CPT code: _____

3. 30 minutes of therapeutic exercise including activities to increase R shoulder ROM and strengthening of R side.

   CPT code: _____ × _____

4. Gait training with comprehensive motion analysis by 3D kinematics, with dynamic plantar pressure measurements during walking.

   CPT code: _____

5. 45 minutes of myofascial release therapeutic massage.

   CPT code: _____ × _____

6. High complexity occupational therapy evaluation with subsequent 20 minutes of training on activities of daily living, including training in adaptive equipment.

   CPT codes: _____ , _____

Speech Therapy Procedures

Codes for speech therapy and speech language pathology services are found in the Medicine section of the CPT code book in the Special Otorhinolaryngologic Services subsection (92502–92700). This section includes a variety of codes that may be performed by SLPs or ENTs. Additional codes from the Surgery section, such as endoscopic examination of the esophagus, may also be reported as necessary, depending on the services provided by the SLP.

Treatments provided by speech language pathologists are designed to rehabilitate and improve swallowing function and communication ability, as well as oral speaking and language ability. They include:

- *Swallowing function.* Swallowing disorders are common conditions, especially in the elderly population, and can cause a range of additional health problems such as weight loss, dehydration, aspiration pneumonia, and obstruction of the airway. Swallowing studies help to diagnose the cause of the patient's **dysphagia** (difficulty swallowing) and improve swallowing ability. Codes for swallowing function studies (92610–92617) identify the method of the test, and whether the SLP provided the full procedure or only the interpretation and report of the test. For example, code 92613, Flexible endoscopic evaluation of swallowing by cine or video recording; interpretation and report only, identifies the type of swallowing study (flexible endoscopic by cine or video recording) and that the therapist only provided the interpretation and report of the study (and did not perform the actual endoscopy). Treatment of a swallowing disorder is coded with 92526, Treatment of swallowing dysfunction and/or oral function for feeding.

- *Augmentative and alternative communication.* **Augmentative and alternative communication (AAC)** is used to communicate with other people and does not include oral communication. For example, an augmentative form of communication includes hand gestures or facial expressions when speaking. These gestures augment and add meaning to the oral words that are spoken. Patients with speech problems rely on AAC to help them communicate with others and may use special devices to further augment their communication and provide alternative communication. Codes for AAC services (92597, 92605–92609) identify the type of service (evaluation or therapeutic service), as well as the type of AAC device. Codes 92605, 92618, 92607, and 92608 are time-based codes that identify the amount of time spent on the evaluation. HCPCS code V5336, Repair/modification of augmentative communicative system or device (excludes adaptive hearing aid), should be reported when the SLP performs either a repair or modification of the AAC device. See figure 16.5 for an example of a speech-generating AAC device.

Figure 16.5. Speech generating AAC device

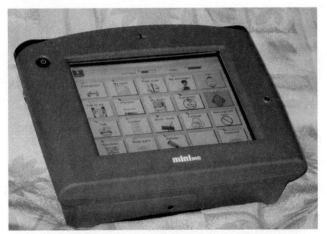

This AAC device allows the user to press the image for the idea or phrase they would like to communicate.

Source: Poule 2009.

- *Speech and language services.* Speech and language services are provided to patients with a range of communication disorders. **Language disorders** are difficulties with understanding or producing oral speech. They include receptive language disorders (when a patient has trouble understanding others) and expressive language disorders (when a patient has trouble sharing his or her thoughts and feelings with others) and may be in either oral or written form. **Social communication disorders** occur when a patient has difficulty understanding social cues in verbal and nonverbal communication, such as sitting down for a formal meal or telling a story from start to finish. **Cognitive communication disorders** include difficulties for patients when organizing thoughts, remembering, paying attention, planning, and problem solving (ASHA n.d.). The way in which an SLP treats a speech and language disorder depends on the type of disorder the patient has. Furthermore, services range from noninvasive evaluations of voice and resonance to minimally invasive procedures, such as a nasopharyngoscopy (an endoscopic examination of the nose and throat). Procedures to treat speech and language disorders include:

- 92507, Treatment of speech, language, voice, communication, and/or auditory processing disorder; *individual*, or 92508, Treatment of speech, language, voice, communication, and/or auditory processing disorder; *group, 2 or more individuals.*
- Endoscopic examinations and function studies (92511–92516).
- Evaluations of hearing loss and rehabilitation status (92626–92633).
- Assessments and testing of aphasia and cognitive development (96105–96111, 96125).
- Techniques to improve sensory and cognitive ability (97127, 97533).
- Telephone and online assessments and management services (98966–98969) and medical team conferences with primary care and other practitioners (99366–99368) (Note that the codes for medical team conferences are in the E/M section of the CPT code book. E/M codes may only be reported by qualified healthcare professionals).

Complete the exercises in There's a Code for That 16.2 to practice reporting codes for speech therapy procedures.

16.2 Speech therapy procedures

There's a Code for That

Read the following documentation of the service and identify the procedure code(s).

1. Treatment of language processing disorder, individual.

   CPT code: _____

2. Evaluation of receptive/expressive language on 5-year-old male patient.

   CPT code: _____

3. 30 minutes of direct patient development of cognitive skills (attention, memory, and problem solving).

   CPT code: _____ × _____

4. Programming and modification of non-speech generating device.

   CPT code: _____

5. Modification of AAC device.

   CPT code: _____

The diagnostic codes used to identify the medical necessity for therapy services are not assigned by therapy providers, as PTs, OTs, and SLPs are not authorized to assign medical diagnoses to patients. However, this does not mean that therapy services do not need ICD-10-CM codes. Rather, the ICD-10-CM codes assigned for therapy services rely on the documentation of the patient's condition by the primary care or referring provider.

Diagnostic Coding for Therapy Services

Therapy services treat a vast range of conditions throughout the human body, from congenital malformations to acquired deformities, traumatic injuries, musculoskeletal conditions, and neurological impairments. Patients undergoing therapy receive a diagnosis from a primary care physician or other treating physician who has determined that the patient needs some sort of therapeutic treatment to help the patient either return to original function or improve function after an injury or other medical condition.

ICD-10-CM codes are used to identify the medical necessity for physical and occupational therapy services, which includes musculoskeletal conditions, injuries, and problems with patient's fine and gross motor functioning. This medical necessity also includes neurological conditions, such as sequela from a stroke or cerebrovascular ~~accident~~ multiple sclerosis (MS). Medical necessity for occupational therapy services also ~~includes~~ behavioral and mental disorders, which may impair a patient's ability to function in a social setting.

Note that when assigning therapy diagnoses, the primary diagnosis code should be the underlying medical necessity for the services. For instance, tear of the anterior cruciate ligament (ACL) of the right knee (S83.511A, Sprain of anterior cruciate ligament of right knee, initial encounter). Additional diagnoses should be assigned to identify any additional impairment, limitation, or disability that necessitates the physical therapy services, such as instability of the right knee (M25.361, Other instability, right knee).

Medical necessity for speech language pathology services includes disorders that impair or inhibit communication and affect the ability to swallow or hear. This includes physical conditions such as malignant neoplasm of the throat or dentofacial anomalies, as well as psychological and behavioral disorders that affect social communication and speaking difficulties.

Ultimately, reporting diagnosis codes for any type of therapy service requires a general knowledge of the ICD-10-CM code book, the ability to assign codes from across many chapters of the ICD-10-CM code book, and interpreting guidelines to ensure correct code selection.

Physical and Occupational Therapy Conditions

Many of the medical conditions treated by physical and occupational therapists result from injuries and musculoskeletal conditions, congenital malformations and anomalies, mental and developmental disorders, and neurological conditions.

Injuries and Musculoskeletal Conditions

Traumatic injuries range from simple fractures that heal without any side effects or necessary treatment or surgical interventions, to severe disfiguring injuries that require surgical interventions, medical treatments, and rehabilitative therapy services. Therefore, coding for injuries and related conditions of the musculoskeletal system (such as joint pain) can also range from reporting symptoms to reporting complex combinations of injuries, musculoskeletal conditions, and side effects.

Injuries are coded from chapter 19 (Injury, Poisoning and Certain Other Consequences of External Causes), and musculoskeletal conditions are coded from chapter 13 (Diseases of the Musculoskeletal System and Connective Tissue) of the ICD-10-CM code book. Medical conditions from these chapters treated by occupational and physical therapists include:

- *Joint pain.* Joint pain (such as back, neck, arm, shoulder, leg, knee, ankle, and foot pain) is a common symptom treated by physical and occupational therapists. It may be a result of a past injury, medical condition, or side effect of surgical treatment. Rehabilitative therapy treatments of joint pain are aimed at reducing the amount of pain and restoring full range of motion of the joint. When searching for a joint pain code, refer to the term *Pain* in the Main Index of the ICD-10-CM code book, then refer to the subterm *joint*, and then the specific joint. Codes for joint pain also identify the laterality of the condition, such as right or left, the codes for which are found in the Tabular List of the codes (for example, M25.561, Pain in right knee).

- *Arthritis and degenerative joint diseases.* The numerous different types of arthritis may also require therapeutic services to reduce pain and restore functionality. Coding for any type of arthritis requires the identification of the spe~~~ of arthritis—such as osteoarthritis, rheumatoid, juvenile, or infect~~ and the specific site involved. Remember that if a definitive diagnosis is identified, then it is not necessary to report the signs or symptoms included in the definitive diagnosis. For example, if the definitive diagnosis were arthritis, then it would not be necessary to report any associated swelling, pain, or reduced range of motion in the arthritic joints. If a patient were treated for severe bilateral osteoarthritis of the hips that caused pain, swelling, lack of range of motion, and caused her to ambulate with a walker, the only diagnosis code reported would be M16.0, Bilateral primary osteoarthritis of hip.

HCC Coding Corner

Note that some, but not all, arthropathies are included in HCC coding, such as pyogenic arthritis, infectious arthritis, reactive arthropathies, inflammatory arthritis (including rheumatoid), and juvenile arthritis.

- *Sports injuries.* Sports injuries occur from either a single instance of a motion or movement resulting in an injury, such as a torn ligament or muscle strain; or an injury resulting from repetitive movements, such as tendinitis of the elbow from playing tennis (tennis elbow). Physical therapists may subspecialize in rehabilitative sports therapy to help restore function to the affected area and make it possible for the patient to resume athletic activities. Some of the more common conditions treated for sports injuries include tears of the anterior cruciate ligament (ACL) in the knee, rotator cuff strains, tendinitis, and various strains and sprains. When searching for a sport-related injury, it is necessary to identify the external causes surrounding the injury, including the patient's activity, place of occurrence, injury mechanism, and the patient status at the time of the injury (for example, code S43.422A, Sprain of left rotator cuff capsule, initial encounter).

- *Amputation.* An **amputation** is the surgical removal of all or a portion of a body part. Often an amputation is performed surgically on an extremity due to a medical condition, such as gangrene, or from a traumatic injury that has either removed the body part or caused so much damage to the body part that it must be removed. Physical and occupational therapy services focus on helping the **amputee**, the patient who has undergone an amputation, learn how to function with a prosthetic device. For example, a lower leg amputee may receive physical therapy services to learn to walk again with the use of a prosthetic leg. Refer to chapter 15 (Orthopedic Services) for the discussion on amputation ICD-10-CM codes.

- *Head injury.* Head injuries can range from a concussion that requires little more than observation to severe and debilitating **traumatic brain injuries (TBI)** requiring invasive surgery and a lifetime of medical treatment and rehabilitative services. Physical and occupational therapists can help patients regain function after a TBI by helping the patient relearn both fine and gross movements. TBI patients may also require the services of a speech therapist as well, depending on the type of injury. TBIs are coded from category S06, Intracranial Injury, and identify:
  - ○ the type of injury (such as cerebral edema, diffuse traumatic brain injury, focal traumatic brain injury, contusion and laceration of cerebrum), and
  - ○ the duration of any loss of consciousness suffered by the patient;
    - ▪ if the patient returned to pre-injury level of consciousness,
    - ▪ if the patient did not return to pre-existing level of consciousness, or
    - ▪ if the patient died (either due to the brain injury or another injury) before regaining consciousness.

An example is code S06.342D, Traumatic hemorrhage of right cerebrum with loss of consciousness of 31 minutes to 59 minutes, subsequent encounter. As with amputation codes, almost all TBI codes are included in HCC coding, so care should be taken to ensure the correct documentation and code selection for these conditions.

- *Spinal cord injuries and paralytic syndromes.* Spinal cord injuries may range in neurological symptoms from tingling and weakness to full paralysis. When coding for a spinal cord injury, identify the specific type of injury, level of the injury (such as cervical or lumbar), and then the specific vertebra(e) involved in the injury. If multiple spinal cord injuries are present, code to the highest level of the injury (for example, code to the cervical level rather than the lumbar level). Paralytic syndromes are coded from categories G81, Hemiplegia and hemiparesis, G82, Paraplegia (paraparesis) and quadriplegia (quadriparesis), and G83, Other paralytic syndromes. Codes from these categories should be reported when the condition is documented without further specification, or if the condition is old or longstanding and the cause is unspecified. These codes may also be used in addition to the code for the original injury, such as spinal cord injury. For example, if the documentation states only that the patient is paraplegic but does not specify the cause of the paraplegia, then report a code from category G82. When coding for paralytic syndromes, codes identify the condition as affecting either the dominant or nondominant side of the body. The **dominant side** is the side that the patient prefers when performing daily functions—writing with the right hand would mean that a person is right-handed. When the dominant side is not identified in the provider's documentation, then code as the following:
  - ○ For ambidextrous patients, report the right side as dominant.
  - ○ If the left side is affected, report the condition as affecting the nondominant side.
  - ○ If the right side is affected, report the condition as affecting the dominant side.

In other words, the right side is the default dominant side. Note that both spinal cord injuries as well as paralytic syndromes are included in HCC coding (see figure 16.6 for the OGCR related to coding for the dominant versus nondominant sides).

Figure 16.6. OGCR I.C.6.a

---

6. Chapter 6: Diseases of the Nervous System (G00-G99)

a. Dominant/nondominant side

Codes from category G81, Hemiplegia and hemiparesis, and subcategories, G83.1, Monoplegia of lower limb, G83.2, Monoplegia of upper limb, and G83.3, Monoplegia, unspecified, identify whether the dominant or nondominant side is affected. Should the affected side be documented, but not specified as dominant or nondominant, and the classification system does not indicate a default, code selection is as follows:

- For ambidextrous patients, the default should be dominant.
- If the left side is affected, the default is non-dominant.
- If the right side is affected, the default is dominant.

Source: CMS 2019.

Episode of Care for Therapy Services

It is necessary to pay special attention to the episode of care for therapy services, especially those related to injuries. A patient may present for therapy services for an injury-related disability or impairment at any time during the injury or healing phase. For example, a patient may receive treatment for a femur fracture during the active phase of treatment for that fracture (and code for the femur fracture with seventh character A, Initial Encounter) to help the patient learn how to use a special walking device. After the healing phase of that fracture is completed and the cast is off, the therapist may see the patient again to help the patient re-learn to walk. In this case, the fracture would be coded with seventh character D, Subsequent Encounter. And finally, the patient may seek physical therapy services for a related sequela of the femur fracture a year or two down the road, for residual pain or limitations in mobility as a result of the femur fracture that occurred a year ago. In this case, the coder would assign the code for the residual condition for which the patient is currently receiving treatment (limitations in mobility), as well as the code for the initial injury with the seventh character S, Sequela. See figure 16.7 for an example of when each episode of care code would be selected.

If the patient's therapy services are not related to an injury or other condition for which an episode of care is not applicable, assign the necessary code(s) for the primary condition and additional code(s) for the related impairment, disability, or limitation that necessitates therapy services.

Figure 16.7. Episode of care for therapy services

Episode of Care	Service Provided	Codes Selected
A, Initial Encounter	Patient receives assistance in learning how to use walking device for femur fracture.	S72.301A, Unspecified fracture of shaft of right femur, initial encounter for closed fracture
D, Subsequent Encounter	Patient receives services to help regain strength in right leg after fracture has healed.	S72.301D, Unspecified fracture of shaft of right femur, subsequent encounter for closed fracture with routine healing
S, Sequela	Patient receives services to treat difficulty walking due to the femur fracture a year ago.	R26.2, Difficulty in walking, not elsewhere classified S72.301S, Unspecified fracture of shaft of right femur, sequela

Aftercare

If the patient's therapy services are provided to help restore movement of a body part after a surgical service or procedure, it may be necessary to report the aftercare diagnosis to indicate the therapy is related to a prior medical procedure. Aftercare is provided as a rehabilitation procedure for a condition that no longer exists. For example, if a patient receives a knee replacement due to severe osteoarthritis of the knee, then this condition no longer exists (as the knee joint was replaced). However, the patient is now receiving therapy directed at the knee joint to restore movement, strength, and flexibility. This procedure would be reported with an aftercare diagnosis, such as Z47.1, Aftercare following joint replacement surgery. The Tabular List includes a note to use additional code to identify the joint, such as Z96.651, Presence of right artificial knee joint. Additional diagnoses should also be added to identify any related disability or debility experienced by the patient.

Aftercare diagnoses are found by searching the term *Aftercare* in the Main Index of the ICD-10-CM code book, and then locating the subterm for the type of medical procedure that was performed on the patient.

Congenital Malformations and Anomalies

A congenital malformation or anomaly is one with which a patient is born. Some congenital malformations may result in musculoskeletal disfigurement to such an extent that the patient requires either physical or occupational therapy (or both) in order to learn how to function.

Congenital malformations are reported from chapter 17 (Congenital Malformations, Deformations and Chromosomal Abnormalities) of the ICD-10-CM code book. These codes may be reported throughout the life of the patient. When searching for a congenital malformation in the ICD-10-CM Index, find the main term to identify the specific type of malformation, and then the subterm for the congenital version of the condition.

Also included in chapter 17 are codes for chromosomal abnormalities, such as Down Syndrome. These are reported with codes from Chromosomal abnormalities, not elsewhere classified (Q90–Q99). Code selection depends on the identification of the specific type of chromosomal abnormality, such as Q95.1, Chromosome inversion in normal individual. Some abnormalities may also be identified by their resulting syndromes, such as Q93.3, Deletion of short arm of chromosome 4 (Wolff-Hirschhorn syndrome). Note that almost all chromosomal abnormalities are included in HCC coding.

Mental and Developmental Disorders

There are a host of mental and developmental disorders that may require therapeutic services to help patients function in a social environment. For example, patients with autism spectrum disorder (ASD) (F84.0, Autistic disorder) may need help learning how to perform everyday tasks without becoming overwhelmed by external influences, such as loud noises or changes in lighting and other environmental factors. Patients with emotional disturbances or mental disorders, such as disruptive mood dysregulation disorder (F34.81, Disruptive mood dysregulation disorder) or excoriation (skin-picking) disorder (F42.4, Excoriation [skin-picking] disorder), may also need therapeutic services in order to function in a social setting or to remove unwanted behaviors.

Codes for mental and developmental disorders may be found in chapter 5 (Mental, Behavioral and Neurodevelopmental Disorders) and chapter 6 (Diseases of the Nervous System) of the ICD-10-CM code book. If the mental disorder is due to a known physiological condition, report the code for the underlying physiological condition in addition to the code for the mental disorder.

Neurological Conditions

Both physical and occupational therapists may treat patients with neurological conditions. These include degenerative neurological conditions such as **multiple sclerosis (MS)**, a disease that affects the central nervous system and causes nerve deterioration and damage, and **amyotrophic lateral sclerosis (ALS)**, also known as Lou Gehrig's Disease, a degenerative disease in which motor neurons slowly die causing muscle weakness, stiffness, and twitching, and for which there is no cure.

Stroke and intracerebral incidents may also result in a range of physical or neurological conditions, such as paralysis and dysphasia. Coding for strokes and intracerebral incidents, such as intracranial hemorrhage and cerebral infarction requires close attention to detail. It is important to understand the difference between a service that is provided to a patient who is currently experiencing a cerebrovascular incident (patient is receiving acute care for the incident), and one who is receiving services for the sequela (late effects) of the incident. Cerebrovascular diseases (I60–I69) are identified as either the current cerebrovascular disease (I60–I66) (the acute incident), or a specific sequela following the cerebrovascular disease (I69) (the late effect of the incident).

For example, if a patient is admitted to the hospital for a cerebral infarction due to an embolism of the basilar artery, then the code reported would be I63.12, Cerebral infarction due to embolism of basilar artery. This diagnosis code would be reported for all services provided to treat the cerebral infarction, such as imaging or surgical services. This is an acute code that is only reported when the cerebral infarction or stroke is actually happening.

Figure 16.8. OGCR I.C.9.d.1 through I.C.9.d.3

---

d. **Sequelae of Cerebrovascular Disease**

    1) Category I69, Sequelae of Cerebrovascular disease

Category I69 is used to indicate conditions classifiable to categories I60-I67 as the causes of sequela (neurologic deficits), themselves classified elsewhere. These "late effects" include neurologic deficits that persist after initial onset of conditions classifiable to categories I60-I67. The neurologic deficits caused by cerebrovascular disease may be present from the onset or may arise at any time after the onset of the condition classifiable to categories I60-I67.

Codes from category I69, Sequelae of cerebrovascular disease, that specify hemiplegia, hemiparesis and monoplegia identify whether the dominant or nondominant side is affected. Should the affected side be documented, but not specified as dominant or nondominant, and the classification system does not indicate a default, code selection is as follows:

• For ambidextrous patients, the default should be dominant.
• If the left side is affected, the default is non-dominant.
• If the right side is affected, the default is dominant.

    2) Codes from category I69 with codes from I60-I67

Codes from category I69 may be assigned on a health care record with codes from I60-I67, if the patient has a current cerebrovascular disease and deficits from an old cerebrovascular disease.

    3) Codes from category I69 and Personal history of transient ischemic attack (TIA) and cerebral infarction (Z86.73)

Codes from category I69 should not be assigned if the patient does not have neurologic deficits.
See Section I.C.21. 4. History (of) for use of personal history codes

---

Source: CMS 2019.

However, therapists only treat the sequela that arise from a stroke—difficulty swallowing or speaking, paralysis, or deficits in cognitive functioning—so it would be incorrect to code for the actual cerebrovascular disease. Instead, report the code for the sequela(e) of the disease, such as cognitive or speech deficits (from category I69). For example, if the patient with the cerebral infarction of the basilar artery suffered hemiplegia due to the infarction, and the patient is receiving physical or occupational therapy to treat the hemiplegia, then the code reported would be I69.351, Hemiplegia and hemiparesis following cerebral infarction affecting right dominant side.

Note that many neurological conditions, because they are life-long and sometimes degenerative diseases, are included in HCC coding and should be coded to the highest specificity possible with complete documentation. See figure 16.8 for the OGCR related to sequela of cerebrovascular diseases.

Key to Success

All codes for sequelae of cerebrovascular diseases are found in category I69 of the ICD-10-CM code book. These codes should not be used to identify the specific type of cerebrovascular disease, but rather the effect resulting from the cerebrovascular disease, like cognitive or speech deficits or paralysis. Pay attention to the guidelines in the Tabular List of the ICD-10-CM code book, as reporting codes for additional or specific types of sequelae may be necessary. If the effects of the cerebrovascular disease are unknown or undocumented, or if there are no sequelae, assign a code from category I60 to I66.

Speech Therapy Conditions

Speech therapy and speech language pathology services are provided to patients who have problems swallowing, speaking, and hearing, as well as patients who need rehabilitation because of a communication disorder. As in diagnosis coding for physical and occupational therapy services, codes that identify the medical necessity for SLP services are found throughout the ICD-10-CM code book. SLPs also treat patients who are experiencing sequela of a stroke or cerebrovascular incident and paralytic syndromes, in addition to those with congenital anomalies and malformations, such as cleft lip or palate. Additional conditions include the following.

- *Neoplasms.* Benign and malignant neoplasms may affect a patient's ability to speak, hear, swallow, or otherwise communicate. They include neoplasms of the lip, tongue, parts of the mouth, tonsil, oropharynx, and esophagus, as well as nasal cavity, middle ear, larynx, and trachea. When coding for neoplasms, remember the basics of neoplasm code selection (refer to chapter 4 for the basics on how to code from the Table of Neoplasms).
    - If the histologic type (morphology) of the neoplasm is known, search for the histologic type of neoplasm in the ICD-10-CM Index. If not, then search the Table of Neoplasms for the site of the neoplasm.
    - Once the site of the neoplasm is located, find the code in the Table of Neoplasms that identifies the type of neoplasm—either malignant, benign, uncertain, or unspecified. Malignant neoplasms are identified as either primary, secondary, or carcinoma in situ (ca in situ).
    - Verify the code for the neoplasm in the Tabular List.
    - If the patient has a history of neoplasm and is no longer undergoing treatment for the condition, then report the code for history of neoplasm.

If the neoplasm has been removed but the patient is still undergoing treatment for the neoplasm (such as chemotherapy), then report the code for the neoplasm as if it still exists. For example, if a patient had undergone a partial glossectomy (removal of the tongue) due to primary malignancy of the tongue, and is now receiving chemotherapy for the treatment of the neoplasm, in addition to SLP services for rehabilitation of speech, then the coder would report the code for the neoplasm (because the patient is still undergoing treatment for the neoplasm, even though it was already excised) and the code(s) for any speech deficits or other problems requiring treatment.

- *Developmental Disorders.* Developmental disorders related to speech and language (F80, Specific developmental disorders of speech and language), scholastic skills (F81, Specific developmental disorders of scholastic skills), motor function (F82, Specific developmental disorder of motor function), and pervasive developmental disorders (F84, Pervasive developmental disorders) may require SLP services to help the patient communicate effectively with others. For example, a patient with F80.0, Phonological disorder, may require SLP services to help with functional speech, remove a lisp, or improve articulation of specific sounds. Report any additional codes for associated hearing loss, medical or neurological condition, or intellectual disability. Note that pervasive developmental disorders (category F84) are included in HCC coding and should be assigned with care.

- *Dentofacial anomalies.* Dentofacial anomalies (M26) are malformations of the jaw and face, resulting from abnormal dental or facial growth. Although they are musculoskeletal in origin, these anomalies can affect the patient's ability to speak or form words and may require speech therapy services.

- *Signs and symptoms.* Speech therapy services may also be required to treat the signs and symptoms of other or undiagnosed disorders. These include category R47, Speech disturbances, not elsewhere classified, which includes codes for dysphasia (difficulty speaking) and other speech disturbances. If an underlying condition is causing the speech disturbance, it should be reported in addition to the fluency or speech disorder. Category R48, Dyslexia and other symbolic dysfunctions, not elsewhere classified, includes the codes for **dyslexia** (difficulty reading) and other symbolic dysfunctions. Category R49, Voice and resonance disorders, includes codes for **aphonia** (loss of voice) and **hypernasality** (excessive nasal tone to the voice). Swallowing disorders are reported with codes from category R13, Aphagia and dysphagia. Dysphagia codes identify the specific phase of dysphagia. When a patient suffers dysphagia due to a stroke or cerebrovascular incident, report the sequela of stroke code and the dysphagia code.

Key to Success

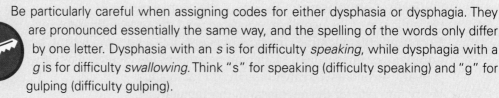

Be particularly careful when assigning codes for either dysphasia or dysphagia. They are pronounced essentially the same way, and the spelling of the words only differ by one letter. Dysphasia with an *s* is for difficulty *speaking*, while dysphagia with a *g* is for difficulty *swallowing*. Think "s" for speaking (difficulty speaking) and "g" for gulping (difficulty gulping).

Complete the exercises in There's a Code for That 16.3 to practice reporting diagnosis codes for physical, occupational, and speech therapy services.

PT, OT, and ST diagnosis coding

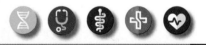

16.3

There's a Code for That

Read the following documentation and assign the appropriate diagnosis code(s) for the patient's condition(s).

1. A 12-year-old male with cerebral palsy and spastic diplegia.

   ICD-10-CM code: _____

2. Late stage Huntington's disease.

   ICD-10-CM code: _____

3. A 70-year-old female with primary osteoarthritis of the right knee with knee stiffness following total right knee arthroplasty presents for physical therapy including range of motion exercises.

   ICD-10-CM codes: _____ , _____ ,

   _____

4. A 50-year-old male with chronic posterior cervicalgia, increasing over the last 6 weeks.

   ICD-10-CM codes: _____ , _____

Putting It All Together: Coding for Therapy Services

Coding correctly for therapy services requires an understanding of the services provided by physical, occupational, and speech therapists, the specific selection of CPT codes they use, and the ability to assign diagnosis codes from various chapters of the ICD-10-CM code book.

Determination of the correct codes relies on the answers to the following questions.

- What type of therapy procedure was performed? If the service was an evaluation, was it an initial or re-evaluation, and what level of service was provided?

- For physical and occupational therapy services, is the service represented by a time-based code or a service-based code? If the code is time based, how much time was spent providing the service?

- Were any additional procedures performed?

- Are there any applicable modifiers for the procedure?

- Is the service related to a prior medical procedure? If so, report the code for aftercare as well as any additional related codes for the prior procedure.

- Is there a debility identified? Is there a definitive diagnosis for the procedure? If so, then code for both the definitive diagnosis and the debility.
  - If multiple therapeutic services were provided, each service must be linked with the appropriate ICD-10-CM codes to identify the medical necessity for the service provided.
- Are there any additional or underlying conditions that need to be reported, such as an underlying mental or neurological disability or intellectual disability?

The following vignette demonstrates how to select the appropriate diagnosis and procedure codes. After reviewing the vignette, complete the exercises in There's a Code for That 16.4 to practice coding for therapy services.

Juan has been working in healthcare billing and coding for a few years and has just moved to a new city where he got a job as a coder in a therapy practice. His new workplace employs about 30 different therapy providers, each of whom performs services at multiple different locations around the city. The therapists who work for his practice include physical, occupational, and speech therapists. Juan is coding for the services provided by the therapists at the therapy group and is working on coding the following physical therapy note: 72-year-old female patient was seen at the clinic for the first time after a subarachnoid hemorrhage (CVA). Sequela from the CVA includes monoplegia of right arm (patient is left-handed), resulting in inability to perform functional ADLs (activities of daily living) and lack of normal mobility. Her healthcare history is also significant for essential hypertension, type II diabetes, and urge incontinence. A high-complexity physical therapy evaluation concluded that the patient's plan of care will include therapeutic exercises to increase the range of motion of the right arm and shoulder, with strengthening exercises of the right side. Functional training to assist in overall mobility and balance, posture, and gait training.

Juan asks himself: What did the therapist do? In this case, the therapist performed a high complexity physical therapy evaluation and developed a plan of care, including therapeutic exercises and functional training. Only the evaluation was performed at this point and no actual therapeutic services were performed. He selects the following code for the physical therapy evaluation:

- *97163, Physical therapy evaluation: high complexity*

Now that Juan has the procedure code, he asks himself: Why did the therapist do it? In this case, the patient has monoplegia of the upper right (nondominant) arm (because the patient is left-handed), due to a subarachnoid hemorrhage, as well as three other significant conditions: essential hypertension, type II diabetes, and urge incontinence. He knows that to code for the sequela of subarachnoid hemorrhage, he needs to use a combination code from category I69 to identify both the hemiplegia as well as the CVA. He selects the following codes for the patient's conditions:

- *I69.033, Monoplegia of upper limb following nontraumatic subarachnoid hemorrhage affecting right nondominant side*
- *I10, Essential (primary) hypertension*
- *E11.9, Type 2 diabetes mellitus without complications*
- *N39.41, Urge incontinence*

He then rechecks the documentation to make sure he has coded everything for the encounter and reports the chosen codes.

Diagnostic and procedural coding for therapy services

Read the following documentation and assign the appropriate CPT, HCPCS, and ICD-10-CM code(s) for the encounter.

1. A 16-year-old male is admitted to inpatient rehab; status post complete spinal cord injury at the T12 level resulting in complete paraplegia below the T12 level. Plan of care was developed at the last encounter and today patient received 40 minutes of wheelchair training including rolling, posture changes, transfers, and wheelchair mobility of different surfaces.

    CPT code: _____ × _____

    ICD-10-CM codes: _____ , _____

2. An 85-year-old male sustained a subarachnoid hemorrhage in his home 3 weeks ago. He now suffers from right-sided hemiparesis, difficulty swallowing, and expressive aphasia. SLP completed an evaluation of oral and pharyngeal swallowing function and diagnosed the patient with oropharyngeal dysphagia.

    CPT code: _____

    ICD-10-CM codes: _____ , _____

3. A 25-year-old female with Down Syndrome received 1 hour of work training, including money management and work task analysis.

    CPT code: _____

    ICD-10-CM codes: _____

Case Study   Physical Therapy Treatment

Physical Therapy Treatment Log

PATIENT: Herbert Simmons

Chief Complaint (C/C):
Patient presents for treatment of gait unsteadiness due to dragging of left foot after CVA two months ago. He reports that since his last treatment he has been able to stand without assistance but is still unstable walking and reports the use of a walker on a daily basis.

Daily Treatment Log:
Patient was seated in chair and was instructed in strengthening exercises for the left lower extremity (LLE), to decrease foot drop during walking. This instruction was provided prior to functional mobility (ambulation) training. During this training, the patient required a minimal number of verbal cues and physical demonstration to complete each exercise, which was completed using 1.5 lb ankle weights for bilateral knee flexion and extension.

Patient was then trained in ankle dorsiflexion, plantar flexion, and inversion/eversion for a 3-second hold per flexion. During this training, the patient required constant maximal verbal and physical cues to reduce compensatory angulation.

Patient then completed standing exercises with aid of the physical therapist, which included bilateral heel raises (with support), using a mirror for visual feedback to ensure proper form.

Total time for combined therapy services was 30 minutes, including time required to allow for therapeutic rest. Patient reports that therapies have consistently helped him strengthen his LLE and walk without dragging his foot as often. Patient still requires the use of his walker for ambulation. Will return to clinic in one week, having instructed patient on how to complete additional strengthening exercises at home.

SIGNED: Santosh Ashokprabhu, PT

Use the following steps to select the appropriate codes for the case study. As you read, look up any medical or procedural terms with which you are unfamiliar.

1. Read through the case study and answer the question: *What did the therapist do?* In this case study, identify the name of the procedure.

   _____

   _____

2. Now that you have identified the procedure, locate the code for the procedure in the CPT code book.
   a. Search the Index for the procedure and search through the options. If there are multiple options, identify the most appropriate code option and refer to the code listed in the Tabular section.

   _____

   _____

   b. In the listing of codes, check for any guidelines, important definitions, or parenthetical notes. Select the code that correctly identifies all of the components of the procedure and list it.

   _____

   _____

   c. Are there any additional procedures that need to be added to identify all of the procedures performed? If yes, follow the previous steps to identify the codes for the additional procedures.

   _____

   _____

   d. Are there any modifiers that need to be added to identify any special circumstance surrounding the procedure(s)? If yes, refer to Appendix A of the CPT code book to assign all appropriate modifiers.

   _____

   _____

3. Now that the procedure(s) and modifier(s) have been identified, refer to the case study and answer the following question: *Why did the therapist do it?* From the case study, identify the patient's diagnosis (note that there may be multiple diagnoses):

_____

_____

4. Now that you have identified the patient's diagnoses, search the ICD-10-CM code book for the correct code for this condition.

a. Search the Main Index for the name of the condition and search through any applicable subterms and cross-references to locate the appropriate code.

_____

_____

b. Verify the codes in the Tabular List. Locate the code identified previously in the Tabular Listing of codes and refer to any applicable guidelines, notes, and symbols. Does the code selected correctly identify the patient's condition? If yes, list the code.

_____

_____

5. Now that the procedure and diagnosis codes have been identified, list them on the CMS-1500 form.

21. DIAGNOSIS OR NATURE OF ILLNESS OR INJURY Relate A-L to service line below (24E)			ICD Ind.	22. RESUBMISSION CODE
A. |_____	B. |_____	C. |_____	D. |_____	
E. |_____	F. |_____	G. |_____	H. |_____	23. PRIOR AUTHORIZATION NU
I. |_____	J. |_____	K. |_____	L. |_____	

24. A. DATE(S) OF SERVICE From / To		B. PLACE OF SERVICE	C. EMG	D. PROCEDURES, SERVICES, OR SUPPLIES (Explain Unusual Circumstances) CPT/HCPCS | MODIFIER	E. DIAGNOSIS POINTER	F. $ CHARGES	G. DAYS OR UNITS
MM DD YY	MM DD YY						
1							
2							
3							

End-of-Chapter Content

Instructions: Indicate whether the following statements are true or false (T or F). For false statements, rewrite the statement on the line below to make the statement true.

1. A physical therapist specializes in procedures on activities of daily living that require fine motor skills.

_____

_____

(Continued on next page)

(Continued)

2. SLPs treat speaking problems such as fluency, problems with voice resonance, and problems with pronunciation.

_____

_____

3. Therapy providers never need a request from a healthcare provider to begin therapy services.

_____

_____

4. Medicare has no limit to the amount of therapy services that can be billed within a calendar year.

_____

_____

5. A treatment modality for physical therapy services is a method of therapeutic treatment.

_____

_____

6. Iontophoresis is a type of electrical stimulation.

_____

_____

7. The 8-minute rule is used for service-based codes.

_____

_____

8. Some of the codes for occupational therapy services can be found in the Special Otorhinolaryngologic Services subsection of the CPT code book.

_____

_____

9. Augmentative and alternative communication (AAC) does not include oral communication.

_____

_____

10. Joint pain is a condition commonly treated by physical therapists.

_____

_____

Instructions: Choose the best answer.

1. Which of the following therapists would perform therapeutic exercises on a patient to help them with swallowing function?
   a. Speech language pathologist
   b. Physical therapist
   c. Occupational therapist
   d. Oral-maxillofacial surgeon

2. Which of the following activities would a physical therapist assist a patient in performing?
   a. Brushing teeth
   b. Speaking
   c. Walking
   d. Eating with a fork

3. Which of the following activities would an occupational therapist help a patient in performing?
   a. Balancing while standing up
   b. Understanding directions
   c. Debriding a wound
   d. Writing with a pencil

4. Which modifier should be used when an ABN may have been required but was not obtained from the patient?
   a. GA
   b. GX
   c. GY
   d. GZ

5. Which of the following is a key component of physical therapy evaluations?
   a. Development of plan of care
   b. Medical evaluation and management
   c. Pharmaceutical management
   d. Prescription of medications

6. Which of the following codes identifies a re-evaluation for occupational therapy services?
   a. 97165
   b. 97164
   c. 97163
   d. 97168

7. Which type of device applies external pressure to the soft tissues and is used to decrease swelling?
   a. Vasopneumatic
   b. Iontophoresis
   c. Diathermy
   d. Whirlpool

8. Using the 8-minute rule, how many units would you report for a therapeutic service that took 43 minutes to complete?
   a. 3
   b. 4
   c. 5
   d. 6

9. Which of the following codes identifies an evaluation for the use of an AAC device to supplement oral speaking?
   a. 92597
   b. 92605
   c. 92609
   d. 92607

10. Which of the following includes problems with understanding or producing oral speech?
    a. Cognitive communication disorders
    b. Social communication disorders
    c. Language disorders
    d. All of the above

11. When searching the ICD-10-CM Index for joint pain of the right hip, which term do you search for first?
    a. Joint
    b. Pain
    c. Right
    d. Hip

12. Which of the following types of anomalies are malformations of the jaw and face?
    a. Oropharyngeal
    b. Dentofacial
    c. Congenital
    d. Hypernasal

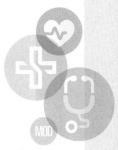

Instructions: Answer the following questions with the appropriate code(s) and modifier(s) when necessary.

1. A 65-year-old male with adhesive capsulitis of the shoulder receives 30 minutes of aquatic therapy with therapeutic exercises. Before therapy begins, PT places hot packs on the affected area for 15 minutes.

   CPT codes: _____ × _____ ,

   _____

   ICD-10 code: _____

2. A 7-year-old male is referred to SLP by his PCP. He was recently begun stuttering in his elementary class and he presents today for evaluation of speech fluency.

   CPT codes: _____

   ICD-10 code: _____

3. A 70-year-old male patient that underwent a bilateral knee replacement due to severe bilateral primary osteoarthritis of the knees now presents to the physical therapist for gait training due to difficulty walking.

   CPT code: _____

   ICD-10-CM codes: _____

References

American Speech-Language-Hearing Association (ASHA). n.d. *Speech-Language Pathologists.* http://www.asha.org/Students/Speech-Language-Pathologists/.

Centers for Medicare and Medicaid Services (CMS). 2019. ICD-10-CM Official Guidelines for Coding and Reporting FY 2020. https://www.cms.gov/Medicare/Coding/ICD10/Downloads/2020-Coding-Guidelines.pdf.

Centers for Medicare and Medicaid Services (CMS). 2018a (December). Medicare Coverage of Therapy Services. https://www.medicare.gov/Pubs/pdf/10988-Medicare-Limits-Therapy-Services.pdf.

Centers for Medicare and Medicaid Services. 2018b (October). Medicare Advance Beneficiary Notices. https://www.cms.gov/Outreach-and-Education/Medicare-Learning-Network-MLN/MLNProducts/downloads/abn_booklet_icn006266.pdf.

Jannenga, H. 2014 (June 3). Founder Letter: 97002 and 97004 (Re-Evaluation) Myths Debunked. https://www.webpt.com/blog/post/founder-letter-97002-and-97004-re-evaluation-myths-debunked.

Poule. 2009. "Minimo.jpg." Digital image. Wikimedia Commons. https://commons.wikimedia.org/wiki/File:Minimo.jpg.

Resources

American Academy of Professional Coders (AAPC). 2018. Build Up Physical and Occupational Therapy Know-how. https://www.aapc.com/blog/40864-build-up-physical-and-occupational-therapy-know-how/.

American Occupational Therapy Association (AOTA). n.d. What is Occupational Therapy? https://www.aota.org/Conference-Events/OTMonth/what-is-OT.aspx.

American Physical Therapy Association (APTA). 2019 (August 14). Identifying the Correct Codes for ICD-10 (ICD-10-CM). http://www.apta.org/ICD10/IdentifyingCodes/.

American Physical Therapy Association (APTA). 2019 (May 24). Who Are Physical Therapists? http://www.apta.org/AboutPTs/.

American Physical Therapy Association (APTA). 2018 (November 13). Coding Interpretations: Group Therapy Patient Scenarios. http://www.apta.org/Payment/Coding/GroupTherapyScenarios/.

American Speech-Language-Hearing Association (ASHA). n.d. Model Superbill for Speech-Language Pathology. http://www.asha.org/uploadedFiles/ModelSuperbillSLP.pdf.

Jannenga, H. 2016 (March 17). Physical Therapists' Guide to Billing. https://www.webpt.com/physical-therapists-guide-to-billing.

Jannenga, H. 2016 (February 2). Physical Therapists' Guide to the 8-Minute Rule. WebPT https://www.webpt.com/8-minute-rule.

Jannenga, H. 2016 (January 25). Physical Therapists' Guide to CPT Codes. https://www.webpt.com/cpt-codes.

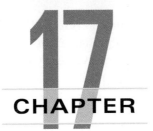

CHAPTER 17

Obstetrics and Gynecology Services

Learning Objectives

- Understand the basics of billing and coding for obstetrics and gynecology services
- Examine procedural codes and guidelines for obstetrics and gynecology services
- Examine diagnosis coding and medical necessity for obstetrics and gynecology services
- Determine and apply ICD-10-CM, CPT, and HCPCS codes to obstetrics and gynecology services

Key Terms

Abortion
Antepartum
Bartholin's glands
Birthing center
Cerclage
Certified nurse midwife (CNM)
Cervix uteri
Cesarean delivery
Conization
Corpus uteri
Diaphragm
Endocervical curettage (ECC)
External os
Fallopian tubes
Gestation
Gestational condition
Gravida
Gynecologists
Incidental pregnancy
Internal os
Intrauterine device (IUD)

Introitus
Labia majora
Labia minora
Last menstrual period (LMP)
Loop electrosurgical excision procedure (LEEP)
Marsupialization
Maternal fetal medicine (MFM) specialist
Maternity services
Non-obstetric
Nuchal cord
Nulligravida
Nulliparous
Obstetric
Obstetricians
Obstetrics and gynecology services
Outcome of delivery code
Ovaries
Oviducts
Parity (or para)

Perinatal
Perinatologist
Perineum
Peripartum
Pessary
Postpartum
Products of conception (POC)
Puerperium
Reproductive endocrinology and infertility (REI) specialist
Reproductive surgery
Sequencing priority
Sexually transmitted infection (STI)
Trimesters
Uterus
Vagina
Vaginal birth after cesarean (VBAC)
Vaginectomy
Vulva

Obstetrics and gynecology services (OB/GYN) are focused on the gynecological and reproductive health of female patients, as well as providing services for pregnant patients and performing deliveries. Obstetrics services are provided to pregnant patients and focus on the reproductive health of the patient, including managing the patient's pregnancy and delivering the fetus at childbirth. Gynecological services focus on the genital and reproductive health of female patients and include services to monitor, diagnose, and treat female patients. Gynecological services may also treat genitourinary conditions of female patients, which include conditions of the female genital and urinary systems, such as urinary tract infections or urinary incontinence.

Obstetrics and gynecology coding includes both gynecological and urinary system treatments and procedures on non-pregnant females, as well as maternity-related procedures on pregnant females. Coding for obstetric and gynecologic services requires an understanding of the medical terminology used and the services included in the global package for maternity care. This chapter discusses the basics of billing and coding for both gynecology and obstetrics, as well as the medical terminology used, and procedural and diagnostic coding for obstetrics and gynecology services.

Obstetrics and Gynecology Basics

Obstetrics and gynecology are often combined into one specialty, called OB/GYN (OB for obstetrics and GYN for gynecology) or OBGYNE. Although they are technically two different healthcare specialties, obstetricians and gynecologists often combine into small or large group practices that treat female patients throughout their life cycles, including during pregnancy.

Proper coding for OB/GYN services requires an understanding of the special services performed by each type of healthcare provider and the unique terminology used in the OB/GYN field.

OB/GYN Providers

Gynecologists are healthcare providers who specialize in the female reproductive system, including the vagina, uterus, and ovaries, as well as the breasts. Gynecologists also help diagnose and treat conditions that affect the urinary system, such as urinary tract infections, sexually transmitted diseases, and urinary incontinence. **Obstetricians** are healthcare providers who specialize in the health of a patient during pregnancy, childbirth, and the postpartum period. This includes managing the health, growth, and development of the pregnant mother and fetus, performing the delivery at childbirth, and providing necessary follow-up care for the mother after delivery. Obstetricians and gynecologists may also specialize in surgical treatments of the female genital and reproductive system, as well as the urinary system, such as surgery to correct urinary incontinence or hysterectomy.

Gynecologists and other primary care physicians or healthcare providers may see patients during pregnancy for non-pregnancy-related conditions (such as an injury), but these visits are to manage a health condition suffered by the pregnant female, and not to manage the pregnancy itself. Coders must interpret whether the services treat or manage the patient's pregnancy, or if the pregnancy is incidental to the patient's treatment. Incidental pregnancy coding is discussed later in this chapter.

As gynecologists and obstetricians specialize in reproductive health of female patients, some healthcare providers are qualified to perform both OB and GYN procedures. However, a major distinction in OB/GYN coding is the difference between obstetric and non-obstetric procedures and conditions. **Obstetric** refers to a procedure performed on a pregnant woman or condition related to a woman's pregnancy, such as a delivery or complication of pregnancy. These services are also referred to as **maternity services**. **Non-obstetric** refers to a procedure performed to treat or manage signs and symptoms, or other encounter for gynecological or genitourinary services, such as reproductive, urinary, and breast health. OB/GYN services are closely related and when coding for OB/GYN services, procedures and diagnosis codes are differentiated based on whether or not the patient in question is pregnant, and if the services were related to the patient's pregnancy. Non-obstetric procedures and treatments are usually performed by a gynecologist, and obstetric procedures are performed by an obstetrician.

Because of the range of OB/GYN services provided, coders should be aware of the different provider types and healthcare settings in which OB/GYN services are provided.

Additional OB/GYN Specialties and Subspecialties

There are a handful of additional healthcare specialists who perform OB/GYN services. Fortunately for the coder, these different specialties do not impact code selection for the services performed.

- **Certified nurse midwife (CNM).** As discussed in chapter 1 (Your Coding Career), a CNM is a mid-level practitioner with an advanced degree as a registered nurse in midwifery, the study of assisting pregnant females in obstetric care and childbirth, including the postpartum period, female care, and birth control. Remember that as a mid-level provider, CNMs must practice under a licensed physician. CNMs may or may not be licensed to perform deliveries, depending on the state in which they practice.

- **Maternal fetal medicine (MFM) specialist.** An MFM specialist, also known as a **perinatologist**, is a medical doctor who specializes in high-risk pregnancies and focuses on the health of the mother and fetus before, during, and after pregnancy. MFM doctors are obstetricians with additional training in managing the health of both the fetus and the mother during risky pregnancies, including additional testing, imaging services, and management of the pregnancy.

- **Reproductive endocrinology and infertility (REI) specialist.** Otherwise known as a fertility specialist, an REI is a medical doctor with additional training and expertise in human reproduction, including the function of hormones in reproduction. A related specialty is **reproductive surgery**, which focuses on surgical treatments to treat infertility. Reproductive surgery services are reported with codes from the Reproductive Medicine Procedures subsection (89250–89398) of the Laboratory and Pathology section of the CPT code book; refer to chapter 14 (Laboratory and Pathology Services).

Place of Service for OB/GYN Services

Depending on the service performed, both gynecologists and obstetricians may perform services in the outpatient office setting or surgeries and deliveries in the inpatient hospital setting. Deliveries may also be performed at a certified **birthing center**, a facility that specializes in providing a comfortable setting for labor, delivery, postpartum care, and immediate newborn care. Birthing centers are not hospitals, but they do have specialized equipment and trained staff to assist with healthcare needs. If a medical emergency occurs during the labor and delivery process, or with the newborn after childbirth, the patient may have to be transported to an inpatient hospital facility for evaluation and treatment. If an obstetrician performs any services at a birthing center, use POS code 25, for a "facility, other than a hospital's maternity facilities or a physician's office, which provides a setting for labor, delivery, and immediate postpartum care as well as immediate care of newborn infants" (AMA 2019).

Pregnancy Timeline and Terminology

When it comes to OB/GYN coding, especially coding for maternity services, it is important to understand the timeline of pregnancy, services involved, and terminology used to discuss pregnancy, childbirth, and the postpartum period. This terminology is used in both CPT and ICD-10-CM coding and is essential in reporting procedural codes for maternity services and diagnosis codes for pregnancy, childbirth, and the puerperium.

Pregnancy Timeline

Pregnancy-related services are reported along a continuum of care (that is, the pregnancy timeline), which begins at the patient's last menstrual period and ends six weeks after childbirth. The **last menstrual period (LMP)** is the first day of the patient's last period; this date is used to estimate the date of conception, and subsequently the estimated date of delivery, 40 weeks after the LMP. The period of pregnancy before childbirth is known as the **antepartum,** or pre-partum, period, and lasts 40 weeks (or until childbirth). The **postpartum** period extends after childbirth to six weeks post-delivery. The postpartum period is also referred to as the **puerperium** (from birth to six weeks after birth). The **peripartum** period pertains to the mother's health and healthcare services and extends from about one month before childbirth to up to five months after childbirth. The **perinatal** period also extends from before until after childbirth but pertains to the health and healthcare services for the fetus (and later newborn). The perinatal period extends from 20 to 28 weeks before childbirth to up to 6 weeks post-delivery. See figure 17.1 for a visual representation of the pregnancy timeline.

Figure 17.1. Pregnancy timeline

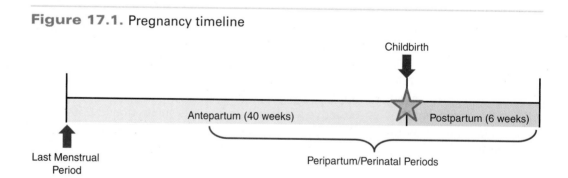

This timeline becomes more important later in this chapter when discussing maternity services and the global maternity package.

Pregnancy Terminology

There are several important terms regarding OB/GYN conditions, and this small section is by no means a full list of the medical terms a coder must know in order to report procedure and diagnosis codes for OB/GYN services. When coding for OB/

GYN services, remember to use a medical dictionary and any other available resources when confronted with an unfamiliar term or phrase.

Pregnant women are often referred to by their gravida status, such as G3P2. The "G" refers to **gravida**, which means pregnant female. The "P" means **parity** (or **para**), the number of previous pregnancies. The numbers between refer to the number of times the patient has been pregnant (after the G) and the number of times the patient has carried to full-term (after the P). For example, a G3P2 patient has been pregnant three times (G3) and carried to full-term twice (P2). This number-and-letter combination is used as a shorthand to refer to patients when they present for OB/GYN services. However, keep in mind that the gravida and parity status of a patient impacts code selection only for patients who are elderly, or if the patient has had multiple miscarriages or abortions (this is discussed later in this chapter). A **nulligravida** female is one who has never been pregnant, and a **nulliparous** female is one who has never carried a pregnancy longer than 20 weeks.

Trimesters of pregnancy are an additional concept that should be fully understood when coding for OB/GYN services. The 40 weeks of pregnancy are divided into three **trimesters**, which are roughly three-month periods into which the 40 weeks of pregnancy are grouped (see figure 17.2). The three trimesters are based on the following timeframes:

- *First trimester:* conception to 13 weeks, 6 days
- *Second trimester:* 14 weeks to 27 weeks, 6 days
- *Third trimester:* 28 weeks to delivery

Figure 17.2. Trimesters of pregnancy

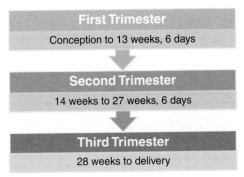

Many codes identify the specific trimester of pregnancy. Also important to understand is the estimated weeks of gestation, which is identified with an additional code. **Gestation** is the time between conception (the moment at which the egg is fertilized) and birth (when the fetus is delivered). There are approximately 40 weeks of gestation for a pregnant human female, divided into three trimesters.

Key to Success

When reporting codes for any type of obstetric or maternity service, keep in mind the difference between the pregnant woman (mother) and the fetus (child). Many terms are similar but refer to either the mother or the baby. For example, the peripartum period refers to the mother's health, while the perinatal period refers to the growth and development of the fetus and eventually the newborn. This is also important to keep in mind when reporting diagnosis codes for the mother versus the baby, as sometimes the codes are similar and difficult to distinguish from one another. Remember, all OB/GYN services are provided on the pregnant female patient. Any services provided to the infant, once born, are provided by a pediatrician or neonatal specialist. A neonatal specialist is a medical doctor who typically works in a Neonatal Intensive Care Unit (NICU) of a hospital to provide intensive care to severely ill or premature infants.

Just as with OB/GYN terminology, there is a difference between OB/GYN services provided to patients who are not pregnant (non-obstetric services) and services provided to pregnant patients. Diagnosis codes also differ based on whether or not the patient is pregnant, and if that pregnancy is related to the service(s) performed or if it is incidental to the services performed.

Procedural Coding for OB/GYN Services

Procedural coding for OB/GYN services depends on whether or not the service was maternity-related. Non-obstetric surgical services are coded from the Female Genital subsection of the CPT code book, and obstetric services are coded from the Maternity subsection of the CPT code book. Evaluation and management (E/M) codes are also commonly reported in the outpatient office setting for gynecological services, as most office visits are reported with an E/M code, using additional codes to identify either procedures performed in the office or surgical procedures performed in the hospital setting.

Key to Success

Many healthcare specialties like OB/GYN report a great deal of E/M codes, as these codes identify outpatient office visits. If the decision for surgery or other medical treatment or diagnostic service is made during an office visit, then additional codes from throughout the CPT code book are used to identify the subsequent services performed.

Gynecology Services

Most gynecology services use E/M codes for outpatient office visits. If a patient is seen and no surgical, medicine, imaging, or laboratory procedures are performed, the encounter should be reported with the appropriate E/M code. For example, if a patient presents to the office of her gynecologist for an annual female examination, this service is reported with the appropriate E/M code. For a reminder of how to correctly select and report and E/M services, refer to chapter 8 (Primary Care).

If, at the E/M encounter, a decision for surgery is made, or if a procedure is performed in addition to the E/M encounter (such as the insertion of an intrauterine device), that service is reported with the appropriate code from the Female Genital subsection of the CPT code book. Note, however, that it is not always appropriate to report an E/M code with the minor surgical procedure code (like the insertion of an IUD). The E/M service must be a significant, separately identifiable service from the minor surgical procedure, as the minor surgical procedure already includes payment for the pre-procedure, intra-procedure, and post-procedure work (refer to chapter 11 for the components of the surgical package).

The Female Genital subsection is organized according to the anatomy of the female genital system, beginning with the vulva, perineum, and introitus; followed by the vagina, cervix uteri, corpus uteri, oviducts; and then the ovaries.

Vulva, Perineum, and Introitus

The external female genitalia are comprised of the vulva, perineum, and introitus (see figure 17.3). The **perineum** is the area between the vagina and the anus. The **vulva** consists of the labia (both labia majora and labia minora), the bulb of the vestibule, vestibule of the vagina, the greater vestibular glands (known as **Bartholin's glands**, which secrete mucus to lubricate the vagina), the lesser vestibular gland, and the vagina orifice, also known as the **introitus**. The **labia majora** is the tissue that surrounds the labia minora and the clitoris. The **labia minora** surrounds the vaginal vestibule and the external urethra.

Figure 17.3. External female genitalia

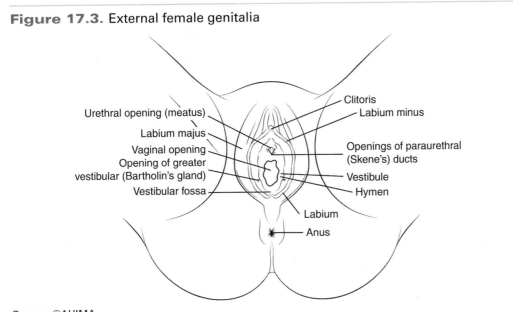

Source: ©AHIMA.

Procedures on the external female genitalia include incision and drainage of abscesses, and marsupialization of Bartholin's gland cysts. **Marsupialization** is a procedure in which a cyst is incised along one edge to form an open pouch, and then sutured open to allow for continuous drainage (see figure 17.4). This procedure is coded with 56440, Marsupialization of Bartholin's gland cyst.

Vulvar lesions may be biopsied, destroyed, or removed. Destruction of vulvar lesions is categorized based on whether the destruction was simple (56501) or extensive (56515), and includes destruction by any method (laser surgery, electrosurgery, cryosurgery, or chemosurgery). Remember that destruction of a lesion is different than *excision* of a lesion. In lesion excision, the tissue or lesion is removed via a scalpel or sharp edge, whereas with destruction, the tissue is destroyed and there is nothing left. There is one code for biopsy of vulvar or perineal lesion, 56605, Biopsy of vulva or perineum (separate procedure); *1 lesion*, with an add-on code for each additional lesion: 56606, Biopsy of vulva or perineum (separate procedure); *each separate additional lesion*.

Figure 17.4. Marsupialization of Bartholin's gland cyst

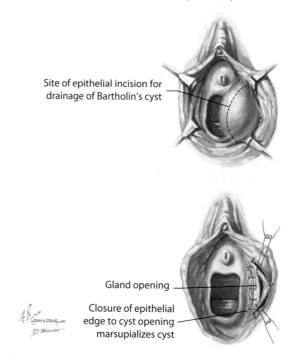

Site of epithelial incision for drainage of Bartholin's cyst

Gland opening

Closure of epithelial edge to cyst opening marsupializes cyst

Excision of vulvar lesions are based on two different principles—the depth of the removal and the extent of the removal. These definitions apply to vulvectomy codes found in codes 56620 through 56640. The depth of a vulvectomy is referred to as either simple or radical:

- A *simple* vulvectomy is the removal of the skin and superficial tissues.
- A *radical* vulvectomy is the removal of the skin and deep subcutaneous tissues.

Vulvectomies are also described according to the extent of the tissue removal, or how large of a surface area of tissue was removed. These are either partial or complete:

- A *partial* vulvectomy is the removal of less than 80 percent of the vulvar area.
- A *complete* vulvectomy is the removal of more than 80 percent of the vulvar area.

When coding for a vulvectomy, both the depth and the extent of the removal must be identified, as in code 56620, Vulvectomy simple; partial. This code reports a simple, partial vulvectomy—the removal of only skin and subcutaneous tissues of less than 80 percent of the vulvar area.

Vagina

The **vagina** is the lower portion of the birth canal, which serves as the conduit for the birth of a fetus, uterine secretions and menstrual flow, and the receptacle for semen from a male during intercourse. The medical prefix for vagina is *colpo-*, and many of the procedural terms in this subheading use this prefix. For example, a *colposcopy* is an endoscopic examination of the vagina, and a *colporrhaphy* is the surgical repair of the vagina.

Procedures on the vagina are more varied in nature and include incision, destruction, excision, introduction, repair, and endoscopy. Incision (57000–57023) procedures performed for drainage of abscesses and hematomas. Note that code 57022, Incision and drainage of vaginal hematoma; *obstetrical/postpartum*, reports the drainage of a hematoma (blood-filled sac) that was related to an obstetric or postpartum condition, whereas code 57023, Incision and drainage of vaginal hematoma; *non-obstetrical (eg, post-trauma, spontaneous bleeding)*, is for the same procedure but due to a non-obstetric condition. Always remember this difference when reporting codes for female genital procedures, as it often results in the selection of a different code.

Additional procedures on the vagina include destruction of vaginal lesions and excisions. Excision codes are divided based on whether the procedure was a biopsy, either simple or extensive (57100, 57105), or a **vaginectomy** (removal of all or part of the vagina). Vaginectomy codes (57106–57135) are categorized based on whether the removal is a partial removal of the vaginal wall (the selective removal of the upper or lower portion of the vagina), or if it was a complete removal of the vaginal wall. Both partial and complete removals have additional codes to identify the removal of paravaginal tissue (radical vaginectomy) with or without bilateral total pelvic lymphadenectomy and para-aortic lymph node sampling (biopsy). Vaginectomy procedures may or may not be followed with plastic repairs of the vagina.

Introduction procedures of the vagina include irrigation or application of therapeutic substances for bacterial, parasitic, or fungoid diseases (57150), as well as the insertion of brachytherapy elements. Brachytherapy is a type of radiation treatment for cancer and is discussed in chapter 18 (Healthcare Specialist Services, Part I). Many of the body systems throughout the CPT surgical section include the insertion of brachytherapy elements, including female genital, male genital, and urinary systems.

Also in the introduction category is code 57160, Fitting and insertion of a pessary or other intravaginal support device. A **pessary** is a small device placed inside the vagina to support the internal structures of the female reproductive system such as the uterus, vagina, bladder, or rectum (see figure 17.5). They can be used to help treat pelvic organ prolapse or stress incontinence, for example. Code 57170, Diaphragm or cervical cap fitting with instructions, is for the manual fitting of a diaphragm. A **diaphragm** is a barrier birth control method in which a small, cup-like device is placed over the cervix during intercourse, along with spermicide, that is later removed (see figure 17.6).

Figure 17.5. Pessary

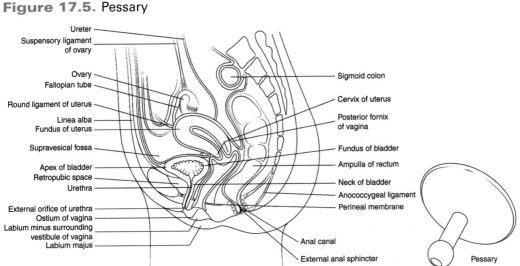

Source: ©AHIMA.

When the procedure for either a pessary or a diaphragm is performed, the pessary or diaphragm is also supplied to the patient. The supply of the actual device is reported with the appropriate HCPCS code, such as A4561, Pessary, rubber, any type, A4562, Pessary, non-rubber, any type, or A4261, Cervical cap for contraceptive use.

Vaginal repairs are reported with codes 57200 through 57335. Codes depend on the specific type of repair, whether the procedure is obstetric or non-obstetric, and the approach to the procedure.

Figure 17.6. Insertion of diaphragm

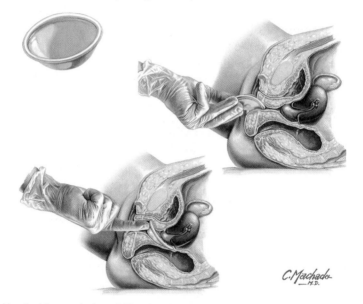

Also included in these codes are procedures for stress incontinence—when physical movement or stress, such as a sneeze or jumping up and down, causes a leakage of urine. Code 57288, Sling operation for stress incontinence (eg, fascia or synthetic), reports an open approach to the procedure. The procedure for stress incontinence performed via a laparoscopic approach is reported with code 51992, Laparoscopy, surgical; sling operation for stress incontinence (eg, fascia or synthetic), which is in the urinary system section of codes.

Endoscopic examinations and procedures of the vagina are reported with codes 57420 through 57426. However, it is important to pay attention to the notes in this section, as they identify additional or more appropriate codes when more than just the vagina is visualized or accessed during the procedure. For example, under code 57421, Colposcopy of the entire vagina, with cervix if present; with biopsy(s) of vagina/cervix, are parenthetical notes including: *For colposcopic visualization of cervix and adjacent upper vagina, use 57452.* This section of codes also includes three laparoscopic procedures of the vagina (57423–57426).

Cervix Uteri

The **cervix uteri**, also known as the cervix, is the lowest part of the uterus, about two to three centimeters long and round in shape, and forms a canal from the upper portion of the vagina to the uterus (see figure 17.7). The lower end of the cervix is called the **external os**, and the upper end, which opens into the uterus, is called the **internal os**.

The cervical canal allows sperm to travel from the vagina to the uterus, and flattens and dilates during vaginal childbirth to open and allow for the passage of the fetus from the uterus through the birth canal.

Procedures on the cervix include biopsies performed to check for malignant cells and removal of cervical tissue (Endoscopy codes located in the range 57452 through 57461; Excision codes located in 57500 to 57558 range). When coding for an excision of cervical tissue, it is necessary to identify the manner in which the procedure was performed—either via endoscope or excision—as well as whether the excision of tissue was for a biopsy, and the manner in which the tissue was removed. Cervical tissue removals are performed via the following procedures.

Figure 17.7. Cervix uteri, corpus uteri, oviducts, and ovaries

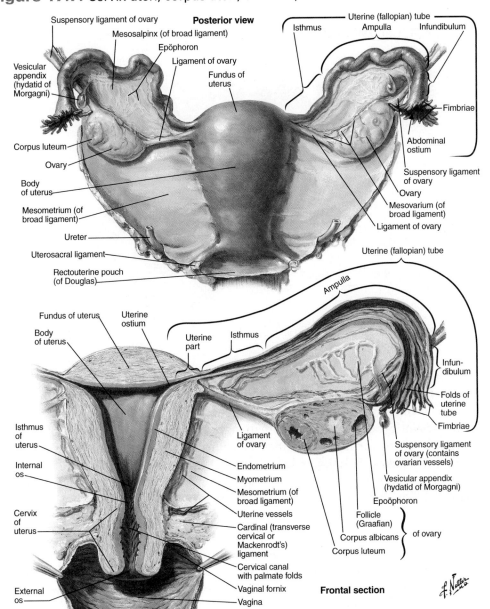

- **Endocervical curettage (ECC).** Procedure in which a curette is used to scrape cells off the cervical canal. For example, code 57505, Endocervical curettage (not done as part of a dilation and curettage).

- **Loop electrosurgical excision procedure (LEEP).** Procedure in which a fine wire with an electrical charge is used to remove cervical tissue. An LEEP may be performed for biopsy or excisional purposes. For example, code 57522, Conization of cervix, with or without fulguration, with or without dilation and curettage, with or without repair; loop electrode excision.

- **Conization.** A procedure that uses either an electrical wire (LEEP), cold knife, or laser to remove a cone of tissue from the cervix, either for diagnostic purposes (biopsy) or to remove cancerous or pre-cancerous cells (see figure 17.8). For example, code 57461, Colposcopy of the cervix including upper/adjacent vagina; with loop electrode conization of the cervix.

Figure 17.8. Conization of the cervix with cold knife

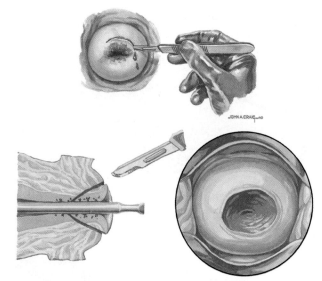

Source: ©2008. Used with permission of Elsevier. All rights reserved.

Additional procedures performed on the cervix uteri include repair, including cerclage of the cervix. A **cerclage** of the cervix is a stitch or band device that helps the cervix remain closed at the external os. It can be done either for cervical incompetence in a non-obstetric case, or during pregnancy in women with history of cervical incompetence or miscarriage. Note that the codes for cerclage reflect whether or not the patient is obstetric: 57700, Cerclage of uterine cervix, nonobstetrical, versus 59320, Cerclage of cervix, during pregnancy; vaginal, or 59325, Cerclage of cervix, during pregnancy; abdominal.

Corpus Uteri

The **corpus uteri**, also known as the uterus, is the body of the uterus above the internal os of the cervix and connects to the fallopian tubes at the fundus at the top of the uterus (refer to figure 17.7). Lined with endometrial cells, the **uterus** is where the fetus develops during gestation.

Procedures on the uterus include excisions, which range from biopsy of endometrial cells in the lining of the uterus to the complete removal of the uterus, cervix, ovaries, and fallopian tubes. When reporting codes for any type of removal procedure, it is important to first determine the components included in the procedure. For example, was the procedure a biopsy and, if so, what tissue was biopsied? If the procedure was an excision of the uterus, what additional components were removed (uterus, cervix, fallopian tubes, or ovaries)? Furthermore, how was the procedure performed? Open excisions of the uterus are reported with codes 58100 through 58294, whereas laparoscopic procedures are reported with codes 58541 through 58579 and 58674. Total hysterectomy codes depend on the weight of the excised organ—250 g or less, or 250 g or more.

There are also introduction procedures in the uterus; for example, the introduction or removal of **intrauterine device (IUD)**—58300, Insertion of intrauterine device (IUD), or 58301, Removal of intrauterine device (IUD). An IUD is a small, T-shaped device inserted into the uterus for birth control purposes (see figure 17.9). Like coding for the fitting or insertion of a pessary or diaphragm, the HCPCS code for the IUD itself is needed when reporting the insertion of an IUD, as in code J7300, Intrauterine copper contraceptive.

Figure 17.9. Intrauterine device

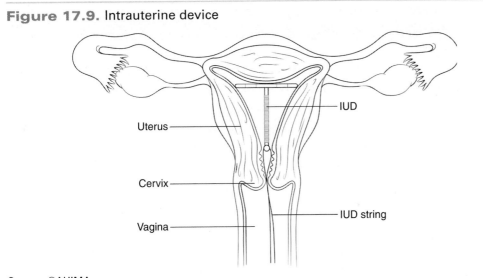

Source: ©AHIMA.

Oviducts and Ovaries

The **oviducts**, also known as the **fallopian tubes**, are the ducts through which eggs released from the ovaries travel. The fallopian tubes are attached to the fundus of the uterus and resemble long tubes, ending with small finger-like fimbriae. The **ovaries** are the glands found on either side of the uterus, below and behind the fallopian tubes, anchored to the uterus with suspensory ligaments. The ovaries form eggs that are released at regular intervals and travel through the fallopian tubes into the uterus where they are either fertilized by sperm or shed by the body (refer to figure 17.7).

Procedures on the oviducts include ligation, transection, or occlusion of the fallopian tubes for birth control purposes (Incision, 58600–58615) and laparoscopic procedures on the fallopian tubes (Laparoscopy 58660–58679). When coding for the excision of fallopian tubes, it is necessary to identify the procedure as either the removal of just the fallopian tubes (58700, Salpingectomy, complete or partial, unilateral or bilateral (separate procedure)) or removal of both the fallopian tubes and the ovaries (58720, Salpingo-oophorectomy, complete or partial, unilateral or bilateral (separate procedure)).

Codes for the removal of ovaries identify the type of removal (biopsy, wedge resection or bisection, cystectomy, or total removal) and additional components included in the excision procedure, such as lymphadenectomy or omentectomy.

Key to Success

When coding for procedures performed on the fallopian tubes or ovaries, remember that these are paired organs, and procedures may be performed either unilaterally or bilaterally. Sometimes codes differ depending on whether the procedure was performed on either one or both sides, so look for this when reporting codes for the fallopian tubes and ovaries.

Complete the exercises in There's a Code for That 17.1 to practice assigning codes for OB/GYN services.

17.1 Coding for OB/GYN services

There's a Code for That

Read the following documentation from OB/GYN encounters and services and assign the appropriate CPT and HCPCS codes. (Note that some of these encounters may require E/M codes, surgical codes, or both).

1. A 23-year-old established patient presents to the office of her gynecologist complaining of fatigue, nausea, and two missed periods. She took a pregnancy test at home, which was positive, and presents today to get a confirmation pregnancy test. E/M service provided includes problem-focused history and examination, and straightforward medical decision-making. Urine pregnancy test performed in office is positive.

   CPT codes: _____ , _____

2. Code for the complete radical vulvectomy with inguinofemoral lymphadenectomy of the left nodes.

   CPT code: _____

3. Perineoplasty to repair traumatic laceration of the perineum.

   CPT code: _____

4. Laparoscopic supracervical hysterectomy with bilateral salpingo-oophorectomy for uterus weighing 278 grams.

   CPT code: _____

5. A 26-year-old female multigravida presents for contraceptive counseling and the insertion of IUD. After 20 minutes spent counseling the patient, Mirena IUD contraceptive (52 mg levonogestrel-releasing) was inserted into cervix without incident.

   CPT codes: _____ , _____ , _____

6. Endoscopic biopsy of the cervix with endometrial sampling.

   CPT codes: _____ , _____

7. Patient with pelvic pain and discomfort for 3 weeks presents for examination. During a detailed history she admits that during her last menstrual period she lost a tampon after insertion. Detailed pelvic examination reveals impacted tampon, near cervical opening. Tampon removed without incident, patient tolerated the procedure well.

CPT code: _____

Maternity and Obstetric Services

Maternity services are reported from the Maternity Care and Delivery (59000–59899) subsection of the CPT code book. This section includes codes for services unrelated to childbirth and delivery but still related to the fetus and care of the mother, as well as services related to routine antenatal, delivery, and postpartum care of the mother.

Maternity Care

Maternity care procedures include Antepartum and Fetal Invasive Services (59000–59076), Excision (59100–59160), Introduction (59200), Repair (59300–59350), Abortion (59812–59857), and Other Procedures (59866–59899).

- Antepartum and fetal invasive services are related to the growth and development of both the mother and the fetus, and include both diagnostic procedures designed to test the health of the fetus, such as 59025, Fetal non-stress test, as well as therapeutic procedures designed to treat the health of the mother or the fetus, such as 59001, Amniocentesis; therapeutic amniotic fluid reduction (includes ultrasound guidance).

- Excision procedures include surgical treatment of ectopic pregnancies. An ectopic pregnancy is one in which the fertilized egg has implanted outside of the uterus. Codes for the surgical removal of an ectopic pregnancy depend on the site of the implantation, such as 59130, Surgical treatment of ectopic pregnancy; abdominal pregnancy, or 59140, Surgical treatment of ectopic pregnancy; cervical, with evacuation.

- Introduction. There is only one code in the introduction category, which is 59200, Insertion of cervical dilator (eg, luminaria, prostaglandin) (separate procedure). A cervical dilator is a small tampon-like device with a small amount of labor-inducing hormones placed against the cervix to help it soften and thin out before inducing labor.

- Repair codes include an episiotomy repair by a healthcare provider other than the one who performed the episiotomy during the delivery (59300), as well as obstetric cerclage (59320–59325) and repair of ruptured uterus (59350).

- **Abortion** procedures are performed to evacuate the uterus of the **products of conception (POC)**. Products of conception are the remaining fetal and placental tissues after either a spontaneous miscarriage or elective pregnancy termination.

- Other procedures include multifetal pregnancy reductions, uterine evacuation and curettage for hydatidiform mole, removal of cerclage sutures under anesthesia, and unlisted maternity care and delivery procedures.

Delivery

Correctly reporting codes for delivery procedures depends on an understanding of the global maternity package. Just like a surgical package, the global delivery package includes several services, ranging from antepartum care to delivery and postpartum care; noted as follows.

- Antepartum services:
  - Initial and subsequent prenatal history and physical examinations
  - Recording of maternal weight, blood pressure, fetal heart tones
  - Routine chemical urinalysis
  - Monthly visits up to 28 weeks of gestation
  - Biweekly visits up to 36 weeks of gestation
  - Weekly visits at week 37 until delivery
- Delivery services:
  - Admission to the hospital, including admission history and physical examination
  - Management of uncomplicated labor
  - Delivery (vaginal or cesarean), including episiotomy and use of forceps
- Postpartum services:
  - Office or other outpatient visits following delivery

When a single provider (or if the patient saw multiple providers from the same group) performed all of the antepartum, delivery, and postpartum services, only one single code identifying the services is reported. For example, if a doctor performed all the antepartum visits, a vaginal delivery, and then the postpartum checkup, he or she would report code 59400, Routine obstetric care including antepartum care, vaginal delivery (with or without episiotomy, and/or forceps) and postpartum care (see figure 17.10). This one code reports the entire package related to the patient's routine antepartum care, delivery, and routine postpartum care, and is often referred to as the global maternity code.

Figure 17.10. The global maternity package

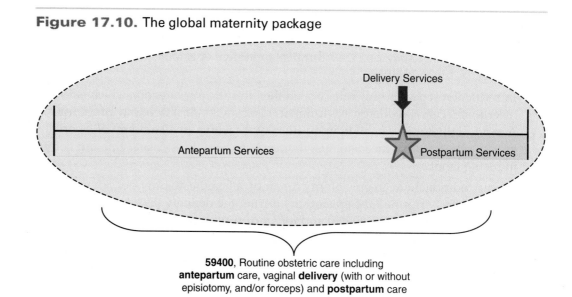

59400, Routine obstetric care including
antepartum care, vaginal **delivery** (with or without
episiotomy, and/or forceps) and **postpartum** care

However, there are several services that are *not* included in routine care. These services should be reported separately, outside of the global maternity package, and include the following:

- Pregnancy confirmation during a problem-oriented or preventive visit. This should be coded with the appropriate E/M code.
- Any visits during the antepartum period that are not routine care related to the patient's pregnancy. For example, a sick visit would not be included in the global maternity package. This would be coded with the appropriate E/M code.
- Medical complications of the pregnancy, such as cardiac problems, neurological problems, diabetes, hypertension, toxemia, hyperemesis (excessive vomiting), preterm labor, premature rupture of membranes, or trauma.
- Medical problems complicating labor and delivery that require additional resources.
- Surgical complications of pregnancy, such as appendectomy, hernia, ovarian cyst, or Bartholin's cyst, that require care during the pregnancy or delivery. These services would be reported with the appropriate surgery codes.

When a healthcare provider performs only a portion of the global maternity service—for example, only the delivery or a portion of the antepartum visits—those specific services are reported according to the exact service the provider performed. For example, if the provider performed only the vaginal delivery because the original doctor was unavailable, he or she would report code 59409, Vaginal delivery only (with or without episiotomy and/or forceps). If the provider performed only antepartum visits, there are two possible codes, one to report 4 to 6 visits (59425, Antepartum care only; 4–6 visits), and one to report over 7 or more antepartum visits (59426, Antepartum care only, 7 or more visits). If the provider performed less than four visits, each of these visits should be reported with the appropriate E/M code according to the level of service that was performed.

Key to Success

When breaking up the global maternity package, remember to code only for the service that your provider performed. For example, if your provider performed only a portion of the antepartum appointments, code for those services only. The remaining services provided by other practitioners will be reported by those practitioners.

Coding for maternity services is further complicated by different types of deliveries as well as multiple births.

Types of Deliveries
The CPT code book identifies four different types of births, each of which are coded with a different range of CPT codes (for individual components and for the global maternity package).

- Vaginal delivery (59400–59414). A vaginal delivery is when the products of conception are delivered through the vaginal canal.
- **Cesarean delivery** (59510–59525). A cesarean delivery is a surgical procedure in which the provider incises the pregnant female's abdomen and uterus to remove the fetus. It is typically performed when a vaginal delivery would put the health of the pregnant female or the fetus at risk.
- **Vaginal birth after cesarean (VBAC)** (59610–59614). A VBAC is when a woman who has previously given birth via cesarean section successfully gives birth vaginally.

- Cesarean delivery after attempted VBAC (59618–59622). This type of delivery is reported when a VBAC is attempted, but for medical reasons must be converted to a cesarean delivery.

When coding for deliveries, first determine the type of delivery (as listed previously) and then the specific service provided (either the global maternity package or a part thereof). Note that codes 59425 through 59430 identify either antepartum care (depending on the number of visits) or postpartum care, not the type of delivery. For these codes, the type of delivery is not relevant because the provider did not perform any of the delivery service.

Multiple Births

Reporting the delivery services for multiple births depends on the type of deliveries and the third-party payer. Unless the insurance has specific reporting requirements, report multiple (twin or more) births as follows (see figure 17.11).

- Multiple birth, all born vaginally. Report code 59400 for the global maternity package with vaginal delivery, in addition to 59409, Vaginal delivery only (with or without episiotomy and/or forceps), appended with modifier -59, Distinct procedural service, to identify the additional procedure as a distinct service.
- Multiple birth, all born via cesarean. Report code 59510 for the global maternity package with cesarean delivery. This code should be reported only once. However, if there was a significant amount of additional work involved, modifier -22, Increased procedural service, should be reported to identify the increased procedural service.
- Multiple births in which one twin is vaginal and the other is born via cesarean. Report code 59510, Routine obstetric care including antepartum care, cesarean delivery, and postpartum care, for the global maternity package for the cesarean delivery (the work involved in the cesarean delivery is higher, so it should be reported as the primary service). Also report code 59409, Vaginal delivery only (with or without episiotomy and/or forceps), appended with modifier -51, Multiple procedures, for the multiple procedures.

Figure 17.11. Multiple births

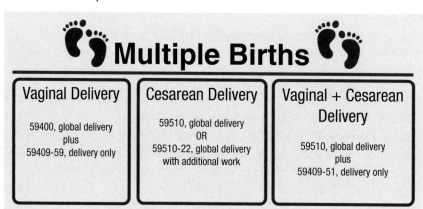

Key to Success

Again, note that these multiple birth delivery guidelines are likely to change. One insurance provider might require modifier -59, Distinct procedural service, while another insurance provider might require modifier -51, Multiple procedures. One insurance provider may allow you to bill the routine delivery code with two or more units, whereas another requires the use of modifier -22, Increased procedural services. Ultimately, report the delivery of multiples according to the guidelines set forth by the payer that is covering the service.

Complete the exercises in There's a Code for That 17.2 to practice reporting maternity and obstetric services.

Coding for maternity and obstetric services

17.2

There's a Code for That

Read the following documentation from maternity encounters and services and assign the appropriate CPT codes.

1. Vaginal cerclage on a pregnant 34-year-old G5P1 with history of incompetent cervix.

   CPT code: _____

2. Cesarean delivery only.

   CPT code: _____

3. A 30-year-old pregnant female received five antepartum visits from Dr. A, and then moved across the state, where Dr. B completed the remaining antepartum care, a cesarean delivery, and the postpartum check.

   Identify the CPT code for Dr. A's services: _____

   Identify the CPT code for Dr. B's services: _____

4. Routine vaginal delivery with episiotomy, including antepartum and postpartum care.

   CPT code: _____

5. Amniocentesis with imaging guidance for fluid reduction.

   CPT code: _____

6. Surgical treatment of septic abortion.

   CPT code: _____

Diagnosis Coding for OB/GYN Services

Diagnosis coding for OB/GYN services generally falls into two broad categories: diseases of the genitourinary system for gynecological services, and codes for pregnancy, childbirth, and the puerperium for obstetric services. A handful of Z-codes for routine examinations, screenings, and additional information for patient encounters are also important to report for OB/GYN services (refer to chapter 8 for a discussion of Z-codes). Codes for abnormal findings and encounters for examinations are also important to understand in OB/GYN coding.

Diseases of the Genitourinary System

Gynecological services are reported primarily with codes from chapter 14 (Diseases of the Genitourinary System) of the ICD-10-CM code book. However, additional codes may be used to identify specific signs and symptoms, such as dysuria or abnormal lab findings. Z-codes may also be reported for healthcare examinations, screenings, personal or family history, or additional pertinent patient information related to the encounter. This chapter includes codes for both the urinary and genital systems for both males and females, and is first organized by urinary conditions, such as Glomerular diseases (N00–N08), Renal tubulo-interstitial diseases (N10-N16), Acute kidney failure and chronic kidney disease (N17–N19), Urolithiasis (N20–N23), Other diseases of the kidney and ureter (N25–N29), and Other diseases of the urinary system (N30–N39). Note that when coding for these categories, there are several valid three-character codes and a handful of notes to report additional code(s) for underlying conditions, an infectious or toxic agent, or a causal condition, when necessary.

Codes in these categories are also applicable to both males and females, as they affect the urinary system. The next category of codes in the chapter, Diseases of male genital organs (N40–N53) pertain specifically to male patients. As with other codes for urinary conditions, pay attention to the notes in the Tabular List that indicate when to include additional codes to identify underlying condition(s), infectious agent, or causal condition. Notice that the codes in this category all have a small male symbol (♂) next to them in the Tabular List, which indicates that these diagnosis codes may only be used for male patients. Additional diagnosis and procedure codes for male genital and urinary systems are discussed in chapter 18.

Remaining categories of codes in this chapter are for Disorders of breast (N60–N65), which may be applicable for either male or female patients, followed by Inflammatory diseases of female pelvic organs (N70–N77) and Noninflammatory diseases of the female genital tract (N80–N98). Note that these last two categories pertain to only female patients. As such, they all each have a small female symbol (♀). (The presence or absence of the male or female symbols depends on the publisher of the ICD-10-CM code book. These symbols may not be present in all code books.)

Abnormal Findings and Encounters for Examinations

OB/GYN providers may also see patients for signs, symptoms, and abnormal findings of the genitourinary system, which are reported with codes from chapter 19 (Symptoms, Signs, and Abnormal Clinical and Laboratory Findings, Not Elsewhere Classified) of the ICD-10-CM code book. Abnormal findings are reported with codes from category R87, Abnormal findings in specimens from female genital organs. These include abnormal findings from Pap smears and cellular changes, which may indicate cancer, among other findings, such as in code R87.610, Atypical squamous cells of undetermined significance on cytologic smear of cervix (ASC-US).

Encounters for examinations and screenings identify that the patient presented for a gynecological examination and are reported with codes from category Z01.4, Encounter for gynecological examination. A code from this category should be reported when a woman presents for a routine gynecological examination. If an abnormal finding is encountered at the examination, such as a genitourinary condition, abnormal laboratory finding, or sign or symptom, report the code for the abnormal finding in addition to the code for the routine screening (with abnormal findings). For example, a woman presenting for a routine gynecological examination with a new diagnosis of endometriosis would be coded as Z01.419, Encounter for gynecological examination (general) (routine) without abnormal findings, with the additional code for the abnormal finding, N80.9, Endometriosis, unspecified.

Encounter codes may also be necessary to identify when a patient receives a contraceptive (Z30, Encounter for contraceptive management) or procreative encounter (Z31, Encounter for procreative management), such as counseling provided to a patient considering a specific type of birth control or regarding fertility. Codes for contraceptive management may also be used when a patient returns for a refill or evaluation and management of a current birth control method, to begin a new birth control method, or to cease a birth control method (such as the removal of an IUD). When coding for contraceptive management, identify the specific type of contraceptive used and the specific contraceptive management service provided. For example, Z30.46, Encounter for surveillance of implantable subdermal contraceptive, identifies the service provided (*surveillance*) and the type of contraceptive (*implantable subdermal*).

Sexually Transmitted Diseases

Codes for sexually transmitted diseases are found in Chapter 1 (Certain Infectious and Parasitic Diseases) of the ICD-10-CM code book. Sexually transmitted diseases or **sexually transmitted infections (STIs)** are infections that usually present with symptoms of the genitourinary system and whose primary mode of transmission is sexual intercourse. OB/GYN providers may diagnose and/or treat sexually transmitted diseases for female patients, whereas a urologist or primary care provider may treat sexually transmitted diseases for male patients.

Coding for laboratory procedures to confirm an STI diagnosis differs from coding for the definitive condition, if present. For example, the STI laboratory screening for a patient who presents with vaginal discharge due to suspected STI would be sent with the sign or symptom code, in this case vaginal discharge. Once the STI is confirmed, the code for the appropriate infection is used. To find the code for an STI, search for the term *Infection* in the Main Index, and then the specific organism. Because infectious organisms may affect different body areas, be sure to assign the diagnosis that most accurately represents the infection. For example, a patient with a vaginal chlamydial infection would be coded with A56.02, Chlamydial vulvovaginitis.

Complete the exercises in There's a Code for That 17.3 to practice assigning OB/GYN diagnosis codes.

Coding for OB/GYN services

17.3

There's a Code for That

Read the following documentation from OB/GYN encounters and services and assign the appropriate ICD-10-CM codes.

1. A 13-year-old female presents complaining of heavy periods. She started her period 2 months ago and her mother is bringing her in today for examination. Impression: pubertal menorrhagia.

   ICD-10-CM code: _____

(Continued on next page)

17.3

Continued

2. Infertility counseling for a 27-year-old G1P2 with polycystic ovarian syndrome (PCOS).

   ICD-10-CM codes: _____ , _____

3. Abnormal Pap smear.

   ICD-10-CM code: _____

4. A 55-year-old female with menopause (started approximately 6 months ago) presents complaining of hot flashes, sleeplessness, and headaches.

   ICD-10-CM codes: _____ , _____. _____

5. Acute vulvovaginitis.

   ICD-10-CM code: _____

6. A 35-year-old female with high-risk heterosexual behavior presents with vaginal discharge. Laboratory test confirms trichomonas of the vagina.

   ICD-10-CM codes: _____ , _____

Pregnancy, Childbirth, and the Puerperium

Conditions related to pregnancy, childbirth, and the puerperium are reported with codes from chapter 15 (Pregnancy, Childbirth, and the Puerperium) and from chapter 21 (Factors Influencing Health Status and Contact with Health Services (Z codes)) of the ICD-10-CM code book.

Codes from chapter 15 begin with the letter *O*, making it easy to remember that O codes are for obstetric services. However, obstetric coding can be a bit more complicated than other types of coding, as the codes in this chapter tend to require additional characters. More codes are also needed to fully identify all of the medical conditions present, as well as the estimated weeks of gestation of the pregnancy. A good rule to follow when assigning codes for obstetric patients is to *code until you can code no longer*. Review the diagnostic statement and ensure that a diagnosis code is assigned for every healthcare condition affecting the patient.

There are also several important guidelines that govern how and when to assign codes for pregnancy, childbirth, and the puerperium. These useful guidelines help coders assign the correct codes and also refer to additional codes, including Z codes, when necessary. Remember that many obstetric cases will contain codes from chapter 15 as well as Z codes from chapter 21. Figure 17.12 provides the OGCR related to obstetrical and reproductive services.

Guidelines for Coding Obstetric Diagnoses

Guidelines for coding obstetric (OB) cases require an understanding of the numerous components and additional codes that should be reported when a patient presents for obstetric services. These include guidelines for sequencing of pregnancy conditions and incidental pregnancy, estimated weeks of gestation, encounters for pregnancy-related services, identification of the fetus in multiple pregnancies, delivery guidelines, and pre-existing versus gestational conditions. Figure 17.13 lists the OGCR related to coding for OB conditions. As you read the following sections, return to this figure to identify the individual OGCR for coding for these conditions.

Figure 17.12. OGCR I.C.21.c.11

11) Encounters for Obstetrical and Reproductive Services

See Section I.C.15. Pregnancy, Childbirth, and the Puerperium, for further instruction on the use of these codes.

Z codes for pregnancy are for use in those circumstances when none of the problems or complications included in the codes from the Obstetrics chapter exist (a routine prenatal visit or postpartum care). Codes in category Z34, Encounter for supervision of normal pregnancy, are always first-listed and are not to be used with any other code from the OB chapter.

Codes in category Z3A, Weeks of gestation, may be assigned to provide additional information about the pregnancy. Category Z3A codes should not be assigned for pregnancies with abortive outcomes (categories O00-O08), elective termination of pregnancy (code Z33.2), nor for postpartum conditions, as category Z3A is not applicable to these conditions. The date of the admission should be used to determine weeks of gestation for inpatient admissions that encompass more than one gestational week.

The outcome of delivery, category Z37, should be included on all maternal delivery records. It is always a secondary code. Codes in category Z37 should not be used on the newborn record.

Z codes for family planning (contraceptive) or procreative management and counseling should be included on an obstetric record either during the pregnancy or the postpartum stage, if applicable.

Z codes/categories for obstetrical and reproductive services:

Z30	Encounter for contraceptive management
Z31	Encounter for procreative management
Z32.2	Encounter for childbirth instruction
Z32.3	Encounter for childcare instruction
Z33	Pregnant state
Z34	Encounter for supervision of normal pregnancy
Z36	Encounter for antenatal screening of mother
Z3A	Weeks of gestation
Z37	Outcome of delivery
Z39	Encounter for maternal postpartum care and examination
Z76.81	Expectant mother prebirth pediatrician visit

Source: CMS 2019.

Sequencing and Incidental Pregnancy

Codes from chapter 15 have sequencing priority over codes from other chapters. **Sequencing priority** means that these codes should be assigned *before* codes from other chapters.

Codes from chapter 15 are commonly assigned with codes from other chapters of the ICD-10-CM code book. In these instances, it is necessary to sequence the O code before the additional codes for the encounter. This guideline overrules other sequencing priority guidelines from other chapters. For example, HIV guidelines state that the code B20 for symptomatic HIV should be sequenced as the first-listed diagnosis on a claim. However, if the HIV-positive patient is pregnant, then a code from subcategory O98.7-, Human immunodeficiency virus [HIV] disease complicating pregnancy, childbirth and the puerperium should be sequenced before the code to identify the type of HIV. In this case, the fact that the patient is pregnant and has HIV is more important than simply the diagnosis of HIV. As such, the obstetric code has sequencing priority. Remember that in this situation, both of the conditions should still be coded, just in a particular order.

However, there is one exception to this rule. When a patient presents for an encounter that is completely unrelated to the pregnancy, such as a finger laceration, the pregnancy should be coded as incidental to the encounter. An **incidental pregnancy** is one that in no way complicates the reason for the healthcare encounter. When a pregnancy is incidental to the encounter, the coder must assign a code detailing the reason for the encounter, such as finger laceration, followed for incidental pregnancy: Z33.1, Pregnant state, incidental.

Key to Success

There are many guidelines to keep in mind when reporting obstetric diagnoses. But don't despair! Remember that all of these guidelines are in the ICD-10-CM code book. You just need to be able to find them when you need them. Read through the OGCR as listed in figure 17.13, and make sure you can locate these guidelines in your code book. Furthermore, remember that additional guidelines and coding conventions are located in the Tabular List at the beginning of each chapter, section, or category of codes, when necessary. Take some time to scan these categories so you can pull out important information about each code before assigning them.

Estimated Weeks of Gestation

Whenever a pregnant patient presents for any type of obstetric service or childbirth, it is necessary to report a code from category Z3A, Weeks of gestation. For example, if a patient reported to the office of her obstetrician for a routine prenatal examination and she was 30 weeks pregnant, then code Z3A.30, 30 weeks gestation of pregnancy, should be reported in addition to any other codes assigned at that visit. According to ICD-10-CM guidelines, category Z3A codes should not be assigned:

- For pregnancies with abortive outcomes (categories O00–O08)
- For elective termination of pregnancy (Z33.32)
- For postpartum conditions (and the patient is no longer pregnant)

Weeks of gestation codes are organized in such a way that they are relatively easy to assign, as the last two digits identify the number of weeks. For example, a patient at 20 weeks gestation is assigned code Z3A.*20*. A patient at 24 weeks gestation is assigned code Z3A.*24*. A patient at 32 weeks gestation is assigned code Z3A.*32*. And so on. The last two digits identify the number of weeks. (Note that this rule does not apply before 8 weeks gestation or after 42 weeks gestation.)

Key to Success

Keep the weeks of gestation guidelines in mind when coding for pregnancy-related services. Unless the patient is in the postpartum period or the pregnancy is aborted or terminated, *every* obstetric case should have at least two codes—one for the reason for the encounter (primary diagnosis) and another from category Z3A to identify the weeks of gestation. If the weeks of gestation are not identified in the documentation, then do not assign a weeks of gestation code.

Encounter for Pregnancy Services

Just like in injury codes, the encounter should be identified for a pregnant patient when she receives pregnancy-related services. However, the encounters do not identify if the service is initial, subsequent, or sequela, but rather where the patient is on the pregnancy timeline.

Figure 17.13. OGCR I.C.15

15. Chapter 15: Pregnancy, Childbirth and the Puerperium (O00-O9A)

a. General Rules for Obstetric Cases

1) Codes from chapter 15 and sequencing priority

Obstetric cases require codes from chapter 15, codes in the range O00-O9A, Pregnancy, Childbirth, and the Puerperium. Chapter 15 codes have sequencing priority over codes from other chapters. Additional codes from other chapters may be used in conjunction with chapter 15 codes to further specify conditions. Should the provider document that the pregnancy is incidental to the encounter, then code Z33.1, Pregnant state, incidental, should be used in place of any chapter 15 codes. It is the provider's responsibility to state that the condition being treated is not affecting the pregnancy.

2) Chapter 15 codes used only on the maternal record

Chapter 15 codes are to be used only on the maternal record, never on the record of the newborn.

3) Final character for trimester

The majority of codes in Chapter 15 have a final character indicating the trimester of pregnancy. The timeframes for the trimesters are indicated at the beginning of the chapter. If trimester is not a component of a code it is because the condition always occurs in a specific trimester, or the concept of trimester of pregnancy is not applicable. Certain codes have characters for only certain trimesters because the condition does not occur in all trimesters, but it may occur in more than just one.

Assignment of the final character for trimester should be based on the provider's documentation of the trimester (or number of weeks) for the current admission/encounter. This applies to the assignment of trimester for pre-existing conditions as well as those that develop during or are due to the pregnancy. The provider's documentation of the number of weeks may be used to assign the appropriate code identifying the trimester.

Whenever delivery occurs during the current admission, and there is an "in childbirth" option for the obstetric complication being coded, the "in childbirth" code should be assigned.

4) Selection of trimester for inpatient admissions that encompass more than one trimester

In instances when a patient is admitted to a hospital for complications of pregnancy during one trimester and remains in the hospital into a subsequent trimester, the trimester character for the antepartum complication code should be assigned on the basis of the trimester when the complication developed, not the trimester of the discharge. If the condition developed prior to the current admission/encounter or represents a pre-existing condition, the trimester character for the trimester at the time of the admission/encounter should be assigned.

5) Unspecified trimester

Each category that includes codes for trimester has a code for "unspecified trimester." The "unspecified trimester" code should rarely be used, such as when the documentation in the record is insufficient to determine the trimester and it is not possible to obtain clarification.

6) 7th character for Fetus Identification

Where applicable, a 7th character is to be assigned for certain categories (O31, O32, O33.3 - O33.6, O35, O36, O40, O41, O60.1, O60.2, O64, and O69) to identify the fetus for which the complication code applies.

Assign 7th character "0":

- For single gestations
- When the documentation in the record is insufficient to determine the fetus affected and it is not possible to obtain clarification.
- When it is not possible to clinically determine which fetus is affected.

b. Selection of OB Principal or First-listed Diagnosis

1) Routine outpatient prenatal visits

For routine outpatient prenatal visits when no complications are present, a code from category Z34, Encounter for supervision of normal pregnancy, should be used as the first-listed diagnosis. These codes should not be used in conjunction with chapter 15 codes.

2) Supervision of High-Risk Pregnancy

Codes from category O09, Supervision of high-risk pregnancy, are intended for use only during the prenatal period. For complications during the labor or delivery episode as a result of a high-risk pregnancy, assign the applicable complication codes from Chapter 15. If there are no complications during the labor or delivery episode, assign code O80, Encounter for full-term uncomplicated delivery.

For routine prenatal outpatient visits for patients with high-risk pregnancies, a code from category O09, Supervision of high-risk pregnancy, should be used as the first-listed diagnosis. Secondary chapter 15 codes may be used in conjunction with these codes if appropriate.

(Continued on next page)

Figure 17.13. *(Continued)*

3) Episodes when no delivery occurs

In episodes when no delivery occurs, the principal diagnosis should correspond to the principal complication of the pregnancy which necessitated the encounter. Should more than one complication exist, all of which are treated or monitored, any of the complications codes may be sequenced first.

4) When a delivery occurs

When an obstetric patient is admitted and delivers during that admission, the condition that prompted the admission should be sequenced as the principal diagnosis. If multiple conditions prompted the admission, sequence the one most related to the delivery as the principal diagnosis. A code for any complication of the delivery should be assigned as an additional diagnosis. In cases of cesarean delivery, if the patient was admitted with a condition that resulted in the performance of a cesarean procedure, that condition should be selected as the principal diagnosis. If the reason for the admission was unrelated to the condition resulting in the cesarean delivery, the condition related to the reason for the admission should be selected as the principal diagnosis.

5) Outcome of delivery

A code from category Z37, Outcome of delivery, should be included on every maternal record when a delivery has occurred. These codes are not to be used on subsequent records or on the newborn record.

c. Pre-existing conditions versus conditions due to the pregnancy

Certain categories in Chapter 15 distinguish between conditions of the mother that existed prior to pregnancy (pre-existing) and those that are a direct result of pregnancy. When assigning codes from Chapter 15, it is important to assess if a condition was pre-existing prior to pregnancy or developed during or due to the pregnancy in order to assign the correct code.

Categories that do not distinguish between pre-existing and pregnancy-related conditions may be used for either. It is acceptable to use codes specifically for the puerperium with codes complicating pregnancy and childbirth if a condition arises postpartum during the delivery encounter.

d. Pre-existing hypertension in pregnancy

Category O10, Pre-existing hypertension complicating pregnancy, childbirth and the puerperium, includes codes for hypertensive heart and hypertensive chronic kidney disease. When assigning one of the O10 codes that includes hypertensive heart disease or hypertensive chronic kidney disease, it is necessary to add a secondary code from the appropriate hypertension category to specify the type of heart failure or chronic kidney disease.

See Section I.C.9. Hypertension.

e. Fetal Conditions Affecting the Management of the Mother

1) Codes from categories O35 and O36

Codes from categories O35, Maternal care for known or suspected fetal abnormality and damage, and O36, Maternal care for other fetal problems, are assigned only when the fetal condition is actually responsible for modifying the management of the mother, i.e., by requiring diagnostic studies, additional observation, special care, or termination of pregnancy. The fact that the fetal condition exists does not justify assigning a code from this series to the mother's record.

2) In utero surgery

In cases when surgery is performed on the fetus, a diagnosis code from category O35, Maternal care for known or suspected fetal abnormality and damage, should be assigned identifying the fetal condition. Assign the appropriate procedure code for the procedure performed.

No code from Chapter 16, the perinatal codes, should be used on the mother's record to identify fetal conditions. Surgery performed in utero on a fetus is still to be coded as an obstetric encounter.

f. HIV Infection in Pregnancy, Childbirth and the Puerperium

During pregnancy, childbirth or the puerperium, a patient admitted because of an HIV-related illness should receive a principal diagnosis from subcategory O98.7-, Human immunodeficiency [HIV] disease complicating pregnancy, childbirth and the puerperium, followed by the code(s) for the HIV-related illness(es).

Patients with asymptomatic HIV infection status admitted during pregnancy, childbirth, or the puerperium should receive codes of O98.7- and Z21, Asymptomatic human immunodeficiency virus [HIV] infection status.

g. Diabetes mellitus in pregnancy

Diabetes mellitus is a significant complicating factor in pregnancy. Pregnant women who are diabetic should be assigned a code from category O24, Diabetes mellitus in pregnancy, childbirth, and the puerperium, first, followed by the appropriate diabetes code(s) (E08- E13) from Chapter 4.

h. Long term use of insulin and oral hypoglycemics

See section I.C.4.a.3 for information on the long term use of insulin and oral hypoglycemic.

i. Gestational (pregnancy induced) diabetes

Gestational (pregnancy induced) diabetes can occur during the second and third trimester of pregnancy in women who were not diabetic prior to pregnancy. Gestational diabetes can cause complications in the pregnancy similar to those of pre-existing diabetes mellitus. It also puts the woman at greater risk of developing diabetes after the pregnancy. Codes for gestational diabetes are in subcategory O24.4, Gestational diabetes mellitus. No other code from category O24, Diabetes mellitus in pregnancy, childbirth, and the puerperium, should be used with a code from O24.4.

The codes under subcategory O24.4 include diet controlled, insulin controlled, and controlled by oral hypoglycemic drugs. If a patient with gestational diabetes is treated with both diet and insulin, only the code for insulin-controlled is required. If a patient with gestational diabetes is treated with both diet and oral hypoglycemic medications, only the code for "controlled by oral hypoglycemic drugs" is required. Code Z79.4, Long-term (current) use of insulin or code Z79.84, Long-term (current) use of oral hypoglycemic drugs,should not be assigned with codes from subcategory O24.4.

An abnormal glucose tolerance in pregnancy is assigned a code from subcategory O99.81, Abnormal glucose complicating pregnancy, childbirth, and the puerperium.

j. Sepsis and septic shock complicating abortion, pregnancy, childbirth and the puerperium

When assigning a chapter 15 code for sepsis complicating abortion, pregnancy, childbirth, and the puerperium, a code for the specific type of infection should be assigned as an additional diagnosis. If severe sepsis is present, a code from subcategory R65.2, Severe sepsis, and code(s) for associated organ dysfunction(s) should also be assigned as additional diagnoses.

k. Puerperal sepsis

Code O85, Puerperal sepsis, should be assigned with a secondary code to identify the causal organism (e.g., for a bacterial infection, assign a code from category B95-B96, Bacterial infections in conditions classified elsewhere). A code from category A40, Streptococcal sepsis, or A41, Other sepsis, should not be used for puerperal sepsis. If applicable, use additional codes to identify severe sepsis (R65.2-) and any associated acute organ dysfunction.

l. Alcohol and tobacco use during pregnancy, childbirth and the puerperium

1) Alcohol use during pregnancy, childbirth and the puerperium

Codes under subcategory O99.31, Alcohol use complicating pregnancy, childbirth, and the puerperium, should be assigned for any pregnancy case when a mother uses alcohol during the pregnancy or postpartum. A secondary code from category F10, Alcohol related disorders, should also be assigned to identify manifestations of the alcohol use.

2) Tobacco use during pregnancy, childbirth and the puerperium

Codes under subcategory O99.33, Smoking (tobacco) complicating pregnancy, childbirth, and the puerperium, should be assigned for any pregnancy case when a mother uses any type of tobacco product during the pregnancy or postpartum. A secondary code from category F17, Nicotine dependence, should also be assigned to identify the type of nicotine dependence.

3) Drug use during pregnancy, childbirth and the puerperium

Codes under subcategory O99.32, Drug use complicating pregnancy, childbirth, and the puerperium, should be assigned for any pregnancy case when a mother uses drugs during the pregnancy or postpartum. This can involve illegal drugs, or inappropriate use or abuse of prescription drugs. Secondary code(s) from categories F11-F16 and F18-F19 should also be assigned to identify manifestations of the drug use.

(Continued on next page)

Figure 17.13. *(Continued)*

m. Poisoning, toxic effects, adverse effects and underdosing in a pregnant patient

A code from subcategory O9A.2, Injury, poisoning and certain other consequences of external causes complicating pregnancy, childbirth, and the puerperium, should be sequenced first, followed by the appropriate injury, poisoning, toxic effect, adverse effect or underdosing code, and then the additional code(s) that specifies the condition caused by the poisoning, toxic effect, adverse effect or underdosing.

See Section I.C.19. Adverse effects, poisoning, underdosing and toxic effects.

n. Normal Delivery, Code O80

1) Encounter for full term uncomplicated delivery

Code O80 should be assigned when a woman is admitted for a full-term normal delivery and delivers a single, healthy infant without any complications antepartum, during the delivery, or postpartum during the delivery episode. Code O80 is always a principal diagnosis. It is not to be used if any other code from chapter 15 is needed to describe a current complication of the antenatal, delivery, or **postnatal** period. Additional codes from other chapters may be used with code O80 if they are not related to or are in any way complicating the pregnancy.

2) Uncomplicated delivery with resolved antepartum complication

Code O80 may be used if the patient had a complication at some point during the pregnancy, but the complication is not present at the time of the admission for delivery.

3) Outcome of delivery for O80

Z37.0, Single live birth, is the only outcome of delivery code appropriate for use with O80.

o. The Peripartum and Postpartum Periods

1) Peripartum and Postpartum periods

The postpartum period begins immediately after delivery and continues for six weeks following delivery. The peripartum period is defined as the last month of pregnancy to five months postpartum.

2) Peripartum and postpartum complication

A postpartum complication is any complication occurring within the six-week period.

3) Pregnancy-related complications after 6 week period

Chapter 15 codes may also be used to describe pregnancy-related complications after the peripartum or postpartum period if the provider documents that a condition is pregnancy related.

4) Admission for routine postpartum care following delivery outside hospital

When the mother delivers outside the hospital prior to admission and is admitted for routine postpartum care and no complications are noted, code Z39.0, Encounter for care and examination of mother immediately after delivery, should be assigned as the principal diagnosis.

5) Pregnancy associated cardiomyopathy

Pregnancy associated cardiomyopathy, code O90.3, is unique in that it may be diagnosed in the third trimester of pregnancy but may continue to progress months after delivery. For this reason, it is referred to as peripartum cardiomyopathy. Code O90.3 is only for use when the cardiomyopathy develops as a result of pregnancy in a woman who did not have pre-existing heart disease.

p. Code O94, Sequelae of complication of pregnancy, childbirth, and the puerperium

1) Code O94

Code O94, Sequelae of complication of pregnancy, childbirth, and the puerperium, is for use in those cases when an initial complication of a pregnancy develops a sequelae requiring care or treatment at a future date.

2) After the initial postpartum period

This code may be used at any time after the initial postpartum period.

3) Sequencing of Code O94

This code, like all sequela codes, is to be sequenced following the code describing the sequelae of the complication.

q. Termination of Pregnancy and Spontaneous abortions

1) Abortion with Liveborn Fetus

When an attempted termination of pregnancy results in a liveborn fetus, assign code Z33.2, Encounter for elective termination of pregnancy and a code from category Z37, Outcome of Delivery.

2) Retained Products of Conception following an abortion

Subsequent encounters for retained products of conception following a spontaneous abortion or elective termination of pregnancy, without complications are assigned O03.4, Incomplete spontaneous, abortion without complication, or codes O07.4, Failed attempted termination of pregnancy without complication. This advice is appropriate even when the patient was discharged previously with a discharge diagnosis of complete abortion. If the patient has a specific complication associated with the spontaneous abortion or elective termination of pregnancy in addition to retained products of conception, assign the appropriate complication **code (e.g., O03.-, O04.-, O07.-)** instead of code O03.4 or O07.4.

3) Complications leading to abortion

Codes from Chapter 15 may be used as additional codes to identify any documented complications of the pregnancy in conjunction with codes in categories in O04, O07 and O08.

r. Abuse in a pregnant patient

For suspected or confirmed cases of abuse of a pregnant patient, a code(s) from subcategories O9A.3, Physical abuse complicating pregnancy, childbirth, and the puerperium, O9A.4, Sexual abuse complicating pregnancy, childbirth, and the puerperium, and O9A.5, Psychological abuse complicating pregnancy, childbirth, and the puerperium, should be sequenced first, followed by the appropriate codes (if applicable) to identify any associated current injury due to physical abuse, sexual abuse, and the perpetrator of abuse.

See Section I.C.19. Adult and child abuse, neglect and other maltreatment.

Source: CMS 2019.

These encounters include the antepartum, childbirth, or puerperal (postpartum) periods. If the patient is in the antepartum period, then identify the specific trimester of the pregnancy. Remember that the first trimester is from conception to less than 14 weeks, 0 days; the second trimester is from 14 weeks, 0 days to less than 28 weeks, 0 days; and the third trimester is from 28 weeks, 0 days until delivery (see figure 17.14).

Figure 17.14. Encounters for pregnancy-related services

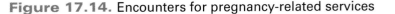
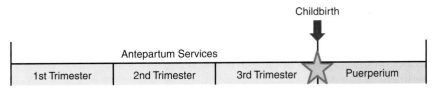

Not all codes identify the encounter for pregnancy-related services. If the condition reported is a condition that always occurs in a specific trimester, then the component of trimester is not included in the code. Some codes have only certain trimesters applicable, because said condition can only occur in specific trimesters. Ultimately, it is important to read the code description thoroughly and always check to see if an additional character is required to identify the trimester of pregnancy, childbirth, or the puerperium.

If the specific trimester is not included in the documentation but the number of weeks is included, it is the coder's responsibility to assign the correct trimester of pregnancy code. If neither the trimester nor the number of weeks of gestation are documented, assign the code for unspecified trimester.

When a pregnant patient presents to routine antepartum care, use the appropriate Z-code for encounter of supervision of pregnancy, assigned from category Z34, Encounter for supervision of normal pregnancy. For example, a pregnant woman in her second trimester at 24 weeks of gestation, who presents for supervision of her normal pregnancy, would be coded as follows:

- Z34.92, Encounter for supervision of normal pregnancy, unspecified, second trimester
- Z3A.24, 24 weeks gestation of pregnancy

Note that there is an Excludes1 note in the Tabular List that category Z34 codes should not be used with any codes from categories O00–O9A. If a patient presents with any type of pregnancy complication or relevant patient history, then do not report the Z code and instead use the code(s) to identify the pregnancy complication(s). For example, a pregnant woman in her second trimester, with a history of pre-term labor, at 24 weeks gestation would be coded as follows:

- O09.212, Supervision of pregnancy with history of pre-term labor, second trimester
- Z3A.24, 24 weeks gestation of pregnancy

To locate the code for routine pregnancy services, search the Main Index for the term *Pregnancy* and then *Supervision of*. For any kind of complications of pregnancy, search the Main Index for the term *Pregnancy* and *Complicated by*, then locate the subterm for each complication.

Identification of Fetus in Multiple Pregnancies

When a patient with a multiple pregnancy (for example, twins or triplets) presents for services, and a specific complication exists for one of the fetuses, it is necessary to assign a complication of pregnancy (O code) to identify the complication for that specific fetus. For example, if fetus 1 in a twin birth is born with a **nuchal cord** (umbilical cord around the neck) without compression, and fetus 2 has no complications, then to the coder must assign code O69.81X1, Labor and delivery complicated by cord around neck, without compression, fetus 1. The seventh character "1" identifies that fetus 1 was affected by the nuchal cord.

The seventh-character "0" for "not applicable" should be used in the following circumstances:

- The pregnancy is a single gestation.
- The documentation does not specify which fetus was affected by the complication.
- When it is not clinically possible to identify which fetus is affected by the complication.

Delivery Guidelines

When coding for pregnancy-related services, coders should identify whether or not a delivery has occurred. The following guidelines apply:

- When no delivery occurs, the first-listed diagnosis should be the primary complication that necessitated the patient encounter. If more than one complication is present, assign one code for each complication.
- When a delivery occurs at a patient admission, the condition that prompted the admission should be sequenced as the first diagnosis. If the patient has multiple conditions, the one that is most related to the patient delivery should be sequenced first. Any additional complication of pregnancy codes should be sequenced after the first-listed code.
- When a delivery occurs, an outcome of delivery code should be assigned. The **outcome of delivery code** identifies the number of births and whether they were

live or stillborn. The outcome of delivery is reported with the appropriate code from category Z37, Outcome of delivery. Note that this code is to be used only on the maternal record, and never on the newborn's record.

- When a delivery occurs, if it is a normal delivery, then code O80, Encounter for full-term uncomplicated delivery, should be assigned. A normal delivery is one that requires minimal or no assistance; occurs with or without episiotomy; occurs without fetal manipulation (such as rotation version); occurs without instrumentation (such as forceps); is a spontaneous, vaginal delivery, single birth of a full-term, liveborn infant.

  Code O80 may not be used with any other code from chapter 15 (O code). The only additional code that may be reported with O80 is the additional code to identify the outcome of delivery (Z37) and weeks of gestation (Z3A).

Category Z37, Outcome of delivery, is used to identify that a pregnant patient presented for delivery and code Z37 identifies the outcome of that delivery, such as a single liveborn. This is similar to the code assigned on the record for a liveborn infant, category Z38, Liveborn infants according to place of birth and type of delivery. A code from category Z38 should be assigned only on the newborn's record to identify the newborn's place of birth, type of delivery, and multiple-birth status. The Z37 code is assigned on the mother's record when she delivers. The Z38 code is assigned on the newborn's record when he or she is born and receives healthcare services. When in doubt regarding which code to assign, look at the notation in the Tabular List that identifies the code as either being applicable to a maternity case or to a newborn case.

Key to Success

Do not confuse the outcome of delivery code (Z37.-), which is used on a maternal record, with the code for liveborn infants according to place of birth and type of delivery (Z38.-), which is assigned on the newborn's record. To help differentiate between these two categories of codes, remember to keep an eye out for the indicators in the Tabular List that identify whether the code should be used on a maternal or a newborn record (such as the little "M" or the little "N").

Pre-existing versus Gestational Conditions

A pre-existing condition is a known condition of the patient before she became pregnant, such as hypertension or type 2 diabetes. On the other hand, a **gestational condition** is one that is a direct result from pregnancy, such as gestational hypertension or gestational diabetes. Gestational conditions are also referred to as pregnancy-induced conditions.

Codes differ based on whether the condition was pre-existing or gestational. For example, category O10, Pre-existing hypertension complicating pregnancy, childbirth, and the puerperium, should be assigned for a patient who had hypertension prior to becoming pregnant. However, category O13, Gestational [pregnancy-induced] hypertension without significant proteinuria, should be assigned for a patient that did not have hypertension before becoming pregnant, and but now has hypertension due to her pregnancy.

It is important to pay attention to the guidelines in the Tabular List for pre-existing conditions, as many guidelines alert the coder that an additional code should be reported to identify the underlying or pre-existing condition. In these cases, the additional condition would not be a complication of pregnancy code, but the code for the specific complication (such as I10, Essential (primary) hypertension).

Complete the exercises in There's a Code for That 17.4 to practice reporting diagnosis codes for maternity and obstetric services.

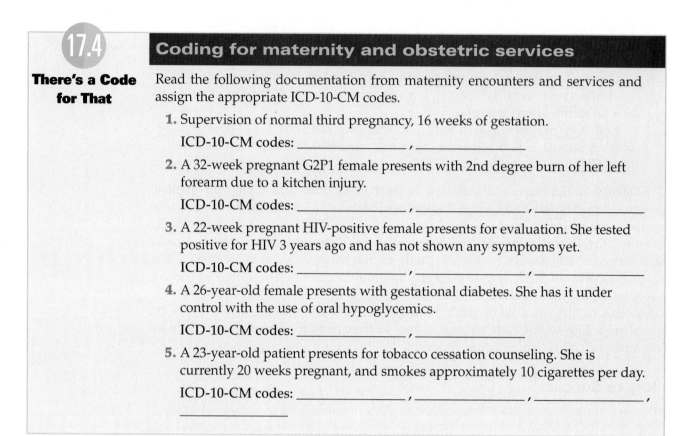

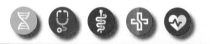

Coding for maternity and obstetric services

There's a Code for That

Read the following documentation from maternity encounters and services and assign the appropriate ICD-10-CM codes.

1. Supervision of normal third pregnancy, 16 weeks of gestation.

    ICD-10-CM codes: _____ , _____

2. A 32-week pregnant G2P1 female presents with 2nd degree burn of her left forearm due to a kitchen injury.

    ICD-10-CM codes: _____ , _____ , _____

3. A 22-week pregnant HIV-positive female presents for evaluation. She tested positive for HIV 3 years ago and has not shown any symptoms yet.

    ICD-10-CM codes: _____ , _____ , _____

4. A 26-year-old female presents with gestational diabetes. She has it under control with the use of oral hypoglycemics.

    ICD-10-CM codes: _____ , _____

5. A 23-year-old patient presents for tobacco cessation counseling. She is currently 20 weeks pregnant, and smokes approximately 10 cigarettes per day.

    ICD-10-CM codes: _____ , _____ , _____ ,
    _____

Putting It All Together: Coding for OB/GYN Services

Coding correctly for OB/GYN services requires an understanding of the differences between gynecological and obstetric services, as well as the guidelines for reporting obstetric diagnosis codes. Determination of the correct codes relies on the answers to the following questions.

- What type of service or procedure was performed, and did the encounter include an E/M service?
    - If so, report the code for the E/M service and any codes for additional procedures (such as the removal of an IUD).
    - If not, report only the code(s) for the service(s) or procedure(s) that were performed.
- Is the service obstetric or non-obstetric?
- Are there any applicable modifiers for the procedure(s)?
- For gynecological services, is there a definitive diagnosis for the encounter? If so, then code for the definitive diagnosis. If not, then report the code for the sign, symptom, or abnormal finding.

- Is the patient presenting for an examination, screening, counseling, or management service? If so, report the Z-code for the encounter type.
- For pregnant patients:
    - Is the pregnancy incidental to the service being provided?
    - Why is the patient presenting to the encounter?
        - Is it a routine examination? If yes, then report the appropriate Z-code.
        - Are there complications of the pregnancy? If yes, assign one code per complication.
        - Where is the patient on the pregnancy timeline?
        - Did a delivery occur? If yes, what type of delivery was it? What was the outcome of delivery?
        - Is it a multiple pregnancy, and which fetus is affected by the complication?
        - What is the estimated week of gestation for the pregnancy?
- Are there any additional conditions that need to be reported, such as pre-existing or underlying conditions?

The following vignette demonstrates how to select appropriate diagnosis and procedure codes. After reviewing the vignette, complete the exercises in There's a Code for That 17.5 to practice coding for OB/GYN services.

Melissa is working as a healthcare coder at a local OB/GYN group practice as she completes her health information management program online. Today she is coding for the deliveries that her OB provided at the hospital over the weekend. She is currently coding the following record: "32-year-old G5P3 high-risk female with history of Factor V deficiency blood clotting disorder presented for induction. Patient is at 36 weeks of gestation. Pitocin was administered at approx. 8 a.m. I checked patient at 12:30 to assess her progress and decided that she was progressing nicely, with 4 cm dilation and 20 percent effacement. Epidural anesthesia was administered by anesthesiologist at approx. 3:30, and labor progressed over the next two hours. At 5:30 I prepped patient for delivery and at 5:47 a male infant with noncompressed triple nuchal cord was delivered vaginally without the use of episiotomy or forceps. I managed this patient throughout her antepartum period (12 visits total) but patient states that she is moving in 2 weeks. Antepartum hospital and delivery records will be forwarded to her new doctor before the postpartum check with the new doctor."

Melissa asks herself: What did the doctor do? In this case, the doctor performed the vaginal delivery of an infant in the hospital. The note also mentions that the same doctor also performed the antepartum care, but that the patient will be moving soon and will receive the postpartum check from a different doctor. In this case, Melissa needs to report the antepartum care as well as the vaginal delivery. She cannot report code 59400, Routine obstetric care including antepartum care, vaginal delivery (with or without episiotomy, and/or forceps) and postpartum care, because the doctor will not be providing the postpartum care. So she reports one code for the antepartum care (for 12 visits), as well as the vaginal delivery:

- *59426, Antepartum care only, 7 or more visits*
- *59409, Vaginal delivery only (with or without episiotomy and/or forceps)*

Melissa does not have to report any of the other services that were performed, because she is only coding for the services that her doctor performed. The anesthesiologist will bill for the epidural, and the hospital will bill for the remaining services.

Now that Melissa has the procedure codes, she asks herself: Why did the doctor do it? In this case, there are several different diagnosis codes that need to be reported to identify the medical necessity for the services performed. Furthermore, she needs to pay attention to how she will link the procedure codes and diagnosis codes.

She decides to report the codes for the delivery first. Melissa remembers that a good measurement for diagnosis coding in OB services is to code until she can code no longer code. Looking at the report, the patient is presenting for delivery, so she knows that she will select the diagnosis codes and identify "delivery" as the encounter for the services. First, the doctor notes that the patient is a high-risk pregnancy due to a Factor V deficiency blood clotting disorder, so she searches the ICD-10-CM Index for Pregnancy, complicated by, *and then* Diseases, *and then* diseases of the blood. *She goes to the Tabular List and verified her code selection with childbirth as the encounter, and selects the code: O99.12, Other diseases of the blood and blood-forming organs and certain disorders involving the immune mechanism complicating childbirth. She now needs to identify the code for the delivery of the infant with noncompressed triple nuchal cord, and finds the code O69.81X0, Labor and delivery complicated by cord around neck, without compression, not applicable or unspecified. She selects "0" as the seventh character because this was a single pregnancy, and so the seventh characters used to identify the fetus in multiple pregnancies is not applicable. The only other code she needs for this visit at this point is to identify the outcome of the delivery (a single live birth), and the weeks of gestation. She reports the following codes for the maternity record:*

- *O99.12, Other diseases of the blood and blood-forming organs and certain disorders involving the immune mechanism complicating childbirth*

- *O69.81X0, Labor and delivery complicated by cord around neck, without compression, not applicable or unspecified*

- *Z37.0, Single live birth*

- *Z3A.36, 36 weeks gestation of pregnancy*

She then rechecks the documentation to make sure she has coded everything for the encounter and reports the chosen codes. Note that the O-codes (obstetric codes) are sequenced first in this scenario, followed by the two Z-codes to identify the outcome of the delivery and the weeks of gestation of the pregnancy. Remember that O-codes have sequencing priority, so they should be sequenced before any other codes reported on the claim. The Z-codes for the outcome of delivery and weeks of gestation should be sequenced after all other codes that may also be included on the claim.

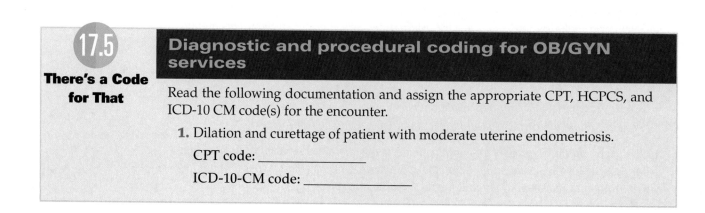

17.5

There's a Code for That

Diagnostic and procedural coding for OB/GYN services

Read the following documentation and assign the appropriate CPT, HCPCS, and ICD-10 CM code(s) for the encounter.

1. Dilation and curettage of patient with moderate uterine endometriosis.

   CPT code: _____

   ICD-10-CM code: _____

2. VBAC delivery of a single female infant, born at 38 weeks of gestation. Patient suffered second degree perineal laceration during delivery.

CPT code: _____

ICD-10-CM codes: _____ , _____ , _____ ,

_____

3. A 17-year-old sexually active female presents with severe abdominal pain and cramping during menstruation. Pelvic examination performed in office revealed numerous ovarian cysts bilaterally. Detailed history and examination with MDM of moderate complexity.

CPT code: _____

ICD-10-CM code: _____ , _____

Case Study   Bilateral Salpingectomy

PATIENT: Alice Simmons

PREOPERATIVE DIAGNOSIS: Symptomatic uterine fibroids

POSTOPERATIVE DIAGNOSIS: Symptomatic uterine fibroids

PROCEDURE: Robotic hysterectomy, bilateral salpingectomy, right ovarian cystectomy

FINDINGS: Enlarged fibroid uterus weighing 224g; right ovarian cyst and endometriotic implants in the posterior pelvis near the bladder.

ESTIMATED BLOOD LOSS: Less than 100 mL

COMPLICATIONS: None; patient tolerated the procedure well.

PROCEDURE IN DETAIL:
The patient was seen in the Holding Room. The risks, benefits, complications, treatment options, and expected outcomes were discussed with the patient. The patient concurred with the proposed plan, giving informed consent. The patient was taken to the operating room, and the procedure was verified as a robotic hysterectomy with bilateral salpingectomy. A time out was held and the above information was confirmed.

After induction of anesthesia, the patient was placed in lithotomy position and prepped and draped in the usual sterile manner. Foley catheter was placed. A v-care uterine manipulator was introduced into the endometrial cavity and secured.

An incision was made above the umbilicus and a 5 mm port introduced. Confirmation of abdominal placement was made with laparoscope. Two additional 8 mm ports were placed in the right and left lower abdomen under direct visualization. The midline was extended for a 12 mm port and a 5 mm port introduced in the nipple line on the left, just below the ribs.

The robot was docked and attention turned to the console.

The uterus was found to be enlarged with multiple fibroids and the ovaries were normal with a hemorrhagic cyst on the right ovary. The ureters were identified and noted to be away from the surgical field. The fallopian tubes were identified, grasped, and followed to the fimbriated ends. They were dissected from their surrounding tissue with harp dissection and cautery. The cyst on the right ovary was dissected from the ovary and removed. The round ligaments were identified, cauterized with bipolar cautery, and cut. The anterior peritoneal reflection was incised and the bladder was dissected off the lower uterine segment. Hemostasis was observed. The uterine vessels were skeletonized, then clamped, and cauterized. Using the v-care as a guide, a posterior colpotomy was made. A circumferential incision was made around the cervix, and the uterus, cervix, and tubes were delivered through the vagina. Vaginal cuff angles as well as the remainder of the vagina cuff were closed using a v-lock suture, incorporating the utero-sacral ligaments for support. Lavage was carried out until clear. Hemostasis was observed.

Interceed was placed in the pelvis due to endometriosis being noted. The robot was undocked, and all instruments removed from the abdomen and the vagina. The midline fascial incision was closed with 0-vicryl suture and all skin incisions were closed with 4-0 vicryl.

A perineal laceration was noted due to the irregular shape of the uterus. This laceration was repaired with 3-0 vicryl suture.

Instrument, sponge, and needle counts were correct prior to abdominal closure and at the conclusion of the case.

SIGNED: Dr. Jordana Morgan, MD

Use the following steps to select the appropriate codes for the case study.

1. Read through the case study and answer the question: *What did the doctor do?* In the case study, identify the name of the procedure.

_____

_____

2. Now that you have identified the procedure, locate the code for the procedure in the CPT code book.
   a. Search the Index for the procedure and search through the options. If there are multiple options, identify the most appropriate code option and refer to the code listed in the Tabular section.

_____

_____

   b. In the listing of codes, check for any guidelines, important definitions, or parenthetical notes. Select the code that correctly identifies all of the components of the procedure and list it.

_____

_____

   c. Are there any additional procedures that need to be added to identify all of the procedures performed? If yes, follow the previous steps to identify the codes for the additional procedures.

_____

_____

   d. Search the Index for the procedure and search through the options. If there are multiple options, identify the most appropriate code option and refer to the code listed in the Tabular section.

_____

_____

   e. In the listing of codes, check for any guidelines, important definitions, or parenthetical notes. Select the code that correctly identifies all of the components of the procedure and list it.

_____

_____

3. Now that the procedure(s) and modifier(s) have been identified, refer to the case study and answer the following question: *Why did the doctor do it?* From the case study, identify the patient's diagnoses.

_____

_____

4. Now that you have identified the patient's diagnoses, search the ICD-10-CM code book for the correct code for this condition.
   a. Search the Main Index for the name of the condition and search through any applicable subterms and cross-references to locate the appropriate code.

      i. _____

      ii. _____

      iii. _____

   b. Verify the codes in the Tabular List. Locate the code identified previously in the Tabular Listing of codes and refer to any applicable guidelines, notes, and symbols. Does the code selected correctly identify the patient's condition? If yes, list the code.

      i. _____

      ii. _____

      iii. _____

   c. Check the procedure note and ICD-10-CM guidelines and conventions to determine the correct sequencing of the diagnosis codes, if applicable. Correctly sequence the diagnosis codes.

_____

_____

5. Now that the procedure and diagnosis codes have been identified, list them on the CMS-1500 form. Be sure to correctly link the procedure and diagnosis codes. Remember to add the number of units as necessary. For this case study, do not calculate the time, base units, or modifying factors. Assign only the ICD-10-CM and CPT codes to the claim with correct code linkage.

21. DIAGNOSIS OR NATURE OF ILLNESS OR INJURY Relate A-L to service line below (24E)				ICD Ind.		22. RESUBMISSION CODE	
A.	B.	C.	D.				
E.	F.	G.	H.			23. PRIOR AUTHORIZATION NU	
I.	J.	K.	L.				

24. A. DATE(S) OF SERVICE From MM DD YY To MM DD YY	B. PLACE OF SERVICE	C. EMG	D. PROCEDURES, SERVICES, OR SUPPLIES (Explain Unusual Circumstances) CPT/HCPCS | MODIFIER	E. DIAGNOSIS POINTER	F. $ CHARGES	G. DAYS OR UNITS
1						
2						
3						

HCC

End-of-Chapter Content

Instructions: Indicate whether the following statements are true or false (T or F). For false statements, rewrite the statement on the line below to make the statement true.

1. A gynecologist is more likely to treat non-obstetric conditions.

_____

_____

2. An obstetric procedure may also be referred to as a maternity procedure.

_____

_____

3. The place of service code for an infant born in a birthing center is 21.

_____

_____

4. The date used to estimate the patient's date of delivery of a fetus is the last menstrual period.

_____

_____

5. A nulliparous female has had multiple pregnancies that were carried to full term.

_____

_____

6. The organization of the female genital subsection of the CPT book begins with the ovaries and ends with the vulva, perineum, and introitus.

_____

_____

7. A conization procedure removes a portion of tissue from the cervix.

_____

_____

8. A pessary is a stitch that helps the cervix remain closed at the external os.

_____

_____

9. A VBAC is a type of delivery in which the pregnant female has had a previous cesarean and is attempting to deliver vaginally.

_____

_____

10. Contraceptive management diagnosis codes should be used when a patient comes in for a refill of her contraceptive prescription.

_____

_____

Instructions: Choose the best answer.

1. Which of the following services would more likely be performed by an obstetrician?
   a. Delivery of a fetus
   b. Treatment of urinary tract infection
   c. Urinary sling procedure for incontinence
   d. Treatment of a sexually transmitted infection

2. Which of the following healthcare providers specializes in fertility?
   a. Certified nurse midwife (CNM)
   b. Reproductive endocrinology and infertility (REI) specialist
   c. Maternal fetal medicine (MFM) specialist
   d. Gynecologist

3. Which of the following periods extends from the date of delivery to the six weeks following delivery?

   a. Antepartum

   b. Perinatal

   c. Postpartum

   d. Peripartum

4. A G4P2 female has carried a pregnancy to full term how many times?

   a. 4

   b. 6

   c. 2

   d. You cannot tell from this gravida/para status

5. Which of the following trimesters encompasses the time between 14 weeks to 27 weeks, 6 days of pregnancy?

   a. First trimester

   b. Second trimester

   c. Third trimester

6. "The incision along the edge of a cyst to form an open pouch for drainage" is which type of procedure?

   a. Centesis

   b. Incision and drainage

   c. Excision

   d. Marsupialization

7. Which of the following vulvectomies involves the removal of skin and deep subcutaneous tissues?

   a. Radical

   b. Simple

   c. Complete

   d. Partial

8. Which of the following devices is used as a cervical cap to cover the cervix for birth control purposes?

   a. Diaphragm

   b. Pessary

   c. IUD

   d. Cerclage

9. Which of the following are included in antepartum services when coding for the global routine delivery package?

   a. Management of labor

   b. Monthly visits with the OB provider

   c. Admission to the hospital

   d. Delivery of the fetus

10. The global delivery package includes which of the following?

    a. Antepartum services

    b. Delivery

    c. Postpartum checkup

    d. Antepartum, delivery, and postpartum services

11. Which of the following best describes the concept of an "incidental pregnancy"?

    a. A pregnancy that was not intended

    b. A pregnancy that occurred out of wedlock

    c. A pregnancy that impacts the medical decision-making of the provider

    d. A pregnancy that does not impact the medical decision-making of the pregnancy

12. Category Z3A codes identify which of the following?

    a. Trimester

    b. Fetus

    c. Weeks of gestation

    d. BMI

13. Which of the following codes would be reported to identify the outcome of delivery on the maternal record?

    a. Z37.1

    b. O80

    c. Z38.00

    d. O82

Instructions: Answer the following questions with the appropriate code(s) and modifier(s).

1. A 40-week pregnant female presents for spontaneous delivery of normal full-term liveborn female infant, delivered vaginally without assistance, no episiotomy, fetal manipulation, or instrumentation used.

   CPT codes: _____

   ICD-10 code: _____ , _____ ,

   _____

2. Total laparoscopic hysterectomy of uterus (307 grams) for intramural uterine fibroids.

   CPT codes: _____

   ICD-10 code: _____

3. Laparoscopic colpopexy for incomplete uterovaginal prolapse.

   CPT codes: _____

   ICD-10 code: _____

References

American Medical Association (AMA). 2019. *CPT 2020 Professional Edition*. Chicago: AMA.

Centers for Medicare and Medicaid Services (CMS). 2019. ICD-10-CM Official Guidelines for Coding and Reporting FY 2020. https://www.cms.gov/Medicare /Coding/ICD10/Downloads/2020-Coding-Guidelines .pdf.

Resources

American Congress of Obstetricians and Gynecologists (ACOG). 2017. Coding Question of the Month. https://www.acog.org/About-ACOG/ACOG -Departments/Coding/Coding-Question-of-the -Month?IsMobileSet=false.

American Medical Association (AMA). 2013. *Advanced Anatomy and Physiology for ICD-10-CM/PCS*. Salt Lake City, UT: Contexo Media.

Centers for Medicare and Medicaid Services (CMS). 2015 (October). ICD-10 Clinical Concepts for OB/GYN. https://www.cms.gov/Medicare/Coding/ICD10 /Downloads/ICD10ClinicalConceptsOBGYN1.pdf.

United Healthcare Oxford. 2017 (October 1). Obstetrical Policy. https://www.oxhp.com/secure/policy /obstetrical_policy.pdf.

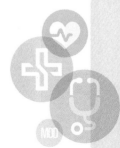

CHAPTER

Healthcare Specialist Services, Part I

Learning Objectives

- Understand the basics of billing and coding for healthcare specialist services, including consultations, hematology and oncology, neurology, and urology and nephrology services
- Examine procedural codes and guidelines, diagnosis coding, and medical necessity for

hematology and oncology, neurology, and urology and nephrology services
- Determine and apply ICD-10-CM, CPT, and HCPCS codes to hematology and oncology, neurology, and urology and nephrology services

Key Terms

Alzheimer's disease
Anemia
Benign prostatic hyperplasia (BPH)
Brachytherapy
Catheterizations
Central nervous system (CNS)
Cerebrospinal fluid (CSF) shunt
Chemodenervation
Chemotherapy
Circumcision
Consultation
Corpora cavernosa
Corpora spongiosum
Craniectomy
Craniotomy
Dementia
Dialysis
Dosimetry
Electroencephalogram (EEG)
Electronic brachytherapy

Epididymis
Epilepsy
Extracorporeal shock wave lithotripsy (ESWL)
Hematologist
Hemodialysis
Hydration
Hydrocele
Infusion
Injection
Intensity Modulated Radiation Treatment Delivery (IMRT)
Interstitial brachytherapy
Intracavitary brachytherapy
Intractable condition
Kidney
Lower urinary tract symptoms (LUTS)
Nephrolithiasis
Nephrolithotomy

Nephrologist
Neurologist
Neuropsychiatry
Neurosurgery
Oncologist
Orchiopexy
Parkinson's disease
Penis
Peripheral nervous system (PNS)
Peritoneal dialysis
Prostate
Push
Radiation oncologist
Scrotum
Seminal vesicles
Spermatic cord
Staghorn calculus
Status epilepticus
Status migrainosus

Stereotactic body radiation treatment (SBRT)

Stereotactic radiosurgery (SRS)

Testes

Transurethral resection of the prostate (TURP)

Tunica vaginalis

Ureters

Urethra

Urinary bladder

Urodynamics

Urologist

Vas deferens

Vasectomy

There are dozens of different healthcare specialties—from general practitioners who care for the entire health of a patient, like a primary care provider (PCP), to subspecialists who treat and manage only a small number of medical conditions, such as a pediatric endocrinologist. Healthcare specialists all focus on a specific body system, medical condition, or treatment type (refer to chapter 1 for a list of healthcare specialties).

Various types of healthcare specialist services have been discussed in this textbook, including obstetrics and gynecology, therapy providers, primary care providers, eye and vision services, and behavioral health services. This chapter discusses three additional specialties—hematology and oncology, neurology, and urology and nephrology. Chapter 19 (Healthcare Specialist Services, Part II) discusses gastroenterology and cardiology. However, this textbook does not address every healthcare specialty in which a coder may practice. It is important to keep in mind that a professional entering the world of coding must be flexible, pay close attention to detail, and follow coding guidelines, all while using a solid understanding of both human anatomy and physiology and medical terminology.

Healthcare Specialist Basics

When coding for services provided by a healthcare specialist, remember that a referral or prior authorization may be required before services can be provided to the patient. Healthcare specialists also provide consultations, which are evaluation and management (E/M) services that have a different set of coding guidelines. Finally, it is important to understand the specific types of services provided by hematologists and oncologists, neurologists, and urologists and nephrologists.

Referrals for Specialist Services

When coding for any type of healthcare specialty, it is important to remember that a healthcare specialist usually does not accept patients who have not been specifically referred to his or her office (see chapter 2 for more information on referrals, including how they function). Patients who see a healthcare specialist most likely have been seen first by a primary care or other provider who has determined that the patient needs specialized care, evaluation, or treatment. For example, a patient cannot determine that he or she has cancer and therefore must see an oncologist. Rather, this patient would be diagnosed first by the PCP, after consulting with a pathologist or radiologist, and then sent to an oncologist for evaluation and treatment.

Remember that the need for a referral depends on the patient's third-party payer (refer to chapter 2), as some policies do not require a referral nor prior authorization before services are provided to the patient. If a referral is required but not obtained prior to service being rendered, or if a referral (or authorization) number is not clearly identified on the CMS-1500 form, the insurance company may deny payment for the claim.

Consultations

A **consultation** is an E/M encounter provided by one healthcare professional, often a specialist, at the request of another healthcare professional such as a primary care provider. The consultant healthcare professional provides an E/M service, which may consist of all of the components of a typical E/M encounter including a history, examination, and medical decision-making, and then provides recommendations regarding the care of the patient. In this way, a consultation is similar to an outpatient office visit, for example, but with the additional element of the service being specifically requested by another provider so that the consulting provider can suggest treatment options or provide recommendations or advice regarding the patient's condition and its management.

A consultation differs from a referral, which is a request for care from one healthcare provider to another. A consultation is requested so that the consulting physician (specialist) can either recommend care for a specific condition or decide if he or she will take over the care of the patient and the specified condition. For example, a patient with an anal fissure may be sent for a consultation with a general surgeon to see if surgical treatment of the fissure is warranted, and to discuss pros, cons, and risks of the surgery. The general surgeon may then render any necessary service, including the surgical treatment.

In order to qualify as a consultation service for billing purposes, it must be formally requested by a healthcare provider (not by the patient or his family); the request must be in writing, and it must be documented in the patient's health record. Furthermore, the consultant's findings must be documented in a written report that is given to the requesting provider once the service is rendered and the consultation is complete. This leads to the three Rs of consultations: request, render, and report (see figure 18.1).

Figure 18.1. Three Rs of consultations

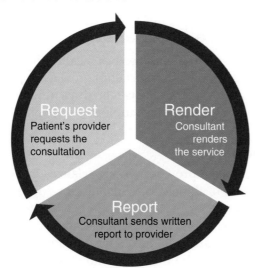

In order to report the code for a consultation service, the consultation must have been formally requested by the patient's healthcare provider. This is the *request*. Then the consultant (the healthcare specialist) provides the service to the patient. If additional procedures or services are necessary to treat, diagnose, or manage the patient, these services may be performed in addition to the consultation and will be coded separately.

This is the *rendering* of the service. After the service is rendered, the consultant must create and send a written report of the findings from the service to the requesting provider. This is the *report*.

If the three components of the consultation are not met, the service may not be billed as a consultation. It is important to understand the necessary components of a consultation and when it is possible to bill for them, as Medicare does not pay for consultation codes (CMS 2011). Other third-party payers may or may not pay for consultations, so it is also important to understand the guidelines for each patient's third-party payer to ensure the claim is coded correctly. If the patient's insurance does not pay for consultations, the service provided should be reported using the appropriate inpatient or outpatient office E/M code. For example, if a surgical consultation is performed in the office setting for a patient requesting a bunionectomy (including the request from the patient's PCP, the rendering of the evaluation and consultation by the surgeon, and the report from the surgeon to the PCP), but the patient's insurance does not cover consultation codes, the coder would need to report the appropriate outpatient office E/M code (99201–99205, 99212–99215) to identify the encounter with the patient, rather than the consultation E/M code.

Key to Success

Note again that Medicare does not pay for consultation services. Other third-party payers may also follow Medicare policy and deny payment for consultation codes. When you are reporting consultation E/M codes, verify with the patient's third-party payer to determine which codes to use. If the third-party payer does not pay for consultation codes (99241–99255), then report the service with the appropriate E/M code from the outpatient/office (99201–99215) or inpatient (99221–99239) E/M encounter codes.

Types of Healthcare Specialists

As mentioned previously, there are dozens of healthcare specialties. As medicine evolves, even more specialties and subspecialties grow as a result of new technologies and healthcare advances. This chapter focuses on three different healthcare specialties: hematology and oncology, neurology, and urology and nephrology.

Hematology and Oncology

A **hematologist** is a healthcare provider who specializes in the diagnosis, treatment, and prevention of diseases of the blood (hematology). An **oncologist** is a healthcare provider who specializes in the development, diagnosis, and treatment of malignant neoplasms and tumors (oncology). These two specialization areas are often combined into one specialty called hematology/oncology, which provides study and treatment for medical conditions of both the blood and tumors. This dual specialty may also be referred to as hem/onc. Similar to OB/GYN providers, providers may choose to specialize only in hematology or oncology but often combine into group practices, as the two specialties are closely related. Other specialists and subspecialists in hematology and oncology include medical or clinical oncologists, who treat cancer with treatments such as chemotherapy; surgical oncologists, who surgically remove tumors; and **radiation oncologists**, also known as interventional radiologists, who specialize in the treatment of cancers via radiation treatments (Cancer.net 2018).

Most of the services rendered by hematology and oncology providers are E/M services to evaluate and manage patients, as well as provide and manage cancer treatments such as chemotherapy, radiation therapy (radiation oncology), and surgical removals. Most of the conditions managed by hematologists and oncologists involve neoplasms and disorders of the blood.

Neurology

A **neurologist** is a medical doctor who specializes in the diagnosis and treatment of neurological disorders, including disorders of the nerves and the nervous system. Neurologists may further specialize in **neuropsychiatry**, treatment of mental or behavioral disturbances as a result of neurological conditions, or **neurosurgery**, surgical treatment of disorders of the nerves and nervous system.

Neurologists treat patients with neurological disorders of both the central nervous system, such as brain or spinal cord injuries, and the peripheral nervous system, such as peripheral neuropathies. Many of the surgical codes for neurological procedures are located in the Nervous system subsection of the CPT code book.

Urology and Nephrology

A medical doctor who specializes in the diagnosis and treatment of conditions of the urinary system, adrenal glands, and the male and female genital systems is a **urologist** (AUA 2018). A **nephrologist** is a medical doctor who focuses on the diagnosis and treatment of conditions of the kidneys, such as chronic kidney disease. Urologists may also treat specific disorders of the kidneys, but nephrologists focus solely on the kidneys.

Because urologists and nephrologists perform numerous surgery-based procedures, the majority of codes for urology and nephrology services are reported from the Urinary and Male Genital System subsections of the CPT code book. Additional codes may be reported from the Female Genital subsection of the CPT code book, when these services are performed by a urologist or nephrologist rather than an OB/GYN provider. Most diagnosis codes reported for medical necessity identify diseases of the genitourinary system.

Consultation Coding for Healthcare Specialist Services

As noted in the previous section, procedure codes for any type of healthcare specialist services depend on the type of specialty and the services provided. This section discusses consultation coding, which may be used by any type of healthcare provider.

To report a code for an office or other outpatient consultation, the service may be provided in any of the following settings:

- Outpatient or other ambulatory facility (like an ASC), including outpatient office
- Hospital observation area
- Home
- Domiciliary or rest home
- Emergency department

Office or other outpatient consultations are reported with codes 99241, Office consultation for a new or established patient, which requires these 3 key components: a problem-focused history; a problem-focused examination; and straightforward medical decision-making, through 99245, Office consultation for a new or established patient, which requires these 3 key components: a comprehensive history; a comprehensive examination; and medical decision-making of high complexity. As long as there is always a request in writing and the service is medically necessary, as many outpatient consultations as necessary may be reported per patient per provider.

Consultations may also be provided in the inpatient setting, to the following patients:

- Hospital inpatients
- Residents of nursing facilities
- Patients in a partial hospital setting (as discussed in chapter 7 [Behavioral Health Services])

In the inpatient setting, only one consultation service may be reported per patient per admission. For example, if a consultation was billed by Dr. Alameda for Patient B, then Dr. Alameda cannot bill for another consultation with the same patient unless Patient B has a new admission to the hospital. For example, if a consultation was provided for a gastrointestinal problem, and the patient was treated and discharged but returned the next day and was admitted again, and the same doctor provided another consultation for the same gastrointestinal problem, then the doctor can report each consultation as they occurred during separate admissions. Inpatient consultations are reported with codes 99251, Inpatient consultation for a new or established patient, which requires these 3 key components: a problem-focused history, a problem-focused examination; and straightforward medical decision-making, through 99255, Office consultation for a new or established patient, which requires these 3 key components: a comprehensive history; a comprehensive examination; and medical decision-making of high complexity.

Key to Success

Consultation codes are located in the E/M section of the CPT code book, after Hospital Inpatient Services (99221–99239).

Codes for consultations are much like the codes for outpatient office or inpatient encounters because they rely on determining the levels of the three key components (history, examination, and medical decision-making) to then determine the level of consultation service provided (as discussed in chapters 7 and 8). However, unlike outpatient office visit encounters, consultation codes do not differ based on whether the service was provided to a new or established patient. Both inpatient and outpatient consultations require all three key components to be at the level described in the code or higher.

Procedural and Diagnostic Coding for Hematology and Oncology

Procedures for hematology and oncology services are found throughout the CPT code book. For example, surgical removal of neoplastic organs and insertion of brachytherapy elements are found in the Surgery section, in each respective subsection; radiation oncology procedures are found in the Radiology section; and infusion procedures for chemotherapy are found in the Medicine section.

Surgical treatment of neoplasms (both benign and malignant) may involve surgical removal. Surgical removal codes are included in the Surgery section of the CPT code book, in their respective body system subsections. For example, the code for the removal of an osteosarcoma (cancer of the bone) would be located in the Musculoskeletal System subsection. To search for the removal of a lesion, organ, or part of an organ, search the CPT Index for the term *Excision* or *Resection* and then search for either the lesion or the type of body tissue or organ that was removed. Using the same example, search for the code for an osteosarcoma of the humerus, then for the term *Resection* in the Index, then *Tumor*, and then find *Humerus*. Next to the term *Humerus*, the coder will find the code for the radical resection of a tumor of the humerus, code 23220, Radical resection of tumor, proximal humerus.

Together with surgical removal of neoplastic tumors, cancers may also be treated in several different ways, and often combine one or more treatment methods. For example, a patient with a malignant neoplasm of the breast might undergo a mastectomy procedure to remove the neoplastic tissue and undergo chemotherapy.

Coding for hematology and oncology requires a strict attention to detail, and an in-depth knowledge of the types of treatments for neoplasms—including brachytherapy, radiation therapy, and chemotherapy. It also requires an in-depth knowledge of diagnosis coding guidelines for neoplasms and the services associated with neoplastic conditions.

Brachytherapy

Brachytherapy, also referred to as clinical brachytherapy, is a cancer treatment method in which small radioactive seeds, capsules, or elements are surgically placed in or near a cancer or cancerous organ (USNLM 2016a). These seeds may also be referred to as *brachytherapy sources* and are specifically designed to treat the neoplasm as best as possible (see figure 18.2). These small seeds emit radiation to the cancerous tissue

Figure 18.2. Brachytherapy seeds

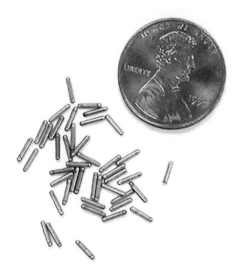

Source: NRC 2012.

while reducing radiation exposure to the remaining tissues at the same time, resulting in a precise treatment directed at the malignant neoplasm. Brachytherapy treatments include several different components, including simulation and planning, which are components of radiation oncology codes (discussed in the following section). Simulation and planning services include the virtual delivery of the brachytherapy treatment to the patient, planning of how the procedure will be performed, and how and where the brachytherapy sources will be implanted into the patient.

Surgical codes for brachytherapy report the actual implantation of the seeds or capsules into the specific organ. These codes are found in the Introduction categories (see chapter 11 [Surgical Services]) in each respective body system because the brachytherapy elements are directly introduced into the body tissues. The placement of brachytherapy elements may be interstitial or intracavitary. **Interstitial brachytherapy** involves placing the radioactive elements directly into the tumor or organ. **Intracavitary brachytherapy** involves placing the radioactive elements into a body cavity, such as the vagina or the bladder. These seeds are typically implanted via the use of radioactive wires, which, under ultrasonic guidance, are used to place the seeds directly where they are needed to treat the cancer. Figure 18.3 illustrates an interstitial brachytherapy procedure to treat prostate cancer.

Figure 18.3. Brachytherapy procedure to treat prostate cancer

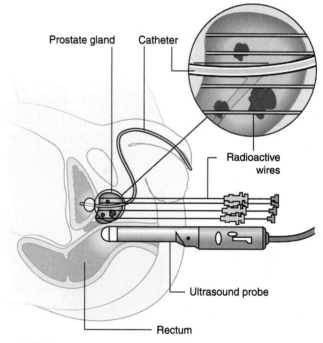

Source: Cancer Research UK 2015.

There are two further distinctions in brachytherapy treatment—clinical and electronic brachytherapy. Clinical brachytherapy is the use of radioactive elements, as described previously. **Electronic brachytherapy** is the use of a small, high-dose x-ray source, applied directly to the malignancy. It is used as an emerging treatment for skin cancer and, as such, codes for electronic brachytherapy treatments are Category III codes.

Key to Success

When coding, do not forget about Category III codes. These codes report new and emerging services and procedures, and all end with the letter *T*. Codes for electronic brachytherapy, for example, include 0394T, High dose rate electronic brachytherapy, skin surface application, per fraction, includes basic dosimetry, when performed.

Codes for the surgical placement of brachytherapy elements differ based on the body area or organ being treated and the method of brachytherapy used (namely, interstitial or intracavitary). For example, code 49411, Placement of interstitial device(s) for radiation therapy guidance (eg, fiducial markers, dosimeter), percutaneous, intra-abdominal, intra-pelvic (except prostate), and/or retroperitoneum, single or multiple, identifies the brachytherapy device placement as in the *intra-abdominal, intra-pelvic, or retroperitoneal* space and the device as *interstitial*. To find the codes for brachytherapy element placement, search for the term *Brachytherapy* in the CPT Index, and then locate the specific service related to the brachytherapy treatment, such as *interstitial application, intracavitary application,* or *planning*.

Because the surgeon is placing a medical device into the patient, it is necessary to report the HCPCS code for the brachytherapy source(s) (the device) in addition to the code for the surgical placement (reported with a CPT code). To search for brachytherapy sources in the HCPCS Index, search under the term *Brachytherapy radioelements,* or *Radioelements for brachytherapy.* The exact phrase for the radioelement source may differ depending on the publisher of the HCPCS code book. HCPCS codes for brachytherapy sources identify the type of source and are per-source codes, meaning that one source is reported per code. So, if 10 sources are used, the HCPCS code should be reported times 10. For example, code C2638, Brachytherapy source, stranded, iodine-125, per source, reports a stranded iodine-125 brachytherapy source. If 10 of these sources were implanted into the patient, the coder would report C2638 × 10 to identify the number of sources used.

In addition to the brachytherapy source insertion and the code for the brachytherapy itself, codes from the radiation oncology subsection of the CPT code book must be reported to identify the brachytherapy planning, simulation, and treatment. Clinical Brachytherapy codes (77750–77799) identify the actual brachytherapy treatment and application of the radioactive elements, solution, or source. They are grouped based on the complexity of the service, such as simple (1 to 4 sources); intermediate (5 to 10 sources); or complex (greater than 10 sources), and the type of brachytherapy treatment performed. For example, code 77761, Intracavitary radiation source application; simple, identifies the complexity of the service (*simple*) and the type of brachytherapy treatment performed (*intracavitary*).

When a brachytherapy service is performed, it is carefully planned and simulated to ensure that the method of treatment and dose are appropriate to treat the cancer while maintaining the surrounding healthy tissues. These services are included in the Radiation Oncology subsection of the CPT code book.

Radiation Oncology

The Radiation Oncology subsection (77261–77799) of the CPT code book reports services that use radioactive treatments for malignant neoplasms. Antineoplastic radiation therapy is a complex, carefully planned, designed, simulated, and delivered treatment that contains numerous components. The first stage of radiation treatment is a clinical consultation with a hematologist or oncologist who determines the need for radiation treatment and begins the radiation oncology service(s). This consultation and any other E/M services are reported with codes from the E/M section.

After the decision to treat the patient via radiation therapy is made, the radiation oncology services begin. The first step is clinical treatment planning and simulation of the treatment. Clinical treatment planning involves:

- Interpreting special tests
- Locating tumors
- Determining treatment volume
- Determining treatment time and dosage
- Choosing the treatment modality
- Determining the number and size of treatment ports
- Selecting treatment devices (AMA 2019)

Simulation is the process of targeting the anatomy to be treated during the procedure and determining the optimal process of radiation treatment for the patient (AMA 2019). These procedures are reported with codes 77261, Therapeutic radiology treatment planning; simple, through 77299, Unlisted procedure, therapeutic radiology clinical treatment planning. Planning and simulation codes are categorized based on whether the service is simple, intermediate, or complex, as defined in the guidelines for each category of codes.

Key to Success

One way to help ensure you are coding from the correct section in the Radiation Oncology subsection is to pay attention to the subheadings in the subsection of codes. Subheadings include Clinical Treatment Planning, Medical Radiation Physics, Dosimetry, Treatment Devices and Special Services, Stereotactic Radiation Delivery, Other Procedures, Radiation Treatment Delivery, and Radiation Treatment Management (among others). Before assigning codes for radiation oncology codes, be sure to review these headings and see how each selection of codes is organized. This will help you keep on track when searching for radiation oncology codes.

After the radiation treatment is planned and simulated, a process called **dosimetry** is performed to calculate the exact dose amount. In order to give the patient the dose of medication determined by the dosimetry calculation, treatment devices—such as patient immobilization devices or radiation-beam modification devices—are designed and created to administer the radiation. Additional consultations are also performed to inform the patient of the dosage and treatment plan. These services are reported with codes 77295, 3-dimensional radiotherapy plan, including dose-volume histograms, through 77370, Special medical radiation physics consultation.

After coding for the planning, simulation, dosimetry, and creation of device, then code for the delivery of different types of radiation treatments. The codes for delivery types are as follows.

- Stereotactic Radiation Treatment Delivery (77371–77373). **Stereotactic radiosurgery (SRS)** is a type of radiation treatment used for intracranial lesions that delivers a precision dose of radiation. SRS services are reported with codes 77371 and 77372. Whole-body SRS treatment, referred to as **stereotactic body radiation treatment (SBRT)**, is a developing type of stereotactic treatment used on body tumors. SBRT is reported with code 77373.

- Radiation Treatment Delivery (77385–77387, 77401–77417, 77424, 77425). Radiation treatment delivery codes depend on the type of radiation treatment delivered and the complexity of the service (simple, intermediate, or complex). Some codes also identify the treatment session for the radiation delivery. Radiation treatment delivery codes in this section include **Intensity Modulated Radiation Treatment Delivery (IMRT)**, a radiation treatment method that uses computer-based mapping to create dosing distributions delivered by a radiotherapy treatment machine.

- Neutron Beam Treatment Delivery (77423). Neutron beam radiation therapy codes identify neutron beam radiation treatments.

- Proton Beam Treatment Delivery (77520–77525). These codes identify radiation therapy services performed with proton beam radiation treatments.

Management of radiation treatments is reported with codes from the Radiation Treatment Management subsection (77427–77499). These codes identify the management services provided by the physician to the patient during the radiation treatment phase. Radiation treatment management services include a minimum of one examination (including assessment of the patient's response to the radiation treatments), coordination of the care and treatment of the patient, and review of each imaging or lab service. All of these services are included in the one radiation treatment management code, as defined by the CPT guidelines before the selection of codes for radiation treatment management.

In sum, radiation oncology coding is a complex subspecialty of coding that requires a comprehensive understanding of the types of treatments and delivery methods, including planning, simulating, and designing the process of radiation treatments for each individual patient.

Infusions

Infusion services for cancer patients are for the delivery of chemotherapy for patients with malignant neoplasms. **Chemotherapy** in general terms is the use of a drug to treat a medical condition. For hematology and oncology, chemotherapy is used to treat patients with malignant neoplasms by administering an infusion of antineoplastic chemotherapeutic agents.

Chemotherapy infusion codes are reported from the Hydration, Therapeutic, Prophylactic, Diagnostic Injections and Infusions, and Chemotherapy and Other Highly Complex Drug or Highly Complex Biologic Agent Administration subsections of codes (96360–96549). Coding for chemotherapy requires the identification of both the infusion service and the drug that was administered during the infusion. The ability to accurately code for infusion services relies on the understanding of a number of important concepts related to infusion services. Note that not all of the following are infusions, but are interrelated types of procedures that entail administering therapeutic, chemotherapeutic, or other substances directly into the patient's blood stream.

- *Hydration.* A **hydration** service is the administration of fluids or electrolytes without the presence of drugs. A hydration line may be started and then later used to administer drugs through the same intravenous (IV) insertion site.

According to CPT guidelines, if a hydration line is started in order to keep the vein open before or after a therapeutic or chemotherapy infusion, then the hydration service is not reported.

- *Injection.* An **injection** is given intramuscularly (into the muscle) to administer a therapeutic substance. Injections in this section of codes are *not* used to report the injection of vaccines, but rather a therapeutic, prophylactic, or diagnostic substance. Unlike a hydration or infusion service, an injection is given in a quick "shot" dose.

- *Infusion.* An **infusion** is the administration of a diagnostic, prophylactic, or therapeutic fluid or drug, given over a period of time longer than 15 minutes. This is the same as a hydration saline drip, except that the substance being administered is therapeutic rather than hydrating.

- *Push.* A **push** is the administration of a therapeutic, prophylactic, or diagnostic substance via an IV line (not an injection). A push can be administered together with an infusion or hydration. The difference between a push and an infusion is the timeframe. A push is an infusion of 15 minutes or less.

When coding for chemotherapy infusion codes, first identify the service as the administration of hydration, a therapeutic substance, or chemotherapy. As a reminder, vaccines are not coded from this category of codes. Refer to chapter 8 for a discussion of vaccine administration coding.

Another important component of infusion coding is the identification of the service as initial, sequential, or concurrent, as the code reported for the infusion service will differ. Note that these guidelines differ depending on whether the service was performed in the inpatient setting or the outpatient setting.

- An initial infusion is the primary reason for the encounter and includes the administration of the first or initial substance.

- A sequential infusion is the infusion or push of a new therapeutic substance after the initial infusion service. In order to qualify as a sequential infusion service, a new substance or drug must be administered through the same injection site.

- A concurrent infusion is the infusion of a new therapeutic substance at the same time as an existing infusion. A concurrent infusion is administered simultaneously with the initial infusion.

When coding for multiple infusions, read the infusion guidelines in the CPT code book to help identify which infusion should be reported as initial, sequential, or concurrent, and to ensure correct code selection. Although these administration codes may be used to report chemotherapy services, they may also be used to report the administration of various other drugs and biological substances, such as injections of antibacterial agents or allergenic extracts.

Key to Success

When coding for multiple infusions, carefully read the guidelines for these services in the CPT code book to ensure you report the infusion services appropriately. This is a long section of guidelines that includes a lot of detailed information. Remember to highlight and make notes in your CPT book to make sure you understand these guidelines and select the correct CPT codes.

Hydrations

Hydration services are reported with codes 96360, Intravenous infusion, hydration; *initial, 31 minutes to 1 hour*, and 96361, Intravenous infusion, hydration; *each additional hour*. Note that these codes identify the amount of time spent providing the hydration service. The first hour should be reported with 96360, with code 96361 added for each additional hour of service provided. For example, if a patient received six hours of hydration therapy, the coder should report 96360 for the first hour, and 96361 × 5 for the additional five hours, equaling six hours total (96360, 96361 × 5). If the patient receives less than 31 minutes of hydration therapy, hydration therapy service codes should not be used.

The parenthetical note under 96361 in the CPT code book specifies to report 96361 for hydration of greater than 30 minutes, up to one hour. In other words, to report the add-on code 96361, the additional time must be *at least* 30 minutes over the hour. For example, if the hydration service lasted for 5 hours 20 minutes, the codes reported would be as follows: 96360, 96361 × 4, equaling five total hours. The last 20 minutes are not counted, as they do not add up to the additional 30 minutes required to report the add-on code 96361 again.

Therapeutic, Prophylactic, and Diagnostic Injections and Infusions

Injections and infusions of therapeutic, prophylactic, and diagnostic substances are reported with codes 96365 through 96379. Note that these codes do not report the injection or infusion of chemotherapy agents; these codes specifically exclude chemotherapeutic substances. When selecting codes from this section, the coder must identify the type of service (injection, infusion, or push), the type of administration (namely, subcutaneous, intramuscular, intra-arterial, intravenous), and the amount of time it took to perform the service. As with hydration codes, the initial hour is reported with the initial code and an add-on code to identify each additional hour (30 minutes or more).

Chemotherapy Injections and Infusions

Chemotherapy administration codes are located in the Chemotherapy and Other Highly Complex Drug or Highly Complex Biologic Agent Administration subsection (96401–96549). This subsection is divided into three sections: Injections and Intravenous Infusions, Intra-arterial Administrations, and Other Injection and Infusion Services. See figure 18.4 for an illustration of chemotherapy administration.

- Injections and Intravenous Infusions report the administration of chemotherapy via an injection or intravenous infusion. Codes differ based on the type of administration (intramuscular, subcutaneous, intralesional, or intravenous), the type of antineoplastic substance, and the time it took to administer the service. Just as with hydration and therapeutic infusions, report the first hour with the code for initial service and then the add-on code for each additional hour (30 minutes or more).

- Intra-arterial Administrations report the administration of a chemotherapeutic agent directly into an arterial structure. Codes identify the time it took to administer the service and the technique used.

- Other Injection and Infusion Services codes report the administration of chemotherapeutic substances into other body structures, such as the pleural or peritoneal cavity, as well as additional services related to the delivery of chemotherapy. An example is code 96440, Chemotherapy administration into pleural cavity, requiring and including thoracentesis.

Figure 18.4. Patient receiving chemotherapy service

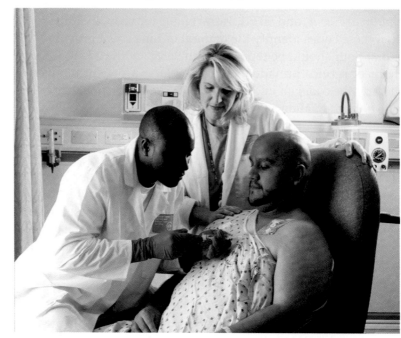

Source: NCI 2010.

Complete the exercises in There's a Code for That 18.1 to practice reporting hematology and oncology procedure codes.

18.1

There's a Code for That

Hematology and oncology procedures

Read the following documentation of the service and identify the CPT procedure code(s).

1. Insertion of vaginal brachytherapy device for female patient with endometrial cancer, with design and construction of simple treatment device.
   CPT codes: _____ , _____

2. Complex simulated field setting for therapeutic radiation treatment.
   CPT code: _____

3. Application of intermediate intracavitary radiation source.
   CPT code: _____

4. Simple radiology treatment planning.
   CPT code: _____

5. Complex radiation treatment delivery.
   CPT code: _____

6. Two hours of IV hydration therapy.
   CPT codes: _____ , _____

7. Intramuscular administration of hormonal anti-neoplastic chemotherapy.

   CPT codes: _____

8. Spinal puncture with intrathecal administration of chemotherapy.

   CPT codes: _____

Hematology and Oncology Diagnoses

Hematologists and oncologists treat both disorders of the blood and neoplasms. When reporting diagnosis codes for neoplasms, there are a number of guidelines that impact code selection and sequencing of which the coder should be aware.

Blood Disorders

Disorders of the blood are reported with codes from Chapter 3 (Diseases of the Blood and Blood-Forming Organs, of the ICD-10–CM) code book. Note that there are no chapter-specific coding guidelines for reporting the conditions in this chapter, so the coder must pay attention to specific instructions in the Tabular List and rely on provider documentation for correct code selection.

Perhaps one of the most common conditions in this chapter is anemia. **Anemia** occurs when a person has abnormally low red blood cells or hemoglobin in the blood. There are several different types of anemia that can be caused by a number of underlying conditions, or it may be idiopathic. Anemic conditions are reported with codes from categories D50 to D53, Nutritional anemias; D55 to D59, Hemolytic anemias; and D60 to D64, Aplastic and other anemias and other bone marrow failure syndromes. When coding for anemias, pay attention to the specific type of anemia, as well as any additional or underlying conditions or external causes. Note that many anemia codes are important in risk adjustment and HCC coding.

Category D63, Anemia in chronic disease classified elsewhere, is a special category of anemia manifestation codes. These codes identify anemia that is a manifestation of a specific disease, which is classified elsewhere in the ICD-10-CM code book. For example, code D63.0, Anemia in neoplastic disease, should be reported for a patient who has a neoplastic disease (such as cancer) that has resulted in anemia. Remember that manifestation codes can *never* be reported by themselves, they must always follow the code for the primary condition (that caused the manifestation). For example, if the patient has chronic kidney disease stage 5, which has resulted in anemia, the coder would select the following codes, in this order: N18.5, Chronic kidney disease, stage 5, and D63.1, Anemia in chronic kidney disease. Note that according to sequencing guidelines, a manifestation code can never be the first listed code on a claim. Instead, code the underlying condition first.

Neoplasms

Neoplasms are all reported with codes from chapter 2 (Neoplasms) of the ICD-10-CM code book. For a refresher on neoplasm coding refer to chapter 4 of this textbook (Learning the ICD-10-CM Code Book) for a description of the different types of neoplasms and how to locate neoplasms on the ICD-10-CM Index.

Neoplasm coding guidelines define the sequencing of neoplasms when a patient has more than one neoplasm, as well as the coding and sequencing of complications, administration of antineoplastic therapies, and current versus personal history of malignancies (see figure 18.5).

Neoplasm Sequencing

According to ICD-10-CM guidelines, when a patient has more than one malignancy, the sequencing depends on the reason for the encounter. Primary malignancies are the originating site of the neoplasm, and secondary malignancies are places to where the cancer has spread. If the patient is being seen for treatment of the primary malignancy, sequence the primary malignancy first, followed by the secondary malignancy. If the patient is being seen for the secondary malignancy, sequence the secondary malignancy first, followed by the code for the primary malignancy.

Coding and Sequencing of Complications

Pay attention to sequencing guidelines when reporting malignancies with complications such as anemia, dehydration, or other complications resulting from the neoplasm, antineoplastic therapy, or surgical procedure.

When a patient presents for treatment of anemia due to a neoplasm, sequence the code for the neoplasm before the code for the anemia. If the anemia is a direct result of antineoplastic therapy—such as chemotherapy or radiation therapy—and the patient is being treated for the anemia, then sequence the code for the anemia first, followed by the code for the malignancy and the adverse effect of antineoplastic therapy code (T45.1X5-, Adverse effect of antineoplastic and immunosuppressive drugs), or the abnormal reaction from radiation therapy code (Y84.2, Radiological procedure and radiotherapy as the cause of abnormal reaction of the patient, or of later complication, without mention of misadventure at the time of the procedure).

If a patient presents for treatment of either dehydration as a result of a malignancy or a complication from a surgical procedure, sequence either the dehydration or the complication first, followed by the code for the malignancy.

Key to Success

When in doubt about neoplasm sequencing, refer to the guidelines. There are many different circumstances to which specific guidelines apply, so make sure that you can locate these in your ICD-10-CM code book. Remember to underline, highlight, and write in your books as reminders about how to use these codes.

Administration of Antineoplastic Therapy

If the patient presents for the administration of antineoplastic chemotherapy, immunotherapy, or radiation therapy, sequence one of the following Z-codes first, followed by the code for the malignancy. If the patient received more than one type of antineoplastic therapy, report one of each of the following Z-codes for each type of antineoplastic therapy performed. These Z-codes are:

- Z51.0, Encounter for antineoplastic radiation therapy
- Z51.11, Encounter for antineoplastic chemotherapy
- Z51.12, Encounter for antineoplastic immunotherapy

If a patient develops complications like nausea or vomiting as a result of the antineoplastic therapy during the encounter, then report the Z-code first, followed by the codes for the complications and the adverse effect of antineoplastic therapy or

Figure 18.5. OGCR I.C.2

---

2. Chapter 2: Neoplasms (C00-D49)

General guidelines

Chapter 2 of the ICD-10-CM contains the codes for most benign and all malignant neoplasms. Certain benign neoplasms, such as prostatic adenomas, may be found in the specific body system chapters. To properly code a neoplasm it is necessary to determine from the record if the neoplasm is benign, in-situ, malignant, or of uncertain histologic behavior. If malignant, any secondary (metastatic) sites should also be determined.

Primary malignant neoplasms overlapping site boundaries

A primary malignant neoplasm that overlaps two or more contiguous (next to each other) sites should be classified to the subcategory/code .8 ('overlapping lesion'), unless the combination is specifically indexed elsewhere. For multiple neoplasms of the same site that are not contiguous such as tumors in different quadrants of the same breast, codes for each site should be assigned.

Malignant neoplasm of ectopic tissue

Malignant neoplasms of ectopic tissue are to be coded to the site of origin mentioned, e.g., ectopic pancreatic malignant neoplasms involving the stomach are coded to malignant neoplasm of pancreas, unspecified (c25.9)

The neoplasm table in the Alphabetic Index should be referenced first. However, if the histological term is documented, that term should be referenced first, rather than going immediately to the Neoplasm Table, in order to determine which column in the Neoplasm Table is appropriate. For example, if the documentation indicates "adenoma," refer to the term in the Alphabetic Index to review the entries under this term and the instructional note to "see also neoplasm, by site, benign." The table provides the proper code based on the type of neoplasm and the site. It is important to select the proper column in the table that corresponds to the type of neoplasm. The Tabular List should then be referenced to verify that the correct code has been selected from the table and that a more specific site code does not exist.

See Section I.C.21. Factors influencing health status and contact with health services, Status, for information regarding Z15.0, codes for genetic susceptibility to cancer.

a. Treatment directed at the malignancy

If the treatment is directed at the malignancy, designate the malignancy as the principal diagnosis.

The only exception to this guideline is if a patient admission/encounter is solely for the administration of chemotherapy, immunotherapy or external beam radiation therapy, assign the appropriate Z51.-- code as the first-listed or principal diagnosis, and the diagnosis or problem for which the service is being performed as a secondary diagnosis.

b. Treatment of secondary site

When a patient is admitted because of a primary neoplasm with metastasis and treatment is directed toward the secondary site only, the secondary neoplasm is designated as the principal diagnosis even though the primary malignancy is still present.

c. Coding and sequencing of complications

Coding and sequencing of complications associated with the malignancies or with the therapy thereof are subject to the following guidelines:

1) Anemia associated with malignancy

When admission/encounter is for management of an anemia associated with the malignancy, and the treatment is only for anemia, the appropriate code for the malignancy is sequenced as the principal or first-listed diagnosis followed by the appropriate code for the anemia (such as code D63.0, Anemia in neoplastic disease).

2) Anemia associated with chemotherapy, immunotherapy and radiation therapy

When the admission/encounter is for management of an anemia associated with an adverse effect of the administration of chemotherapy or immunotherapy and the only treatment is for the anemia, the anemia code is sequenced first followed by the appropriate codes for the neoplasm and the adverse effect (T45.1X5, Adverse effect of antineoplastic and immunosuppressive drugs).

When the admission/encounter is for management of an anemia associated with an adverse effect of radiotherapy, the anemia code should be sequenced first, followed by the appropriate neoplasm code and code Y84.2, Radiological procedure and radiotherapy as the cause of abnormal reaction of the patient, or of later complication, without mention of misadventure at the time of the procedure.

3) Management of dehydration due to the malignancy

When the admission/encounter is for management of dehydration due to the malignancy and only the dehydration is being treated (intravenous rehydration), the dehydration is sequenced first, followed by the code(s) for the malignancy.

(Continued on next page)

Figure 18.5. *(Continued)*

4) Treatment of a complication resulting from a surgical procedure

When the admission/encounter is for treatment of a complication resulting from a surgical procedure, designate the complication as the principal or first-listed diagnosis if treatment is directed at resolving the complication.

d. Primary malignancy previously excised

When a primary malignancy has been previously excised or eradicated from its site and there is no further treatment directed to that site and there is no evidence of any existing primary malignancy, a code from category Z85, Personal history of malignant neoplasm, should be used to indicate the former site of the malignancy. Any mention of extension, invasion, or metastasis to another site is coded as a secondary malignant neoplasm to that site. The secondary site may be the principal or first-listed with the Z85 code used as a secondary code.

e. Admissions/Encounters involving chemotherapy, immunotherapy and radiation therapy

1) Episode of care involves surgical removal of neoplasm

When an episode of care involves the surgical removal of a neoplasm, primary or secondary site, followed by adjunct chemotherapy or radiation treatment during the same episode of care, the code for the neoplasm should be assigned as principal or first-listed diagnosis.

2) Patient admission/encounter solely for administration of chemotherapy, immunotherapy and radiation therapy

If a patient admission/encounter is solely for the administration of chemotherapy, immunotherapy or external beam radiation therapy assign code Z51.0, Encounter for antineoplastic radiation therapy, or Z51.11, Encounter for antineoplastic chemotherapy, or Z51.12, Encounter for antineoplastic immunotherapy as the first-listed or principal diagnosis. If a patient receives more than one of these therapies during the same admission more than one of these codes may be assigned, in any sequence.

The malignancy for which the therapy is being administered should be assigned as a secondary diagnosis.

If a patient admission/encounter is for the insertion or implantation of radioactive elements (e.g., brachytherapy) the appropriate code for the malignancy is sequenced as the principal or first-listed diagnosis. Code Z51.0 should not be assigned.

3) Patient admitted for radiation therapy, chemotherapy or immunotherapy and develops complications

When a patient is admitted for the purpose of external beam radiotherapy, immunotherapy or chemotherapy and develops complications such as uncontrolled nausea and vomiting or dehydration, the principal or first-listed diagnosis is Z51.0, Encounter for antineoplastic radiation therapy, or Z51.11, Encounter for antineoplastic chemotherapy, or Z51.12, Encounter for antineoplastic immunotherapy followed by any codes for the complications.

When a patient is admitted for the purpose of insertion or implantation of radioactive elements (e.g., brachytherapy) and develops complications such as uncontrolled nausea and vomiting or dehydration, the principal or first-listed diagnosis is the appropriate code for the malignancy followed by any codes for the complications.

f. Admission/encounter to determine extent of malignancy

When the reason for admission/encounter is to determine the extent of the malignancy, or for a procedure such as paracentesis or thoracentesis, the primary malignancy or appropriate metastatic site is designated as the principal or first-listed diagnosis, even though chemotherapy or radiotherapy is administered.

g. Symptoms, signs, and abnormal findings listed in Chapter 18 associated with neoplasms

Symptoms, signs, and ill-defined conditions listed in Chapter 18 characteristic of, or associated with, an existing primary or secondary site malignancy cannot be used to replace the malignancy as principal or first-listed diagnosis, regardless of the number of admissions or encounters for treatment and care of the neoplasm.

See section I.C.21. Factors influencing health status and contact with health services, Encounter for prophylactic organ removal.

h. Admission/encounter for pain control/management

See Section I.C.6. for information on coding admission/encounter for pain control/management.

i. Malignancy in two or more noncontiguous sites

A patient may have more than one malignant tumor in the same organ. These tumors may represent different primaries or metastatic disease, depending on the site. Should the documentation be unclear, the provider should be queried as to the status of each tumor so that the correct codes can be assigned.

j. Disseminated malignant neoplasm, unspecified

Code C80.0, Disseminated malignant neoplasm, unspecified, is for use only in those cases where the patient has advanced metastatic disease and no known primary or secondary sites are specified. It should not be used in place of assigning codes for the primary site and all known secondary sites.

k. Malignant neoplasm without specification of site

Code C80.1, Malignant (primary) neoplasm, unspecified, equates to Cancer, unspecified. This code should only be used when no determination can be made as to the primary site of a malignancy. This code should rarely be used in the inpatient setting.

l. Sequencing of neoplasm codes

1) Encounter for treatment of primary malignancy

If the reason for the encounter is for treatment of a primary malignancy, assign the malignancy as the principal/first-listed diagnosis. The primary site is to be sequenced first, followed by any metastatic sites.

2) Encounter for treatment of secondary malignancy

When an encounter is for a primary malignancy with metastasis and treatment is directed toward the metastatic (secondary) site(s) only, the metastatic site(s) is designated as the principal/first-listed diagnosis. The primary malignancy is coded as an additional code.

3) Malignant neoplasm in a pregnant patient

When a pregnant woman has a malignant neoplasm, a code from subcategory O9A.1-, Malignant neoplasm complicating pregnancy, childbirth, and the puerperium, should be sequenced first, followed by the appropriate code from Chapter 2 to indicate the type of neoplasm.

4) Encounter for complication associated with a neoplasm

When an encounter is for management of a complication associated with a neoplasm, such as dehydration, and the treatment is only for the complication, the complication is coded first, followed by the appropriate code(s) for the neoplasm.

The exception to this guideline is anemia. When the admission/encounter is for management of an anemia associated with the malignancy, and the treatment is only for anemia, the appropriate code for the malignancy is sequenced as the principal or first-listed diagnosis followed by code D63.0, Anemia in neoplastic disease.

5) Complication from surgical procedure for treatment of a neoplasm

When an encounter is for treatment of a complication resulting from a surgical procedure performed for the treatment of the neoplasm, designate the complication as the principal/first-listed diagnosis. See the guideline regarding the coding of a current malignancy versus personal history to determine if the code for the neoplasm should also be assigned.

6) Pathologic fracture due to a neoplasm

When an encounter is for a pathological fracture due to a neoplasm, and the focus of treatment is the fracture, a code from subcategory M84.5, Pathological fracture in neoplastic disease, should be sequenced first, followed by the code for the neoplasm.

If the focus of treatment is the neoplasm with an associated pathological fracture, the neoplasm code should be sequenced first, followed by a code from M84.5 for the pathological fracture.

m. Current malignancy versus personal history of malignancy

When a primary malignancy has been excised but further treatment, such as an additional surgery for the malignancy, radiation therapy or chemotherapy is directed to that site, the primary malignancy code should be used until treatment is completed.

When a primary malignancy has been previously excised or eradicated from its site, there is no further treatment (of the malignancy) directed to that site, and there is no evidence of any existing primary malignancy at that site, a code from category Z85, Personal history of malignant neoplasm, should be used to indicate the former site of the malignancy. Subcategories Z85.0-Z85.7 should only be assigned for the former site of a primary malignancy, not the site of a secondary malignancy. Codes from subcategory Z85.8-, may be assigned for the former site(s) of either a primary or secondary malignancy included in this subcategory.

See Section I.C.21. Factors influencing health status and contact with health services, History (of)

n. Leukemia, Multiple Myeloma, and Malignant Plasma Cell Neoplasms in remission versus personal history

The categories for leukemia, and category C90, Multiple myeloma and malignant plasma cell neoplasms, have codes indicating whether or not the leukemia has achieved remission. There are also codes Z85.6, Personal history of leukemia, and Z85.79, Personal history of other malignant neoplasms of lymphoid, hematopoietic and related

(Continued on next page)

Figure 18.5. *(Continued)*

tissues. If the documentation is unclear, as to whether the leukemia has achieved remission, the provider should be queried.

See Section I.C.21. Factors influencing health status and contact with health services, History (of)

o. **Aftercare following surgery for neoplasm**

See Section I.C.21. Factors influencing health status and contact with health services, Aftercare

p. **Follow-up care for completed treatment of a malignancy**

See Section I.C.21. Factors influencing health status and contact with health services, Follow-up

q. **Prophylactic organ removal for prevention of malignancy**

See Section I.C. 21, Factors influencing health status and contact with health services, Prophylactic organ removal

r. **Malignant neoplasm associated with transplanted organ**

A malignant neoplasm of a transplanted organ should be coded as a transplant complication. Assign first the appropriate code from category T86.-, Complications of transplanted organs and tissue, followed by code C80.2, Malignant neoplasm associated with transplanted organ. Use an additional code for the specific malignancy.

Source: CMS 2019.

abnormal reaction to radiation therapy code. Again, refer to the OGCR (listed above) to make sure that all codes are assigned correctly and in the correct order.

Current versus Personal History of Neoplasm

Neoplasms should be reported as current until the patient is no longer undergoing any type of treatment toward that specific neoplasm (even if that neoplasm has been surgically removed).

Once the malignancy has been excised or successfully treated, there is no longer any treatment directed at the site, and there is no evidence of existing malignancy, then report the code for personal history of malignant neoplasm (from category Z85). For example, if a patient with breast cancer has a mastectomy, but is still undergoing chemotherapy treatments, then the coder should report the code for the breast cancer even though the patient has received a mastectomy. Once the patient completes the chemotherapy regimen and is no longer receiving any type of treatment for that breast cancer, then the coder should report the history of breast cancer code.

Complete the exercises in There's a Code for That 18.2. to practice reporting diagnosis codes for hematology and oncology services.

 18.2

Hematology and oncology diagnosis coding

There's a Code for That

Read the following documentation and assign the appropriate diagnosis code(s) for the patient's condition(s).

1. Iron deficiency anemia, NOS.

   ICD-10-CM code: _____

2. Anemia due to cancer of the pancreas.

   ICD-10-CM codes: _____ , _____

3. Primary malignant neoplasm of the tongue, frenulum linguae.

   ICD-10-CM code: _____

4. A 36-year-old female with family history of breast cancer is BRCA1 gene mutation positive, presents today for biopsy of lump in the upper outer quadrant of the right breast.

   ICD-10-CM codes: _____ , _____ , _____

5. Metastatic cancer of the left lung.

   ICD-10-CM code: _____

6. A 42-year-old patient presents for antineoplastic chemotherapy for angiosarcoma of the liver.

   ICD-10-CM codes: _____ , _____

Procedural and Diagnostic Coding for Neurology

Codes for nervous system procedures are found in two sections of the CPT code book: Surgery and Medicine. Codes in the Nervous System subsection of the Surgery section identify invasive surgical procedures like placement of a cerebrospinal fluid shunt, whereas codes in the Medicine section identify mostly noninvasive procedures and studies of the neurological system, such as routine electroencephalography (EEG). Diagnoses commonly seen by neurologists and neurosurgeons include mental and behavioral disorders, as well as medical conditions of the nervous system.

Nervous System Surgical Procedures

The nervous system surgery codes are divided into two main divisions, which correspond with the two main divisions in the human nervous system—the **central nervous system (CNS)** and the **peripheral nervous system (PNS)**. The central nervous system is comprised of all of the nerves of the brain and the spinal cord. The peripheral nervous system is comprised of all the other nerves throughout the body (USNLM 2016b). Procedures on the central nervous system are reported with codes from the Skull, Meninges, and Brain (61000–62258) and Spine and Spinal Cord (62263–63746) subsections, and procedures on the peripheral nervous system are reported with codes from the Extracranial Nerves, Peripheral Nerves, and Autonomic Nervous System (64400–64999).

Skull, Meninges, and Brain

Procedures on the skull, meninges, and brain include the creation of an access point into the skull, such as a subdural tap through a fontanelle (the soft spot on the head of an infant), a twist drill hole, burr hole, trephine, or craniectomy or craniotomy (see figure 18.6). Twist drill, burr hole, and trephine procedures are all used to create a small opening into the skull, either for diagnostic or therapeutic purposes. Code selection depends on the type of opening created and the purpose of the procedure, as seen in code 61105, Twist drill hole for subdural or ventricular puncture.

Figure 18.6. Craniotomy

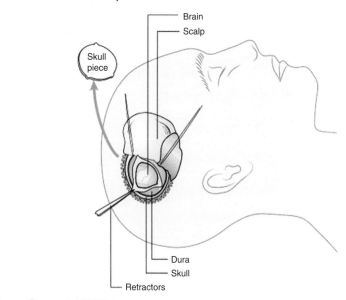

Source: Cancer Research UK 2014a.

Craniectomy and Craniotomy codes (61304–61576) are more numerous and identify the specific type of procedure (craniectomy or craniotomy), area of the procedure, and purpose of the procedure or any additional services performed (for example, code 61510, Craniectomy, trephination, bone flap craniotomy; for excision of brain tumor, supratentorial, except meningioma). Craniectomies are performed to remove a portion of skull for an indicated reason, such as a lesion of the skull or damaged area, or to allow for a therapeutic procedure. Craniotomies are performed to remove a portion of the skull to allow access into the cranium or for therapeutic reasons, such as to relieve pressure or allow for drainage.

Key to Success

Do not get confused between craniectomies and craniotomies. A **craniectomy** is the removal of a portion of the skull. A **craniotomy** is an incision into the skull. The difference between the two is that in a craniotomy, the piece of skull is removed for therapeutic or diagnostic reasons, then placed back in its original location, whereas in a craniectomy, the fragment of bone is not replaced.

Surgeries of the skull base (61580–61619) are detailed procedures that require a number of qualified surgeons working as a team to complete the surgery. There are three different components to a surgery of the skull base: the approach procedure, the definitive procedure, and the repair/reconstructive procedure. The approach and the definitive procedures are always coded separately, with different CPT codes. The approach procedure describes the way in which the skull base is dissected open to reveal the lesion, as well as any additional procedures performed to gain access to the lesion, such as removal of sinuses or removal of facial bones. The definitive procedure describes the service that was performed on the lesion once access was gained, such as resection or excision of the lesion. The repair or reconstruction procedure is only

remember that vertebrae have two sides. If a procedure is performed on both sides of the vertebra, it should be reported as a bilateral service (modifier -50). Read code descriptions thoroughly to ensure correct code selection and the application of any necessary modifiers. For example, code 63020, Laminotomy (hemilaminectomy), with decompression of nerve root(s), including partial facetectomy, foraminotomy and/or excision of herniated intervertebral disc; 1 interspace, cervical, describes the spinal area (*cervical*), and describes a unilateral procedure. In the parenthetical notes under the code description, it states: *For bilateral procedure, report 63020 with modifier 50.* This means that code 63020 describes a unilateral procedure, so if the procedure was performed on both sides, it should be reported with modifier -50.

Key to Success

Remember that when coding for procedures on the vertebrae or spinal column, some codes describe the number of interspaces or vertebral segments involved in the procedure. For more than one interspace or vertebral segment, check for the add-on code that is used to identify each additional interspace or segment. For example, if the provider performed the procedure described by code 63020 on three interspaces in the cervical region, then the coder should report code 63020 once for the first segment, and then the add-on code 63035, Each additional interspace, cervical or lumbar, twice for the additional two segments: 63020, 63035 × 2.

Extracranial Nerves, Peripheral Nerves, and Autonomic Nervous System

Procedures on the extracranial, peripheral, and autonomic nerves include injections of anesthetic and therapeutic substances, implantation of neurostimulators, and destruction of nerves. When coding for any kind of service on a nerve, it is necessary to identify the specific nerve involved in the procedure, as in code 64405, Injection(s), anesthetic agent(s) and/or steroid; greater occipital nerve. In many of the categories, nerves are grouped by their type, such as somatic nerves, paravertebral spinal nerves and branches, autonomic nerves, and sympathetic nerves.

Codes 64600 through 64681 report destruction by neurolytic agent (for example, chemical, thermal, electrical, or radiofrequency), and chemodenervation procedures. **Chemodenervation** is the injection of botulinum toxin, a potent neurotoxin, to an affected nerve for various reasons including pain management and reduction of muscle spasticity. Like nerve injection procedures, chemodenervation codes identify the specific nerve or muscle being treated. Check for add-on codes in this section to fully report each injection performed.

Additional procedures in this section include:

- Neuroplasty (Exploration, Neurolysis or Nerve Decompression) codes (64702–64727), which report plastic surgical decompression or freeing of intact nerves from scar tissue.

- Transection or Avulsion codes (64732–64772), which report the actual transection (cutting of the nerve) or avulsion (tearing away) of nerves for therapeutic purposes.

- Excision codes (64774–64823) report the surgical removal of either nerves or tumors on specific nerves.

- Neurorrhaphy codes (64831–64876) report the surgical repair of nerves via suture or anastomosis.

- Neurorrhaphy With Nerve Graft, Vein Graft, or Conduit codes (64885–64913) report surgical repair of nerves using a graft for the repair.

Neurology Medicine Procedures

There are also several neurology procedures in the Medicine section of the CPT code book. These include specialized tests and treatments to help diagnose, treat, and assist with surgical procedures. These procedures include:

- Sleep Medicine (95782, 95783, 95800–95811) .
- Routine Electroencephalography (EEG) (95812–95827, 95830). An **electroencephalogram (EEG)** is a diagnostic study of the electrical impulses of the brain. EEGs are useful in diagnosing neurological conditions such as epilepsy, brain tumors, encephalitis, encephalopathy, strokes, sleep disorders, and dementia.
- Range of Motion Testing (95851–95852, 95897).
- Electromyography (95860–95872, 95885–95887).
- Muscle Testing and Guidance (95873–95875).
- Nerve Conduction Studies (95905–95913).
- Intraoperative Neurophysiology (95940, 9594).
- Autonomic Function Tests (95921–95924, 95943).
- Evoked Potentials and Reflex Tests (95925–95939).
- Special EEG Tests (95954–95967, 95700-95726). Like routine EEGs, special EEGs are recordings of the brain's electrical impulses. However, these EEGs are extended or performed in a different manner than routine EEGs.
- Neurostimulators, Analysis-Programming (95970–95984).
- Motion Analysis (96000–96004).
- Functional Brain Mapping (96020).

As a tool to help support correct code selection, Appendix J of the CPT code book includes an Electrodiagnostic Medicine Listing of Sensory, Motor, and Mixed Nerves. This appendix, as first mentioned in chapter 5, identifies nerves that may be assigned to nerve conduction studies (95907–95913), as well as electromyography (EMG) (95860–95864, 95867–95870, 95885–95887), and neuromuscular junction testing (95937). As with coding for all CPT codes, reporting neurology medicine procedures requires a strict attention to detail and understanding of how to report CPT codes properly.

Complete the exercises in There's a Code for That 18.3 to practice reporting neurology procedure codes.

18.3

There's a Code for That

Neurology procedures

Read the following documentation of the service and identify the CPT procedure code(s).

1. Infratentorial trephine.

   CPT code: _____

2. Craniectomy of the posterior fossa of the skull for excision of meningioma.

   CPT code: _____

3. Simple dural repair of intracranial arteriovenous malformation.

   CPT code: _____

4. Creation of subdural-pleural CSF shunt.

   CPT code: _____

5. Cervical laminectomy with exploration and decompression of spinal cord without discectomy, of three vertebral segments.

   CPT code: _____

6. Thoracic discectomy and decompression of spinal cord and nerve roots, T3 to T6.

   CPT code: _____ , _____

Neurology Diagnoses

The majority of diagnosis codes reported by neurologists are located in chapter 5 (Mental, Behavioral, and Neurodevelopmental Disorders) and chapter 6 (Diseases of the Nervous System) of the ICD-10-CM code book. However, keep in mind that neurology conditions may present with additional comorbidities or complications that would be coded from other chapters of the ICD-10-CM code book. Also, neurologists will see patients who have suffered traumatic brain injuries or stroke victims. Refer to chapter 16 for guidance on how to report strokes and cerebrovascular incidents, as well as traumatic brain injuries.

Mental, Behavioral, and Neurodevelopmental Disorders

The only coding guidelines that pertain to coding for conditions from the Mental, Behavioral, and Neurodevelopmental Disorders chapter are for the reporting of pain disorders due to psychological factors and mental disorders due to psychoactive substance use.

One commonly seen condition coded from this chapter is dementia. **Dementia** is the term for loss of memory and mental abilities due to an underlying physical change in the brain. Codes for dementia are located in categories F01, Vascular dementia, F02, Dementia in diseases classified elsewhere, and F03, Unspecified dementia. For both vascular and dementia in diseases classified elsewhere, there is a note in the Tabular List to code first for the underling physiological condition, such as cerebrovascular incident (stroke) or Alzheimer's disease. Note that dementia codes are included in HCC and special attention should be paid to the documentation and reporting of the most specified dementia codes.

Chapter 5 of the ICD-10-CM code book also includes codes for mental disorders such as schizophrenia, mood disorders, and depression. Many of these conditions are discussed in chapter 7 of this textbook regarding behavioral health services. As a rule of thumb, neurologists treat mental diagnoses that are a result of an underlying physiological condition, such as vascular dementia—dementia caused by a vascular disease of the brain. However, these conditions do sometimes present in conjunction with mental disorders often treated by a behavioral healthcare practitioner.

Diseases of the Nervous System

Neurologists treat a wide range of neurological conditions, most of which are included in chapter 6 (Diseases of the Nervous System) of the ICD-10-CM code book. Note that the guidelines for this chapter pertain to dominant and nondominant sides and pain, discussed in chapters 16 and 12 of this textbook, respectively. Conditions treated by neurologists in this chapter of the ICD-10-CM book include the following (note that many of these conditions are also classified as HCC codes, so it is important to ensure that these codes are documented fully and coded to the highest level of specificity).

- Extrapyramidal and movement disorders (G20–G26), including Parkinson's disease (G20, Parkinson's disease). **Parkinson's disease** is a progressive disorder of the central nervous system that causes tremors, rigidity, and postural problems.

- Other degenerative diseases of the nervous system (G30–G32), including Alzheimer's disease (G30.-). **Alzheimer's disease** is a progressive form of dementia that causes loss of memories and cognitive abilities that interfere with activities of daily living. Codes for Alzheimer's disease specify whether the condition is early-onset (before the age of 65), late onset, or other form. Note the guidelines in the Tabular List to use an additional code to identify Alzheimer's dementia with or without behavioral disturbance (F02.80, Dementia in other diseases classified elsewhere without behavioral disturbance, or F02.81, Dementia in other diseases classified elsewhere with behavioral disturbance). According to ICD-10-CM Tabular notes, the appropriate code for dementia or delirium should always accompany the code for Alzheimer's disease. When sequencing Alzheimer's disease and dementia, sequence the Alzheimer's code first, followed by the code for the dementia (either with or without behavioral disturbance) or delirium.

- Episodic and Paroxysmal Disorders (G40–G47), including Epilepsy and recurrent seizures (G40). **Epilepsy** is a neurological condition that manifests in sensory disturbances, loss of consciousness, and seizures (convulsions) as a result of abnormal electrical activity in the brain. Codes for epilepsy identify various components, which make them some of the more complex codes in ICD-10-CM. These include:
  - *The type of epilepsy.* For example, localization-related (focal) (partial) symptomatic epilepsy, generalized idiopathic epilepsy, or juvenile myoclonic epilepsy.
  - *The type of seizures.* For example, seizures of localized onset, simple partial seizures, or complex partial seizures.
  - *Intractability status.* An **intractable condition** is one that does not respond to medical treatment. For example, an intractable migraine is one that does not respond to migraine pain medication. Intractable epilepsy is difficult or impossible to control with treatment. Codes for epilepsy identify whether the condition is intractable or not.
  - *Status epilepticus.* **Status epilepticus** is a type of epilepsy in which the seizures occur too close together for the patient to fully recover in-between seizures, or when a seizure lasts for a long period of time. Codes for epilepsy also identify whether the condition presents with status epilepticus or not.

For example, code G40.019, Localization-related (focal) (partial) idiopathic epilepsy and epileptic syndromes, with seizures of localized onset, intractable, without status epilepticus, identifies the type of epilepsy (*localization-related*), type of seizures (*localized onset*), intractability status (*intractable*), and with or without status epilepticus (*without status epilepticus*).

- Migraine (G43) codes are similar in complexity to epilepsy codes, as they identify the following elements:
  - *The type of migraine.* These types include with aura (sensory disturbances such as seeing haloes around objects), without aura, hemiplegic migraine, persistent migraine aura without cerebra infarction, and persistent migraine aura with cerebral infarction.
  - *Intractability status.* Just as in epileptic syndromes, migraines that are intractable do not respond to medication. A non-intractable migraine is one that does respond to pain medication.
  - *Status migrainosus.* **Status migrainosus** migraines are long-lasting migraines, which can last 72 hours or more.

For example, code G43.401, Hemiplegic migraine, not intractable, with status migrainosus, identifies the type of migraine (*hemiplegic*), intractability status (*not intractable*), and with or without status migrainosus (*with status migrainosus*).

Additional conditions in this chapter include nerve disorders, neuropathies, and paralytic syndromes.

Complete the exercises in There's a Code for That 18.4 to practice reporting neurology diagnosis codes.

Neurology diagnosis coding

18.4

There's a Code for That

Read the following documentation and assign the appropriate diagnosis code(s) for the patient's condition(s).

1. Parkinson's disease with dementia with aggressive and combative behavior.

   ICD-10-CM code: _____ , _____

2. Congenital nonprogressive ataxia.

   ICD-10-CM code: _____

3. Parkinsonism due to vascular malformation.

   ICD-10-CM code: _____

4. Lewy body dementia without behavioral disturbance.

   ICD-10-CM code: _____ , _____

5. Multiple sclerosis.

   ICD-10-CM code: _____

6. Intractable absence epileptic syndrome, without status epilepticus.

   ICD-10-CM code: _____

7. Persistent migraine aura without cerebral infarction, without refractory migraine, with status migrainosus.

   ICD-10-CM code: _____

Procedural and Diagnostic Coding for Urology and Nephrology

Coding for urology and nephrology services requires an understanding of at least two subsections of the CPT code book: the Urinary System and Male Genital System. Remember that urologists may also perform some procedures on the female urinary system (such as a sling operation for stress incontinence), which are located in the Female Genital System subsection. Dialysis is performed for patients with chronic kidney disease and end-stage renal disease, and codes for dialysis and end-stage renal disease services are found in the Medicine section of the CPT code book.

Urinary System Procedures

Surgical procedures on the urinary system are all located in the Urinary System subsection of the CPT code book. This subsection is organized into four main sections, according to the four main organs in the urinary system—kidneys, ureters, bladder, and urethra.

The **kidneys** are two bean-shaped organs that function to filter waste products from the blood and to control electrolyte balance and the body's balance of fluid. In this process, the kidneys create urine, which passes through the urinary system through the **ureters**—two thin tubes that connect the kidneys to the urinary bladder. The **urinary bladder**, also known as the bladder, is a hollow muscular organ that holds urine until it is emptied from the body through the urethra. The **urethra** is the last part of the

Figure 18.9. Urinary system anatomy

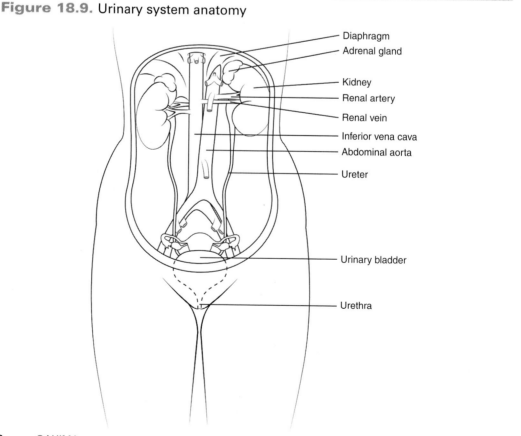

urinary system, through which urine passes during elimination from the bladder. In females, the urethra is about 1 to 1.5 inches long, ending directly in front of the vaginal opening and located between the labia. In males, the urethra is about 7 to 8 inches long, beginning at the bladder and ending at the urethral orifice at the tip of the penis. The **prostate** is a gland only found in males that stores and assists in making seminal fluid, and sits under the urinary bladder surrounding part of the urethra. See figure 18.9 for an overview of urinary system anatomy.

Kidney

Surgical procedures on the kidneys are reported with codes from the Kidney subheading (50010–50593). Note that nephrologists, as specialists in the diagnosis and treatment of kidney disorders, are more likely to perform procedures on the kidneys, although some minor procedures may be performed by urologists as well. This depends on the resources, training, and availability of the healthcare specialists.

Figure 18.10. Renal calculi

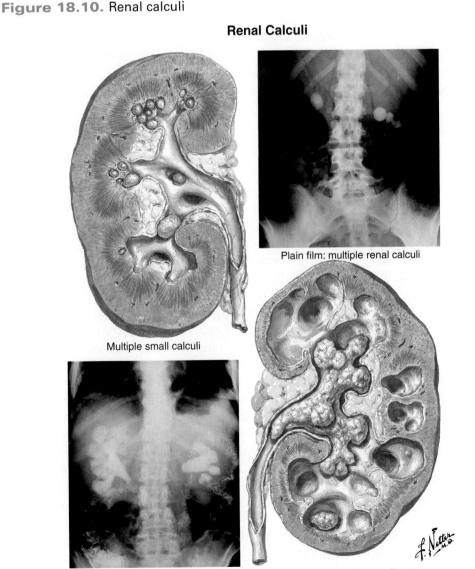

Renal Calculi

Plain film: multiple renal calculi

Multiple small calculi

Bilateral staghorn calculi

Staghorn calculus plus smaller stone

Many of the surgical procedures on the kidneys are for the treatment of **nephrolithiasis**, or kidney stones. Kidney stones—also known as renal calculi—are usually small, condensed deposits of minerals and other solids that form in the kidneys (see figure 18.10). To expel the stone from the urinary tract, it passes through the urinary system, down the ureters, through the bladder, and out through the urethra. This is a painful and sometimes lengthy process. However, if the stone is too large to pass naturally through the urinary tract, or if it becomes obstructed (stuck), it must be treated surgically. A large nephrolithiasis, known as **staghorn calculus**, completely fills the renal pelvis (the area within the kidney), and is too big to pass naturally through the urinary system and may require surgical treatment.

Codes for the open incision of the kidneys are located in the Incision category (50010–50135) and include codes for the incision and drainage of renal abscesses, as well as **nephrolithotomy**—incision into the kidney for the removal of a kidney stone. Nephrolithotomy codes identify the type of operation and the type of calculus. For example, code 50075, Nephrolithotomy; removal of large staghorn calculus filling renal pelvis and calyces (including anatrophic pyelolithotomy), reports an incisional procedure to remove a staghorn calculus from the kidney.

MOD

Because kidneys are bilateral organs, the coder must identify the laterality of the procedure by appending modifier -RT or -LT, for right or left side. Unless there are specific notations in the CPT code book, if the procedure was performed bilaterally, append modifier -50 to report the bilateral service. Note that the way unilateral or bilateral codes are reported may depend on the third-party payer; always check the payer requirements to ensure correct modifier selection.

Excision codes (50200–50290) identify excisional procedures performed in the kidneys, such as renal biopsies and excision of kidneys. If the excision of the kidney is part of a kidney transplantation procedure, it is coded from the Renal Transplantation subsection (50300–50380). Remember that there are three main components to any major organ transplant—organ removal, backbench work, and recipient transplantation (refer to chapter 11). Note that a donated kidney may come from either a living or cadaver donor, and kidney transplants may be performed with or without the removal of the recipient's kidney. Both of these components impact code selection, as seen in code 50365, Renal allotransplantation, implantation of graft; with recipient nephrectomy.

Kidney Introduction procedures (50382–50435) include the placement and removal of catheters (both internally dwelling as well as externally accessible) in the renal pelvis, and the creation of nephrostomies and injection procedures.

Laparoscopic procedures of the kidney are reported with codes 50541 through 50549. Many of these procedures are also located in other procedural categories, with the exception that codes in this section all identify laparoscopic procedures. For example, code 50547, Laparoscopy, surgical; donor nephrectomy (including cold preservation), from living donor, is the same procedure as code 50320, Donor nephrectomy (including cold preservation); open, from living donor, with the exception that code 50547 is performed via the laparoscopic approach, and code 50320 is performed via the open approach.

Codes for Endoscopy (50551–50580) of the kidneys differ depending on the approach to the endoscopic procedure (through nephrostomy or nephrotomy), and the definitive procedure performed during the endoscopy (such as removal of calculus).

The Other Procedures category of codes (50590–50593) contain the code 50590, Lithotripsy, extracorporeal shock wave. **Extracorporeal shock wave lithotripsy (ESWL)** is a procedure in which shock waves are sent through the patient's body to break up a nephrolithiasis into tiny fragments. Once the stone is broken up, it naturally passes through the urinary system (see figure 18.11).

Figure 18.11. Extracorporeal shockwave lithotripsy (ESWL)

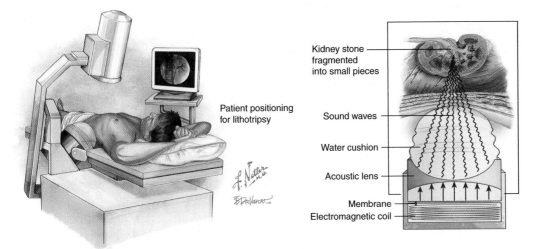

Patient positioning for lithotripsy

Kidney stone fragmented into small pieces

Sound waves

Water cushion

Acoustic lens

Membrane
Electromagnetic coil

Ureter

Procedures on the ureters include Incision (50600–50630), Excision (50650–50660), Introduction (50684–50695), Repair (50700–50940), Laparoscopy (50945–50980), and Endoscopy (50951–50980). When coding for ureteral procedures, identify the procedure as being performed on the right or left side, or if the procedure was performed bilaterally. Note that these components are not included in the code descriptions. For example, code 50605, Ureterotomy for insertion of indwelling stent, all types, does not identify the procedure as either unilateral or bilateral. In this case, the documentation should identify the laterality of the procedure, and the coder should append modifier -50 if the procedure was performed bilaterally, or modifier -LT or -RT to identify the laterality of the procedure for unilateral procedures.

Bladder

There are more procedures on the bladder than for any other organ in the urinary system. These include procedures for the removal of calculi, destruction and removal of lesions and tissue, introduction procedures, and repair procedures.

Key to Success

The medical prefix for the bladder is *cyst/o-*, and numerous procedures in this subheading refer to *cystotomy*, *cystectomy*, or *cystostomy*. If you think of a cyst as a fluid-filled sac, it is easy to remember that *cyst/o-* refers to the bladder—a sac that holds urine.

Procedures on the bladder include:

- Incision (51020–51080) codes identify surgical incisions into the bladder to remove calculi, insert radioactive material as a treatment for cancer, or for drainage.
- Removal (51100–51102) codes report the surgical aspiration of bladder contents via needle, trocar or intracatheter, or with insertion of suprapubic catheter.
- Excision (51500–51597) codes identify the removal of the bladder or additional urinary components. When coding for cystectomies, identify the components removed and any additional procedures performed.
- Introduction (51600–51720) codes report the introduction of a catheter, injected substance, or cystostomy tube. This subheading includes codes for urinary catheterizations. Catheterizations are common procedures that involve the insertion of a catheter tube in through the urethra and into the bladder to drain urine. There are two types of catheterizations—straight and indwelling:
  - Straight catheterization, coded with 51701, Insertion of non-indwelling bladder catheter (eg, straight catheterization for residual urine), is performed by inserting a catheter through the urethra and into the bladder to drain urine from the bladder. This procedure is performed to either completely drain the bladder or to collect a urine sample. Once the urine is drained, the catheter is removed.
  - Indwelling catheterization, coded with 51702, Insertion of temporary indwelling bladder catheter; simple (eg, Foley), or 51703, Insertion of temporary indwelling bladder catheter; complicated (eg, altered anatomy, fractured catheter/balloon), is performed by inserting a catheter with a small balloon at the tip through the urethra and into the bladder, where the balloon is inflated so that it stays in place (see figure 18.12). This allows the urine to drain from the bladder for a longer period of time, into a collection bag. Indwelling catheters are used for continuous drainage for patients who are undergoing surgery, bedridden, or are otherwise unable to move themselves to the toilet. Indwelling catheters may stay in place for several days, depending on the patient's medical condition and the safety implications of a long-term bladder catheterization.

Figure 18.12. Indwelling catheterization

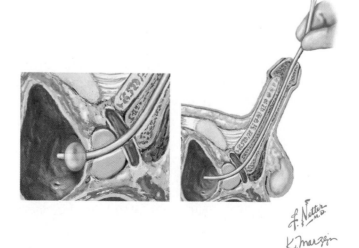

- Urodynamics codes (51725–51798) report a variety of procedures. Urodynamics is the study of the motion and flow of urine. These codes identify procedures designed to study urinary flow and pressure, as well as additional studies on the nerve conduction of the anal or urethral sphincter, and measurement of urinary post-voiding.

- Repair codes (51800–51980) report the surgical repair of the bladder and associated components, as well as closure of fistulas. Some of these procedures include repair of components located in the female genital system, so it is important to pay attention to the parenthetical notes in the Tabular List to ensure correct code selection.

- Laparoscopy codes (51990–51999) report two different types of sling operations for stress incontinence in which sutures are placed near the bladder to support the neck of the urethra. If this procedure is performed via the open approach, it is reported with the appropriate code from the female vaginal system. When performed via the open approach, urinary incontinence surgeries for males are coded from the Urethra subheading of codes in the Repair category. Again, it is important to pay attention to the parenthetical notes in the Tabular List to ensure correct code selection.

- Endoscopy—Cystoscopy, Urethroscopy, Cystourethroscopy codes (52000–52010) identify endoscopic procedures of the urinary system. This subsection includes Transurethral Surgery of the Urethra and Bladder (52204–52318) and of the Ureter and Pelvis (52320–52356), as well as endoscopic procedures of the Vesical Neck and Prostate (52400–52700). Procedures on the vesical neck and prostate include transurethral procedures on the prostate. One of the most common medical conditions of the prostate is benign prostatic hyperplasia (BPH), a condition in which the prostate gland is enlarged, causing urinary frequency and urgency, nocturia (urinating at night), and urinary retention (among other symptoms). As a treatment for BPH and the lower urinary tract symptoms, prostatic tissue can be surgically removed to reduce obstruction and pressure on the bladder and urethra. One of the ways in which this tissue is removed is via a procedure called a transurethral resection of the prostate (TURP) (see figure 18.13). Coded with 52601, Transurethral electrosurgical resection of the prostate, including control of postoperative bleeding, complete (vasectomy, meatotomy, cystourethroscopy, urethral calibration and/or dilation, and internal urethrotomy are included), TURP involves the insertion of a resectoscope through the male urethra, which is threaded to the area of the prostate tissue to be removed. An electrocautery knife is then used to cut away at the enlarged prostatic tissue. Transurethral excision or destruction of prostatic tissue may also be performed via laser coagulation of the prostate (52647), laser vaporization of the prostate (52648), and laser enucleation of the prostate (52649). Open procedures of the prostate are reported with codes from the Male Genital System subsection under the heading Prostate (55700–55899).

Key to Success

Do not get confused between a *cystoscopy* and a *cystourethroscopy*, though these two procedures are similar. A cystourethroscopy is the endoscopic examination of both the urethra and the bladder, whereas a cystoscopy is the examination of just the bladder. However, because an imaging procedure of the bladder typically passes through the urethra (to gain access to the bladder), endoscopic examinations of the bladder may be referred to as cystourethroscopies (including the urethra and the bladder). Thus, endoscopic examinations of the bladder are listed in the section of codes for cystourethroscopies in the CPT code book. If you read the parent code for each procedure in the endoscopy section of the bladder, you will see that all these procedures are described as cystourethroscopies. When the documentation of a healthcare procedure identifies the procedure as a *cystoscopy*, you should select the appropriate *cystourethroscopy* code. Although these two procedures are technically different, the terms are used interchangeably in the CPT book.

Key to Success

Transurethral excisions of prostatic tissue are technically prostatectomies, as they remove the tissue of the prostate. This is confusing, as prostatectomy codes are also included in the Male Genital System subsection. The difference between the two is that prostatectomies in the Urinary System subsection are all performed through the transurethral approach, whereas prostatectomies in the Male Genital System are all performed via an open excisional approach.

Figure 18.13. Transurethral resection of the prostate (TURP)

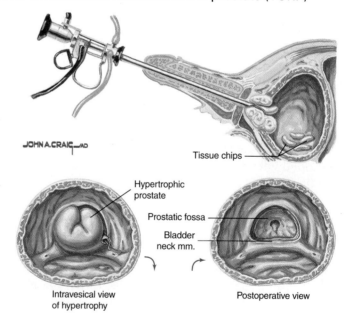

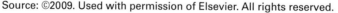

Source: ©2009. Used with permission of Elsevier. All rights reserved.

Urethra

Procedures on the urethra include Incision (53000–53085), Excision (53200–53275), Repair (53400–53520), Manipulation (53600–53665), and Other Procedures (53850–53899). Some of these procedures indicate patient gender, as the male and female urethra differ. Note that three of the procedures in the Other Procedures category (53850–53855) are additional procedures that may be performed to remove prostatic tissue (via microwave or radiofrequency thermotherapy) and to insert an indwelling prostatic urethral stent.

Male Genital Procedures

Surgical procedures on the male genital system are all located in the Male Genital System subsection of the CPT code book. This subsection is divided based on the specific anatomy of the male genital system including the penis, testis, epididymis, tunica vaginalis, scrotum, vas deferens, spermatic cord, seminal vesicles, and prostate.

The **penis** is the main male reproductive organ and is made up of two types of tissue: **corpora cavernosa**, which is made up of erectile tissue, and **corpora spongiosum**, which lies under the corpora cavernosa and forms the internal shape of the penis with a bulbous shape at the end of the penis and helps to prevent urethral compression during erection. The **testes**, glands of the reproductive and endocrine systems, produce and store sperm and male sex hormones. In healthy males, there are two testes (or testicles) located behind the penis in a pouch of skin called the **scrotum**. The **tunica vaginalis** is a layer of tissue covering the testes in the shape of a pouch. The **epididymis** is a duct behind the testes, in which newly created sperm cells mature and then move into the vas deferens. The **vas deferens** (also referred to as the vas or ductus deferens) are made of smooth muscle and are located in the **spermatic cord**, a cord-like structure made up of the vas deferens and surrounding tissues. The vas deferens transport sperm from the epididymis to the urethra, which is later ejaculated through the urethral orifice. The **seminal vesicles** are small male accessory sex glands that help to form the lubricating fluid of semen. The prostate is a gland, located under the urinary bladder and in front of the rectum, helps in making and storing seminal fluid. See figures 18.14 and 18.15 for an overview of the male genital and reproductive systems.

Key to Success

The male genital system is made up of numerous anatomical components. However, the number of procedures that can be performed on those components is relatively small. If you are having problems finding codes in the Male Genital System subsection, locate the subheading for the anatomical area on which the procedure is being performed (such as the tunica vaginalis), and then try searching the available codes for the procedure that was performed.

Penis

The Penis subheading (54000–54450) contains the largest number of codes in the Male Genital System subsection. These procedures include incision, destruction, and excision procedures. Keep in mind that when performing a procedure on the penis, the surgeon is not working on the skin of the penis, but rather the deep tissues of the penis. For example, instead of the destruction of a lesion on the skin of the penis, code 54050, Destruction of lesion(s), penis (eg, condyloma, papilloma, molluscum contagiosum, herpetic vesicle), simple; chemical, should be reported for the destruction of a lesion of the penile tissue under the subcutaneous layer of skin. This is a common distinction in surgical coding—if the procedure was performed on the skin of an organ or on the deeper structure.

A common excision procedure performed on the penis is a circumcision, often performed on newborn males and coded with 54150, Circumcision, using clamp or other device with regional dorsal penile or ring block, through 54161, Circumcision, surgical excision other than clamp, device, or dorsal slit; older than 28 days of age. A **circumcision** is the surgical removal of the foreskin at the tip of the penis. When coding

Figure 18.14. Male genital system

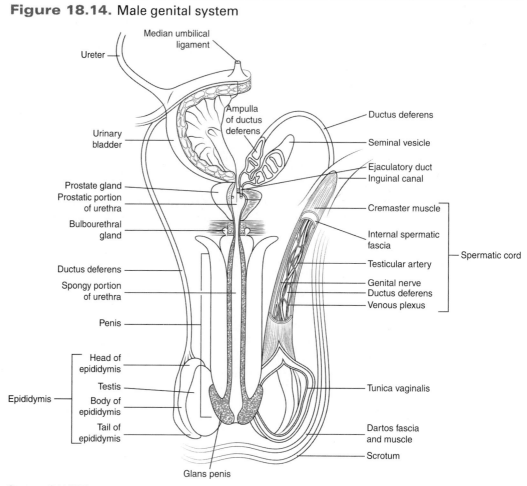

Source: ©AHIMA.

Figure 18.15. Cross-section of male genital system

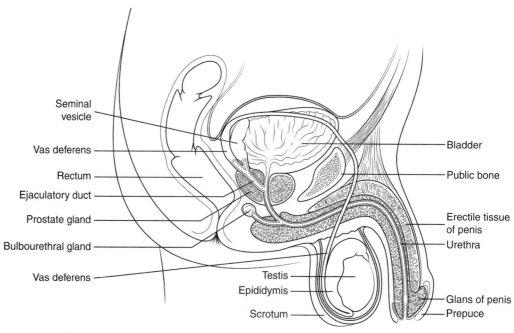

Source: ©AHIMA.

for circumcisions, identify the method of circumcision (clamp or device) and whether a penile ring block was used for anesthesia. If a penile ring block was not used, then the age of the patient must be identified (a neonate 28 days or less, or older than 28 days of age).

Additional procedures on the penis include Introduction (54200–54250), Repair (54300–54400), and Manipulation (54450).

Testis

Testis codes (54500–54699) report procedures for the biopsy and excision of testis (both via open approach and laparoscopically), exploration, and repair. Exploration codes (54550–54560) are reported for the exploration of undescended testes. Undescended testes may need to be surgically fixated in the scrotal sac in a procedure known as an **orchiopexy**. Orchiopexy codes are located in both the Repair (54600–54680) and Laparoscopy (54690–54699) categories, depending on the approach to the procedure.

Epididymis

Epididymis codes (54700–54901) identify procedures to incise and drain abscess or hematoma of the epididymis, biopsy or excision of lesion of the epididymis, exploration, and repair.

Tunica Vaginalis

Tunica Vaginalis codes (55000–55060) identify the treatment of hydrocele of the tunica vaginalis. A **hydrocele** is a fluid-filled sac that can cause pain and discomfort. Treatment includes puncture aspiration, excision, or repair of a tunica vaginalis hydrocele.

Scrotum

Scrotum codes (55100–55180) identify procedures performed on the scrotal sac (not the skin of the scrotum), such as removal of foreign bodies, drainage of abscess, resection, and repair.

Vas Deferens

The most common procedure performed in the Vas Deferens subheading of codes (55200–55400) is a vasectomy, coded with 55250, Vasectomy, unilateral or bilateral (separate procedure), including postoperative semen examination(s). **Vasectomy** is an outpatient procedure commonly performed for elective sterilization. In the procedure, a small section of the vas deferens are cut and removed, so that semen does not flow through the vas to the urethra during ejaculation. This is a procedure that can be reversed through a vasovasostomy or vasovasorrhaphy, connecting the vas back together again.

Spermatic Cord

Spermatic Cord codes (55500–55559) report procedures on the spermatic cord, including excision of lesions, hydroceles, or varicocele. Note that these procedures can be performed either via open incision or laparoscopically.

Seminal Vesicles

Seminal Vesicles procedures (55600–55680) include either incision or excision procedures, with a specific code for the excision of a Mullerian duct cyst, which can cause urinary urgency, frequency, dysuria, and urinary obstruction, among other symptoms. The code for the excision of the Mullerian duct cyst is 55680, Excision of Mullerian duct cyst.

Prostate

Prostate procedures (55700–55899) include biopsy of the prostate, and drainage of prostatic abscesses, as well as excision of the prostate via open or laparoscopic approaches. Prostatectomy codes located in this section include the removal of the entire prostate, rather than a small section of prostatic tissue (as in transurethral resection of the prostate). Open prostatectomy codes differ depending on the approach to the procedure (open, laparoscopic, perineal, suprapubic, retropubic), and the elements included in the excision procedure.

Dialysis

Dialysis is the process of filtering waste products from the blood, which replaces the function of the kidneys for patients with end-stage renal disease or renal failure. There are two types of dialysis—hemodialysis and peritoneal dialysis. **Hemodialysis** is the process of filtering the blood of waste products using a dialyzer machine that removes the waste products from the blood. **Peritoneal dialysis** involves the placement of a dialyzing solution into the peritoneal cavity in the abdomen, where it removes waste products from the body and is then drained, removing extra fluid and waste products.

Codes for dialysis are found in the Medicine section of the CPT code book, in the Dialysis subsection (90935–90999). There are four subheadings of codes.

- Hemodialysis (90935–90940). Hemodialysis procedure codes identify the actual dialysis service performed per date of service.
- Miscellaneous Dialysis Procedures (90945–90947). Miscellaneous dialysis procedure codes are used for dialysis procedures other than hemodialysis, such as peritoneal dialysis.
- End-Stage Renal Disease Services (90951–90970). End-stage renal disease (ESRD) service codes are reported once per month to identify the services provided to the patient in relation to the patient's ESRD. These services include the establishment of a dialyzing cycle, outpatient E/M of the dialysis visits, telephone calls, and other patient management reported on a monthly basis. Codes 90951 through 90966 report a full month of services, whereas codes 90967 through 90970 report ESRD-related services per day. Code selection for ESRD-related services requires identification of the age of the patient, and the number of face-to-face visits between the patient and healthcare provider per month. For example, code 90961, End-stage renal disease (ESRD) related services monthly, for patients 20 years of age and older; with 2–3 face-to-face visits by a physician or other qualified healthcare professional per month, identifies the age of the patient (*20 years of age or older*) as well as the number of face-to-face visits with the healthcare provider (2–3).
- Other Dialysis Procedures (90989, 90999). Other dialysis procedure codes include patient training on use of dialysis equipment as well as an unlisted dialysis services code.

Complete the exercises in There's a Code for That 18.5 to practice reporting codes for urology and nephrology procedures.

Urology and nephrology procedures

18.5

Read the following documentation of the service and identify the CPT procedure code(s).

1. Nephrolithotomy with removal of calculus, complicated by congenital kidney malformation.

   CPT code: _____

2. Simple Foley Y-pyeloplasty with pyelostomy and ureteral splinting.

   CPT code: _____

3. ESWL.

   CPT code: _____

4. Complex cystometrogram with voiding pressure studies and simple uroflowmetry.

   CPT code: _____ - _____ , _____

5. Removal of plastic implant from penile tissue.

   CPT code: _____

6. Bilateral vesiculectomy.

   CPT code: _____ - _____

7. Retropubic radical prostatectomy performed with nerve sparing and laparoscopic robotic assistance.

   CPT code: _____

8. ESRD related services for 25-year-old female, including two face-to-face visits per month.

   CPT code: _____

9. Peritoneal dialysis with single evaluation and management encounter with healthcare provider.

   CPT code: _____

Urology and Nephrology Diagnosis Codes

Diagnosis codes reported by urologists and nephrologists are located in chapter 14 (Diseases of the Genitourinary System) of the ICD-10-CM code book. Coding guidelines for this chapter discuss coding situations for chronic kidney disease, a common nephrology diagnosis. Additional, important diagnoses for urology and nephrology include nephrolithiasis and benign prostatic hyperplasia.

Chronic Kidney Disease

Chronic kidney disease (CKD) and acute kidney failure are all coded from the section Acute Kidney Failure and Chronic Kidney Disease (N17–N19). Codes for CKD, located in category N18, identify the stage of the CKD and if the patient is in end-stage renal disease. All codes in category N18 for chronic kidney disease are classified as HCC codes, so pay special attention when selecting these codes to ensure they are coded to the highest level of specificity. According to ICD-10-CM coding guidelines, when coding for CKD, use an additional code to identify either diabetic or hypertensive CKD, whether the patient has previously received a kidney transplant (Z94.0, Kidney transplant status), or if the patient is currently on dialysis (Z99.2, Dependence on renal dialysis). See figure 18.16 for the guidelines related to CKD coding. For example, if a patient with hypertensive stage 5 CKD and hypertensive heart failure who is currently dependent on renal dialysis presented for treatment, the codes reported would be as follows:

- I13.2, Hypertensive heart and chronic kidney disease with heart failure and with stage 5 chronic kidney disease, or end-stage renal disease
- I50.9, Heart failure, unspecified
- N18.5, Chronic kidney disease, stage 5
- Z99.2, Dependence on renal dialysis

Figure 18.16. OGCR I.C.14

14. **Chapter 14: Diseases of the Genitourinary System (N00-N99)**

   a. **Chronic kidney disease**

   1) **Stages of chronic kidney disease (CKD)**

   The ICD-10-CM classifies CKD based on severity. The severity of CKD is designated by stages 1-5. Stage 2, code N18.2, equates to mild CKD; stage 3, code N18.3, equates to moderate CKD; and stage 4, code N18.4, equates to severe CKD. Code N18.6, End stage renal disease (ESRD), is assigned when the provider has documented end-stage-renal disease (ESRD).

   If both a stage of CKD and ESRD are documented, assign code N18.6 only.

   2) **Chronic kidney disease and kidney transplant status**

   Patients who have undergone kidney transplant may still have some form of chronic kidney disease (CKD) because the kidney transplant may not fully restore kidney function. Therefore, the presence of CKD alone does not constitute a transplant complication. Assign the appropriate N18 code for the patient's stage of CKD and code Z94.0, Kidney transplant status. If a transplant complication such as failure or rejection or other transplant complication is documented, see section I.C.19.g for information on coding complications of a kidney transplant. If the documentation is unclear as to whether the patient has a complication of the transplant, query the provider.

   3) **Chronic kidney disease with other conditions**

   Patients with CKD may also suffer from other serious conditions, most commonly diabetes mellitus and hypertension. The sequencing of the CKD code in relationship to codes for other contributing conditions is based on the conventions in the Tabular List.

   See I.C.9. Hypertensive chronic kidney disease.

   See I.C.19. Chronic kidney disease and kidney transplant complications.

Source: CMS 2019.

Nephrolithiasis

Nephrolithiasis and urinary calculi are all reported with codes from section Urolithiasis (N20–N23). These codes identify the location of the stone—in kidney, ureter, kidney with ureter, or such. If the calculus is due to an underlying condition, report the code for the underlying condition first.

Benign Prostatic Hyperplasia

As mentioned previously, benign prostatic hyperplasia (BPH) is one of the most common conditions affecting the prostate. BPH is reported with the appropriate code from category N40, Benign prostatic hyperplasia, and code selection depends on whether the condition is BPH or nodular prostate, and if it presents with or without lower urinary tract symptoms. **Lower urinary tract symptoms (LUTS)** include the various symptoms that can present with BPH, such as urinary frequency, urinary retention, or urinary urgency. Note that these symptoms can also present without BPH, but when they are present with BPH, then add one code per symptom. For example, if a 60-year-old male patient with BPH presented with the LUTS of urinary obstruction and a weak urinary system, the codes reported would be as follows:

- N40.1, Benign prostatic hyperplasia with lower urinary tract symptoms
- N13.8, Other obstructive and reflux uropathy
- R39.12, Poor urinary stream

Key to Success

Coding for BPH is one instance in which you code for both the definitive diagnosis and the symptoms of the disease. In this case, when a patient presents with BPH with LUTS, it is not only acceptable but required to code for *both* the definitive diagnosis and the symptoms.

Complete the exercises in There's a Code for That 18.6. to practice reporting diagnosis codes for urology and nephrology conditions.

Urology and nephrology diagnosis coding

There's a Code for That

Read the following documentation and assign the appropriate diagnosis code(s) for the patient's condition(s).

1. Patient with ESRD is on daily dialyzing schedule and kidney transplant list.
   ICD-10-CM codes: _____ , _____

2. Overactive bladder.
   ICD-10-CM code: _____

3. Erectile dysfunction due to hypogonadism.
   ICD-10-CM codes: _____ , _____

4. BPH with straining upon urination.
   ICD-10-CM codes: _____ , _____

5. Prostate cancer.
   ICD-10-CM code: _____

6. A 35-year-old multigravida presents with both urge and stress incontinence.
   ICD-10-CM code: _____

Putting It All Together: Coding for Healthcare Specialist Services, Part I

Coding for healthcare specialist services requires reading the documentation of the service provided carefully, then accessing each code book to find the procedure or service provided and the corresponding diagnosis or diagnoses to support the medical necessity for the service. Procedural and supply codes are found in the CPT and HCPCS code books, and diagnosis codes are found in the ICD-10-CM code book.

Determination of the correct codes relies on the answers to the following questions.

- What services were provided to the patient?
  - Was an E/M service provided?
    - If the service provided was a consultation, determine if the consultation code may be reported, based on the patient's third-party payer. If the third-party payer does not reimburse for consultation codes, report the appropriate E/M code for the service provided.
  - Were any additional procedures performed, such as labs, x-rays or other imaging services, or any additional medical or surgical procedures?
- Are there any applicable modifiers or add-on codes?
- Is there a definitive diagnosis for the encounter? If yes, this should be the first-listed diagnosis code. If not, then use the code for the signs or symptoms.
- Include any additional diagnosis codes for comorbidities or complications, if necessary.

The following vignette demonstrates how to select the appropriate diagnosis and procedure codes. After reviewing the vignette, complete the exercises in There's a Code for That 18.7 to practice coding for healthcare specialist services.

Maria is studying for her coding examination and she is currently coding the case for a 67-year-old male patient. This patient went to his primary care provider complaining of urinary urgency and frequency. The PCP performed a digital rectal examination and found that the patient's prostate was significantly enlarged, and sent the patient to a urologist for a consultation. Maria is now coding for the services performed by the urologist: After a detailed history and examination and moderate complexity MDM consultation, the urologist performed a total prostate-specific antigen (PSA) test, which revealed an abnormally high PSA. He then performed a needle biopsy of the prostate, which revealed malignant cells. The urologist diagnosed the patient with malignant neoplasm of the prostate, and referred the patient to an oncologist to discuss antineoplastic treatment, including surgery. The urologist then compiled his findings and prepared a report for the PCP regarding the findings from the encounter and suggested treatment.

First, Maria asks herself: What did the healthcare provider do? The physician performed a consultation service, as well as a total PSA and then needle biopsy of the prostate. After the urologist performed the E/M service (the consultation), he decided to perform a biopsy (a surgical procedure), and so she knows that modifier -57, Decision for surgery, should be appended to the E/M code. Maria also knows that many payers do not reimburse for consultation services, so after verifying that the patient's insurance will pay for the consultation code, she reports the following procedure codes:

- *99243-57, Office consultation for a new or established patient, which requires these 3 key components: a detailed history; a detailed examination; and medical decision-making of low complexity*
- *84153, Prostate specific antigen (PSA); total*
- *55700, Biopsy, prostate; needle or punch, single or multiple, any approach*

Now that she has the procedure codes, Maria asks herself: Why did the healthcare provider do it? The patient was referred to the urologist because the PCP found an enlarged prostate and the patient was complaining of urinary symptoms. The urologist performed the PSA test and found an abnormally high PSA level and the biopsy confirmed the diagnosis of malignant neoplasm of the prostate. Maria needs to report two diagnosis codes—one for the prostate cancer and one for the high PSA levels. She refers to the Table of Neoplasms and selects the code for primary malignant neoplasm of the prostate (because the neoplasm is not specified as secondary or carcinoma in situ, she uses the default code for primary malignant cancer). She then finds the code for elevated PSA, and verifies both codes in the Tabular List. She then reports the following codes:

- *C61, Malignant neoplasm of prostate*
- *R97.20, Elevated prostate specific antigen [PSA]*

She then rechecks the documentation to make sure she has coded everything for the encounter and reports the chosen codes on the claim for the service.

Diagnostic and procedural coding for healthcare specialist services

18.7

There's a Code for That

Read the following documentation and assign the appropriate CPT, HCPCS, and ICD-10 CM code(s) for the encounter.

1. Outpatient office consultation for a 45-year-old female patient with estrogen-receptor positive (ER+) cancer of the upper-outer quadrant of left female breast. Comprehensive history and examination with high complexity MDM. Patient medical history reveals a significant family history of breast cancer and she has elected for a radical double mastectomy.

   CPT code: _____

   ICD-10-CM code: _____ , _____ , _____

2. Surgical oncologist treated osteosarcoma of the femur of the left leg via surgical resection.

   CPT code: _____

   ICD-10-CM code: _____

3. Suture of sciatic nerve for injury of the sciatic nerve at the left hip.

   CPT code: _____

   ICD-10-CM code: _____

(Continued on next page)

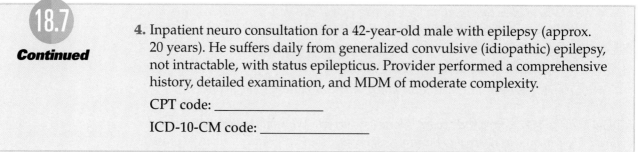

4. Inpatient neuro consultation for a 42-year-old male with epilepsy (approx. 20 years). He suffers daily from generalized convulsive (idiopathic) epilepsy, not intractable, with status epilepticus. Provider performed a comprehensive history, detailed examination, and MDM of moderate complexity.

CPT code: _____

ICD-10-CM code: _____

Case Study | Xiaflex Injection

PATIENT: Joseph Yando

PROCEDURE: Xiaflex injection

INDICATIONS: Peyronie's Disease

PROCEDURE NOTE:
A 65-year-old male presents to the office today for treatment of Peyronie's disease. He completed his first round of Xiaflex and saw no significant change. He is here today for the first injection of cycle number 2.

Consent was obtained after discussing the risk and indications for the procedure. The patient was placed in the supine position, and prepped and draped appropriately. The penis was then prepped with Betadine. 20 mL of lidocaine 1% without epinephrine was infused into the suprapubic adipose tissue and then the subcutaneous tissue at the base of the penis for a penile block. The plaque was easily palpable. Using the closed syringe and needle system, 0.9 mL of reconstituted Xiaflex was injected directly into the plaque where maximal curvature occurs. There was appropriate resistance during injection indicating that the medication was being injected into the plaque. The needle was then removed. Gauze and Coban dressing was placed around the penis to prevent hematoma. Patient was counseled on restrictions and no sex for 3 weeks.

COMPLICATIONS: None, patient tolerated the procedure well.

SIGNED: Dr. Chandra Yang, MD

Use the following steps to select the appropriate codes for the case study.

1. Read through the case study and answer the question: *What did the doctor do?* In the case study, identify the name of the procedure.

_____

_____

2. Now that you have identified the procedure, locate the code for the procedure in the CPT code book.

   a. Search the Index for the procedure and search through the options.

   b. Refer to the code listed in the Tabular section and identify the correct code range. In the listing of codes, check for any guidelines, important definitions, or parenthetical notes. Select the appropriate codes and list them.

   _____

   _____

   c. Are there any additional procedures that need to be added to identify all of the procedures performed? If yes, follow the previous steps to identify the codes for the additional procedures.

   _____

   _____

   d. Are there any modifiers that need to be added to identify any special circumstance surrounding the procedure(s)? If yes, refer to Appendix A of the CPT code book to assign all appropriate modifiers.

   _____

   _____

3. Now that the procedure(s) and modifier(s) have been identified, review the case study and answer the following question: *Why did the doctor do it?*

   _____

   _____

4. Now that you have identified the patient's diagnoses, search the ICD-10-CM code book for the correct codes for these conditions. Follow these steps for each of the diagnoses identified.

   a. Search the Main Index for the name of each condition and search through any applicable subterms and cross-references to locate the appropriate code.

   _____

   _____

   b. Verify the code in the Tabular List. Locate the code identified previously in the Tabular Listing of codes and refer to any applicable guidelines, notes, and symbols. Does the code selected correctly identify the patient's condition? If yes, list the code.

   _____

   _____

   c. Check the procedure note and ICD-10-CM guidelines and conventions to determine the correct sequencing of the diagnosis codes, if applicable. Correctly sequence the diagnosis codes.

_____

_____

5. Now that the procedure and diagnosis codes have been identified, list them on the CMS-1500 form. Be sure to correctly link the procedure and diagnosis codes. Remember to add the number of units as necessary.

21. DIAGNOSIS OR NATURE OF ILLNESS OR INJURY Relate A-L to service line below (24E)				ICD Ind.		22. RESUBMISSION CODE	
A. L_____	B. L_____	C. L_____	D. L_____				
E. L_____	F. L_____	G. L_____	H. L_____			23. PRIOR AUTHORIZATION NU	
I. L_____	J. L_____	K. L_____	L. L_____				

24. A. DATE(S) OF SERVICE						B. PLACE OF SERVICE	C. EMG	D. PROCEDURES, SERVICES, OR SUPPLIES (Explain Unusual Circumstances) CPT/HCPCS | MODIFIER	E. DIAGNOSIS POINTER	F. $ CHARGES	G. DAYS OR UNITS
From MM	DD	YY	To MM	DD	YY						
1											
2											
3											

End-of-Chapter Content

Instructions: Indicate whether the following statements are true or false (T or F). For false statements, rewrite the statement on the line below to make the statement true.

1. Once a consultation is complete, the consulting provider must provide the requesting provider with a report of his or her findings.

_____

_____

2. If the patient's insurance does not reimburse for consultation codes, then E/M codes should be used in their place.

_____

_____

3. A neurologist treats conditions of the urinary tract, including the kidneys.

_____

_____

4. A push is given in a period of time under 15 minutes.

_____

_____

5. A personal history of neoplasm code should be used when the patient is undergoing treatment for a neoplasm.

_____

_____

6. Chemodenervation is the injection of a therapeutic substance to a nerve.

_____

_____

7. Status epilepticus occurs when the patient is unresponsive to treatment.

_____

_____

8. The prostate gland is only found in males.

_____

_____

9. Codes in the Penis (54000–54450) subheading include procedures on the skin of the penis.

_____

_____

10. Dialysis is often performed on patients with little or no liver function.

_____

_____

Instructions: Choose the best answer.

1. Which of the following parties may request a consultation for a patient?

a. The patient's healthcare provider
b. The patient's family
c. The surgeon
d. The patient's employer

2. Which of the following describes the rendering of a consultation service?

a. The healthcare provider requesting the service from the consultation
b. The consultant providing the healthcare service to the patient
c. The consultant providing a written report of findings form the consultation
d. The referral request sent to the insurance company

3. Which of the following types of providers would provide a brachytherapy service?

   a. Urologist
   b. OB/GYN
   c. Oncologist
   d. Nephrologist

4. Which of the following types of healthcare providers would perform a renal transplant?

   a. Neurologist
   b. Hematologist
   c. Urologist
   d. Nephrologist

5. Which of the following is a surgical treatment for a neoplasm?

   a. Chemotherapy infusions
   b. Brachytherapy
   c. Excision
   d. Radiation treatment

6. Which of the following is the intravenous administration of diagnostic, therapeutic, or prophylactic substance, given over a period of time longer than 15 minutes?

   a. Infusion
   b. Push
   c. Drip
   d. Injection

7. Which of the following codes would be used when a patient presents for antineoplastic chemotherapy?

   a. Z99.2
   b. Z51.0
   c. Z51.11
   d. Z51.12

8. Which of the following procedures removes a piece of skull without replacing it?

   a. Trephine
   b. Craniotomy
   c. Craniectomy
   d. Incision

9. When reporting codes for procedures on the spine, what should the coder always check for?

   a. The type of excision performed
   b. The area of the spine and whether it was unilateral or bilateral
   c. The spinal instrumentation used in the procedure
   d. Whether or not there was a neurostimulator placed

10. Which type of procedure is the repair of a nerve via suture or anastomosis?

    a. Excision
    b. Avulsion
    c. Neuroplasty
    d. Neurorrhaphy

11. Which of the following is an organ that filters waste products from the blood?

    a. Ureter
    b. Bladder
    c. Urethra
    d. Kidney

12. Which type of calculus completely fills the renal pelvis?

    a. Nephrolithiasis
    b. Staghorn calculus
    c. Cholelithiasis
    d. Choledocholithiasis

13. Which of the following codes would be reported for the transurethral coagulation of the prostate?

    a. 52601
    b. 52648
    c. 52647
    d. 52649

14. Codes for male circumcisions are found in which of the following subheadings in the Male Genital System subsection?

    a. Penis
    b. Integumentary
    c. Scrotum
    d. Vas deferens

Instructions: Answer the following questions with the appropriate code(s) and modifier(s).

1. Extradural resection of metastatic lesion of the left temporal lobe, using infratemporal pre-auricular approach to middle cranial fossa, including disarticulation of the mandible and parotidectomy.

   CPT codes: _____- _____ , _____

   ICD-10 code: _____

2. Suture of kidney laceration performed on patient who suffered a moderate laceration to the right kidney.

   CPT codes: _____

   ICD-10 code: _____

3. Patient with sepsis without septic shock and with acute kidney failure is undergoing hemodialysis, requiring multiple evaluations by the healthcare provider and revision of the dialyzing schedule.

   CPT codes: _____

   ICD-10 code: _____ , _____ ,

   _____ , _____

4. Initial dilation of urethral stricture by passage of urethral dilator, in a male with post-traumatic anterior urethral stricture.

   CPT codes: _____

   ICD-10 code: _____

References

American Medical Association (AMA). 2019. *CPT 2020 Professional Edition*. Chicago: AMA.

American Urological Association (AUA). 2018. Urology. https://www.auanet.org/guidelines/urology.

Cancer.net. 2018 (March). Types of Oncologists. https://www.cancer.net/navigating-cancer-care/cancer-basics/cancer-care-team/types-oncologists.

Cancer Research UK. 2015 (January). "Diagram showing how you have high dose brachytherapy for prostate cancer CRUK 419.svg." Digital image. Wikimedia Commons. https://commons.wikimedia.org/wiki/File:Diagram_showing_how_you_have_high_dose_brachytherapy_for_prostate_cancer_CRUK_419.svg.

Cancer Research UK. 2014a. Diagram Showing a Craniotomy CRUK 063.svg. Digital image. Wikimedia Commons. https://en.wikipedia.org/wiki/Craniotomy#/media/File:Diagram_showing_a_craniotomy_CRUK_063.svg.

Cancer Research UK. 2014b. Diagram Showing a Brain Shunt CRUK 052.svg. Digital image. Wikimedia Commons. https://en.wikipedia.org/wiki/Cerebral_shunt#/media/File:Diagram_showing_a_brain_shunt_CRUK_052.svg.

Centers for Medicare and Medicaid Services (CMS). 2011 (November 8). Revisions to Consultation Services Payment Policy. https://www.cms.gov/Outreach-and-Education/Medicare-Learning-Network-MLN/MLNMattersArticles/downloads/mm6740.pdf.

National Cancer Institute (NCI). Created by Rhoda Baer. 2010 (May). "Patient receives chemotherapy.jpg." Digital image. Wikimedia Commons. https://commons.wikimedia.org/wiki/File:Patient_receives_chemotherapy.jpg.

Nuclear Regulatory Commission (NRC). 2012 (August). "Radioactive Seeds (7845754328).jpg." Digital image. Wikimedia Commons. https://commons.wikimedia.org/wiki/File:Radioactive_Seeds_(7845754328).jpg.

OpenStax College. 2013. 705 Lateral View of Skull-01.jpg. Digital image. Wikimedia Commons. https://commons.wikimedia.org/wiki/Category:Anatomical_plates_and_drawings_of_the_human_skull#/media/File:705_Lateral_View_of_Skull-01.jpg.

US National Library of Medicine (USNLM). 2016a (December 30). Brachytherapy. https://www.ncbi.nlm.nih.gov/pubmedhealth/PMH0072483/.

US National Library of Medicine (USNLM). 2016b (August 19). How Does the Nervous System Work? https://www.ncbi.nlm.nih.gov/pubmedhealth/PMH0072574/.

Resources

Alzheimer's Association. 2019. Types of Dementia. http://www.alz.org/dementia/types-of-dementia.asp.

Alzheimer's Association. 2019. What Is Alzheimer's? http://www.alz.org/alzheimers_disease_what_is_alzheimers.asp.

American Association of Medical Dosimetrists (AAMD). 2016 (June 15). Deciphering Brachytherapy Coding and Documentation. http://atlanta2016.medicaldosimetry.org/2016AnnualConference/assets/File/Wednesday/Brown.pdf.

American Medical Association (AMA). 2013. *Advanced Anatomy and Physiology for ICD-10-CM/PCS*. Salt Lake City, UT: Contexo Media.

Devaraju, S., R. Nerli, and M Hiremath. 2012 (Autumn). A large Mullerian duct cyst presenting as an abdominal mass with ipsilateral renal agenesis: An unusual presentation. *Nephrourology Monthly* 4(4):640–643. https://www.ncbi.nlm.nih.gov/pmc/articles /PMC3614304/.

Endicott, M. 2012 (November). Taking the sting out of injection and infusion coding. *Journal of AHIMA* 83(11):74–76. http://bok.ahima.org/doc?oid=105755# .WVKPvmgrI2w.

Flewelling, C.2015 (June). Injection and infusion coding offers high stakes: Outpatient coders must play their cards right. *Journal of AHIMA* 86(6): extended online version. http://bok.ahima.org/doc?oid=107707# .WVKP0GgrI2w.

Mayo Clinic. 2018 (December 7). EEG (electroencephalogram). http://www.mayoclinic.org /tests-procedures/eeg/basics/definition/prc-20014093.

Parkinson's Disease Foundation (PDF). 2019. Understanding Parkinson's. https://www.parkinson.org /understanding-parkinsons.

RadiologyInfo.org. 2019 (May 28). Stereotactic Radiosurgery (SRS) and Stereotactic Body Radiotherapy (SBRT). https://www.radiologyinfo.org/en/info .cfm?pg=stereotactic.

US National Library of Medicine (USNLM). 2017. Dialysis. https://www.ncbi.nlm.nih.gov/pubmedhealth /PMHT0022165/.

US National Library of Medicine (USNLM). 2017. Hemodialysis. https://www.ncbi.nlm.nih.gov /pubmedhealth/PMHT0022166/.

US National Library of Medicine (USNLM). 2017. Peritoneal Dialysis. https://www.ncbi.nlm.nih.gov /pubmedhealth/PMHT0022170/.

US National Library of Medicine (USNLM). 2017. Status Epilepticus. https://meshb.nlm.nih.gov/record /ui?ui=D013226.

Wheeler, A. 2017 (May 5). Therapeutic Injections for Pain Management. http://emedicine.medscape.com /article/1143675-overview#a9.

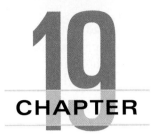

CHAPTER

Healthcare Specialist Services, Part II

Learning Objectives

- Examine procedural codes and guidelines, diagnosis coding, and medical necessity for gastroenterology and cardiology services

- Determine and apply ICD-10-CM, CPT, and HCPCS codes to gastroenterology and cardiology services

Key Terms

Abdominal aortic aneurysm (AAA)

Aneurysm

Angiography

Atherosclerosis

Bariatric surgery

Cardiac electrophysiology

Cardiologist

Cardiopulmonary bypass (CPB)

Cardiothoracic surgery

Central venous access devices (CVAD)

Colonoscopy

Colorectal surgery

Coronary artery bypass grafts (CABG)

Coronary artery disease

Deep vein thrombosis (DVT)

Dissecting aneurysm

Diverticulitis

Diverticulosis

Embolus

Endoscopic retrograde cholangiopancreatography (ERCP)

Endovascular procedure

Esophagogastroduodenoscopy (EGD)

Fundoplasty

Gastric bypass

Gastroenterologist

Gastroesophageal reflux disease (GERD)

Hemorrhoids

Implantable cardiac defibrillator (ICD)

Non-ruptured aneurysms

Pacemaker

Percutaneous transluminal coronary angioplasty (PTCA)

Pericardium

Proctosigmoidoscopy

Pulmonary embolism

Ruptured aneurysm

Sigmoidoscopy

Thrombosis

Transluminal procedure

Varicose vein

This chapter discusses two additional healthcare specialties—gastroenterology and cardiology services. Coding professionals must pay close attention to detail, follow coding guidelines, and use their understanding of medical terminology and human anatomy and physiology when coding for these specialties.

Procedural and Diagnostic Coding for Gastroenterology

A **gastroenterologist** is a healthcare provider who specializes in the diagnosis and treatment of disorders of the digestive system, including but not limited to disorders of the esophagus, stomach, intestines, colon, and rectum and anus. Gastroenterologists can further specialize in surgical gastroenterology, or **bariatric surgery** (surgery performed on the stomach or intestines to induce weight loss), or **colorectal surgery** (surgery of the colon, rectum, and anus).

The majority of the surgical codes reported by gastroenterologists are located in the Digestive System subsection of the CPT code book, with a small selection of codes located in the Medicine section. Diagnosis codes for gastroenterology services are located mainly in the chapter for diseases of the digestive system—chapter 11 of the ICD-10-CM code book. The following sections discuss procedural and diagnostic coding for gastroenterology procedures.

Key to Success

Note that gastroenterologists are commonly referred to as GI doctors, as they treat the gastrointestinal system (gastro=G, intestinal=I).

Gastroenterology Procedures

Gastroenterology procedures range from medical studies of the function of the gastrointestinal system to invasive surgical procedures. Noninvasive gastroenterology procedures (91010–91299), such as acid perfusion tests for esophageal reflux, are found in the Medicine section of the CPT code book. Gastroenterology surgical procedures are located in the Digestive System subsection of the Surgery section of the CPT code book. This section includes codes for all components of the digestive system, beginning with the lips and vestibule of the mouth, through the alimentary tract to the rectum and anus (see figure 19.1). It also includes procedures on organs that assist in the digestive process, such as the liver, biliary tract, and pancreas, as well as the abdomen, peritoneum, and omentum. These sections are as follows: Lips; Vestibule of Mouth; Tongue and Floor of Mouth; Dentoalveolar Structures; Palate and Uvula; Salivary Gland and Ducts; Pharynx, Adenoids, and Tonsils; Esophagus; Stomach; Intestines (Except Rectum); Meckel's Diverticulum and the Mesentery; Appendix; Colon and Rectum; Anus; Liver; Biliary Tract; Pancreas; and Abdomen, Peritoneum, and Omentum.

Upper Alimentary Tract

Gastroenterologists focus on diagnosis and treatment of disorders of the esophagus, stomach, intestines, colon, and rectum/anus (see figure 19.2), even though additional anatomical structures are technically included in this body system.

Many of the anatomical structures located in the Digestive System subsection are outside of the realm of treatment for a gastroenterologist, which include those performed on the upper alimentary tract: lips; vestibule of mouth; tongue and floor of mouth; dentoalveolar structures; palate and uvula; salivary gland and ducts; and pharynx, adenoids, and tonsils. Procedures on the Lips (40490–40799) are likely to be performed by plastic or reconstructive surgeons who specialize in working with the soft tissues of the face. Procedures on the Vestibule of the Mouth (40800–40899), Tongue and Floor of Mouth (41000–41599), Dentoalveolar Structures (41800–41899), Palate and Uvula (42000–42299), and Salivary Gland and Ducts (42300–42699), are likely to be performed by oral/maxillofacial surgeons who focus on the surgical treatment of the mouth and jaw, such as cleft lip or cleft palate repair. Finally, procedures on the Pharynx, Adenoids, and Tonsils (42700–42999), are often performed by otorhinolaryngologists— ear, nose, and throat (ENT) doctors—who focus on the diagnosis and treatment of conditions in the throat, and who perform procedure on the tonsils and adenoids, like tonsillectomies (refer to chapter 11[Surgical Services]).

Figure 19.1. Gastrointestinal system

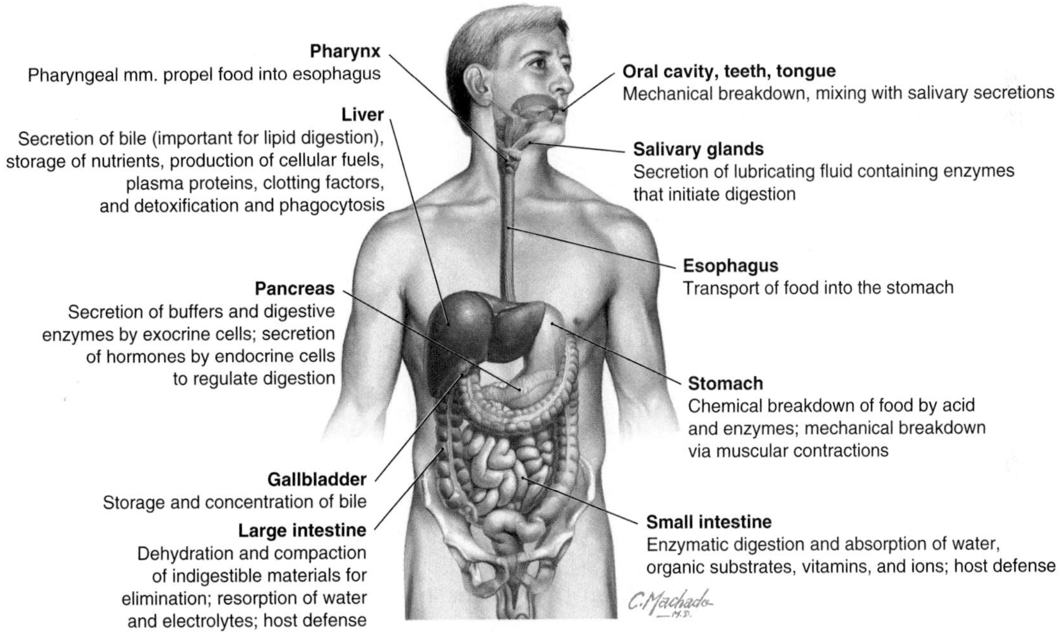

Pharynx
Pharyngeal mm. propel food into esophagus

Liver
Secretion of bile (important for lipid digestion), storage of nutrients, production of cellular fuels, plasma proteins, clotting factors, and detoxification and phagocytosis

Pancreas
Secretion of buffers and digestive enzymes by exocrine cells; secretion of hormones by endocrine cells to regulate digestion

Gallbladder
Storage and concentration of bile

Large intestine
Dehydration and compaction of indigestible materials for elimination; resorption of water and electrolytes; host defense

Oral cavity, teeth, tongue
Mechanical breakdown, mixing with salivary secretions

Salivary glands
Secretion of lubricating fluid containing enzymes that initiate digestion

Esophagus
Transport of food into the stomach

Stomach
Chemical breakdown of food by acid and enzymes; mechanical breakdown via muscular contractions

Small intestine
Enzymatic digestion and absorption of water, organic substrates, vitamins, and ions; host defense

Esophagus

Procedures on the esophagus include Incision (43020–43045) and Excision (43100–43135), but by far the majority of procedures on the esophagus are Endoscopy (43180–43278). Because the esophagus is a large, natural opening that allows access to the upper part of the gastrointestinal system, endoscopic examinations and procedures are a common procedure.

Remember that there are three components to endoscopy coding—approach, extent, and surgical versus diagnostic services (see chapter 11). These three components play a large part in coding for endoscopies. For example, an esophagoscopy is the examination of the esophagus. The term used to identify the endoscopy usually indicates where the endoscope stopped and did not proceed any further (an *esophagoscopy* stopped in the *esophagus*). An esophagogastrostomy is the examination of the esophagus and stomach, which does not extend to the duodenum. An **esophagogastroduodenoscopy (EGD)** is the examination of the esophagus and the stomach, which extends to the duodenum.

Figure 19.2. Digestive system

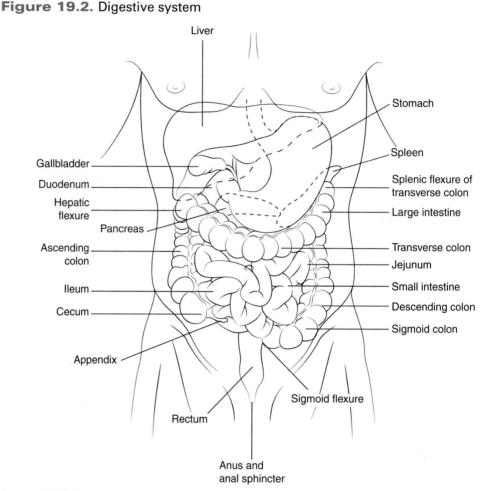

Source: ©AHIMA.

EGDs are a common type of endoscopic examination of the digestive system, as they are a complete examination from the esophagus to the duodenum at the end of the stomach.

Once the endoscope is inserted, several different procedures may be performed. There are many bundled codes in this section, and one code may include procedures that are described by different codes. The coder must pay close attention to the parenthetical notes in the codes in this section, as they describe when specific codes may or may not be used with each other, or when alternative codes may be appropriate in given situations. For example, under code 43235, Esophagogastroduodenoscopy, flexible, transoral; diagnostic, including collection of specimen(s) by brushing or washing, when performed (separate procedure), is the following parenthetical note: *Do not report 43235 in conjunction with 43197, 43198, 43210, 43236–43259, 43266, 43270, 44360, 44361, 44363, 44364, 44365, 44366, 44369, 44370, 44372, 44373, 44376, 44377, 44378, 44379.* In this example, the parenthetical notes identify specific codes that may not be reported with the previously referenced code.

Key to Success

Codes for esophageal endoscopies can be challenging, as there are only one or two standalone parent codes for the endoscopy procedures and countless pages of indented codes. To help make sure you do not get lost, consider highlighting or underlining the parent codes, or using a straight edge or ruler when reviewing the codes, to ensure that you do not miss the next parent code and that you select the most appropriate code available.

Another common procedure performed through the natural opening of the esophagus is an **endoscopic retrograde cholangiopancreatography (ERCP)**. An ERCP is a procedure performed to both diagnose and treat, when necessary, blockages of the pancreatic and bile ducts. During an ERCP, a thin flexible catheter is extended through the duodenum into the bile and pancreatic ducts, where a contrast medium is injected and x-rays taken. These x-rays are then examined to determine where, if any, blockages exist, so that the provider may dilate blocked ducts, remove calculi, or insert a stent, for example (see figure 19.3) (NIDDK 2016). ERCP codes (43260–43265, 43273–43278) are similar in nature to endoscopic procedures on the esophagus, as they identify any additional procedures performed during the endoscopic examination. A diagnostic ERCP would be reported with 43260, Endoscopic retrograde cholangiopancreatography (ERCP); diagnostic, including collection of specimen(s) by brushing or washing, when performed (separate procedure). A surgical ERCP code, on the other hand, would be 43265, Endoscopic retrograde cholangiopancreatography (ERCP); with destruction of calculi, any method (eg, mechanical, electrohydraulic, lithotripsy). Note that there are many parenthetical notes throughout the ERCP section of codes to help with accurate code selection.

Figure 19.3. ERCP

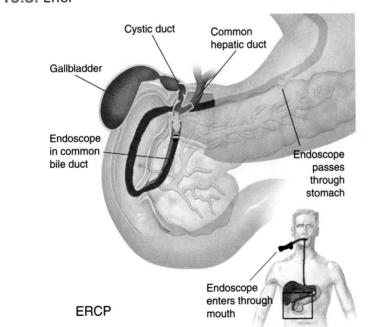

Source: Drus1a 2018.

Commonly performed to surgically treat gastroesophageal reflux disease (GERD), a fundoplication, and referred to as a **fundoplasty**, is a procedure in which the fundus of the stomach (the top bulging part of the stomach) is wrapped around the lower end of the esophagus, underneath the diaphragm. This helps to re-create pressure at the lower end of the diaphragm and this relieve symptoms of GERD, due to reflux from the contents of the stomach into the lower end of the esophagus (Seeras 2018). Fundoplasty codes depend on the surgical technique, as in code 43280, Laparoscopy, surgical, esophagogastric fundoplasty (eg, Nissen, Toupet procedures).

Remaining procedural categories of codes in the Esophagus subheading include Laparoscopy (43279–43289), Repair (43300–43425), Manipulation (43450–434600), and Other Procedures (43496–43499).

Stomach

Code categories for procedures on the stomach include Incision (43500–43520), Excision (43605–43641), and Introduction (43752–43763) procedures. Laparoscopy (43644–43659), Bariatric Surgery (43770–43775), and Other Procedures (43800–43999) codes report, among other things, bariatric surgeries as a treatment for morbid obesity. Bariatric surgery is a type of surgery that focuses on reducing the size of the stomach and the patient feeling full faster than he or she normally would. Ultimately the patient would then eat less and lose weight (ASMBS 2017).

One form of bariatric surgery is a **gastric bypass** procedure, also called a Roux-en-Y procedure, in which a small stomach pouch is created by separating the top of the stomach from the rest of the stomach. This pouch is attached to a part of the small intestine, in essence creating a small stomach out of the larger stomach. Codes for gastric bypass depend on whether the procedure was performed laparoscopically or via an open approach. For example, compare codes 43644, Laparoscopy, surgical, gastric restrictive procedure; with gastric bypass and Roux-en-Y gastroenterostomy (roux limb 150 cm or less), and 43846, Gastric restrictive procedure, with gastric bypass for morbid obesity; with short limb (150 cm or less) Roux-en-Y gastroenterostomy. See figure 19.4 for an illustration of different gastric surgery procedures.

Figure 19.4. Gastric surgeries for obesity

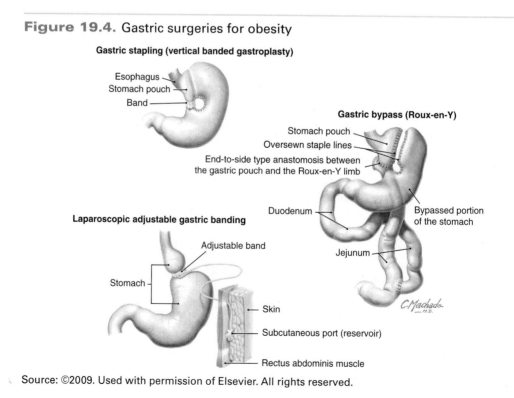

Intestines

Procedures on the intestines include Incision (44005–44055); Excision (44100–44160), including codes for intestinal donation and transplantation; Laparoscopy (44180–44238); and Enterostomy (44300–44346). Codes for endoscopic examinations of the intestines specifically highlight one of the components of endoscopies—the coder should report the code according to the *approach* to the procedure. Endoscopy codes for the intestines are categorized depending on the approach to the procedure: Endoscopy, Small Intestine (44360–44379), and Endoscopy, Stomal (44380–44408). Endoscopies in the small intestine category are ones that have extended through the esophagus, stomach, and the duodenum into the first portion of the small intestine. Note the approach described in the code description (in italics): 44376, Small intestinal endoscopy, *enteroscopy beyond second portion of duodenum, including ileum*; diagnostic, with or without collection of specimen(s) by brushing or washing (separate procedure). Alternatively, read the approach for a Stomal endoscopy (in italics): 44382, Ileoscopy, *through stoma*; with biopsy, single or multiple. In the first example, the approach was through the duodenum, whereas in the second example, the approach was through a stoma.

Meckel's Diverticulum and the Mesentery

There are only four codes total for Meckel's Diverticulum, a rare bulge in the small intestine that is a remnant of the umbilical cord, and the Mesentery, the membrane that connects the intestines with the walls of the internal abdominal cavity. These codes report Excision (44800–44820), Suture (44850), and Other Procedures (44899).

Appendix

Procedures on the Appendix include Incision (44900), Excision (44950–44960), and Laparoscopy (44970–44979). The one incision procedure is coded with 44900, Incision and drainage of appendiceal abscess, open. The excision and laparoscopy procedure codes all describe different forms of appendectomies, previously described more in depth in chapter 11. When coding for appendectomies, identify whether the procedure was open or laparoscopic; and for open procedures, identify why the procedure was performed and if the appendix was ruptured.

Colon and Rectum

Procedures on the colon and rectum include Incision (45100–45020), Excision (45100–45172), and Destruction (45190). However, by far the most common procedures of the colon are Endoscopy (45300–45393, 45398).

The colon is divided into the ascending, transverse, descending, and sigmoid portions (see figure 19.5). The ascending portion is the most distal portion from the anus. The ascending colon extends to the transverse portion, which stretches lengthwise to form the descending colon that descends downward toward the anus. The sigmoid colon is the closest to the rectum and anus and forms an S-shaped loop. To code for an endoscopic examination of the colon properly, coders should use all three components of endoscopy codes.

- *Extent*: Colonoscopy codes are divided based on how far the endoscope was inserted into the colon. A **proctosigmoidoscopy** is the examination of the rectum and may include a portion of the sigmoid colon. A **sigmoidoscopy** is the examination of the entire rectum and sigmoid colon, and may include an examination of the descending colon. A **colonoscopy** is the examination of the entire colon, from the rectum to the cecum at the end of the ascending colon, and may include an examination of the ileum.

- *Approach*: Colonoscopies may be performed through a stoma, an artificial opening from the colon to the outside of the body (such as a colostomy).
- *Surgical versus diagnostic*: Colonoscopy codes are divided based on whether the procedure was solely diagnostic or if a surgical procedure was performed during the colonoscopy, such as biopsy or destruction of colonic polyps.

Figure 19.5. Colon

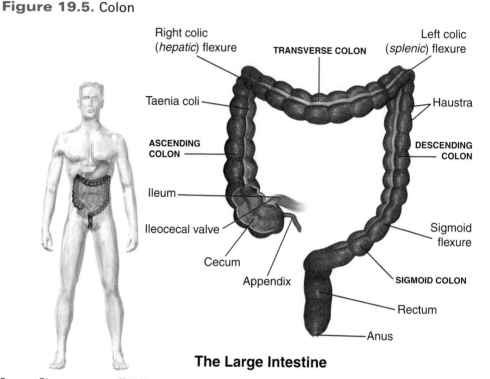

Right colic (*hepatic*) flexure

TRANSVERSE COLON

Left colic (*splenic*) flexure

Taenia coli

Haustra

ASCENDING COLON

DESCENDING COLON

Ileum

Ileocecal valve

Sigmoid flexure

Cecum

Appendix

SIGMOID COLON

Rectum

Anus

The Large Intestine

Source: Blausen.com staff 2013a.

For example, a full diagnostic colonoscopy is extended through the entire colon (from the rectum to the cecum or terminal ileum), and no other procedures are performed during the procedure (such as a biopsy or destruction of a lesion). The diagnostic colonoscopy code is 45378, Colonoscopy, flexible; diagnostic, including collection of specimen(s) by brushing or washing, when performed. If any other procedures were performed during the colonoscopy, then code 45378 would be replaced by the code(s) that identify the surgical procedure(s). For example, if the doctor identified a colonic polyp during the diagnostic colonoscopy and then used a snare technique to remove the lesion, then the code reported would be 45385, Colonoscopy, flexible; with removal of tumor(s), polyp(s), or other lesion(s) by snare technique. Note that the CPT professional edition includes a flowchart that aids in the decision process for colonoscopies.

Anus

Procedures on the anus include Incision (46020–46083), Excision (46200, 46220–46221, 46230, 46250–46288, 46945–46946), Introduction (46500–46505), Endoscopy (46600–46615), Repair (46700–46761, 46947), Destruction (46900–46942), and Other Procedures (46999). The excision category includes codes for hemorrhoidectomy, the removal of hemorrhoids. These codes depend on whether the hemorrhoids are internal or external, as well as the number of columns or groups that were excised, and if the procedures were performed along with a fissurectomy (excision of anal fissure) or fistulectomy (removal of anal fistula).

Liver, Biliary Tract, Pancreas, Abdomen, Peritoneum, and Omentum

Procedures on the Liver (47000–47399), Biliary Tract (47400–47999), Pancreas (48000–48999), and Abdomen, Peritoneum, and Omentum (49000–49999) are likely to be performed by both gastroenterology surgeons and general surgeons (hernia repair, for example). Refer to chapter 11 for guidelines on coding for these procedures.

Complete the exercises in There's a Code for That 19.1 to practice reporting gastroenterology procedures.

Gastroenterology procedures

19.1

There's a Code for That

Read the following documentation of the service and identify the CPT procedure code(s).

1. Endoscope was extended through the rectum and into sigmoid colon, and two polyps were removed via snare technique.

   CPT code: _____

2. Diagnostic proctosigmoidoscopy.

   CPT code: _____

3. Diagnostic EGD.

   CPT code: _____

4. Excision of esophageal lesion through cervical incision.

   CPT code: _____

5. Transoral esophagoscopy with band ligation of esophageal varices.

   CPT code: _____

6. Laparoscopic fundoplasty with repair of esophageal hernia and implantation of synthetic mesh.

   CPT code: _____

7. Surgical closure of gastrostomy opening.

   CPT code: _____

8. Laparoscopic resection of two separate sections of small intestine, with anastomosis.

   CPT code: _____ , _____

9. Diagnostic colonoscopy through stoma with removal of foreign body.

   CPT code: _____

10. ERCP with surgical ablation of two polyps.

    CPT code: _____

Gastroenterology Diagnoses

Diagnosis codes for gastroenterology conditions are found mostly in chapter 11 (Diseases of the Digestive System) of the ICD-10-CM code book. There are no guidelines for this chapter, so appropriate code selection depends on provider documentation and careful reading of the notations in the Tabular List. Note that this chapter is similar to the Digestive System subsection of the CPT code book because it includes codes for conditions beginning with the lips, teeth, gums, and mouth, and includes codes for conditions through the alimentary tract to the anus and rectum. Common conditions include esophageal reflux, colonic polyps and screening colonoscopies, diverticulitis and diverticulosis, and hemorrhoids.

Figure 19.6. Colon cancer screening techniques

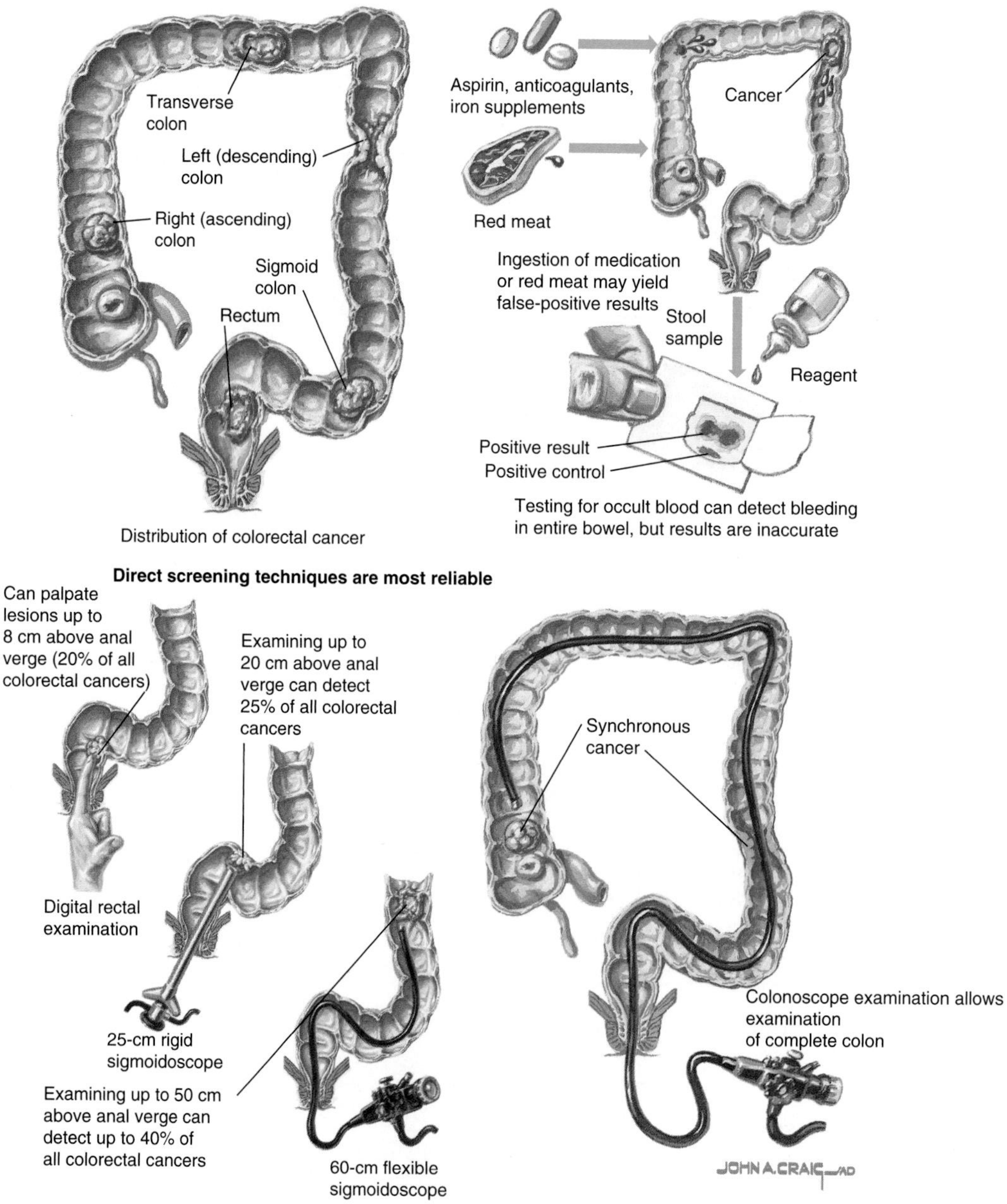

Transverse colon

Left (descending) colon

Right (ascending) colon

Sigmoid colon

Rectum

Distribution of colorectal cancer

Aspirin, anticoagulants, iron supplements

Cancer

Red meat

Ingestion of medication or red meat may yield false-positive results

Stool sample

Reagent

Positive result

Positive control

Testing for occult blood can detect bleeding in entire bowel, but results are inaccurate

Direct screening techniques are most reliable

Can palpate lesions up to 8 cm above anal verge (20% of all colorectal cancers)

Examining up to 20 cm above anal verge can detect 25% of all colorectal cancers

Synchronous cancer

Digital rectal examination

25-cm rigid sigmoidoscope

Examining up to 50 cm above anal verge can detect up to 40% of all colorectal cancers

60-cm flexible sigmoidoscope

Colonoscope examination allows examination of complete colon

JOHN A. CRAIG—AD

Esophageal Reflux

Gastroesophageal reflux disease (GERD) is a common condition that causes heartburn, indigestion, and chest pain in affected individuals. There are only two codes for GERD, which differ depending on whether the condition presents with or without esophagitis (inflammation of the esophagus): K21.0, Gastroesophageal reflux disease with esophagitis, and K21.9, Gastroesophageal reflux disease without esophagitis.

Colon Screenings and Colonic Polyp

Routine colonoscopies are a regular part of preventive healthcare procedures and are referred to as screening colonoscopies. When a patient presents for a routine screening colonoscopy, the primary diagnosis code should be Z12.11, Encounter for screening for malignant neoplasm of colon. If any abnormal findings, such as a polyp, are encountered, then an additional code should be reported to identify the polyp. See figure 19.6 for an illustration of colon screening techniques.

Colonic polyps are coded from a few different areas in the ICD-10-CM code set, including:

- K63.5, Polyp of colon. Use this code to report an unspecified polyp of the colon.
- K51.4-, Inflammatory polyps of colon. These codes identify polyps that are inflammatory in nature, and any additional complications like rectal bleeding, intestinal obstruction, fistula, abscess, or other specified complication.
- D12.6, Benign neoplasm of colon, unspecified. Use this code when a colonic polyp has been determined to be benign in nature.

Diverticulitis and Diverticulosis

Diverticulitis and diverticulosis are both coded from category K57, Diverticular disease of intestine. Diverticulitis is the inflammation of the diverticula, which are small pockets lining the inside of the intestines (see figure 19.7). Diverticulosis is a condition in which diverticula begin forming within the intestines (see figure 19.8). Although these conditions are closely related, code selection depends on the ability to differentiate between the two.

Code selection depends on the identification of the condition as:

- Either diverticulitis or diverticulosis
- The location of the condition (small intestine, large intestine, or both large and small intestine)
- With or without perforation or abscess
- With or without bleeding.

For example, code K57.51, Diverticulosis of both small and large intestine without perforation or abscess with bleeding, identifies whether the condition is diverticulosis or diverticulitis (*diverticulosis*), the location of the condition (*both small and large intestine*), with or without perforation or abscess (*without perforation or abscess*), and with or without bleeding (*with bleeding*).

Hemorrhoids

Hemorrhoids, sometimes referred to as piles, are inflamed or swollen veins located near the anus or lower rectum, inside the rectal canal. Codes for hemorrhoids (located in category K64) depend on the clinical severity of the hemorrhoids, either first (least severe), second, third, or fourth (most severe) degree. Additional codes exist for hemorrhoidal skin tags, perianal venous thrombosis, and other and unspecified hemorrhoids.

Figure 19.7. Diverticulitis

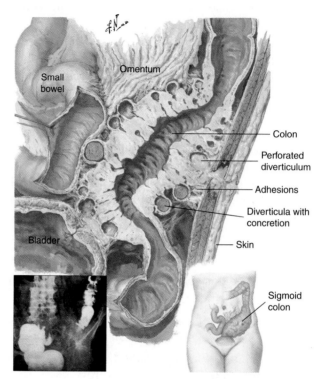

Figure 19.8. Diverticulosis

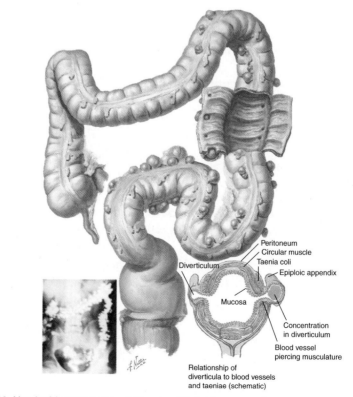

Complete the exercises in There's a Code for That 19.2 to practice assigning diagnosis codes to gastroenterology conditions.

Gastroenterology diagnosis coding

Read the following documentation and assign the appropriate diagnosis code(s) for the patient's condition(s).

There's a Code for That

1. A 45-year-old male presents with esophagitis and GERD. He has been dependent on daily alcohol consumption for the last 25 years.

   ICD-10-CM code: _____ , _____

2. A 65-year-old male presents for routine colonoscopy, which reveals five 1–2 mm polyps of the transverse colon.

   ICD-10-CM code: _____ , _____

3. Adenocarcinoma of the rectosigmoid junction.

   ICD-10-CM code: _____

4. Acute ulcer of the stomach with hemorrhage and perforation.

   ICD-10-CM code: _____

5. Crohn's disease of large intestine with intestinal obstruction.

   ICD-10-CM code: _____

6. Patient presents with severe diarrhea in irritable bowel syndrome.

   ICD-10-CM code: _____

7. Intestinal malabsorption following gastrointestinal surgery.

   ICD-10-CM code: _____

Procedural and Diagnostic Coding for Cardiology

A **cardiologist** is a healthcare provider who specializes in the diagnosis and treatment of the diseases of the heart, coronary vessels, and cardiovascular system. There are numerous subspecialties in the field of cardiology, which includes cardiologists who specialize in invasive or noninvasive cardiology, as well as cardiology treatment strategies and **cardiac electrophysiology** (the study of the electrical system of the heart). Surgical cardiology specialties include cardiac and **cardiothoracic surgery**, which focuses on the surgical treatment of the heart and organs in the thorax (such as the lungs). Because the cardiovascular system runs throughout the entire body, additional subspecialties may focus on peripheral vascular diseases that affect the extremities of the body.

Because cardiovascular services are so varied, codes for these services are located in different sections of the CPT code book. Just as in other specialties, evaluation and management (E/M) codes are used to identify services such as office visits and consultations. Surgical services are coded from the Cardiovascular System subsection of the CPT code book. Additional cardiology services are found in both the Radiology and Medicine sections. The Radiology section includes codes for diagnostic imaging of the cardiovascular system and imaging guidance for cardiovascular procedures; and the Medicine section includes noninvasive or minimally invasive procedures of the cardiovascular system, such as electrocardiograms (ECGs). When coding for cardiovascular services, codes from many different sections of the CPT code book may need to be reported, depending on the service that was performed. The coder must remain flexible and pay attention to parenthetical notes to determine accurate code selection.

Coding for cardiology requires an understanding of the numerous areas in which cardiovascular procedures are found in the CPT code book—cardiovascular surgery, cardiovascular radiology procedures, and cardiovascular medicine procedures. Diagnosis codes for cardiovascular services are found in chapter 9 (Diseases of the Circulatory System) of the ICD-10-CM code book. Note that cardiology patients may present with additional conditions and comorbidities, so it is still important to use all necessary chapters of the ICD-10-CM code book.

Cardiology Procedures

There are three areas of the CPT code book in which cardiovascular codes are found, depending on the type of procedure performed: cardiovascular surgery, cardiovascular radiology, and cardiovascular medicine procedures. Codes in the cardiovascular surgery section identify invasive procedures on the cardiovascular system, such as open-heart surgery or venipuncture. Cardiovascular radiology procedures are performed to produce images to help inform a provider about a patient's cardiovascular medical condition and assist providers in performing cardiovascular surgical and medical procedures. Cardiovascular medicine procedures include all the noninvasive tests and procedures (such as ECGs and cardiovascular stress tests) that may be performed on the patient, as well as some minimally invasive procedures like insertions of cardiac catheters. Although these procedures are in different sections of the CPT code book, they may be reported together, as cardiovascular services sometimes entail all three surgical, radiological, and medical components.

Cardiovascular Surgery

Surgical procedures performed on the cardiovascular system are located in the Cardiovascular System subsection of the CPT code book. This subsection lists invasive surgical procedures on all areas of the cardiovascular system, including the heart and pericardium as well as the arteries and veins throughout the human body.

There is some overlap between the services listed in the Surgery subsection and those listed in both the Radiology and Medicine sections. For example, cardiac catheterizations are found in both the Surgery and Medicine sections. When coding for cardiology services, pay close attention to the guidelines, definitions, and parenthetical notes to ensure correct code selection. Parenthetical notes sometimes supply invaluable information, such as when or when not to use a specific code, which services may be bundled into a specific code or when they must be reported separately, and when to use an additional code or alternative code from a different section of the CPT code book.

Heart and Pericardium

The procedures listed in the Heart and Pericardium subheading (33016–33999) include surgical procedures on the heart, including the coronary valves and vessels, and the pericardium—the sac that holds the heart.

Among these procedures are codes for the reporting of Pacemaker and Implantable Defibrillator services (33202–33275). A **pacemaker** is a small, battery-powered device that is implanted in the patient's chest or abdomen and helps maintain a normal heart rhythm (see figure 19.9). An **implantable cardiac defibrillator (ICD)** is a small device similar to a pacemaker that monitors the heart rate and delivers a small shock to the heart when it detects heart-threatening arrhythmias (see figure 19.10). Both devices send electrical impulses directly into the heart through a series of leads placed in certain areas in the heart, as needed by the patient's condition. Leads are made up of one or more electrodes, conductor wires, insulation, and a fixation mechanism. The leads are attached to a pulse generator and battery pack that provides the electrical stimulation. The pulse generator is placed in a small pocket of skin (subcutaneous pocket), either under the collarbone, above the heart, or above the abdominal muscles below the ribcage. Leads are either inserted into the heart via a vein (transvenous) or placed on the surface of the heart (epicardial).

Codes for pacemaker and ICDs differ, depending on the service performed, type of device, and type of system.

Figure 19.9. Dual-chamber pacemaker

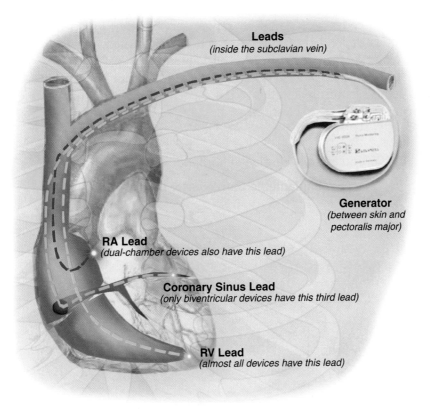

Source: Npatchett 2016.

- A *single chamber* system, also referred to as a single-lead system, includes a pulse generator and one electrode, which is inserted in either the atrium or the ventricle of the heart.
- A *dual chamber* system, also referred to as a dual-lead system, includes a pulse generator and two leads, one of which is inserted into the right atrium, and the other is inserted into the right ventricle.
- A *bi-ventricular pacing* system, or multiple-lead system, is a dual chamber system in which an additional lead is inserted into the left ventricle. This results in three leads—right atrium, left ventricle, and right ventricle (NHLBI n.d.).

Services provided include insertion of the system, leads, and components; replacement of the system or any component parts; upgrade of the system and components; removal of the system or components; removal and replacement of the system; and conversion of the existing system to a different system. For example, code 33234, Removal of transvenous pacemaker electrode(s); single lead system, atrial or ventricular, identifies the service (*removal of electrodes*), type of device (*pacemaker*), and type of system (*single lead system*).

An important component of several cardiovascular procedures is cardiopulmonary bypass, which may impact code selection. **Cardiopulmonary bypass (CPB)** is a technique in which a machine takes over the function of the heart and lungs during surgery, maintaining the circulation and oxygenation of the blood during the procedure. Many of the codes for procedures on the heart differ depending on whether or not cardiopulmonary bypass was used. For example, code 33300, Repair of cardiac wound; without bypass, reports the procedure performed *without* bypass, whereas code 33305, Repair of cardiac wound; with cardiopulmonary bypass, identifies the same procedure but performed *with* bypass.

Cardiac Valve codes (33361–33478) report services performed on the valves of the heart. Codes depend on the type of service performed, as well as the specific valve(s) involved in the procedure: Aortic Valve (33361–33417, 33440), Mitral Valve (33418–33430), Tricuspid Valve (33460–33468), or Pulmonary Valve (33470–33478). The guidelines in this section are lengthy, so it is especially important to read through all of them to ensure correct code selection.

Figure 19.10. Implantable cardiac defibrillator with dual leads

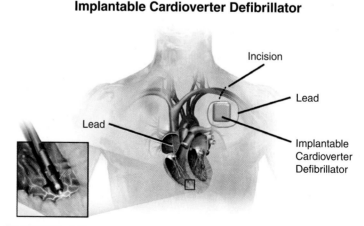

Implantable Cardioverter Defibrillator

Incision

Lead

Lead

Implantable
Cardioverter
Defibrillator

Tip of lead in right
ventricle of Heart

Source: Blausen.com staff 2013b.

Coronary artery bypass grafts (CABG—sounds like "cabbage") are procedures in which a small piece of vein or artery is used to bypass a coronary artery (see figure 19.11). CABGs are commonly performed for atherosclerosis and arteriosclerosis of the arteries, which reduce blood flow and can cause infarctions among other serious heart problems. Codes for coronary artery bypass grafts depend on the vessel used in the repair.

Figure 19.11. Coronary artery bypass graft (CABG)

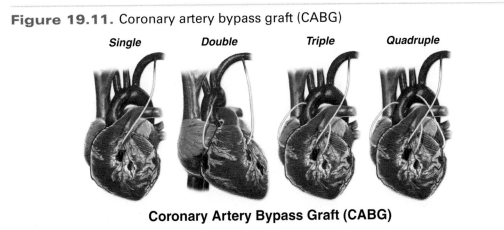

Coronary Artery Bypass Graft (CABG)

Source: Blausen.com staff 2013c.

- A venous graft is one in which a vein is used for the procedure. Venous grafts are reported with codes from the subheading Venous Grafting Only for Coronary Artery Bypass (33510–33516). Codes identify the number of veins used in the CABG. For example, a CABG using three venous grafts would be coded with 33512, Coronary artery bypass, vein only; 3 coronary venous grafts.

- An arterial graft is one in which an artery is used for the procedure. Arterial grafts are reported with codes from the subheading Arterial Grafting for Coronary Artery Bypass (33533–33548). These codes identify the number of arteries used in the CABG. For example, CABG using two arterial grafts would be reported with code 33534, Coronary artery bypass, using arterial graft(s); 2 coronary arterial grafts.

- If both an artery and a vein are used in the CABG, the procedure is reported with at least two codes—one code to identify the arterial grafts and then an add-on code to report the venous grafting. These add-on codes are found under the subheading Combined Arterial-Venous Grafting for Coronary Bypass (33517–33530). Note that these are all add-on codes and cannot be used alone—they must be added to the code for the primary procedure, the arterial graft. For example, a CABG using two arterial grafts and three venous grafts would be reported with 33534, Coronary artery bypass, using arterial graft(s); 2 coronary arterial grafts, and 33519, Coronary artery bypass, using venous graft(s) and arterial graft(s); 3 venous grafts. In this example, the number of arterial and venous grafts is the same in the previous two examples, but the code for the venous grafts changed. Instead of using 33512, Coronary artery bypass, vein only; 3 coronary venous grafts, the correct code is 33519, Coronary artery bypass, using venous graft(s) and arterial graft(s); 3 venous grafts, identifying that the venous grafts were performed in addition to the arterial grafts.

The last component of CABGs is the procurement of the vessel used in the grafting procedure. The procurement (also called harvesting) of the vessel is the procedure performed to obtain the vessel (vein or artery) to be used in the procedure. Coding for the harvesting of the vessel depends on the vessel, as follows:

- Harvesting of the saphenous vein is included in the code for venous CABG, and should not be coded separately.

- Harvesting of an upper extremity vein should be reported with 35500, Harvest of upper extremity vein, 1 segment, for lower extremity or coronary artery bypass procedure.

- Harvesting of a femoropopliteal vein segment should be reported with 35572, Harvest of femoropopliteal vein, 1 segment, for vascular reconstruction procedure (eg, aortic, vena caval, coronary, peripheral artery).

- Harvesting of an upper extremity artery should be reported with 35600, Harvest of upper extremity artery, 1 segment, for coronary artery bypass procedure.

As usual, pay special attention to the parenthetical notes and guidelines in the CPT code book, as they help to guide the coder to the correct code.

Arteries and Veins

The Arteries and Veins subheading of codes (34001–37799) is large, as it identifies procedures on the vascular system throughout the body (with the exception of the heart, coronary vessels, and pericardium).

There are numerous endovascular procedures in this section of codes. An **endovascular procedure** is one in which a catheter is inserted into the body to perform a procedure. Literally, the procedure is performed "inside the vessel" (*endo-* meaning *inside*, and *vascular* pertaining to the vessel). A common endovascular procedure is the repair of aneurysms, such as the repairs listed in the subheading for Endovascular Repair Abdominal Aorta and/or Iliac Arteries (34701–34834), and Endovascular Repair of Iliac Aneurysm (34900).

Bypass grafts can be performed on areas other than the coronary arteries. Bypass grafts of the vascular system are reported with Bypass Graft (35500–35671) codes. These codes identify the beginning and end site of the bypass graft. For example, a bypass graft from the subclavian to the brachial artery would be reported with code 35512, Bypass graft, with vein; subclavian-brachial. Once again, code selection depends on the vessel used for the graft—either Vein (35500–35587) or Other Than Vein (35600–35671). Grafts using arteries or synthetic grafts are reported with Other Than Vein codes.

An **angiography** is the x-ray examination of blood vessels after the administration of a contrast material (see figure 19.12). Codes for angiographies are found in two sections of the CPT code book: Surgery (discussed here) and Radiology (discussed in chapter 13 of this textbook). Codes for angiographies in the Cardiovascular Surgery section report the catheterization of the vessel, the angiography procedure, and the radiological supervision and interpretation of the procedure. Rather than having one code for the catheterization and one for the radiological supervision and interpretation (S&I), these codes are combination codes that combine the components and are reported with 36221 through 36228. It is important to read through these code descriptions carefully, as well as all parenthetical notes and guidelines, to ensure correct code selection.

Central venous access procedures (36555–36598) are performed on **central venous access devices (CVAD)**, which are flexible tubes inserted in patients who require frequent access to the bloodstream. They can stay in place for up to a year and can be used to deliver chemotherapy, parenteral nutrition, blood and blood products,

Figure 19.12. Coronary angiography

Coronary Angiography

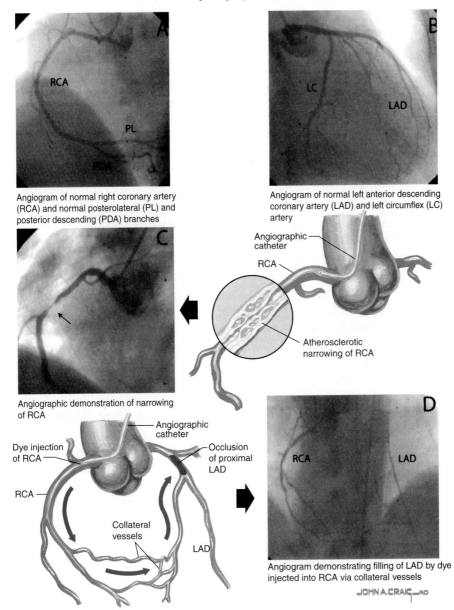

Angiogram of normal right coronary artery (RCA) and normal posterolateral (PL) and posterior descending (PDA) branches

Angiogram of normal left anterior descending coronary artery (LAD) and left circumflex (LC) artery

Angiographic catheter

RCA

Atherosclerotic narrowing of RCA

Angiographic demonstration of narrowing of RCA

Dye injection of RCA

Angiographic catheter

Occlusion of proximal LAD

RCA

Collateral vessels

LAD

Angiogram demonstrating filling of LAD by dye injected into RCA via collateral vessels

JOHN A. CRAIG—AD

antibiotics, and other medicinal substances (USNLM 2017). Procedures on central venous access devices include:

- Insertion (36555–36573). Codes identify the specific type of device (non-tunneled or tunneled, with or without subcutaneous port), and the age of the patient.
- Repair (36575, 36576).
- Partial replacement (36578).
- Complete Replacement (36580–36585).
- Removal (36589, 36590).
- Other Procedures (36591–36598).

Cardiovascular Radiology

Within the Radiology section, there are codes that report vascular procedures on the aorta and arteries and veins and lymphatics. There is also a selection of codes for transcatheter procedures.

Procedures on the Aorta and Arteries (75600–75756, 75774) include aortography (imaging of the aorta) and angiography (imaging of the arteries). These procedures provide detailed images of the vascular structures that allow healthcare providers to diagnose and treat vascular conditions (see figure 19.13 for an example of a thoracic aortography). The procedures listed in this subsection of codes are diagnostic and are used to provide an image to assist the provider in making a diagnosis. Therapeutic procedures are reported with codes in the Transcatheter Procedures subheading.

Procedures on the Veins and Lymphatics (75801–75893) are similar in nature to those for the aorta and arteries, with the exception that the procedures reported are lymphangiography (imaging of the lymph system) and venography (imaging of the veins). Again, these codes identify diagnostic procedures. Therapeutic procedures on the veins and lymphatics are reported with transcatheter procedures codes.

Transcatheter Procedures (75894–75989) identify the radiological component of catheterizations, in which specific procedures were performed. These codes include the injection of contrast material, angiography and venography, roadmapping, fluoroscopic guidance, and vessel measurement, so these components should not be reported separately. It is important to pay close attention to detail when reporting codes from this section, as parenthetical notes alert the coder to the appropriate code(s) for the surgical service performed in conjunction with the radiological procedure. For example, code 75901, Mechanical removal of pericatheter obstructive material (eg, fibrin sheath) from central venous access device via separate venous access, radiologic supervision and interpretation, is followed by a parenthetical note: *For procedure, use 36595*. Code 36595, Mechanical removal of pericatheter obstructive material (eg, fibrin sheath) from central venous device via separate venous access, identifies the actual procedure to remove the obstructive material. Code 75901 reports the radiology imaging service performed with the surgical removal of the obstructive device, to provide imaging guidance during the procedure. In this case, if the provider performed both the imaging service as well as the removal of the device, then both codes should be reported.

Cardiovascular Medicine Procedures

Cardiovascular procedures in the Medicine section of the CPT code book include coronary therapeutic services and procedures, cardiovascular monitoring services, cardiac device evaluations, cardiac catheterizations, electrophysiologic evaluations, and noninvasive vascular diagnostic studies. The codes in the Medicine section for cardiovascular services are primarily noninvasive or minimally invasive. This means that they may invade the body cavity, but only percutaneously (through the skin). Although some of the procedures in the Medicine section sound similar to those in the Surgery section, as a whole they are less invasive than those in the Surgery section.

Coronary Therapeutic Services and Procedures (92920–92979) report an array of different procedures performed transluminally. A **transluminal procedure** is one that is performed within a vessel. One common procedure listed here is a **percutaneous transluminal coronary angioplasty (PTCA)**. In this procedure, a catheter is threaded into the body through an incision in the femoral artery in the groin, to the site of the angioplasty (usually an area clogged by atherosclerosis). Then a small balloon at the tip of the catheter is slowly inflated, stretching the sides of the vessel and creating a wider opening through which blood can flow (see figure 19.14). Code 92920, Percutaneous

Figure 19.13. Thoracic aortography

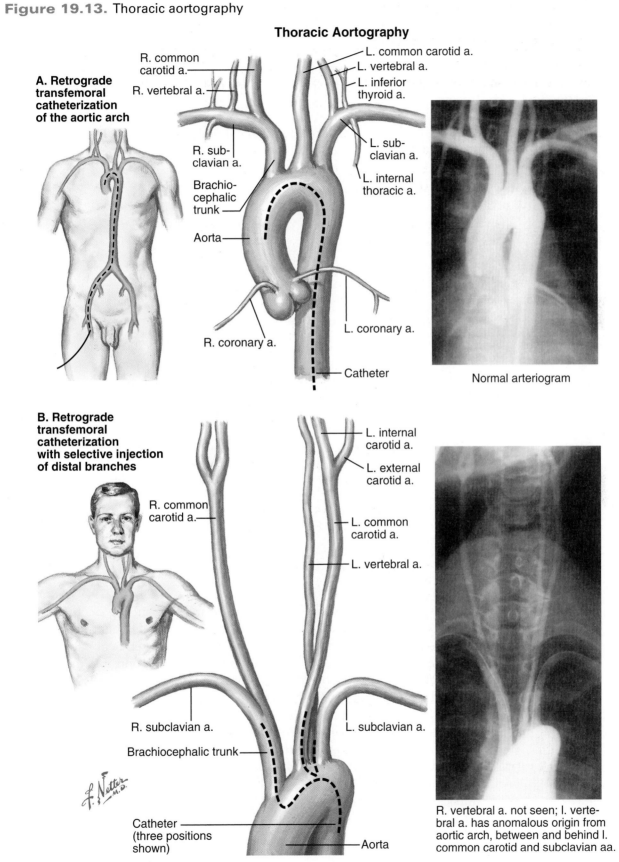

Thoracic Aortography

A. Retrograde transfemoral catheterization of the aortic arch

R. common carotid a.
R. vertebral a.
L. common carotid a.
L. vertebral a.
L. inferior thyroid a.
R. sub-clavian a.
Brachio-cephalic trunk
L. sub-clavian a.
L. internal thoracic a.
Aorta
R. coronary a.
L. coronary a.
Catheter

Normal arteriogram

B. Retrograde transfemoral catheterization with selective injection of distal branches

R. common carotid a.
L. internal carotid a.
L. external carotid a.
L. common carotid a.
L. vertebral a.
R. subclavian a.
L. subclavian a.
Brachiocephalic trunk
Catheter (three positions shown)
Aorta

R. vertebral a. not seen; l. vertebral a. has anomalous origin from aortic arch, between and behind l. common carotid and subclavian aa.

transluminal coronary angioplasty; single major coronary artery or branch, is reported for the first site of balloon inflation. If additional branches of the same major coronary artery are also treated, then report code 92921, Percutaneous transluminal coronary angioplasty; each additional branch of a major coronary artery. Note that codes in this section report PTCA when performed with additional procedures, such as atherectomy (removal of fatty substance from the artery), or placement of intracoronary stent.

Figure 19.14. Percutaneous transluminal coronary angioplasty (PTCA)

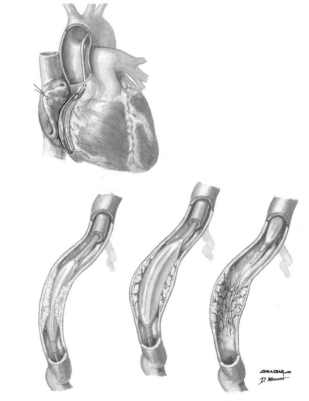

Source: ©2017. Used with permission of Elsevier. All rights reserved.

Implantable and Wearable Cardiac Device Evaluations (93264, 93279–93298) report the additional services performed with pacemaker and implantable defibrillators. In the Surgery section, pacemaker and implantable defibrillator codes identify the surgical services involved in the procedure, such as implantation or removal. However, the codes in the Medicine section identify the programming, evaluation, and management of the pacemaker or implantable defibrillator system. Codes identify the service performed and the patient's type of system.

Cardiac Catheterization (93451–93592) codes identify the direct catheterization of the heart. This procedure involves the introduction, positioning, and repositioning (when necessary) of the catheter within the vascular system; recoding of intravascular pressures; and final evaluation and report of the catheterization procedure. When coding for heart catheterizations, it is important to identify three components, all of which impact code selection:

- Was the catheterization performed for congenital cardiac anomalies?
- Which area of the heart was accessed—right, left, coronary artery, bypass graft, or a combination thereof?

- Was there a definitive procedure, test, or vascular study performed during the catheterization? If so, then an additional code should be reported to identify the add-on procedure. Examples of additional procedures include transseptal or transapical puncture; pharmacological studies; exercise studies; injection procedures for selective right ventricular of right atrial angiography; injection procedures for supravalvular aortography; and injection procedures for pulmonary angiography.

For example, code 93455, Catheter placement in coronary artery(s) for coronary angiography, including intraprocedural injection(s) for coronary angiography, imaging supervision and interpretation, with catheter placement(s) in bypass graft(s) (internal mammary, free arterial, venous grafts) including intraprocedural injection(s) for bypass graft angiography, identifies the area(s) of the heart that were accessed (*coronary artery and bypass grafts*). If an additional injection procedure was performed, then it would be reported in addition to the primary code for the procedure, such as code 93567, Injection procedure during cardiac catheterization including imaging supervision, interpretation, and report; for supravalvular aortography (in this case the additional procedure was an injection for supravalvular aortography performed in addition to the injection(s) for bypass graft angiography as described in the primary procedure code). The professional edition of the CPT code book includes a helpful decision-making chart that aids in the selection of the heart catheterization code(s) that include all necessary elements.

Additional procedures in the Medicine section of cardiovascular codes include electrophysiological studies (Intracardiac Electrophysiological Procedures/Studies, 93600–93662) that study the electrical conduction system of the heart, as well as additional Noninvasive Vascular Diagnostic Studies (93880–93998) of the vascular system throughout the body.

Complete the exercises in There's a Code for That 19.3 to practice reporting codes for cardiology procedures.

Cardiology procedures

19.3

There's a Code for That

Read the following documentation of the service and identify the CPT procedure code(s).

1. Patient underwent a pericardiocentesis.

   CPT code: _____

2. Valvuloplasty via leaflet reconstruction with transmyocardial laser revascularization.

   CPT codes: _____ , _____

3. Open-heart valvotomy with CPB.

   CPT code: _____

4. CABG of three coronary vessels using femoropopliteal vein (harvested at same surgical session by surgical assistant).

   CPT codes: _____ , _____ - _____

5. Coronary artery bypass graft using 2 venous and 1 arterial grafts.

   CPT codes: _____ , _____

(Continued on next page)

19.3
Continued

6. Aortofemoral bypass graft, using upper extremity vein harvested at same surgical session.

    CPT codes: _____ , _____

7. Routine venipuncture.

    CPT code: _____

8. Insertion of implantable defibrillator system with dual transvenous leads and insertion of pacing electrode for left ventricular pacing.

    CPT codes: _____ , _____

9. CT angiography of abdominal aorta and bilateral iliofemoral runoff, with and without contrast.

    CPT code: _____

10. Injection of contrast material and venography of bilateral posterior tibial veins.

    CPT codes: _____ , _____

11. Percutaneous transluminal balloon angioplasty of two pulmonary arteries.

    CPT codes: _____ , _____

Cardiology Diagnoses

Diagnosis codes for cardiovascular conditions are located in chapter 9 (Diseases of the Circulatory System) of the ICD-10-CM code book. In this chapter there are a number of guidelines that apply to hypertension, sequela of vascular diseases, and myocardial infarctions. Hypertension, myocardial infarction, and sequela of cerebrovascular disease are discussed in chapter 8 (Primary Care) and chapter 16 (Therapy Services), respectively. Additional important cardiovascular conditions include atherosclerosis and arteriosclerosis, cerebrovascular diseases, thrombosis, arrhythmias, aneurysms, and varicose veins and varices.

Atherosclerosis

Atherosclerosis (a form of arteriosclerosis, the hardening of the walls of the arteries), is the hardening of fatty substances within the blood vessels that leads to a buildup of plaque. This narrows the diameter of the blood vessel and reduces blood flow and causes the formation of blood clots that can travel through the vessels and cause further obstruction of blood flow (see figure 19.15). Atherosclerosis is one of the most common conditions affecting the arteries and is treated through a variety of surgically invasive and minimally invasive strategies (as described previously).

Atherosclerosis is reported with codes from category I70, Atherosclerosis. Codes for atherosclerosis contain several components. First, the codes identify the blood vessel affected by the condition. Most codes identify the vessel as either native or a bypass graft. Atherosclerosis can occur in the vessel that had been used previously in a bypass procedure. If the atherosclerosis is in a bypass graft, codes differ depending on whether the graft is an autologous vein, nonautologous biological, nonbiological, or other type of bypass graft. Codes also specify the body area (such as leg, thigh, or calf) and the laterality of the condition (right, left, or bilateral). Furthermore, the codes identify any

Figure 19.15. Atherosclerosis

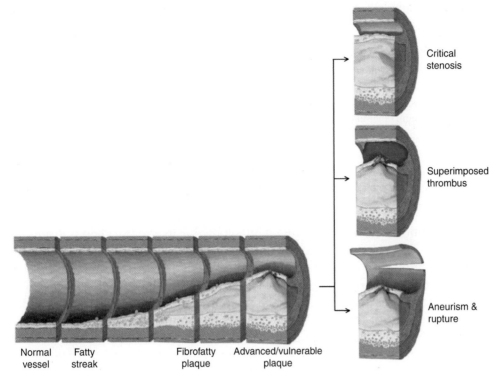

Normal   Fatty   Fibrofatty   Advanced/vulnerable
vessel   streak   plaque   plaque

Source: Npatchett 2015.

complications that present with the atherosclerosis, such as intermittent claudication, rest pain, ulceration, or gangrene.

For example, code I70.421, Atherosclerosis of autologous vein bypass graft(s) of the extremities with rest pain, right leg, identifies the site of the atherosclerosis (*bypass graft*), type of bypass graft (*autologous vein*), specific body area (*leg*) and laterality (*left*), and any further complications (*rest pain*). Note also that atherosclerosis codes are included in HCCs, which means that these components must be identified clearly in the documentation with the most specific ICD-10-CM code.

Atherosclerosis of the coronary arteries is a commonly diagnosed condition and one of the leading causes of death of both men and women in the United States. This condition, often called coronary artery disease or CAD, is when atherosclerotic changes are detected in the arteries of the heart (coronary arteries) (Boudi 2016). Healthcare providers often document this condition as CAD, rather than coronary atherosclerosis, although these two conditions are essentially the same. To search for CAD in the ICD-10-CM code book, look up the term *Disease*, and then refer to the subterm *artery*, which should lead you to the subterm *coronary*. If the patient also presents with angina pectoris in addition to the CAD, then report the combination code for the CAD with angina. See the related OGCR in figure 19.16.

Cerebrovascular Diseases

Cerebrovascular diseases codes (I60–I69) are reported for intracerebral and subdural incidents, including nontraumatic subarachnoid hemorrhage and cerebral infarction, also referred to as a stroke. As mentioned in chapter 16, codes for cerebrovascular diseases identify the current condition and sequela from the cerebrovascular incident. This is an important distinction to make, as a healthcare provider or surgeon treating the current infarction, hemorrhage, or other vascular condition would code for the

Figure 19.16. OGCR I.C.9.b

---

b. Atherosclerotic Coronary Artery Disease and Angina

ICD-10-CM has combination codes for atherosclerotic heart disease with angina pectoris. The subcategories for these codes are I25.11, Atherosclerotic heart disease of native coronary artery with angina pectoris and I25.7, Atherosclerosis of coronary artery bypass graft(s) and coronary artery of transplanted heart with angina pectoris.

When using one of these combination codes it is not necessary to use an additional code for angina pectoris. A causal relationship can be assumed in a patient with both atherosclerosis and angina pectoris, unless the documentation indicates the angina is due to something other than the atherosclerosis.

If a patient with coronary artery disease is admitted due to an acute myocardial infarction (AMI), the AMI should be sequenced before the coronary artery disease.

See Section I.C.9. Acute myocardial infarction (AMI)

Source: CMS 2019.

current condition, such as I63.6, Cerebral infarction due to cerebral venous thrombosis, nonpyogenic. These codes identify the current condition only, and not any sequela from the condition such as dysphagia or hemiparesis.

Sequela from cerebrovascular diseases are reported with codes from category I69, Sequela of cerebrovascular disease, and are reported when the healthcare provider is treating the sequela of the disease, such as partial paralysis or difficulty swallowing (refer to chapter 16). For example, I69.131, Monoplegia of upper limb following nontraumatic intracerebral hemorrhage affecting right dominant side. See figure 19.17 for the OGCR related to coding for cerebrovascular diseases.

Codes for cerebrovascular diseases fall into HCCs, so it is important to be careful when assigning these codes to patient cases and ensure the selection of each code is supported by clear documentation in the health record.

Thrombosis

A **thrombosis**, otherwise known as a blood clot, is a formation of blood cells, fatty deposits, or other particles that form a clot within the blood vessel. Thrombosis can form in either an artery or a vein, and codes differ depending on which vessel is impacted by the clot. The most common type of thrombosis is a **deep vein thrombosis (DVT)**, which forms in the deep veins of the lower extremities. If the thrombosis dislodges from the vessel and begins to travel through the blood, it is referred to as an **embolus**. This embolus can then travel through the blood vessel and get lodged in a smaller vessel, where it can obstruct blood flow. A **pulmonary embolism** is an embolus that may be the result of a DVT becoming dislodged and traveling into the lungs.

Codes for both emboli and thromboses differ depending on the type of vessel impacted by the clot (either a vein or artery), the specific vessel impacted, and the acuity of the condition. For example, code I82.513, Chronic embolism and thrombosis of femoral vein, bilateral, identifies the type of vessel impacted (*vein*), the specific vessel impacted (*femoral*), and the acuity of the condition (*chronic*). For paired organs the code also identifies the laterality of the condition, as in the example code (*bilateral*). Note that these conditions also fall into HCCs, and so care must be taken to ensure they are coded to the utmost level of specificity.

Aneurysm

An **aneurysm** is the bulging or ballooning of a small portion of an artery, caused by weakening or degeneration of the wall of the vessel. Aneurysms are classified according to three characteristics: non-ruptured, ruptured, and dissecting. **Non-ruptured aneurysms** are often symptomless and are usually found during a radiological imaging

Figure 19.17. OGCR I.C.9.d

---

d. Sequelae of Cerebrovascular Disease

1) Category I69, Sequelae of Cerebrovascular disease

Category I69 is used to indicate conditions classifiable to categories I60-I67 as the causes of sequela (neurologic deficits), themselves classified elsewhere. These "late effects" include neurologic deficits that persist after initial onset of conditions classifiable to categories I60-I67. The neurologic deficits caused by cerebrovascular disease may be present from the onset or may arise at any time after the onset of the condition classifiable to categories I60-I67.

Codes from category I69, Sequelae of cerebrovascular disease, that specify hemiplegia, hemiparesis and monoplegia identify whether the dominant or nondominant side is affected. Should the affected side be documented, but not specified as dominant or nondominant, and the classification system does not indicate a default, code selection is as follows:

- For ambidextrous patients, the default should be dominant.
- If the left side is affected, the default is non-dominant.
- If the right side is affected, the default is dominant.

2) Codes from category I69 with codes from I60-I67

Codes from category I69 may be assigned on a health care record with codes from I60-I67, if the patient has a current cerebrovascular disease and deficits from an old cerebrovascular disease.

3) Codes from category I69 and Personal history of transient ischemic attack (TIA) and cerebral infarction (Z86.73)

Codes from category I69 should not be assigned if the patient does not have neurologic deficits.

See Section I.C.21. 4. History (of) for use of personal history codes

---

Source: CMS 2019.

procedure. If the walls of the aneurysm burst, it is referred to as a **ruptured aneurysm**. This is a dangerous condition that causes hemorrhaging into the surrounding body cavity or tissues. A **dissecting aneurysm** is one that contains a small tear in the inner lining of the arterial walls, in which blood is beginning to accumulate. Dissecting aneurysms typically result in a rupture of the aneurysm. A common medical condition, an **abdominal aortic aneurysm (AAA)** is an aneurysm located in the abdominal aorta, which can be life-threatening if it bursts (see figure 19.18).

Figure 19.18. Abdominal aortic aneurysm (AAA)

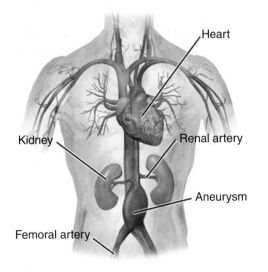

Source: BruceBlaus 2016.

Codes for aneurysms are located in categories I71, Aortic aneurysm and dissection, and I72, Other aneurysm. Category I71 codes identify the site of the aneurysm and if it is dissecting or ruptured. Aneurysm codes qualify as HCC codes and so care should be taken to ensure the code is reported to the highest level of specificity and supported by documentation in the health record.

Varicose Veins and Varicosities

Varicose veins are a result of an insufficiency in the valves of the lower veins to push blood upward toward the heart, causing a buildup of blood (see figure 19.19). Management of varicose veins ranges from wearing compression stockings to surgical intervention. Codes for varicose veins (located in category I83, Varicose veins of lower extremities) depend on the site of the varicosity (the affected vein), including the laterality, and any complications due to the varicose veins. Complications include ulcer, inflammation, both ulcer and inflammation, or other specified complication such as pain, edema, or swelling. For example, code I83.225 Varicose veins of left lower extremity with both ulcer other part of foot and inflammation, identifies the site, including laterality (*left lower extremity, other part of foot*), and complications (*ulcer and inflammation*).

Figure 19.19. Varicose veins

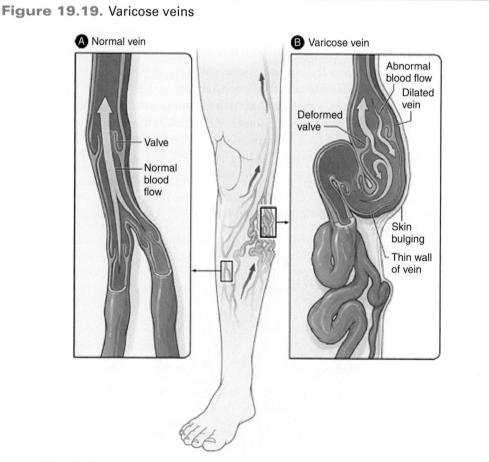

Source: NHLBI 2017.

Key to Success

Note that many cardiovascular conditions fall into HCC categories. This is because many of them identify chronic health conditions that require continuous healthcare treatment, follow-up, or observation. When coding for cardiovascular conditions, ensure that provider documentation is complete and all additional pertinent conditions are captured and reported.

Complete the exercises in There's a Code for That 19.4 to practice assigning diagnosis codes for cardiology conditions.

Cardiology diagnosis coding

19.4

There's a Code for That

Read the following documentation and assign the appropriate diagnosis code(s) for the patient's condition(s).

1. Prinzmetal angina.

ICD-10-CM code: _____

2. Persistent longstanding atrial fibrillation.

ICD-10-CM code: _____

3. Cardiomegaly.

ICD-10-CM code: _____

4. Cerebral infarction due to embolism of bilateral vertebral arteries.

ICD-10-CM code: _____

5. Atherosclerosis of autologous vein bypass graft of lower left extremity with ulceration of calf with exposure of fat layer.

ICD-10-CM codes: _____ , _____

6. Acute DVT of left calf.

ICD-10-CM code: _____

7. Patient on long-term use of oral anticoagulants presents for evaluation of chronic pulmonary embolism.

ICD-10-CM codes: _____ , _____

8. Abdominal aortic aneurysm.

ICD-10-CM code: _____

9. An 82-year-old female presents complaining of pain and inflammation of bilateral varicose veins of the lower extremities.

ICD-10-CM codes: _____ , _____ , _____

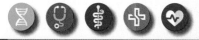

Putting It All Together: Coding for Healthcare Specialist Services, Part II

Coding for healthcare specialist services requires reading the documentation of the service given carefully, then accessing each code book to find the procedure or service provided and the corresponding diagnosis or diagnoses to support the medical necessity for the service. Procedural and supply codes are found in the CPT and HCPCS code books, and diagnosis codes are found in the ICD-10-CM code book. Refer to chapter 18 (Healthcare Specialist Services, Part I) for tips on how to determine the correct code(s) for healthcare specialist services.

The following vignette demonstrates how to select the appropriate diagnosis and procedure codes. After reviewing the vignette, complete the exercises in There's a Code for That 19.5 to practice for healthcare specialist services.

Maria is studying for her coding examination and she is currently coding the case for a 38-year-old female patient. This patient has been overweight most of her life, and is now weighing in at 348 pounds. Her current BMI is 49.9, making her morbidly obese (due to excess calories). Her clinical history is also significant for type 2 diabetes mellitus with neuropathy, controlled with daily use of insulin, and essential hypertension, controlled with daily use of ACE inhibitor. After careful consideration of her weight loss options, including non-surgical interventions, she has decided to undergo a gastric bypass procedure. Surgeon performed Roux-en-Y gastroenterostomy with small intestine reconstruction without complications.

First, Maria asks herself: What did the healthcare provider do? The surgeon performed a Roux-en-Y gastroenterostomy with a small intestine reconstruction. Maria checks to make sure that there were no complications or additional procedures noted on the documentation of the procedure, so no additional procedure codes or modifiers are necessary. She then reports the following procedure code:

- *43847, Gastric restrictive procedure, with gastric bypass for morbid obesity; with small intestine reconstruction to limit absorption*

Now that she has the procedure codes, Maria asks herself: Why did the healthcare provider do it? This female had multiple medical conditions in addition to the obesity. She has a current health history of both diabetes with mononeuropathy, which is controlled by insulin (each of which will be reported with diagnosis codes), and hypertension (which will be reported with another diagnosis code). Maria also needs to assign additional diagnosis codes for the patient's morbid obesity and her body mass index measurement (49.9). After accessing the Main Index to find her codes and verifying them in the Tabular List, she reports the following codes:

- *E11.41, Type 2 diabetes mellitus with diabetic mononeuropathy*
- *I10, Essential (primary) hypertension*
- *E66.01, Morbid (severe) obesity due to excess calories*
- *Z68.42, Body mass index (BMI) 45.0-49.9, adult*
- *Z79.4, Long-term (current) use of insulin*

She then rechecks the documentation to make sure she has coded everything for the encounter and reports the chosen codes on the claim for the service.

Diagnostic and procedural coding for healthcare specialist services

19.5

There's a Code for That

Read the following documentation and assign the appropriate CPT, HCPCS, and ICD-10 CM code(s) for the encounter.

1. Diagnostic flexible EGD performed on 45-year-old male revealed Barrett esophagus with low grade dysplasia.

   CPT code: _____

   ICD-10-CM code: _____

2. Dr. Hidalgo was called out to the emergency department to perform a gastric intubation on a patient who was experiencing severe generalized stomach pains, vomiting, and elevated blood pressure due to ingestion of noxious berries.

   CPT code: _____

   ICD-10-CM code: _____ , _____ , _____ ,

   _____

3. Cardiothoracic surgeon was called into the ER to perform an emergency surgery for a ruptured abdominal aortic aneurysm (AAA) on a 50-year-old male patient with stage 3 chronic kidney disease due to hypertension. Patient is a current cigarette smoker and smokes about one pack per day. Surgeon performed an endovascular repair of the infrarenal abdominal and visceral aorta with fenestrated visceral aortic endograft and two visceral artery endoprostheses of the superior mesenteric arteries.

   CPT code: _____

   ICD-10-CM code: _____ , _____ , _____ ,

   _____

Case Study   Flexible Sigmoidoscopy

PATIENT: Lawrence Egbert

PROCEDURE: Flexible Sigmoidoscopy with Anesthesia

PREOPERATIVE DIAGNOSIS: History of rectal cancer, status post colon resection, rectal incontinence

POSTOPERATIVE DIAGNOSIS: History of rectal cancer, status post colon resection, rectal incontinence

FINDINGS: Anastomotic stenosis

ESTIMATED BLOOD LOSS: Minimal

DRAINS: None

DISPOSITION: Awakened from anesthesia and taken to recovery room in stable condition, having suffered no untoward event.

COMPLICATIONS: None

TECHNIQUE:

After informed consent was obtained, this patient with mild systemic disease was placed in the left lateral position. General anesthesia was administered by the anesthesiologist. A time out was performed and the patient and procedure were confirmed. A digital rectal exam was performed. Fibrosis was noted at the anastomosis. No masses were palpable. This was followed by flexible sigmoidoscopy. The endoscope was introduced through the anastomosis and up to the sigmoid colon. The quality of prep was poor with heavy stool burden within the sigmoid and rectal area. This was irrigated to visualize the anastomosis. A posterior recess was noted consistent with patient's history of perirectal sinus that had healed well. No evidence of recurrent malignant disease was noted. A guidewire was then passed through the scope into the sigmoid colon and the scope was withdrawn. The anastomotic area was then dilated using Savary dilators starting at 45 French dilating it up to 60 French. The dilators were removed and a repeat endoscopy was performed. There is no evidence of injury or bleeding from the anastomosis. No evidence of perforation was noted. The procedure was terminated and patient was taken to the recovery room in stable condition. There were no immediate complications and the estimated blood loss was minimal.

SIGNED: Dr. Topher Crawley, MD

Use the following steps to select the appropriate codes for the case study.

1. Read through the case study and answer the question: *What did the doctor do?* (Note that this case is the same case that was presented in chapter 12, but now it is necessary to identify the procedure performed by the surgeon, rather than the anesthesiologist.) Identify the name of the procedure.

   _____

   _____

2. Locate the code for the anesthesia procedure in the CPT code book.
   a. Search the Index for the procedure and search through the options.
   b. In the listing of codes, check for any guidelines, important definitions, or parenthetical notes. Select the appropriate code and list it.

   _____

   _____

3. Now that the procedure(s) and modifier(s) have been identified, review the case study and answer the following question: *Why did the doctor do it?*

_____

_____

4. Now that you have identified the patient's diagnoses, search the ICD-10-CM code book for the correct codes for these conditions. Follow these steps for each of the diagnoses identified.

  a. Search the Main Index for the name of each condition and search through any applicable subterms and cross-references to locate the appropriate code.

    i. _____

    ii. _____

    iii. _____

    iv. _____

  b. Verify the code in the Tabular List. Locate the code identified previously in the Tabular Listing of codes and refer to any applicable guidelines, notes, and symbols. Does the code selected correctly identify the patient's condition? If yes, list the code.

    i. _____

    ii. _____

    iii. _____

    iv. _____

  c. Check the procedure note and ICD-10-CM guidelines and conventions to determine the correct sequencing of the diagnosis codes, if applicable. Correctly sequence the diagnosis codes.

_____

_____

5. Now that the procedure and diagnosis codes have been identified, list them on the CMS-1500 form. Be sure to correctly link the procedure and diagnosis codes. Remember to add the number of units as necessary. For this case study, do not calculate the time, base units, or modifying factors. Assign only the ICD-10-CM and CPT codes to the claim, with correct code linkage.

End-of-Chapter Content

Instructions: Indicate whether the following statements are true or false (T or F). For false statements, rewrite the statement on the line below to make the statement true.

1. A gastroenterologist is a healthcare provider who specializes in the treatment and management of genitourinary diseases.

   _____

   _____

2. A bariatric surgeon performs surgeries on the genitourinary system.

   _____

   _____

3. The lips are included in the gastroenterology subsection of the CPT code book.

   _____

   _____

4. A Roux-en-Y procedure is performed for weight loss.

   _____

   _____

5. A cardiologist treats conditions of the heart and surrounding vessels.

   _____

   _____

6. A pacemaker helps to maintain normal heart rhythm.

   _____

   _____

7. CPB is a technique in which a machine takes over the function of the heart and lungs during surgery.

   _____

   _____

8. When only veins are used during CABG surgery, use a code from 33510 to 33516.

_____

_____

9. Coronary artery bypass grafts that use both arteries and veins are coded from 33533 to 33548.

_____

_____

10. An angiography is the x-ray examination of only the aorta.

_____

_____

Instructions: Choose the best answer.

1. Which of the following types of healthcare providers performs surgeries meant to assist with weight loss?

a. Bariatric surgeon
b. Colorectal surgeon
c. Gastroenterologist
d. Surgical urologist

2. An EGD is the endoscopic examination of which of the following?

a. Esophagus, duodenum, and rectum
b. Esophagus, stomach, and duodenum
c. Stomach, duodenum, and small intestine
d. Anus, rectum, and colon

3. Which of the following is a rare bulge in the small intestine that is a remnant of the umbilical cord?

a. Bartholin's gland
b. Meckel's diverticulum
c. Seminal vesicle
d. Mesentery

4. Which of the following conditions causes heartburn and indigestion?

a. Vesicoureteral reflux
b. Angina
c. Esophageal varices
d. GERD

5. Which of the following types of colon polyps are inflammatory in nature?

a. K63.5
b. D12.6
c. K51.40
d. D37.4

6. Which of the following types of cardiovascular providers would treat cardiovascular conditions that affect the extremities of the body?

a. Cardiothoracic surgeon
b. Cardiac electrophysiologist
c. Interventional cardiologic specialist
d. Peripheral vascular surgeon

7. Noninvasive cardiovascular procedures and studies are found in which section of the CPT code book?

a. Surgery
b. Radiology
c. Medicine
d. Anesthesia

8. Which of the following is an ICD system in which two leads are placed into the heart, in the right atrium and right ventricle?

a. Dual chamber pacemaker
b. Single chamber implantable cardiac defibrillator
c. Bi-ventricular pacemaker
d. Dual chamber implantable cardiac defibrillator

9. Harvesting of which of the following vessels is included in a CABG procedure?

    a. Upper extremity artery
    b. Saphenous vein
    c. Femoropopliteal vein
    d. Brachial artery

10. Which of the following best describes cardiovascular procedures found in the Radiology section?

    a. Injection of contrast material
    b. Imaging of peripheral vessels
    c. Noninvasive cardiovascular studies
    d. Cardiovascular surgery

11. Which of the following conditions is a hardening of the fatty substances within a vessel?

    a. Arteriosclerosis
    b. Deep vein thrombosis
    c. Pulmonary embolism
    d. Atherosclerosis

12. Which of the following is a blood clot that has dislodged and is moving through the blood stream?

    a. Peripheral vascular disease
    b. Deep vein thrombosis
    c. Pulmonary nodule
    d. Embolus

Instructions: Answer the following questions with the appropriate code(s) and modifier(s).

1. Percutaneous catheter inserted with imaging guidance for fluid collection from a 40-year-old male with abscessed appendix.

    CPT codes: _____

    ICD-10 code: _____

2. A 43-year-old new patient with severe GERD presents for surgical consultation. Comprehensive history and evaluation with moderate complexity MDM. Diagnostic transoral esophagoscopy performed in office revealed significant reflux esophagitis. Decision for surgery was made and patient scheduled for laparoscopic fundoplasty in two weeks.

    CPT codes: _____- _____ , _____

    ICD-10 code: _____

3. Cardiopulmonary resuscitation performed on patient with acute cardiac arrest.

    CPT codes: _____

    ICD-10 code: _____

4. Right heart catheterization for atrial septal defect.

    CPT codes: _____

    ICD-10 code: _____

5. Venipuncture of scalp vein in an 18-month-old female with severe dehydration.

    CPT codes: _____

    ICD-10 code: _____

References

American Society for Metabolic and Bariatric Surgery (ASMBS). 2017. Bariatric Surgery Procedures. https://asmbs.org/patients/bariatric-surgery-procedures.

Blausen.com staff. 2013a. Blausen 0604 LargeIntestine2.png. Digital image. Wikimedia Commons. https://en.wikipedia.org/wiki/Large_intestine#/media/File:Blausen_0604_LargeIntestine2.png.

Blausen.com staff. 2013b. Blausen 0543 ImplantableCardioverterDefibrillator InsideLeads.png. Digital image. Wikimedia Commons. https://en.wikipedia.org/wiki/Implantable_cardioverter-defibrillator#/media/File:Blausen_0543_ImplantableCardioverterDefibrillator_InsideLeads.png.

Blausen.com staff. 2013c. Blausen 0152 CABG All.png. Digital image. Wikimedia Commons. https://en.wikipedia.org/wiki/Coronary_artery_bypass_surgery#/media/File:Blausen_0152_CABG_All.png.

Boudi, F. B. 2016 (April 25). Coronary Artery Atherosclerosis. https://emedicine.medscape.com/article/153647-overview.

BruceBlaus. 2016. Abdominal Aortic Aneurysm Location.png. Digital image. Wikimedia Commons. https://en.wikipedia.org/wiki/Abdominal_aortic_aneurysm#/media/File:Abdominal_Aortic_Aneurysm_Location.png.

Centers for Medicare and Medicaid Services (CMS). 2019. ICD-10-CM Official Guidelines for Coding and Reporting FY 2020. https://www.cms.gov/Medicare/Coding/ICD10/Downloads/2020-Coding-Guidelines.pdf.

Drus1a. 2018 (March). "ERCP.png." Digital image. Wikimedia Commons. https://commons.wikimedia.org/wiki/File:ERCP.png.

National Heart Lung and Blood Institute (NHLBI). 2017. Varicose veins-en.svg. Digital image. National Heart Lung and Blood Institute. https://commons.wikimedia.org/wiki/File:Varicose_veins-en.svg.

National Heart Lung and Blood Institute (NHLBI). n.d. Pacemakers. Accessed Dec. 13, 2019. https://www.nhlbi.nih.gov/health-topics/pacemakers.

National Institute of Diabetes and Digestive and Kidney Diseases (NIDDK). 2016 (June). Endoscopic Retrograde Cholangiopancreatography (ERCP). https://www.niddk.nih.gov/health-information/diagnostic-tests/endoscopic-retrograde-cholangiopancreatography.

Npatchett. 2016. "PPM.png." Digital image. Wikimedia Commons. https://en.wikipedia.org/wiki/Artificial_cardiac_pacemaker#/media/File:PPM.png.

Npatchett. 2015. "Late Complications of Atherosclerosis.png." Digital image. Wikimedia Commons. https://en.wikipedia.org/wiki/Atherosclerosis#/media/File:Late_complications_of_atherosclerosis.PNG.

Seeras, K. and M. A. Siccardi. 2019. Nissen Fundoplication (Anti-reflux Procedure). https://www.ncbi.nlm.nih.gov/books/NBK519521/

US National Library of Medicine (USNLM). 2017 (August 16). Central Venous Catheters–Ports. https://medlineplus.gov/ency/patientinstructions/000491.htm.

Resources

American Heart Association. 2016 (September 30). Cardiac Event Recorder. http://www.heart.org/HEARTORG/Conditions/Arrhythmia/PreventionTreatmentofArrhythmia/Cardiac-Event-Recorder_UCM_447317_Article.jsp#.WVVY3GgrLb0.

DecisionHealth. 2013. *Advanced Anatomy and Physiology for ICD-10-CM/PCS*. Salt Lake City, UT: Contexo Media.

Johns Hopkins Medicine. 2019. Percutaneous Transluminal Angioplasty. http://www.hopkinsmedicine.org/interventional-radiology/procedures/pta/.

MedlinePlus. 2019 (November 1). Pacemakers and Implantable Defibrillators. https://medlineplus.gov/pacemakersandimplantabledefibrillators.html.

Texas Heart Institute. n.d. Cardiovascular Glossary. Accessed Dec. 13, 2019. http://www.texasheart.org/HIC/Gloss/.

University of California San Francisco (UCSF). 2019. Endovascular Surgery. https://www.ucsfhealth.org/treatments/endovascular_surgery/.

US Department of Health and Human Services (HHS). n.d. What Are Varicose Veins? Accessed Dec. 13, 2019. https://www.nhlbi.nih.gov/health-topics/varicose-veins.

US National Library of Medicine (USNLM). 2017. Meckel Diverticulum. https://www.ncbi.nlm.nih.gov/pubmedhealth/PMHT0022924/.

US National Library of Medicine (USNLM). 2017. Mesentery. https://www.ncbi.nlm.nih.gov/pubmedhealth/PMHT0028174/.

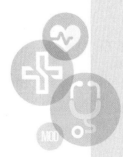

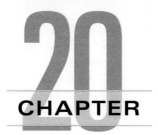

CHAPTER

Inpatient Hospital Services

Learning Objectives

- Identify ICD-10-PCS codes and explain their use in the healthcare setting
- Examine the structure of ICD-10-PCS codes and code book

- Use general ICD-10-PCS coding guidelines to create ICD-10-PCS codes

Key Terms

Alteration
Approach
Bypass
Change
Character
Code table
Complication/Comorbidity (CC)
Control
Creation
Delivery
Destruction
Detachment
Device
Diagnosis-related groups (DRGs)
Dilation
Division
Drainage

Excision
Extirpation
Extraction
Fragmentation
Fusion
Hospital-acquired condition (HAC)
Inpatient prospective payment system (IPPS)
Insertion
Inspection
Major complication/comorbidity (MCC)
Map
Multiaxial structure
Occlusion
Prospective payment system (PPS)
Qualifier

Reattachment
Release
Removal
Repair
Replacement
Reposition
Resection
Restriction
Revision
Root operation
Supplement
Transfer
Transplantation
UB-04
Uniform Hospital Discharge Data Set (UHDDS)

Inpatient hospital facility services are reported with ICD-10-PCS codes, which are seven-character alphanumeric codes used to identify services provided to patients in the inpatient facility setting. As previously discussed in chapter 3 (Basics of Coding), ICD-10-PCS codes represent procedures or services and are similar in nature to CPT and HCPCS codes, as they identify the service that was provided to the patient. However, ICD-10-PCS codes (also referred to as PCS codes) identify services performed in the inpatient or facility setting only. For example, if a patient received an appendectomy (removal of the appendix) in an inpatient hospital, the hospital would use a PCS appendectomy code to report the procedure.

As discussed in chapter 1 (Your Coding Career), inpatient services are provided to patients who have been admitted to an acute-care facility where they receive around-the-clock healthcare services in addition to medical and surgical procedures. Inpatient coding differs from outpatient coding in that the healthcare facility does not report the procedure codes directly for reimbursement, as is the case in professional billing (in which CPT or HCPCS codes are directly tied to the services provided). In inpatient billing, PCS codes are reported to identify the service(s) the healthcare provider performed on the patient. The PCS code is added to the claim for the service and compiled into a diagnostic-related group (DRG) to determine the amount of payment that will be received for the services. Reimbursement for the services provided by the inpatient facility is therefore based on the diagnosis code(s)—the medical necessity, in addition to any comorbid conditions or complications—for the patient's stay, as well as the procedures performed and other factors (such as the patient's gender and discharge status). Refer to chapters 1 and 3 for more information on the difference between inpatient and outpatient coding.

In addition to learning a new code set and method of coding (ICD-10-PCS), it is important to keep in mind that inpatient facility ICD-10-CM coding for diagnoses is also a bit different. For example, unlike in outpatient coding, in which it is never acceptable to report a suspected condition, inpatient coding guidelines do allow the coder to report a suspect condition (one that has not been confirmed).

Furthermore, it is important to understand the importance of data collection for inpatient stays and procedures, governed by performance measures and federal guidelines such as the Uniform Hospital Discharge and Data Set (UHDDS).

ICD-10-PCS coding requires an in-depth understanding of the multiaxial structure of the codes themselves, which must be built according to the procedure that was performed. In the case of ICD-10-PCS coding, this multiaxial structure is based on coding tables that contain options for each of the seven characters in the code (characters 1 through 7). To build the code, the coder must carefully select one character from the table for each of the seven required characters. This allows the coder to create a code that precisely describes the procedure performed. Rather than simply selecting a PCS code from the Tabular List (as in CPT or HCPCS coding), PCS codes must be built character by character, depending on what, where, and how each procedure was performed. Coders must be able to locate the tables for each procedure type and create the code based on the documentation of the procedure.

This chapter briefly discusses inpatient coding in general, including ICD-10-CM guidelines for inpatient diagnoses, and UHDDS and data collection. It also discusses ICD-10-PCS coding in general, what it is used for, how to use the ICD-10-PCS code book to create a PCS code, and finally how to create a PCS code for the documented procedure.

ICD-10-CM Inpatient Coding Guidelines

The majority of ICD-10-CM diagnosis coding guidelines apply to both inpatient and outpatient reporting, with special sections that pertain specifically to coding in either the inpatient or outpatient setting. Among the guidelines that do not change based on the setting are the following:

- Use of the Alphabetic Index and Tabular List
- Use of coding conventions such as *"code first"* and *"use additional code"*
- Etiology and manifestation coding
- Use of ICD-10-CM codes to identify the medical necessity of services provided
- Coding to the highest level of specificity for each condition

Nevertheless, it is important to understand the specific ICD-10-CM coding guidelines for the inpatient setting and how they differ from similar guidelines for outpatient coding. See figure 20.1 for the ICD-10-CM guidelines that impact inpatient code selection.

Key to Success

ICD-10-CM guidelines pertaining to inpatient services are not referred to as "OGCR." This is because they are not *outpatient* guidelines for coding and reporting, as they are used only in the inpatient setting. You may think of the "O" in OGCR as referring to "outpatient."

The guidelines shown in figure 20.1 pertain to the selection of the principal diagnosis, which is, according to the UHDDS definition (discussed in the following section), "that condition established after study to be chiefly responsible for occasioning the admission of the patient to the hospital for care" (HHS 1985). One of the biggest differences between inpatient and outpatient diagnosis reporting is that in the outpatient setting the coder must report only confirmed diagnoses (or the signs and symptoms for an unconfirmed diagnosis). Unlike outpatient coding, inpatient coding allows the reporting of "suspected," "probable," or "rule out" diagnoses. In inpatient coding, in other words, it is acceptable to report a diagnosis that was not confirmed by the provider. The reason for this, as stated in the guidelines, is due to the fact that a suspected diagnosis may be the reason for workup, arrangements for further workup, or observation (see figure 20.1, ICD-10-CM Guidelines Section II.H. Uncertain Diagnosis).

Other than the principal diagnosis, all other conditions that require or impact patient care should also be reported in the inpatient setting. These include conditions that, during the admission, required:

- Clinical evaluation
- Therapeutic treatment
- Diagnostic procedures
- Extended length of hospital stay
- Increased nursing care
- Monitoring (CMS 2019a)

Figure 20.1. ICD-10-CM guidelines for inpatient reporting

Section II. Selection of Principal Diagnosis

The circumstances of inpatient admission always govern the selection of principal diagnosis. The principal diagnosis is defined in the Uniform Hospital Discharge Data Set (UHDDS) as "that condition established after study to be chiefly responsible for occasioning the admission of the patient to the hospital for care."

The UHDDS definitions are used by hospitals to report inpatient data elements in a standardized manner. These data elements and their definitions can be found in the July 31, 1985, Federal Register (Vol. 50, No, 147), pp. 31038–40.

Since that time the application of the UHDDS definitions has been expanded to include all non-outpatient settings (acute care, short term, long term care and psychiatric hospitals; home health agencies; rehab facilities; nursing homes, etc). The UHDDS definitions also apply to hospice services (all levels of care).

In determining principal diagnosis, coding conventions in the ICD-10-CM, the Tabular List and Alphabetic Index take precedence over these official coding guidelines.

(See Section I.A., Conventions for the ICD-10-CM)

The importance of consistent, complete documentation in the medical record cannot be overemphasized. Without such documentation the application of all coding guidelines is a difficult, if not impossible, task.

A. Codes for Symptoms, Signs, and Ill-Defined Conditions

Codes for symptoms, signs, and ill-defined conditions from Chapter 18 are not to be used as principal diagnosis when a related definitive diagnosis has been established.

B. Two or More Interrelated Conditions, Each Potentially Meeting the Definition for Principal Diagnosis

When there are two or more interrelated conditions (such as diseases in the same ICD-10-CM chapter or manifestations characteristically associated with a certain disease) potentially meeting the definition of principal diagnosis, either condition may be sequenced first, unless the circumstances of the admission, the therapy provided, the Tabular List, or the Alphabetic Index indicate otherwise.

C. Two or More Diagnoses that Equally Meet the Definition for Principal Diagnosis

In the unusual instance when two or more diagnoses equally meet the criteria for principal diagnosis as determined by the circumstances of admission, diagnostic workup and/or therapy provided, and the Alphabetic Index, Tabular List, or another coding guidelines does not provide sequencing direction, any one of the diagnoses may be sequenced first.

D. Two or More Comparative or Contrasting Conditions

In those rare instances when two or more contrasting or comparative diagnoses are documented as "either/or" (or similar terminology), they are coded as if the diagnoses were confirmed and the diagnoses are sequenced according to the circumstances of the admission. If no further determination can be made as to which diagnosis should be principal, either diagnosis may be sequenced first.

E. A Symptom(s) Followed by Contrasting/Comparative Diagnoses

GUIDELINE HAS BEEN DELETED EFFECTIVE OCTOBER 1, 2014.

F. Original Treatment Plan not Carried out

Sequence as the principal diagnosis the condition, which after study occasioned the admission to the hospital, even though treatment may not have been carried out due to unforeseen circumstances.

G. Complications of Surgery and Other Medical Care

When the admission is for treatment of a complication resulting from surgery or other medical care, the complication code is sequenced as the principal diagnosis. If the complication is classified to the T80–T88 series and the code lacks the necessary specificity in describing the complication, an additional code for the specific complication should be assigned.

H. Uncertain Diagnosis

If the diagnosis documented at the time of discharge is qualified as "probable", "suspected", "likely", "questionable", "possible", or "still to be ruled out," **"compatible with," "consistent with,"** or other similar terms indicating uncertainty, code the condition as if it existed or was established. The bases for these guidelines are the diagnostic workup, arrangements for further workup or observation, and initial therapeutic approach that correspond most closely with the established diagnosis.

Note: This guideline is applicable only to inpatient admissions to short-term, acute, long-term care and psychiatric hospitals.

I. Admission from Observation Unit

1. Admission Following Medical Observation

When a patient is admitted to an observation unit for a medical condition, which either worsens or does not improve, and is subsequently admitted as an inpatient of the same hospital for this same medical condition, the principal diagnosis would be the medical condition which led to the hospital admission.

2. Admission Following Post-Operative Observation

When a patient is admitted to an observation unit to monitor a condition (or complication) that develops following outpatient surgery, and then is subsequently admitted as an inpatient of the same hospital, hospitals should apply the Uniform Hospital Discharge Data Set (UHDDS) definition of principal diagnosis as "that condition established after study to be chiefly responsible for occasioning the admission of the patient to the hospital for care."

J. Admission from Outpatient Surgery

When a patient receives surgery in the hospital's outpatient surgery department and is subsequently admitted for continuing inpatient care at the same hospital, the following guidelines should be followed in selecting the principal diagnosis for the inpatient admission:

- If the reason for the inpatient admission is a complication, assign the complication as the principal diagnosis.
- If no complication, or other condition, is documented as the reason for the inpatient admission, assign the reason for the outpatient surgery as the principal diagnosis.
- If the reason for the inpatient admission is another condition unrelated to the surgery, assign the unrelated condition as the principal diagnosis.

K. Admissions/Encounters for Rehabilitation

When the purpose for the admission/encounter is rehabilitation, sequence first the code for the condition for which the service is being performed. For example, for an admission/encounter for rehabilitation for rightsided dominant hemiplegia following a cerebrovascular infarction, report code I69.351, Hemiplegia and hemiparesis following cerebral infarction affecting right dominant side, as the first-listed or principal diagnosis.

If the condition for which the rehabilitation service is being provided is no longer present, report the appropriate aftercare code as the first-listed or principal diagnosis, unless the rehabilitation service is being provided following an injury. For rehabilitation services following active treatment of an injury, assign the injury code with the appropriate seventh character for subsequent encounter as the first-listed or principal diagnosis. For example, if a patient with severe degenerative osteoarthritis of the hip, underwent hip replacement and the current encounter/admission is for rehabilitation, report code Z47.1, Aftercare following joint replacement surgery, as the first-listed or principal diagnosis. If the patient requires rehabilitation post hip replacement for right intertrochanteric femur fracture, report code S72.141D, Displaced intertrochanteric fracture of right femur, subsequent encounter for closed fracture with routine healing, as the first-listed or principal diagnosis.

See Section I.C.21.c.7, Factors influencing health states and contact with health services, Aftercare.

See Section I.C.19.a for additional information about the use of 7th characters for injury codes.

Source: CMS 2019a.

For the guidelines pertaining to reporting additional diagnoses, refer to figure 20.2.

Additional components of inpatient diagnosis coding include complication/comorbidity (CC) and major complication/comorbidity (MCC) codes. In inpatient coding and reporting, a **complication/comorbidity (CC)** is a condition, either a complication (a medical condition that arises during the hospital stay) or a comorbidity (a pre-existing medical condition), that requires additional resources, affects treatment to the patient, or prolongs the patient's inpatient stay (HMSA 2014). A **major complication/comorbidity (MCC)** is similar in nature to a CC but with a higher severity, which may require more resources, treatment, or prolonged stay. CCs and MCCs become important when discussing reimbursement for inpatient hospital services, as inpatient services are reimbursed by some payers on a prospective basis, using the IPPS system discussed in the following section. CCs and MCCs identify a

Figure 20.2. ICD-10-CM guidelines for reporting additional diagnoses

Section III. Reporting Additional Diagnoses

GENERAL RULES FOR OTHER (ADDITIONAL) DIAGNOSES

For reporting purposes the definition for "other diagnoses" is interpreted as additional conditions that affect patient care in terms of requiring:

- clinical evaluation; or
- therapeutic treatment; or
- diagnostic procedures; or
- extended length of hospital stay; or
- increased nursing care and/or
- monitoring

The UHDDS item #11-b defines Other Diagnoses as "all conditions that coexist at the time of admission, that develop subsequently, or that affect the treatment received and/or the length of stay. Diagnoses that relate to an earlier episode which have no bearing on the current hospital stay are to be excluded." UHDDS definitions apply to inpatients in acute-care, short-term, long term care and psychiatric hospital setting. The UHDDS definitions are used by acute-care shortterm hospitals to report inpatient data elements in a standardized manner. These data elements and their definitions can be found in the July 31, 1985, *Federal Register* (Vol. 50, No, 147), pp. 31038–40.

Since that time the application of the UHDDS definitions has been expanded to include all nonoutpatient settings (acute-care, short-term, long-term care and psychiatric hospitals; home health agencies; rehab facilities; nursing homes, etc). The UHDDS definitions also apply to hospice services (all levels of care).

The following guidelines are to be applied in designating "other diagnoses" when neither the Alphabetic Index nor the Tabular List in ICD-10-CM provide direction. The listing of the diagnoses in the patient record is the responsibility of the attending provider.

A. Previous Conditions

If the provider has included a diagnosis in the final diagnostic statement, such as the discharge summary or the face sheet, it should ordinarily be coded. Some providers include in the diagnostic statement resolved conditions or diagnoses and status-post procedures from previous admission that have no bearing on the current stay. Such conditions are not to be reported and are coded only if required by hospital policy.

However, history codes (categories Z80–Z87) may be used as secondary codes if the historical condition or family history has an impact on current care or influences treatment.

B. Abnormal Findings

Abnormal findings (laboratory, x-ray, pathologic, and other diagnostic results) are not coded and reported unless the provider indicates their clinical significance. If the findings are outside the normal range and the attending provider has ordered other tests to evaluate the condition or prescribed treatment, it is appropriate to ask the provider whether the abnormal finding should be added.

Please note: This differs from the coding practices in the outpatient setting for coding encounters for diagnostic tests that have been interpreted by a provider.

C. Uncertain Diagnosis

If the diagnosis documented at the time of discharge is qualified as "probable", "suspected", "likely", "questionable", "possible", or "still to be ruled out," **"compatible with," "consistent with,"** or other similar terms indicating uncertainty, code the condition as if it existed or was established. The bases for these guidelines are the diagnostic workup, arrangements for further workup or observation, and initial therapeutic approach that correspond most closely with the established diagnosis.

Note: This guideline is applicable only to inpatient admissions to short-term, acute-care, long-term care and psychiatric hospitals.

Source: CMS 2019a.

more patient with more complex medical needs, which required more treatment, and thus which should be reimbursed at a higher rate.

Depending on the publisher of your ICD-10-CM code book, MCCs and CCs may be identified with colored highlighting or a footnote in the Tabular List. In the American Health Information Management Association (AHIMA) ICD-10-CM code book, MCC and CC codes are flagged in the Tabular List with a purple MCC or CC for easier identification.

The Importance of Data in the Inpatient Setting

Both new and experienced inpatient coders should understand the importance of data collected from inpatient stays. This data can be used to monitor the outbreak of medical conditions, manage health resources, and make changes in medical care, all based on the codes submitted. A major factor in the collection of data from inpatient stays is the **Uniform Hospital Discharge Data Set (UHDDS)**. This data set was originally created in 1974 to "improve the uniformity and comparability of hospital discharge data" for the Medicare and Medicaid programs (HHS 1985). The UHDDS was revised in 1985 to specify data requirements for all inpatient admissions, as well as to clarify guidance on patient diagnoses, which is still included in the ICD-10-CM guidelines (see figures 20.1 and 20.2).

The UHDDS consists of the following data elements, which must be included on the UB-04 form for inpatient claims:

- Personal identification
- Date of birth
- Sex
- Race and ethnicity
- Residence
- Hospital identification
- Admission date
- Discharge date
- Attending physician
- Operating physician
- Diagnoses
- Procedures and dates
- Disposition of patient
- Expected payer (anticipated financial guarantor for services)

Data from inpatient admissions, diagnoses, and procedures, are used to identify the performance of each inpatient facility by quantifying patient diagnoses, causes of death or treatment, and the treatments performed. An example of a performance measurement program is one that identifies and tracks hospital-acquired conditions (HACs). A **hospital-acquired condition (HAC)** is a condition that a patient acquires at a hospital, such as a urinary tract infection from catheterization, that results in additional resources being required to care for that patient. In other words, HACs are a direct result of the hospital stay. HACs are tracked as part of identifying the performance of an inpatient facility and:

- Are high cost or high volume or both,
- Result in the assignment of a case to a DRG that has a higher payment when present as a secondary diagnosis, and

- Could reasonably have been prevented through the application of evidence-based guidelines (CMS 2019b).

Ultimately, the more HACs that a facility reports, the lower the quality of care it is implied to provide, as patients of that facility are subject to additional conditions caused by their inpatient stay. Hospitals may be subject to penalties or lower reimbursement rates due to high incidences of HACs.

Like CCs and MCCs, HACs may be flagged the ICD-10-CM code book with color-coordinated highlighting, a footnote in the Tabular List, or another convention, depending on the publisher. For example, the AHIMA ICD-10-CM code book highlights HAC codes in an orange color in the Tabular List for easier identification.

Complete the exercises in There's A Code for That 20.1 to practice coding in the inpatient setting.

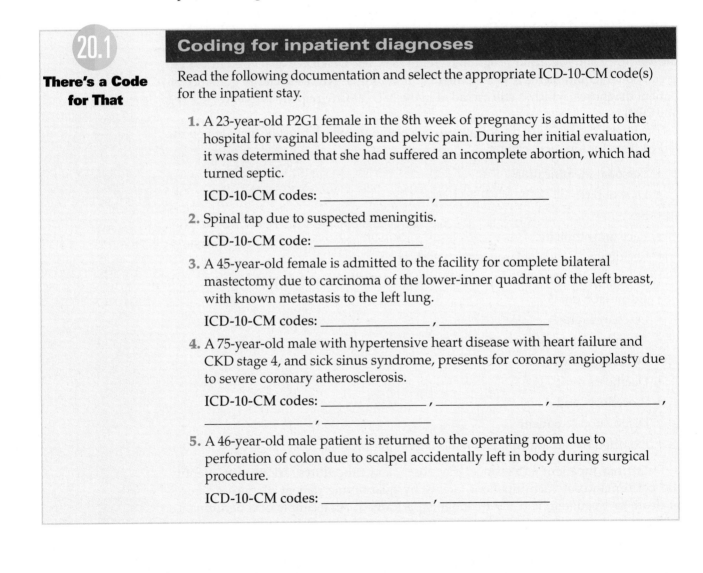

20.1

There's a Code for That

Coding for inpatient diagnoses

Read the following documentation and select the appropriate ICD-10-CM code(s) for the inpatient stay.

1. A 23-year-old P2G1 female in the 8th week of pregnancy is admitted to the hospital for vaginal bleeding and pelvic pain. During her initial evaluation, it was determined that she had suffered an incomplete abortion, which had turned septic.

   ICD-10-CM codes: _____ , _____

2. Spinal tap due to suspected meningitis.

   ICD-10-CM code: _____

3. A 45-year-old female is admitted to the facility for complete bilateral mastectomy due to carcinoma of the lower-inner quadrant of the left breast, with known metastasis to the left lung.

   ICD-10-CM codes: _____ , _____

4. A 75-year-old male with hypertensive heart disease with heart failure and CKD stage 4, and sick sinus syndrome, presents for coronary angioplasty due to severe coronary atherosclerosis.

   ICD-10-CM codes: _____ , _____ , _____ , _____ , _____

5. A 46-year-old male patient is returned to the operating room due to perforation of colon due to scalpel accidentally left in body during surgical procedure.

   ICD-10-CM codes: _____ , _____

ICD-10-PCS Coding

There are numerous differences between coding for services performed in the inpatient facility setting, as reported with ICD-10-PCS codes, and outpatient professional coding, as reported with CPT codes. Unlike CPT or HCPCS codes, PCS codes are not directly used for reimbursement. Furthermore, facility services are reported on the UB-04 form (as opposed to the CMS-1500 form used in professional billing). Payment for facility services is based on a prospective payment system, rather than fee-for-service.

Inpatient Facility Coding and Prospective Payment System

As previously mentioned, PCS codes are used only in the inpatient or facility setting to identify the services performed by the healthcare provider(s). This is in contrast to *professional* services, which are typically reported on a fee-for-service basis—that is, the procedure codes(s) assigned for the procedure are attached to a fee for that service. For example, an evaluation and management (E/M) code for an office visit charge may be $100. However, *facility* procedures reported with PCS codes are *not* reported with specific charges per procedure. ICD-10-PCS coding is part of a **prospective payment system (PPS)**, a type of reimbursement system based on preset payment levels rather than actual charges billed after the service has been provided. Payment is based on predetermined payment rates or periods and linked to the anticipated intensity of services delivered as well as the beneficiary's condition (as identified by the patient's diagnosis codes, CCs and MCCs, procedures performed in the facility setting, and additional factors).

In the **Inpatient Prospective Payment System (IPPS)**, the prospective payment system used in the inpatient facility setting, the diagnosis code(s) and procedure code(s) are combined using **diagnosis-related groups (DRGs)** to identify the predetermined amount of payment for hospital services. DRG classification is a system that groups patients according to diagnosis, type of treatment, age, and other relevant criteria. Under the IPPS, hospitals are paid a set fee for treating patients in a single DRG category.

An inpatient coder is responsible for reporting ICD-10-CM and ICD-10-PCS codes for each admission, which are linked to the appropriate DRG via the facility's practice management software program, to obtain a prospective payment amount for the services performed. This allows the hospital facility to bill for the services that were provided during the procedure (such as hospital bed, staff, nursing services, meals, the use of equipment such as x-rays, and surgical supplies), but not actually bill for the procedure itself (the procedure is billed by the performing provider using the appropriate CPT or HCPCS codes).

Procedures represented by PCS codes must still be supported with medical necessity, which means that both ICD-10-CM and PCS codes may be reported on the same claim. Keep in mind that PCS codes are only used for *facility* billing—such as inpatient hospital services, skilled nursing facility services, or inpatient mental hospital services. They also may be used to report outpatient hospital services, if the outpatient hospital participates in facility reporting. See figure 20.3 for a refresher of the different types of codes.

Key to Success

The codes reported by the hospital are *facility* codes (ICD-10-CM and ICD-10-PCS), and the codes reported by the healthcare provider are the *professional* codes for the services performed (ICD-10-CM, CPT, and HCPCS).

UB-04 Claim Form

Another difference between inpatient and outpatient coding is the form used for billing third-party insurance payers. In professional coding, the CMS-1500 form is used. In facility inpatient and outpatient reporting, the **UB-04**, also known as the CMS-1450, form is the hardcopy claim form used for billing services (see figure 20.4). Note that the UB-04 form includes more than twice as many informational fields as the CMS-1500 form used for outpatient billing; these fields are for information regarding inpatient services, such as discharge information, information regarding the hospital services, and the providers who performed the services, as required by the UHDDS.

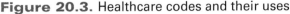

Figure 20.3. Healthcare codes and their uses

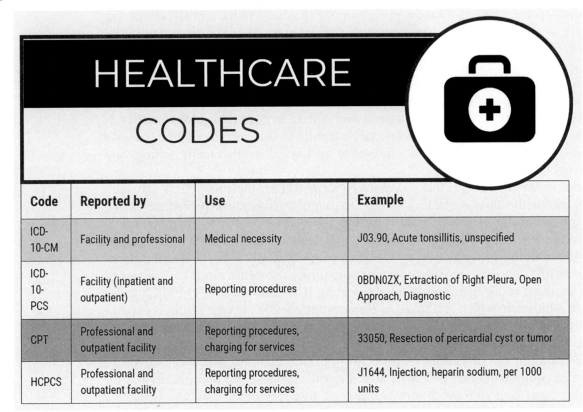

Code	Reported by	Use	Example
ICD-10-CM	Facility and professional	Medical necessity	J03.90, Acute tonsillitis, unspecified
ICD-10-PCS	Facility (inpatient and outpatient)	Reporting procedures	0BDN0ZX, Extraction of Right Pleura, Open Approach, Diagnostic
CPT	Professional and outpatient facility	Reporting procedures, charging for services	33050, Resection of pericardial cyst or tumor
HCPCS	Professional and outpatient facility	Reporting procedures, charging for services	J1644, Injection, heparin sodium, per 1000 units

While the CMS-1500 form has 12 lines on which a coder may enter ICD-10-CM diagnosis codes, the UB-04 form has over 20 lines. ICD-10-CM codes are entered in form locator (FL) 67 through 67.Q, FL 69, and FLs 70.a, 70.b, and 70.c, as necessary (see figure 20.5). Remember that ICD-10-CM diagnosis coding guidelines for inpatient services are different from those used in the outpatient setting. When reporting diagnosis codes for inpatient services, it is important to understand the coding guidelines related to inpatient coding and pay attention to notations in the Tabular List of the ICD-10-CM code book.

PCS codes identify the procedure(s) performed during the patient's admission, necessitated as indicated by the diagnosis code(s) (CM codes). There is room on the UB-04 form for up to six individual PCS codes, in FLs 74 through 74.e (see figure 20.6). One PCS code should be entered on the left under the word CODE, and the date the procedure was performed in the box under the word DATE. If more than six codes need to be reported, an additional form or forms would be included.

Facility services include all the services that may be performed on the patient, such as surgical treatments, face-to-face encounters, maternal care and delivery, and chiropractic services. Due to their multiaxial structure, PCS codes are more variable than CPT codes, so coders can report an additional level of specificity by adjusting the code to report exactly what procedure was performed and how it was performed. In PCS coding, the coder builds the code to report the specifics of how the procedure was performed.

Figure 20.4. UB-04 form

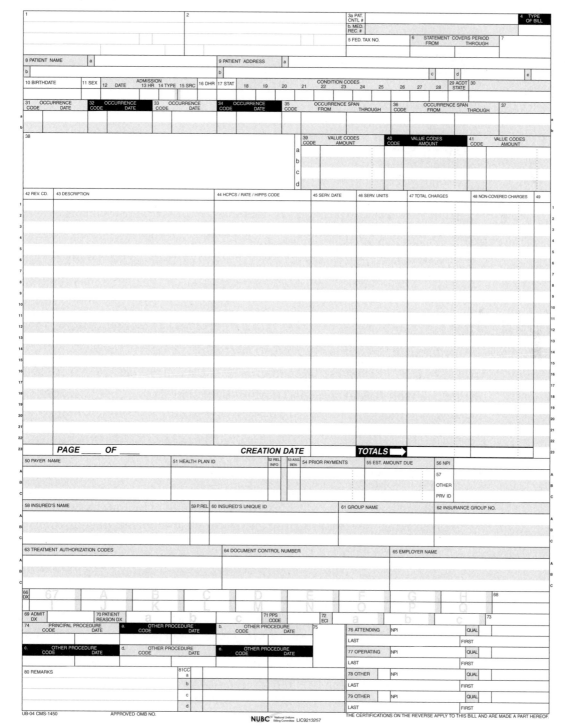

Source: CMS 2019c.

Figure 20.5. UB-04 FL 67 through 67.Q, 69, 70.a through 70.c

66 DX	67	A	B	C	D	E	F	G	H	68
		J	K	L	M	N	O	P	Q	
69 ADMIT DX		70 PATIENT REASON DX	a	b	c	71 PPS CODE	72 ECI	a	b	c	73

Source: CMS 2019c.

Figure 20.6. UB-04 FL 74 through 74.e

74	PRINCIPAL PROCEDURE CODE DATE	a.	OTHER PROCEDURE CODE DATE	b.	OTHER PROCEDURE CODE DATE
c.	OTHER PROCEDURE CODE DATE	d.	OTHER PROCEDURE CODE DATE	e.	OTHER PROCEDURE CODE DATE

Source: CMS 2019c.

Key to Success

Assigning codes for facility services (just as for professional services), requires an in-depth understanding of medical terminology, anatomy and physiology, and the various procedure types and treatment strategies for patient conditions. It is helpful to use as many resources as possible when learning PCS coding, like a medical dictionary, a medical terminology textbook, or an anatomy and physiology textbook.

ICD-10-PCS Code Structure and Code Book

ICD-10-PCS codes were built to accommodate a completely new procedural coding system. Instead of preset codes that approximated the service performed, PCS codes were built with certain structural attributes to allow for the creation of an expandable, flexible, and functional code set. These structural attributes are the following:

- *Multiaxial structure.* PCS codes are built with a **multiaxial structure**, meaning that each individual character within the code can represent a specific detail of the procedure performed. The term **character** refers to each of the individual numbers or letters within an ICD-10-PCS code. Each of the characters in the code are built upon a specific structure, as defined by the code table for each procedure type. This structure allows for flexibility and functionality.

- *Completeness.* The PCS code structure and guidelines allow for complete reporting of all components of the procedure performed. This includes coding for each individual procedure that was performed, using unique codes for each procedure.

- *Expandability.* The PCS code structure also allows for expandability for future code development, by easily adding new characters or meanings to the code tables without disrupting the existing code set.

PCS codes are seven characters in length and contain both numbers and letters. For example, the incision and drainage of an abscess on the skin of the abdomen is reported with code 0H97X0Z, Drainage of Abdomen Skin with Drainage Device, External Approach. Each character in the code identifies a specific detail of the procedure and must be selected by accessing the appropriate table in the PCS code set. For example, in the characters of the code 0H97X0Z:

1. 0 identifies the procedure as medical and surgical in nature.

2. H identifies that the procedure was performed on the skin and breast.

3. 9 identifies the procedure as drainage.

4. 7 identifies the area of the procedure as on the skin of the abdomen.

5. X describes the approach to the procedure as external.

6. 0 describes the device used as a drainage device.

7. Z identifies that there are no further qualifying characteristics of the procedure.

The following section of this chapter discusses the ICD-10-PCS code structure and how to use PCS code tables to build a PCS code. The last section discusses the organization of the ICD-10-PCS code book.

ICD-10-PCS Code Structure

PCS codes have seven characters, each of which depend on the section of the code book from which the code is being reported. Each character has a different meaning, based on the section of the code book from which it is selected. For example, the code for an open appendectomy is 0DTJ0ZZ, Resection of Appendix, Open Approach (see table 20.1). These characters are presented in a **code table**—a table of all of the character options. Note that the code tables are based on the first three characters only; the additional four characters are then selected from the code table in the ICD-10-PCS code book. Coders use the code table to build the additional characters into the code until all seven characters have been selected, according to how the procedure was performed.

Key to Success

As you learn about PCS codes and their structure, refer to the tables in your ICD-10-PCS code book. As you read through the following sections, follow along in your PCS book for a better understanding of these codes and how the code tables work.

Table 20.1. Open appendectomy PCS code

Character 1	Character 2	Character 3	Character 4	Character 5	Character 6	Character 7
0	D	T	J	0	Z	Z
Medical and Surgical	Gastro-intestinal	Resection	Appendix	Open	No Device	No Device

Each character in the code is carefully selected to identify a specific component of the procedure—such as that it was performed with an open approach or that the procedure was performed on the appendix. Coders must access the code tables in each section of the code book and carefully select the characters to build the code out to seven total characters. Review the following character components, their descriptions, and the code structure provided (see also table 20.2). This list identifies what each character means based on its placement (position one through seven).

Table 20.2. PCS characters and locations

Character 1	Character 2	Character 3	Character 4	Character 5	Character 6	Character 7
Section	Body System	Root Operation	Body Part	Approach	Device	Qualifier

1. The first character identifies the Section, which is the general type of procedure.

2. The second character identifies the Body System, which is the general physiological or anatomical region on which the procedure is performed.

3. The third character identifies the Root Operation or Type, which is the type and objective of the procedure.

4. The fourth character identifies the Body Part or Region, which is the specific organ or anatomical region involved in the procedure.

5. The fifth character identifies the Approach to the procedure, which is the technique used to gain access to the surgical site.

6. The sixth character identifies the **Device** that was used in the procedure, which is any material or appliance that remains after the procedure is performed.

7. The seventh character identifies the **Qualifier** for the procedure, which identifies any additional attributes of why or how the procedure was performed.

The sixth and seventh characters—device and qualifier—are not applicable for many procedures. As such, if no device or qualifier is applicable, use the character Z for no device or qualifier. This is noted in the code table.

The characters are listed in a set of tables from which the coder identifies each individual character and thus build a seven-character code. Tables are arranged based on the first three characters for each code—the section, body system, and root operation. The section that makes up the greatest deal of the PCS code book is comprised of these tables. The table in the Medical and Surgical section for resection of the gastrointestinal system is shown in table 20.3.

To create a PCS code, the coder must select the appropriate component of the procedure and build the code character by character, according to the table. To find the correct table, the coder must locate the first three characters of a code, as all tables are listed by their first three characters. It is helpful to rely on the Index, as well as knowledge of the root operation definitions, to identify the first three characters of a code, then access that code table to build the rest of the code.

Figure 20.7 illustrates how to build the code for an open appendectomy, as follows:

- The first three characters are located at the top of the table: 0DT.
- The fourth character is located in the first column on the left, under Body Part. Locate the word *Appendix* and select the character to which it corresponds: J.
- The fifth character is selected from the next column, under the heading Approach. Locate the word *Open* and assign the character to which it corresponds: 0.
- The last two characters are located in the last two columns. In this case, there is only one option for each: Z, for no device and no qualifier.

This builds the complete code 0DTJ0ZZ, Resection of Appendix, Open Approach.

Table 20.3. 0DT table in the Medical and Surgical section

Section	0	Medical and Surgical
Body System	D	Gastrointestinal System
Operation	T	**Resection:** Cutting out or off, without replacement, all of a body part

Body Part (4th)	Approach (5th)	Device (6th)	Qualifier (7th)
1 Esophagus, Upper 2 Esophagus, Middle 3 Esophagus, Lower 4 Esophagogastric Junction 5 Esophagus 6 Stomach 7 Stomach, Pylorus 8 Small Intestine 9 Duodenum A Jejunum B Ileum C Ileocecal Valve E Large Intestine F Large Intestine, Right H Cecum J Appendix K Ascending Colon P Rectum Q Anus	0 Open 4 Percutaneous Endoscopic 7 Via Natural or Artificial Opening 8 Via Natural or Artificial Opening Endoscopic	Z No Device	Z No Qualifier
G Large Intestine, Left L Transverse Colon M Descending Colon N Sigmoid Colon	0 Open 4 Percutaneous Endoscopic 7 Via Natural or Artificial Opening 8 Via Natural or Artificial Opening Endoscopic F Via Natural or Artificial Opening With Percutaneous Endoscopic Assistance	Z No Device	Z No Qualifier
R Anal Sphincter U Omentum	0 Open 4 Percutaneous Endoscopic	Z No Device	Z No Qualifier

Source: Casto 2018, 618.

Key to Success

To verify that the code that you have built is valid and complete, flip past the tables in each section to find the code listing for each code section. This is a list of the codes that can be created using the tables in that section. For example, if you want to verify that code 0DTJ0ZZ is valid, locate the code in the Gastrointestinal System Code Listing section at the end of the section to find: 0DJT0ZZ Resection of Appendix, Open Approach. Note that these lists are available in the AHIMA version of the ICD-10-PCS code book but may not be available in all code books.

Key to Success

When reporting PCS codes, be careful to differentiate between the letter *O* and the number 0 as they are very similar. The letter *O* is always listed as a capital letter, so it closely resembles the number 0. However, the letter *O* is rounder—more circular—than the number 0. The number 0 is more elongated—like an oval—than

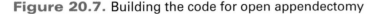

the letter *O* and may sometimes have a line through it (Ø) to indicate that it is a number rather than a letter.

Figure 20.7. Building the code for open appendectomy

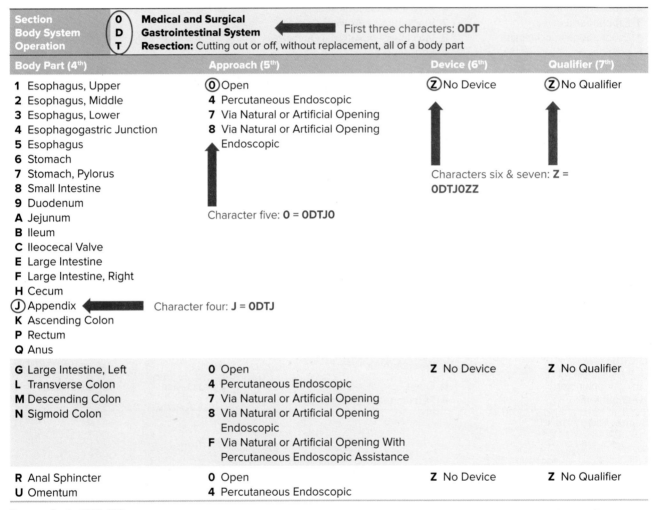

Source: Casto 2019, 620.

When using PCS tables, note that some tables are too large to be included in full on one page, so they may be continued on the following page. Some tables are so large that they may span *multiple* pages. It helps to look past the table referenced to ensure that it either has or has not been continued to the next page. Note that some publishers may include a "continued" note at the bottom of a table, or a small arrow, to indicate that the table continues on the next page.

Not all options are available for all procedures. For example, in the previous table, the Approach column (fifth character) does not include all seven approach types. In this case, the External (character X), Percutaneous (character 3), and Via Natural or Artificial Opening with Percutaneous Endoscopic Assistance (character F) are not listed. This is because none of the procedures in that section, body system, operation, and body area may be performed in that manner and, therefore, those approaches are not applicable.

ICD-10-PCS Code Book

The ICD-10-PCS code book is organized in a similar fashion to the ICD-10-CM code book. Coders should first access the Index at the beginning of the book to help find procedure codes, which are then verified in the Tabular List in the remainder of the book. However, there are striking differences between CM and PCS coding, and the organization of the book is really the only similarity. The major difference between ICD-10-CM and ICD-10-PCS code books is that instead of including a Tabular List that identifies individual codes, each with code descriptions (as in the CM code book), the PCS code book's Tabular List is comprised of tables that the coder must use to build a code.

In this sense, PCS coding is much more interactive and requires attention to details identified by each character in the code. Coders may find that the PCS code table includes body areas, organs, devices, or other details specific to only certain types of procedures. In these instances, using available reference materials—including medical terminology and anatomy and physiology resources—may be valuable, especially as a beginning coder.

The following sections identify each of the respective sections of the ICD-10-PCS code book: front matter, index, sections and code tables, and appendices.

Key to Success

As you read through the following sections, open your PCS code book and locate each individual area and note the details of how to use that section of the book.

Front Matter

The first part of the PCS code book is the Introductory material, which includes an overview of the code set, a description of the code structure, ICD-10-PCS organization and conventions, and the ICD-10-PCS Official Guidelines for Coding and Reporting for the current year's book. Note that there are not nearly as many coding guidelines for PCS procedural coding as there are for CM diagnosis coding, which makes it easier to access appropriate guidelines for the procedures being coded. Depending on the publisher of the code book, these guidelines may also be included before each respective section in the code tables for easy reference. Note that the PCS code set is published by the Centers for Medicare and Medicaid Services (CMS), and all of the codes and code tables are accessible via the CMS website.

The front matter of each code book is likely to differ from publisher to publisher. Therefore, it is always helpful to become familiar with the front matter, as it may include information regarding how to use the book, how to select the codes, or how to use the guidelines. Note that the AHIMA version of the ICD-10-PCS code book includes the full ICD-10-PCS Official Guidelines for Coding and Reporting for reference.

Index

After the introductory material is the ICD-10-PCS Index. The PCS Index works in the same way as the indices to the other code books. Coders should reference the Index to find the procedural description, which refers the coder to a code or cross-reference. It is important to still verify the code in the code tables and add all necessary characters to the code to create a seven-character code.

When searching the Index, locate the procedure type, such as *Destruction*, *Excision*, or *Replacement*. Once a procedural description is found, identify the body area or organ

Table 20.4. ICD-10-PCS sections and characters

Character	Section	Definition
0	Medical and Surgical	This character identifies invasive and noninvasive procedures performed on patients and compiles the vast majority of procedures reported with PCS codes.
1	Obstetrics	This character identifies procedures performed on the products of conception only, including the fetus, amnion, umbilical cord, and placenta. Procedures performed on the pregnant female are identified with codes from the Medical and Surgical section (character "0").
2	Placement	This character identifies procedures that involve placing an external device in or on a body part in order to protect, immobilize, stretch, compress, or for packing purposes.
3	Administration	This character identifies procedures that involve putting in or on a substance used as a therapeutic, diagnostic, nutritional, physiological, or prophylactic.
4	Measurement and Monitoring	This character identifies procedures that determine the level of a physical or physiological function.
5	Extracorporeal or Systemic Assistance and Performance Section	This character identifies procedures that utilize equipment outside of the body to assist or perform a physiological function.
6	Extracorporeal Therapies	This character identifies procedures that utilize equipment outside of the body for therapeutic purposes that do not assist or perform a physiological function.
7	Osteopathic	This character identifies procedures that involve the manual treatment of alleviating somatic dysfunction and related disorders.
8	Other Procedures	This character identifies a miscellaneous range of procedures that do not fall into any other section, including acupuncture, in vitro fertilization, and suture removal.
9	Chiropractic	This character identifies procedures that involve a direct thrust to a joint for the purpose of moving it as a therapeutic treatment.
B	Imaging	This character identifies procedures that involve creating images of the patient's anatomical structures, including plain radiography (x-ray), fluoroscopy, CT, MRI, and ultrasound. This does not include nuclear imaging studies (reported with character "C") or radiation oncology procedures (reported with character "D").
C	Nuclear Medicine	This character identifies procedures that introduce radioactive material into the patient in order to create an image of the patient's anatomical structures, such as PET.
D	Radiation Therapy	This character identifies procedures that utilize radiation to treat cancerous disorders (radiation oncology).
F	Physical Rehabilitation and Diagnostic Audiology	This character identifies procedures that identify physical, occupational, and speech language pathology services.
G	Mental Health	This character identifies procedures that are focused on treating the emotional and behavioral health of the patient, and includes crisis intervention and educational and vocational counseling.
H	Substance Abuse	This character identifies procedures aimed at eliminating substance use, abuse, and dependence, and includes detoxification services and individual counseling.
X	New Technology	This character identifies procedures that are not classified elsewhere in the ICD-10-PCS code set, and identify procedures that utilize a new device substance, or technology.

Source: CMS 2016.

on which the procedure was performed, or follow all cross-references until the Index identifies a code or code beginning. For example, if coding an incision and drainage procedure on an abscess of the skin of the abdomen, the coder would first search for *Drainage*, then *skin*, and then *abdomen*, which leads the coder to the code beginning 0H97. However, this is not a valid PCS code, as PCS codes are all seven characters in length. Once the coder finds the beginning characters, he or she must then build the rest of the code based on the appropriate table.

Unlike the CPT or HCPCS code books, the ICD-10-PCS code books do not include eponyms in either the Index or the code tables. Instead, the coder must identify the specifics of how the procedure was performed rather than relying on a name by which the procedure may be referred.

Sections and Code Tables

The PCS code sections, including the code tables used to build the codes, follow the Index. There are 17 different sections of codes, each of which begins with a different character. For example, all the codes in the Medical and Surgical section begin with the number 0, and all of the codes in the Mental Health section begin with the character G. The 17 sections are listed in table 20.4.

Each one of these sections includes the code tables for those specific types of procedures. Code tables are used to identify the remaining characters so that each code can be built and total seven characters. The first character of a code is the section identifier (see table 20.5).

Table 20.5. PCS code character 1

Character 1	Character 2	Character 3	Character 4	Character 5	Character 6	Character 7
0						
Medical and Surgical						

Key to Success

It is a good idea to place tabs in your PCS code book for easy access to sections in the book. For example, have one tab for the Obstetrics section, another for the Placement section, and so on. Depending on the publisher, your PCS code book may contain a page of blank tabs that can be used for this purpose. Also, note that each individual section in the ICD-10-PCS code book may have a colored outer edge, which helps to differentiate sections of the book.

The largest section of PCS codes is the Medical and Surgical section, which includes 31 different body systems, each of which has a selection of tables that apply to that specific body system. The body systems in the Medical and Surgical section are listed in table 20.6.

Each body system is identified by a corresponding character (letter or number) as identified in table 20.6. This is a glimpse of how to build PCS codes. For example, an appendectomy—the surgical removal (resection) of the appendix—would be coded from the Medical and Surgical section because it is a surgery, so the code would start with the character 0. The next character would correspond to the body system, in this

Table 20.6. ICD-10-PCS Medical and Surgical section body systems and characters

Body System	Character
Central Nervous System	0
Peripheral Nervous System	1
Heart and Great Vessels	2
Upper Arteries	3
Lower Arteries	4
Upper Veins	5
Lower Veins	6
Lymphatic and Hemic Systems	7
Eye	8
Ear, Nose, Sinus	9
Respiratory System	B
Mouth and Throat	C
Gastrointestinal System	D
Hepatobiliary System and Pancreas	F
Endocrine System	G
Skin and Breast	H
Subcutaneous Tissue and Fascia	J
Muscles	K
Tendons	L
Bursae and Ligaments	M
Head and Facial Bones	N
Upper Bones	P
Lower Bones	Q
Upper Joints	R
Lower Joints	S
Urinary System	T
Female Reproductive System	U
Male Reproductive System	V
Anatomical Regions, General	W
Anatomical Regions, Upper Extremities	X
Anatomical Regions, Lower Extremities	Y

Table 20.7. PCS code character 2: body system

Character 1	Character 2	Character 3	Character 4	Character 5	Character 6	Character 7
0	D					
Medical and Surgical	Gastro-intestinal					

case the gastrointestinal system, so the next character in the code would be D. So, the PCS code for an appendectomy would begin with the characters 0D (see table 20.7). The following sections discuss how to build the rest of this code.

Appendices

Appendices follow the PCS code sections and contain additional information on terminology definitions, body parts, medical and surgical devices, and substances. They may include the following: Root Operations; Type and Qualifier Definitions; Approach Definitions; Medical and Surgical Body Parts; Medical and Surgical Device Table (Device Key) and Device Aggregation Table; and Substance Qualifier Table. These appendices may differ depending on the code book publisher.

Root Operations Definitions Appendix

The Root Operations Definitions lists the definitions for the root operations for the first 10 sections of the PCS code book (Medical and Surgical through Chiropractic). **Root operations** are the type of surgery, operation, or procedure that was performed.

It is important to read through and thoroughly study the definitions of the root operations in this section, especially after learning CPT and HCPCS coding. The terminology for some procedures in the CPT or HCPCS code books may differ from the procedural terminology used in PCS coding. For example, in the CPT code book, the term *excision* is sometimes used to report the complete removal of an organ or body part, such as excision of a kidney (nephrectomy). However, in PCS coding, the term *excision* is used only when a *portion* of an organ or body part is removed, and the term *resection* is used to identify the *complete* removal of an organ or body part. It is imperative to understand the root operation terms to ensure correct code selection, so this appendix is a useful tool when learning PCS coding.

There are 31 different root operations for codes in the Medical and Surgical section. Table 20.8 lists the root operation name, character value, definition, and an example of the procedure.

Table 20.8. Root operations in Medical and Surgical sections

Root Operation	Character	Definition	Example
Alteration	0	Modifying the anatomic structure of a body part without affecting the function of the body part	Face lift, breast augmentation
Bypass	1	Altering the route of passage of the contents of a tubular body part	CABG, formation of colostomy
Change	2	Taking out or off a device from a body part and putting back an identical or similar device in or on the same body part without cutting or puncturing the skin or a mucous membrane	Urinary catheter change, gastrostomy tube change
Control	3	Stopping, or attempting to stop, postprocedural or other acute bleeding	Control of subdural hemorrhage or bleeding ulcer
Creation	4	Putting in or on biological or synthetic material to form a new body part that to the extent possible replicates the anatomic structure or function of an absent body part	Creation of right and left atrioventricular (AV) valve from common AV valve
Destruction	5	Physical eradication of all or a portion of a body part by the direct use of energy, force, or a destructive agent	Fulguration of a polyp
Detachment	6	Cutting off all of a portion of the upper or lower extremities	Amputation of the leg below knee

(Continued on next page)

Table 20.8. *(Continued)*

Root Operation	Character	Definition	Example
Dilation	7	Expanding an orifice of the lumen of a tubular body part	PTCA
Division	8	Cutting into a body part, without draining fluids and/or gases from the body part, in order to separate or transect a body part	Spinal cordotomy, osteotomy
Drainage	9	Taking or letting out fluids and/or gases from a body part	Incision and drainage
Excision	B	Cutting out or off, without replacement, a portion of a body part	Liver biopsy
Extirpation	C	Taking or cutting out solid matter from a body part	Thrombectomy
Extraction	D	Pulling or stripping out or off all or a portion of a body part by the use of force	Dilation and curettage
Fragmentation	E	Breaking solid matter in a body part into pieces	Transurethral lithotripsy
Fusion	G	Joining together portions of an articular body part rendering the articular body part immobile	Ankle arthrodesis
Insertion	H	Putting a nonbiological appliance that monitors, assists, performs, or prevents a physiological function but does not physically take the place of a body part	Central line insertion
Inspection	J	Visually and/or manually exploring a body part	Exploratory laparotomy
Map	K	Locating the route of passage of electrical impulses and/or locating functional areas in a body part	Cardiac mapping
Occlusion	L	Completely closing an orifice or the lumen of a tubular body part	Fallopian tube ligation
Reattachment	M	Putting back in or on all or a portion of a separated body part to its normal location or other suitable location	Reattachment of hand
Release	N	Freeing a body part from an abnormal physical constraint by cutting or by the use of force	Carpal tunnel release
Removal	P	Taking out or off a device from a body part	Cardiac pacemaker removal
Repair	Q	Restoring, to the extent possible, a body part to its normal anatomic structure and function	Suture of laceration
Replacement	R	Putting in or on biological or synthetic material that physically takes the place and/or function of all or a portion of a body part	Total hip replacement
Reposition	S	Moving to its normal location or other suitable location, all or a portion of a body part.	Fracture reduction
Resection	T	Cutting out or off, without replacement, all of a body part	Total nephrectomy
Restriction	V	Partially closing an orifice of the lumen of a tubular body part	Cervical cerclage
Revision	W	Correcting, to the extent possible, a portion of a malfunctioning device or the position of a displaced device to the extent possible	Re-cementing of hip prosthesis
Supplement	U	Putting in or on biological or synthetic material that physically reinforces and/or augments the function of a portion of a body part	Herniorrhaphy using mesh
Transfer	X	Moving, without taking out, all or a portion of a body part to another location to take over the function of all or a portion of a body part	Skin flap transfer
Transplantation	Y	Putting in or on all or a portion of a living body part taken from another individual or animal to physically take the place and/or function of all or a portion of a similar body part	Kidney transplant, heart transplant

Source: CMS 2016.

There are additional root operation terms unique to each particular section of the PCS code book. For example, the root operation **delivery**, which is assisting the passage of the products of conception from the genital canal, is unique to the obstetrics section. The definitions for these additional root operations are included with the Root Operations Definitions appendix, after the Medical and Surgical Root Operation Definitions (listed previously), as well as in the guidelines at the beginning of each section of code tables.

Root operations are listed in the third character location of PCS codes. So if the first two characters of the PCS code for an appendectomy are 0D, then the root operation character is added as the third character. An appendectomy is the complete removal of the appendix, which is classified as the root operation *resection* and represented with the character *T*. Therefore, the first three characters for an appendectomy are 0DT (see table 20.9).

Table 20.9. PCS code character 3: root operation

Character 1	Character 2	Character 3	Character 4	Character 5	Character 6	Character 7
0	D	T				
Medical and Surgical	Gastro-intestinal	Resection				

Key to Success

Read through the root operation terms, definitions, explanations, and examples located in the appendix of the PCS code book. These are terms under which procedures are listed in the Index. As mentioned before, PCS terms differ from the way these same terms may be used in either CPT or HCPCS coding. Do not forget to access this appendix when you are coding with ICD-10-PCS, especially if you are confused about a specific type of operation and under which root operation term it would be classified.

Type and Qualifier Definitions Appendix

The Type and Qualifier Definitions appendix contains the definitions of the type and qualifier characters found in five of the last seven sections of the PCS code book: Imaging; Nuclear Medicine; Physical Rehabilitation and Diagnostic Audiology; Mental Health; and Substance Abuse Treatment. These lists include the terms and definitions for the third, fourth, or fifth characters found in the codes for these sections, as well as the character values. The third characters in these code tables take the place of the root operation characters for these specific procedure types because these procedure types, such as substance abuse treatment, do not include an operation per se. Instead, these procedures are nonsurgical, and so the third character identifies a different component of the procedure. For example, the term *Computerized Tomography* (CT scan) (in the Imaging section) is identified by the number 2 and defined as a computer reformatted digital display of multiplanar images developed from the capture of multiple exposures of external ionizing radiation. Just as with the previous appendix, these characters are located in the third character value of the PCS code.

Approach Definitions Appendix

The Approach Definitions appendix lists the descriptions for the different types of approaches to a procedure. The **approach** of a procedure identifies the manner in which the provider accessed the area in order to perform the procedure. Appendix C lists the different approaches and the definitions for each, within each respective section of the PCS code book. The approaches for the Medical and Surgical section are as follows in table 20.10.

Table 20.10. Approaches for the Medical and Surgical section

Approach	Character	Definition	Example
External	X	Procedures performed directly on the skin or mucous membrane and procedures performed indirectly by the application of external force through the skin or mucous membrane.	Excision of skin lesion, closed reduction of fracture
Open	0	Cutting through the skin or mucous membrane and any other body layers necessary to expose the site of the procedure.	Open CABG, open abdominal appendectomy
Percutaneous	3	Entry, by puncture or minor incision, of instrumentation through the skin or mucous membrane and any other body layers necessary to reach the site of the procedure.	Liposuction, needle biopsy
Percutaneous Endoscopic	4	Entry, by puncture or minor incision, of instrumentation through the skin or mucous membrane and any other body layers necessary to reach and visualize the site of the procedure.	Laparoscopic appendectomy, arthroscopy of knee
Via Natural or Artificial Opening	7	Entry of instrumentation through a natural or artificial external opening to reach the site of the procedure.	Placement of urinary catheter, endotracheal intubation
Via Natural or Artificial Opening Endoscopic	8	Entry of instrumentation through a natural or artificial opening to reach *and visualize* the site of the procedure.	Colonoscopy, EGD
Via Natural or Artificial Opening with Percutaneous Endoscopic Assistance	F	Entry of instrumentation through a natural or artificial external opening and entry, by puncture or minor incision, of instrumentation through the skin or mucous membrane and any other body layers necessary to aid in the performance of the procedure.	Laparoscopic-assisted bariatric surgery

Source: CMS 2016.

Key to Success

When looking at the different types of approaches for surgical procedures, pay attention to those used with the aid of an endoscope versus those used without the aid of an endoscope, as the definitions are similar. For example, the only difference between the approaches Percutaneous and Percutaneous Endoscopic is the addition of "and visualize" in the definition of the approach. This is because an endoscope is used for visualization during the procedure.

Again, the first three characters of an appendectomy code are 0DT to identify the procedure as Medical and Surgical (0), on the Gastrointestinal System (D), and the procedure type as Resection (T). Once the coder has located the first three characters in a code, he or she can turn to that specific code table in the ICD-10-PCS code book to determine the remaining characters and complete the code. In the code table for 0DT, the first column identifies the characters for each specific body part in the gastrointestinal system. It is here that the coder would find the character *J* is used to identify the body part that was removed as the appendix.

The character for the approach to a surgical procedure is placed in the fifth location of a PCS code. For example, if the procedure was performed via an open incision, then the fifth character *0* should be selected to identify the procedure as open. All five of these characters are added together to create the code 0DTJ0. Note that this is only a five-character code, and therefore it is not complete. To complete the code, two more characters are still needed (see table 20.11).

Table 20.11. PCS code character 4 and 5: body part and approach

Character 1	Character 2	Character 3	Character 4	Character 5	Character 6	Character 7
0	D	T	J	0		
Medical and Surgical	Gastro-intestinal	Resection	Appendix	Open		

Medical and Surgical Body Parts Appendix

The Medical and Surgical Body Parts appendix includes tables that list the specific body parts identified by the fourth character for medical and surgical codes. These tables are helpful when trying to determine which specific body part belongs to which character. For example, if the description of the procedure were identified as being on the body part *hallux*, then the coder could refer to this table in the appendix of the ICD-10-PCS code book to make sure that the hallux is included in the character for first toe, left; or first toe, right (see figure 20.8).

Figure 20.8. Medical and Surgical Body Parts appendix

Section 0 - Medical and Surgical — Character 4 - Body Part	
1st Toe, Left **1st** Toe, Right	**Includes:** Hallux
Abdomen Muscle, Left **Abdomen** Muscle, Right	**Includes:** External oblique muscle Internal oblique muscle Pyramidalis muscle Rectus abdominis muscle Transversus abdominis muscle
Abdominal Aorta	**Includes:** Inferior phrenic artery Lumbar artery Median sacral artery Middle suprarenal artery Ovarian artery Testicular artery

Source: Casto 2019, 1491.

Medical and Surgical Device Table (Device Key) and Device Aggregation Table Appendix

The Medical and Surgical Device Table (Device Key) and Device Aggregation Table appendix lists the devices that may be used in medical and surgical codes, as well as additional devices and where they may be identified by a specific PCS character. This list also includes brand-name devices, and to which device character they should apply. For example, a feeding device in gastrointestinal system includes a PEG/J (percutaneous endoscopic gastrojejunostomy tube) (see figure 20.9).

Figure 20.9. Medical and Surgical Device table

Section 0 - Medical and Surgical — Character 6 - Device	
Extraluminal Device	**Includes:** AtriClip LAA Exclusion System LAP-BAND® adjustable gastric banding system REALIZE® Adjustable Gastric Band

Feeding Device in
Gastrointestinal System
	Includes:
	Percutaneous endoscopic
	  gastrojejunostomy (PEG/J) tube
	Percutaneous endoscopic gastrostomy
	  (PEG) tube

Hearing Device in Ear, Nose, Sinus	**Includes:** Esteem® implantable hearing system

Source: Casto 2019, 1506.

The sixth character location of a PCS code is used to specify the device. For example, in the code table for 0DT, there are no options for the sixth character other than *Z* for *No Device*. An open appendectomy does not use any type of device, so the letter *Z* is used in the sixth character location to identify that no device was placed during the procedure. The addition of the letter *Z* expands the code to six characters: 0DTJ0Z. At this point, this code still requires one additional character to become a valid seven-character PCS code (see table 20.12).

To make the code for appendectomy complete, the coder would have to add character 7 to identify the qualifier. Referencing the code table in the PCS book reveals that no qualifier is applicable, so character *Z* for *no qualifier* would be added in the seventh character location, thus completing the code: 0DTJ0ZZ, Resection of Appendix, Open Approach.

Table 20.12. PCS code character 6: device

Character 1	Character 2	Character 3	Character 4	Character 5	Character 6	Character 7
0	D	T	J	0	Z	
Medical and Surgical	Gastro- intestinal	Resection	Appendix	Open	No Device	

Key to Success

The PCS code set uses the character Z when no other character is applicable for the procedure reported. For example, if a procedure does not involve a device, or if no qualifier (as reported by character 7) is applicable, then the character Z is added for *No Device* or *No Qualifier*.

Key to Success

If there is no device placed during the procedure, and if no qualifier is applicable for the procedure, then the last two characters will be ZZ, for no device and no qualifier. This is a quick way to remember to "Z it out" if neither a device nor a qualifier are options for the procedure. However, be sure to always check your code tables to determine whether these characters are an option.

Substance Qualifier Table Appendix

The Substance Qualifier Table appendix lists the substances that are included in the substance character descriptions for two sections: Administration (section 3) and New Technology (section X). This appendix is used in the same manner as the previous two appendices, except it lists the substances included with the character descriptions for the code table. Coders can use this information to help identify specific substances used in procedures as well as the character(s) that identify those substances. For example, if the procedure description referenced a substance used or administered as Seprafilm, the coder could access this appendix and determine the character for Adhesion Barrier applies (see figure 20.10).

Figure 20.10. Substance Qualifier table

Section 3 – Administration Character 6 – Substance	
4-Factor Prothrombin Complex Concentrate	**Includes:** Kcentra
Adhesion Barrier	**Includes:** Seprafilm
Anti-Infective Envelope	**Includes:** AIGISRx Antibacterial Envelope Antibacterial Envelope (TYRX) (AIGISRx) Antimicrobial envelope TYRX Antibacterial Envelope
Clofarabine	**Includes:** Clolar

Source: Casto 2019, 1514.

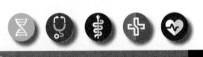

Putting It All Together: Building PCS Codes

The following vignette demonstrates how to select the appropriate procedure codes. After reviewing the vignette, complete the exercises in There's a Code for That 20.2 to practice coding for inpatient services

Helen is a new coding professional at a 200-bed inpatient hospital in a Midwestern town. She has just graduated from a coding program at a local vocational college. After receiving brief training in ICD-10-PCS coding, she is practicing coding facility inpatient charts. She is coding the following case: a 50-year-old female patient presented to the operating room with a herniated disc of the T4 level. Surgeon performed a partial discectomy via open incision.

To find the codes for the surgical service, Helen asks herself: What did the doctor do? In this case, the doctor removed part of a herniated disc from the patient. She has to build the PCS code for the service according to the specifics of how the procedure was performed. First, she must determine the first three characters of the code so she can locate the code table and build the rest of the code. She knows that the procedure was a partial removal of a vertebral disc, which is classified in PCS as an excision procedure. She searches for Excision in the PCS Index, and then locates the subterm Disc. Under the subterm Disc she locates the term Thoracic Vertebral, which gives her the first four characters for her code: 0RB9.

Now that she has the first four characters for her code, Helen accesses the Tabular List to find the code table for her first three characters. See figure 20.11 to view the code table.

Helen verifies the character 9 for the fourth character, as the procedure was performed on the disc of a thoracic vertebra, which brings her to the following: 0RB9. For the fifth character, she selects 0 as the approach, because the procedure was performed via an open incision. This brings her to the following: 0RB90. For the sixth character, she selects the character Z for no device. Not only is this the only option according to the code table, but there was no device left in place after the surgery (remember that a device is any material or appliance that remains after the procedure is performed). This leads her to the code 0RB90Z, which still needs one more character before it is complete. The last character she selects is Z for no qualifier, as the only other option is diagnostic and this was not a diagnostic procedure. This leads her to the following complete code:

- *0RB90ZZ, Excision of Thoracic Vertebral Disc, Open Approach*

Figure 20.11 0RB code table

Section	0	**Medical and Surgical**
Body System	R	**Upper Joints**
Operation	B	**Excision:** Cutting out or off, without replacement, a portion of a body part

Body Part (4th)	Approach (5th)	Device (6th)	Qualifier (7th)
0 Occipital-cervical Joint 1 Cervical Vertebral Joint 3 Cervical Vertebral Disc 4 Cervicothoracic Vertebral Joint 5 Cervicothoracic Vertebral Disc 6 Thoracic Vertebral Joint 9 Thoracic Vertebral Disc A Thoracolumbar Vertebral Joint B Thoracolumbar Vertebral Disc C Temporomandibular Joint, Right D Temporomandibular Joint, Left E Sternoclavicular Joint, Right F Sternoclavicular Joint, Left G Acromioclavicular Joint, Right H Acromioclavicular Joint, Left J Shoulder Joint, Right K Shoulder Joint, Left L Elbow Joint, Right M Elbow Joint, Left N Wrist Joint, Right P Wrist Joint, Left Q Carpal Joint, Right R Carpal Joint, Left S Carpometacarpal Joint, Right T Carpometacarpal Joint, Left U Metacarpophalangeal Joint, Right V Metacarpophalangeal Joint, Left W Finger Phalangeal Joint, Right X Finger Phalangeal Joint, Left	0 Open 3 Percutaneous 4 Percutaneous Endoscopic	Z No Device	X Diagnostic Z No Qualifier

Source: Casto 2019, 1009.

Now that she has her PCS code, she needs to find the CM code for the service. According to the documentation, the procedure was performed because of a herniated T4 disc. She selects the following code:

- *M51.24, Other intervertebral disc displacement, thoracic region*

She then rechecks the documentation to make sure she has coded everything for the encounter and reports the chosen codes.

Coding for inpatient services

20.2

There's a Code for That

Read the following documentation and select the appropriate ICD-10-CM and ICD-10-PCS code(s) for the procedure.

1. A 45-year-old female underwent an open left kidney allotransplantation due to ESRD.

    ICD-10-PCS code: _____

    ICD-10-CM code: _____

2. Chest tube for drainage was changed in a patient with left primary spontaneous pneumothorax.

    ICD-10-PCS code: _____

    ICD-10-CM code: _____

3. Esophagogastroduodenoscopy performed on patient with dyspepsia and dysphagia.

    ICD-10-PCS code: _____

    ICD-10-CM code: _____ , _____

4. An 8-year-old male underwent a repair of umbilical hernia. The contents of the hernia were reduced into the abdominal cavity and the abdominal wall was sutured.

    ICD-10-PCS code: _____

    ICD-10-CM code: _____

Case Study | Hysterectomy, Bilateral Salpingectomy, Excision of Ovarian Cyst

PATIENT: Alice Simmons

PREOPERATIVE DIAGNOSIS: Symptomatic uterine fibroids

POSTOPERATIVE DIAGNOSIS: Symptomatic uterine fibroids

PROCEDURE: Robotic hysterectomy, bilateral salpingectomy, right ovarian cystectomy

FINDINGS: Enlarged fibroid uterus weighing 224 g; right ovarian cyst and endometriotic implants in the posterior pelvis near the bladder.

ESTIMATED BLOOD LOSS: Less than 100 mL

COMPLICATIONS: None; patient tolerated the procedure well

PROCEDURE IN DETAIL:
The patient was seen in the Holding Room. The risks, benefits, complications, treatment options, and expected outcomes were discussed with the patient. The patient concurred with the proposed plan, giving informed consent. The patient was taken to the operating room, and the procedure was verified as a robotic hysterectomy with bilateral salpingectomy. A time out was held, and the above information was confirmed.

After induction of anesthesia, the patient was placed in lithotomy position and prepped and draped in the usual sterile manner. Foley catheter was placed. A v-care uterine manipulator was introduced into the endometrial cavity and secured.

An incision was made above the umbilicus and a 5-mm port introduced. Confirmation of abdominal placement was made with laparoscope. Two additional 8-mm ports were placed in the right and left lower abdomen under direct visualization. The midline was extended for a 12-mm port and a 5-mm port introduced in the nipple line on the left, just below the ribs.

The robot was docked and attention turned to the console.

The uterus was found to be enlarged with multiple fibroids and the ovaries were normal with a hemorrhagic cyst on the right ovary. The ureters were identified and noted to be away from the surgical field. The fallopian tubes were identified, grasped, and followed to the fimbriated ends. They were dissected from their surrounding tissue with harp dissection and cautery. The cyst on the right ovary was dissected from the ovary and removed. The round ligaments were identified, cauterized with bipolar cautery, and cut. The anterior peritoneal reflection was incised and the bladder was dissected off the lower uterine segment. Hemostasis was observed. The uterine vessels were skeletonized, then clamped, and cauterized. Using the v-care as a guide, a posterior colpotomy was made. A cicumferential incision was made around the cervix, and the uterus, cervix and tubes were delivered through the vagina. Vaginal cuff angles as well as the remainder of the vagina cuff were closed using a v-lock suture, incorporating the utero-sacral ligaments for support. Lavage was carried out until clear. Hemostasis was observed.

Interceed was placed in the pelvis due to endometriosis being noted. The robot was undocked, and all instruments removed from the abdomen and the vagina. The midline fascial incision was closed with 0-vicryl suture and all skin incisions were closed with 4-0 vicryl.

A perineal laceration was noted due to the irregular shape of the uterus. This laceration was repaired with 3-0 vicryl suture.

Instrument, sponge, and needle counts were correct prior to abdominal closure and at the conclusion of the case.

SIGNED: Dr. Jordana Morgan, MD

Use the following steps to select the appropriate codes for the case study. This case study was already presented in chapter 17 (Obstetrics and Gynecology Services); however, in this case, you will need to assign the ICD-10-PCS codes for the procedures, rather than CPT codes.

1. Read through the case study and answer the question: *What did the doctor do?* Identify the name of the procedures performed.

_____

_____

2. Now that you have identified the procedure, locate the code for the procedure in the ICD-10-PCS code book.

   a. Search the Index for the procedure and search through the options for each procedure.

      i. _____

      ii. _____

      iii. _____

3. Now that the procedure codes have been identified, review the case study and answer the following question: *Why did the doctor do it?* Identify the patient's diagnoses.

_____

_____

4. Now that you have identified the patient's diagnoses, search the ICD-10-CM code book for the correct code for this condition.

   a. Search the Main Index for the name of the condition and search through any applicable subterms and cross-references to locate the appropriate code.

      i. _____

      ii. _____

      iii. _____

   b. Verify the codes in the Tabular List. Locate the code identified previously in the Tabular Listing of codes and refer to any applicable guidelines, notes, and symbols. Does the code selected correctly identify the patient's condition? If yes, list the code here:

      i. _____

      ii. _____

      iii. _____

   c. Check the procedure note and ICD-10-CM guidelines and conventions to determine the correct sequencing of the diagnosis codes, if applicable. Correctly sequence the diagnosis codes.

_____

_____

5. Now that the procedure and diagnosis codes have been identified, list them on the UB-04 form template provided. Be sure to correctly link the procedure and diagnosis codes. Remember to add the number of units as necessary. For this case study, do not calculate the time, base units, or modifying factors. Assign only the ICD-10-CM and PCS codes to the claim.

End-of-Chapter Content

Instructions: Indicate whether the following statements are true or false (T or F). For false statements, rewrite the statement on the line below to make the statement true.

1. ICD-10-CM codes are reported for inpatient services in addition to ICD-10-PCS codes.

_____

_____

2. Facility inpatient services are reported on the CMS-1500 paper claim form.

_____

_____

3. Facility inpatient services are paid on a fee-for-service basis.

_____

_____

4. ICD-10-PCS codes have seven alphabetical characters.

_____

_____

5. A device is any material or appliance that remains after the procedure is performed.

_____

_____

6. The Medical and Surgical section is identified by the character 0.

_____

_____

7. The PCS code book does not include an index; coders must rely only on their knowledge of the procedure performed to find the code.

_____

_____

8. The procedure qualifier is the type of surgery, operation, or procedure performed.

_____

_____

9. A percutaneous endoscopic procedure is performed by cutting into the skin or mucous membrane in order to gain entrance into the body area.

_____

_____

Instructions: Choose the best answer.

1. Which of the following codes would an inpatient facility report to identify an appendectomy procedure?

a. ICD-10-PCS
b. ICD-10-CM
c. CPT
d. HCPCS

2. Which of the following codes would the healthcare provider report to identify an appendectomy procedure?

a. ICD-10-PCS
b. ICD-10-CM
c. CPT
d. HCPCS

3. In prospective payment, what is used to identify the predetermined amount of payment?

a. PPS
b. Fee-for-service
c. PCS codes
d. DRGs

4. How many ICD-10-CM codes can be reported on the UB-04 form?

a. 4
b. 12
c. Over 20
d. Over 30

5. A valid ICD-10-PCS code is how many characters?

   a. 5
   b. 3
   c. 3 to 7
   d. 7

6. The first character of a PCS identifies which of the following?

   a. Section
   b. Body system
   c. Root operation
   d. Body part or region

7. Which of the following identifies any additional attributes of why or how the procedure was performed?

   a. Qualifier
   b. Device
   c. Root operation
   d. Body system

8. Which of the following characters is used for the Chiropractic section?

   a. A
   b. X
   c. 9
   d. 7

9. Which of the following root operations is altering the route of passage of the contents of a tubular body part?

   a. Alteration
   b. Restriction
   c. Transfer
   d. Bypass

10. Which of the following root operations is cutting out or off, without replacement, all of a body part?

   a. Excision
   b. Resection
   c. Transplantation
   d. Extirpation

11. Which of the following root operations is breaking solid matter in a body part into pieces?

   a. Extirpation
   b. Extraction
   c. Fragmentation
   d. Occlusion

12. Which of the following types of approaches to a procedure is an incisional abdominal appendectomy?

   a. External
   b. Open
   c. Percutaneous
   d. Via natural opening

Instructions: Answer the following questions with the appropriate code(s) and modifier(s).

1. A 60-year-old male with primary malignant neoplasm of the prostate underwent total prostatectomy via open approach.

   ICD-10-PCS code: _____

   ICD-10-CM code: _____

2. Amputation of right lower leg at the mid-calf-level of an 83-year-old female with DM2, with ulcer of the calf with necrosis of bone.

   ICD-10-PCS code: _____

   ICD-10-CM code: _____

3. A 42-year-old male suffered a traumatic amputation of his right arm during a mechanical accident at work. Arm was reattached at the mid-humerus level.

   ICD-10-PCS code: _____

4. Patient with intestinal perforation underwent an open colostomy formation of the transverse colon.

   ICD-10-PCS code: _____

5. Bilateral mastectomy performed for breast cancer.

   ICD-10-PCS code: _____

6. Biopsy of the skin of the right breast for suspected melanoma.

   ICD-10-PCS code: _____

References

Casto, A.B. 2019. *ICD-10-PCS Code Book*. Chicago: AHIMA.

Centers for Medicaid Services (CMS). 2019a. ICD-10-CM Guidelines for Coding and Reporting FY 2020. https://www.cms.gov/Medicare/Coding/ICD10/Downloads/2020-Coding-Guidelines.pdf.

Centers for Medicare and Medicaid Services (CMS). 2019b. Hospital-Acquired Conditions. https://www.cms.gov/Medicare/Medicare-Fee-for-Service-Payment/HospitalAcqCond/Hospital-Acquired_Conditions.html.

Centers for Medicare and Medicaid Services (CMS). 2019c. CMS 1450. https://www.cms.gov/Medicare/CMS-Forms/CMS-Forms/CMS-Forms-Items/CMS1196256.html.

Centers for Medicare and Medicaid Services (CMS). 2016. Development of the ICD-10 Procedure Coding System (ICD-10-PCS). https://www.cms.gov/Medicare/Coding/ICD10/Downloads/2016-Developmentofthe-ICD-10-Procedure-Coding-System.pdf.

HMSA. 2014. Complications and Comorbidities. https://hmsa.com/portal/provider/zav_pel.fh.COM.600.htm.

US Department of Health and Human Services (HHS). 1985. Health Information Policy Council; 1984 Revision of the Uniform Hospital Discharge Data Set. *Federal Register* 50(147): 31048–31040.

Resources

Barta, A., K. DeVault, and M. Endicott. 2014. *2014 ICD-10-PCS Coder Training Manual*. Chicago: AHIMA.

Centers for Medicare and Medicaid Services (CMS). 2019. ICD-10-PCS Official Guidelines for Coding and Reporting FY 2020. https://www.cms.gov/Medicare/Coding/ICD10/Downloads/2020-ICD-10-PCS-Guidelines.pdf.

Centers for Medicare and Medicaid Services (CMS). 2019. Pub 100-04. *Medicare Claims Processing Manual*. https://www.cms.gov/Regulations-and-Guidance/Guidance/Manuals/Internet-Only-Manuals-IOMs-Items/CMS018912.

Centers for Medicare and Medicaid Services (CMS). 2017 (July 26). 2018 ICD-10 PCS and GEMs. https://www.cms.gov/Medicare/Coding/ICD10/2018-ICD-10-PCS-and-GEMs.html.

Centers for Medicare and Medicaid Services (CMS). 2016. Using the ICD-10-PCS New Technology Section Codes. https://www.cms.gov/Medicare/Coding/ICD10/Downloads/2016-Section-X-New-Technology-.pdf.

DecisionHealth. 2013. *Advanced Anatomy and Physiology for ICD-10-CM/PCS*. Salt Lake City, UT: Contexo Media.

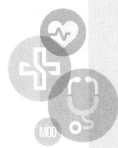

Appendix A: Coding Certifications and Professional Coding Organizations

Professional certifications are one of the best measures of one's ability, and as such are highly regarded within the world of health information management (HIM), billing, and coding. Going through the rigorous demands of the certification process is a great way to prove your coding prowess to potential employers and as a way to move up the career ladder.

There are dozens of different healthcare certifications, including specialty-specific coding, general billing practices, compliance, auditing, and other special topics. It is helpful to become familiar with a few of the more prominent certifications you may encounter as a professional coder. In addition, many educational coding and billing programs require students to take a certification exam to complete the course. Certain certifications may also be a requirement for employment at healthcare coding or billing organizations.

The following is a list of some of the certifications you can obtain after completing your coding education, as well as a selection of certifications that you can obtain after you gain more professional experience in medical billing and a number of additional areas within HIM.

Coding Certifications

The following are the more prominent coding certifications and are commonly the focus of medical coding programs. As you can see, there are general coding certifications that cover all areas of coding as well as other certifications that are very specific to certain areas of coding. Many HIM employers require one of the following coding certifications as a requirement for hire.

- **Certified Coding Associate (CCA):** The CCA credential offered by the American Health Information Management Association (AHIMA) is a nationally recognized HIM certification that focuses on inpatient and outpatient settings. CCA-certified individuals are committed, competent, and qualified to be professionals within the field of HIM and have basic ICD diagnostic and procedural and CPT coding knowledge (AHIMA 2017a).

- **Certified Coding Specialist (CCS):** The CCS credential, offered by AHIMA, is a highly regarded credential across both hospital and physician office settings. It indicates that a coder is proficient in ICD-10-CM, CPT, medical terminology, disease processes, pharmacology, and is familiar with the relationship between codes and their impact on practice revenues and patient health outcomes (AHIMA 2017b).

- **Certified Professional Coder (CPC):** The CPC credential is offered by the American Academy of Professional Coders (AAPC) for coders reporting professional services performed in both outpatient and inpatient settings. Individuals who obtain this certification demonstrate proficiency in ICD-10-CM, CPT, and HCPCS codes across a wide range of services and comprehend coding guidelines and regulations, including compliance and reimbursement for medical services. For coders interested in inpatient coding, the AAPC also offers the Certified Inpatient Coder (CIC) certification (AAPC 2017b).

- **Certified Billing and Coding Specialist (CBCS):** The CBCS, offered by the National Healthcareer Association (NHA), demonstrates a basic knowledge of billing and coding in the outpatient setting only. This includes the gathering and verification of patient demographics, a working knowledge of fraud and abuse in the medical setting, assigning ICD-10-CM, CPT, and HCPCS codes, and working with healthcare providers to receive optimal reimbursement for services provided (NHA 2017b).

Additional Certifications

Additional certifications in the field of HIM and health information technology are plentiful, to say the least. From medical billing to clinical documentation, informatics, and electronic health records, there are many career avenues that you can explore by obtaining a certification in a healthcare field other than coding. It is a good idea to start with a basic coding or billing certification, work in the industry for a few years to get experience, and then find a niche in which you can excel. Once you find this niche, you can pursue a certification in this field to prove to your employer, or to potential employers, that you are an expert in that area.

Figure A.1. Additional professional certifications

Professional Organization	Coding	Billing & Health Information Management	Practice Management & Administration	Health Information Technology	Other
American Health Information Management Association (AHIMA)	Certified Coding Associate (CCA), Certified Coding Specialist (CCS)	Registered Health Information Associate (RHIA), Registered Health Information Technician (RHIT)	Registered Health Information Associate (RHIA)	Certified Healthcare Technology Specialist (CHTS), Certified Professional in Health Informatics (CPHI)	Certified Health Data Analyst (CHDA), Certified in Healthcare Privacy and Security (CHPS), Certified Documentation Improvement Practitioner (CDIP)
American Academy of Professional Coders (AAPC)	Certified Professional Coder (CPC), Specialty Coding Certifications	Certified Professional Biller (CPB)	Certified Professional Practice Manager (CPPM)		Certified Professional Medical Auditor (CPMA), Certified Risk Adjustment Coder (CRC)
National Healthcareer Association (NHA)	Certified Billing and Coding Specialist (CBCS)	Certified Billing and Coding Specialist (CBCS)		Certified Electronic Health Records Specialist (CEHRS)	
Association of Clinical Documentation Improvement Specialists (ACDIS)					Certified Clinical Documentation Specialist (CCDS)
Medical Group Management Association (MGMA)			Certified Medical Practice Executive (CMPE)		

There is no glass ceiling with medical billing and coding. You can truly go as far as you want to go, and one of the best ways to move up is to get an additional certification. Figure A.1 shows many common and desirable certifications in multiple areas of billing, coding, and HIM, and the professional organization that offers each.

Professional Organizations

Certifications within the fields of billing, coding, and HIM are offered by professional organizations such as those listed below. Whether you obtain a certification from one of these organizations or not, it pays to be a member of the corresponding organization as you typically receive a number of benefits, such as monthly or quarterly publications with insights from the field, and access to networking forums where you can discuss important topics with others in the industry. As a student of medical billing and coding, there are three main professional organizations of which you need to be aware:

- **American Health Information Management Association (AHIMA)**. AHIMA is an organization for HIM professionals and is a respected leader in the management of health data, health records, and delivery of quality healthcare. They offer cutting-edge programs, professional development opportunities, continuing education, textbooks, credentials, online education, newsletters, monthly publications, and more. AHIMA is also significant as it is one of the four cooperating parties that collaborates to create and revise ICD-10 guidelines (AHIMA 2017c).

- **American Academy of Professional Coders (AAPC)**. The AAPC was originally founded with the purpose of providing education and certifications to medical coders, but has expanded to elevate the entire profession of medical coding. It now provides training, 32 different certifications, networking opportunities, job opportunities, and monthly publications. Training and certifications provided by the AAPC cover not only medical coding, but also billing, medical auditing, clinical documentation, medical compliance, and practice management (AAPC 2017a).

- **National Healthcareer Association (NHA)**. The NHA provides training and certifications for eight allied health careers including medical assistants, medical administrative assistants; phlebotomy, EKG, pharmacy, and patient care technicians; and medical billing, coding, and HIM professionals. The NHA's entry-level billing and coding credential, the CBCS, is an entry-level credential of choice for medical billing, coding, and HIM programs at vocational colleges (NHA 2017a).

Once you enter the world of healthcare, you might encounter additional professional organizations, such as the Association of Clinical Documentation Improvement Specialists (ACDIS) or the Medical Group Management Association (MGMA), to which you may become a member, depending on your job title and responsibilities. No matter which organization you choose, it is a good idea to become a member of at least one of these organizations to remain up to date in your field of expertise, as well as to improve your chances of career success.

Membership in a professional organization typically requires an annual membership fee, and if you have a certification, you must maintain continuing education units (CEUs). As discussed in chapter 1, a CEU is a unit of measurement used in continuing education programs, and a certified coder must attain a certain number of CEUs each year to maintain his or her certification. CEUs are earned by engaging in educational training, webinars, or in-field activities that show that you are keeping up to date with your profession. Depending on your type and number of certifications, you may need to complete more or less CEUs. It pays to do your research, determine the medical setting in which you want to work, join the right professional organization for you, and set your sights toward the future!

References

AAPC. 2017a. About Us. https://www.aapc.com/aboutus/.

AAPC. 2017b. Certified Professional Coder (CPC®). https://aapc.com/certification/cpc/.

AHIMA. 2017a. Overview of Certified Coding Associate (CCA®). http://www.ahima.org/certification/CCA.

AHIMA. 2017b. Overview Certified Coding Specialist (CCS®). http://www.ahima.org/certification/CCS.

AHIMA. 2017c. Who We Are. http://www.ahima.org/about/aboutahima.

NHA. 2017a. About NHA. https://www.nhanow.com/about-nha.

NHA. 2017b. Certified Billing & Coding Specialist (CBCS). https://www.nhanow.com/certifications/billing-coding.

Appendix B: Answer Key to There's a Code for That Exercises

Chapter 3 Basics of Coding

There's a Code for That 3.1

1. Procedure: Psychoanalysis and physical examination
   Diagnosis: Depression

2. Procedure: Appendectomy
   Diagnosis: Ruptured appendix (includes the diagnosis of severe abdominal pain, fever, and vomiting)

3. Procedure: Evaluation and management service
   Diagnosis: Asthma

4. Procedure: Extended evaluation and management service
   Diagnosis: Asthma with acute exacerbation (includes the diagnosis of wheezing and trouble breathing)

5. Procedure: Chest x-ray
   Diagnosis: Pneumonia, left lower lobe

There's a Code for That 3.2

1. Visual screening linked to blurry vision. Joint injection linked to knee pain.

2. Routine pregnancy check-up linked to pregnancy. Incision and drainage of abscess linked to abscess of right upper shoulder.

3. Suture of wound linked to laceration of left leg. X-ray examination and fracture care with casting linked to fracture of left ankle.

4. Evaluation and management office visit linked to COPD and emphysema. Skin biopsy linked to mole on left torso.

Chapter 4 Learning the ICD-10-CM Code Book

There's a Code for That 4.1

1. Pain
2. Disease
3. Difficulty
4. Degeneration
5. Hernia

There's a Code for That 4.2

1. Nonessential
2. Essential
3. Nonessential
4. Nonessential
5. Essential

There's a Code for That 4.3

1. ICD-10 Code: J13
2. ICD-10 Code: L22
3. ICD-10 Code: R13.12

4. ICD-10 Code: R48.8
5. ICD-10 Code: M04.2
6. ICD-10 Code: Q45.9

There's a Code for That 4.4

1. ICD-10 Code: D12.2
2. ICD-10 Code: C44.41
3. ICD-10 Code: C00.0
4. ICD-10 Code: C78.7
5. ICD-10 Code: D01.7
6. ICD-10 Code: C68.0

There's a Code for That 4.5

1. ICD-10 Code: T59.891
2. ICD-10 Code: T43.1X5
3. ICD-10 Code: T62.0X2
4. ICD-10 Code: T60.1X1
5. ICD-10 Code: T62.2X3
6. ICD-10 Code: T40.2X4

There's a Code for That 4.6

1. Injury mechanism: Struck by soccer ball
   ICD-10 Code: W21.02

2. Place of occurrence: soccer field
   ICD-10 Code: Y92.322

3. Activity: Soccer
   ICD-10 Code: Y93.66

4. Patient status: Recreational or sport, not for income
   ICD-10 Code: Y99.8

There's a Code for That 4.7

1. E
2. A
3. B
4. H
5. D
6. G
7. C
8. I
9. F
10. J

There's a Code for That 4.8

1. A-initial
   D-subsequent
   S-sequela
2. A-initial encounter for closed fracture
   B-initial encounter for open fracture
   D-subsequent encounter for fracture with routine healing
   G-subsequent encounter for fracture with delayed healing
   K-subsequent encounter for fracture with nonunion
   S-sequela
3. 0-not applicable or unspecified
   1-mild stage
   2-moderate stage
   3-severe stage
   4-indeterminate stage
4. 0-not applicable or unspecified
   1-fetus 1
   2-fetus 2
   3-fetus 3
   4-fetus 4
   5-fetus 5
   9-other fetus

There's a Code for That 4.9

1. A-initial
2. D-subsequent

3. S-sequela
4. A-initial (patient is still in active treatment phase for the injury)

There's a Code for That 4.10

1. C
2. ICD-10 code: W54.0XXA
3. ICD-10 code: S60.00XD
4. ICD-10 code: W35.XXXA

Chapter 5 Learning the CPT and HCPCS Code Books

There's a Code for That 5.1

1. C. Category III
2. A. Category I
3. A. Category I
4. B. Category II
5. B. Category II

There's a Code for That 5.2

1. Appendix A
2. Appendix F
3. Appendix E
4. Appendix C
5. Appendix D
6. Appendix P

There's a Code for That 5.3

1. Procedure name: Calculus, removal, gallbladder; Index entry: 47544
2. Procedure name: Salpingectomy, with vaginal hysterectomy; Index entry: 58262, 58263, 58291, 58292
3. Procedure name: Salpingectomy, with vaginal hysterectomy, laparoscopic; Index entry: 58552, 58554
4. Procedure name: Amputation, leg, lower; Index entry: 27598, 27880-27882

There's a Code for That 5.4

1. No, 32562
2. No, 61538
3. Yes
4. Yes
5. No, 58956

There's a Code for That 5.5

1. Index entry: G8417–G8422
2. Index entry: G0009
3. Index entry: A4650–A4927
4. Index entry: V5030–V5060
5. Index entry: G0127
6. Index entry: Q0477, Q0480–Q0505

There's a Code for That 5.6

1. No, E1615
2. Yes
3. Yes
4. No, Q0112
5. No, K0007

Chapter 6 Supplies and Services

There's a Code for That 6.1

1. HCPCS code: A0431
2. HCPCS modifier: SH
3. HCPCS code: A0431-SI
   HCPCS code: A0436 × 15
4. HCPCS code: A0431-SH
   HCPCS code: A0436 × 13
   Transportation Indicator: D2
   ICD-10 code: S41.111A
5. HCPCS code: A0130-RN
   HCPCS code: A0380 × 7
   ICD-10 code: G82.50
   ICD-10 code: Z99.11

There's a Code for That 6.2

1. HCPCS modifier: A5
2. HCPCS modifier: T3
3. HCPCS modifier: RT

4. HCPCS modifier: NU

5. HCPCS modifier: KL

6. HCPCS modifier: LM

7. HCPCS modifier: JA

8. HCPCS modifier: E1

There's a Code for That 6.3

1. HCPCS code: A4620
   HCPCS code: A4616 × 2
   ICD-10 code: J43.9

2. HCPCS code: K0019 × 2

3. HCPCS code: A4376

4. HCPCS code: A6412 × 5

5. HCPCS code: S8451

There's a Code for That 6.4

1. HCPCS code: J0135

2. HCPCS code: J0400 × 2
   ICD-10 code: F31.9

3. HCPCS code: J1650
   ICD-10 code: D68.2

4. HCPCS code: J7610 × 2
   ICD-10 code: J45.21

Chapter 7 Behavioral Health

There's a Code for That 7.1

1. 11, Office

2. 42, Ambulance—Air or Water

3. 81, Independent Laboratory

4. 14, Group Home

5. 09, Prison/Correctional Facility

There's a Code for That 7.2

1. Type of service: office visit
   Patient status: new
   Place of service: outpatient office
   E/M codes: 99201–99205
   POS code: 11, Office

2. Type of service: subsequent care
   Patient status: N/A
   Place of service: nursing facility
   E/M codes: 99307–99310
   POS code: 32, Nursing Facility

3. Type of service: behavior change intervention (individual)
   Patient status: new
   Place of service: N/A (office)
   E/M codes: 99406–99409
   POS code: 11, Office

4. Type of service: initial care
   Patient status: inpatient
   Place of service: hospital
   E/M codes: 99221–99223
   POS code: 21, Inpatient Hospital

5. Type of service: emergency department visit
   Patient status: N/A (in the emergency department setting, patients are not identified as either new or established, see CPT guidelines)
   Place of service: emergency department
   E/M codes: 99281–99285
   POS code: 23, Emergency Room—Hospital

There's a Code for That 7.3

1. E/M Code: 99202

2. E/M Code: 99215

3. E/M Code: 99212

4. E/M Code: 99222

5. E/M Code: 99231

6. E/M Code: 99243

7. E/M Code: 99308

8. E/M Code: 99284

There's a Code for That 7.4

1. CPT Code: 90839

2. CPT Code: 90876

3. CPT Code: 90832-95

4. CPT Code: G0397

5. CPT Code: 90837, 90785

6. CPT Code: 90867

There's a Code for That 7.5

1. ICD-10 Code: F32.0

2. ICD-10 Code: F41.1, F33.1 Z62.819

3. ICD-10 Code: F50.02

4. ICD-10 Code: F91.3

5. ICD-10 Code: F11.21

6. ICD-10 Code: F43.12, Z65.5

There's a Code for That 7.6

1. CPT Code: 90867
   ICD-10 Code: F33.2

2. CPT Code: 90865
   ICD-10 Code: F10.24

3. CPT Code: 99205
   ICD-10 Code: F10.150

4. CPT Code: 99223
   ICD-10 Code: F20.0

5. CPT Code: 90832, 90863
   ICD-10 Code: F31.12, F40.11

Chapter 8 Primary Care

There's a Code for That 8.1

1. **8 elements** (location, right knee; quality, aching; severity, 4/10; duration, three days ago; timing, constant; modifying factors, when he lifts his leg; associated signs and symptoms, numbness, tingling, or redness of skin), level of HPI is **extended**

2. **5 systems** (constitutional, generally fine; allergic/immunologic, no problems; integumentary, no rash/no bruising; musculoskeletal, muscle cramps pain in knee joint; neurological; no

tingling), level of ROS is **extended**

3. **Established, 1 element from each type of history** (past medical, no known drug allergies, no joint or immunologic problems or past injuries; family history, no history of osteoarthritis; social history, patient is active in football), level of PFSH is **complete**

4. **Detailed** (extended HPI, extended ROS, and complete PFSH bring the level of history to detailed. If the ROS was complete, then the level of history would be comprehensive, but because the level of ROS was extended, then it is the lowest common denominator, and it brings down the levels of HPI and PFSH to detailed.)

Level of History	HPI	ROS	PFSH
Problem focused	Brief	N/A	N/A
Expanded problem focused	Brief	Problem pertinent	N/A
Detailed	Extended	(Extended)	Pertinent
Comprehensive	(Extended)	Complete	(Complete)

There's a Code for That 8.2

1. **5 body areas/organ systems** (cardiovascular, respiratory, lymphatic, musculoskeletal, integumentary), level of exam is **expanded problem focused** (limited exam of affected area and other related/symptomatic organ systems)

There's a Code for That 8.3

1. **4 points**, level of this element is **extensive**

2. **1 point**, level of this element is **minimal**

3. Level of this element is **low**

4. Low

There's a Code for That 8.4

1. Detailed

2. Expanded problem-focused

3. Low

4. 99213 (comprehensive history, expanded problem focused exam, low complexity MDM)

There's a Code for That 8.5

1. CPT Code: 99381

2. CPT Code: 99396

3. CPT Codes: 99392, 99212-25

4. CPT Code: 99396-32

5. Modifier: -57

6. CPT Code: 90832-95
   ICD-10-CM Code: F40.00

7. CPT Code: 77067-33
   ICD-10-CM Code: Z12.31

8. CPT Code: G0402

There's a Code for That 8.6

1. CPT Codes: 90471, 90657

2. CPT Codes (DTaP admin): 90460, 90461 × 2
   CPT Code (DTaP): 90700
   CPT Code (Varicella admin): 90460
   CPT Code (Varicella): 90716

3. CPT Codes (HPV admin and serum): 90471, 90649
   CPT Codes (Meningococcal admin and serum): 90472, 90619

4. CPT Code (E/M service): 99392
   CPT Codes (rotavirus admin and serum): 90471, 90680
   CPT Codes (Hep B admin and serum): 90472, 90744
   CPT Codes (IPV admin and serum): 90474, 90713
   CPT Codes (influenza admin and serum): 90474, 90660

There's a Code for That 8.7

1. CPT Code (E/M service): 99203-25
   CPT Code (urinalysis): 81005
   CPT Code (catheterization):
   51701

2. CPT Code: 17110

3. CPT Codes: 99392, 99173

There's a Code for That 8.8

1. ICD-10 Code: J11.1

2. ICD-10 Codes: R50.9, R51, J02.9

3. ICD-10 Codes: R10.31, R11.2

4. ICD-10 Codes: Z00.110

5. ICD-10 Codes: Z00.00, Z23, Z85.3, Z90.11

6. ICD-10 Code: R07.2

7. ICD-10 Codes: Z00.01, I10

8. ICD-10 Codes: E66.01, Z68.41

There's a Code for That 8.9

1. ICD-10 Code: E11.9

2. ICD-10 Codes: E11.3293, E11.36, Z79.84

3. ICD-10 Codes: E24.9, E08.9

4. ICD-10 Codes: E11.9, I10, E78.5, E66.09, Z68.34

5. ICD-10 Code: E10.9

6. ICD-10 Codes: I11.0, I50.21

7. ICD-10 Codes: I12.9, N18.3, E11.40, I50.9

8. ICD-10 Codes: J44.0, J20.9

9. ICD-10 Codes: J45.41, Z77.22

10. ICD-10 Codes: J45.40

11. ICD-10 Codes: I10, E11.9, J44.9, E78.00

12. ICD-10 Codes: P59.9

There's a Code for That 8.10

1. CPT Codes: 99213-25, 69210
   ICD-10 Codes: H61.22, H66.011

2. CPT Code: 99212
   ICD-10 Codes: N39.0, B95.62

3. CPT Codes: 99214, 85025
   ICD-10 Codes: N18.3, D63.1

4. CPT Codes: 99215, 99173
   ICD-10 Codes: E11.321, E11.36, Z79.4

5. CPT Codes: 99396, 90471, 90658
   ICD-10 Codes: Z00.00, Z23

Chapter 9 Eye and Vision Services

There's a Code for That 9.1

1. CPT Codes: 92014, 92015

2. CPT Codes: 92004, 76514, 92132, 92083

3. CPT Codes: S0621, V2020, V2100-RT, V2100-LT, V2750

4. CPT Codes: 99213-57, 65222

There's a Code for That 9.2

1. CPT Code: 67210-RT

2. HCPCS Code: S0800

3. CPT Code: 65820, 66990

4. CPT Code: 66984

5. CPT Code: 67801-E4

There's a Code for That 9.3

1. ICD-10 Code: Z01.00

2. ICD-10 Codes: Z01.01, H52.221

3. ICD-10 Codes: E11.3511, E11.3592

4. ICD-10 Code: Q12.0

5. ICD-10 Code: H40.1131

6. ICD-10 Codes: H26.122, W21.210S

7. ICD-10 Code: H35.30

There's a Code for That 9.4

1. CPT Code: 92225
   ICD-10 Codes: H53.149, H53.19, H43.392

2. CPT Codes: 67312-LT, 67314-LT, 67334-LT
   ICD-10 Code: H50.012

3. CPT Code: 67105-RT
   ICD-10 Code: H33.011

Chapter 10 Urgent Care and Emergency Department Services

There's a Code for That 10.1

1. CPT Codes: 99202, 73110, S9088

2. CPT Codes: 99214, 87880, 85025, 99051

3. CPT Codes: 12032, 12052-59, 12004-59, S9088

4. CPT Codes: 99214, 87850, 99051, S9088

There's a Code for That 10.2

1. CPT Codes: 99283-25, 30320, 99151

2. CPT Codes: 31500

3. CPT Code: 30901

4. CPT Code: 20103

5. CPT Code: 99285-25, 62270

There's a Code for That 10.3

1. ICD-10 Code: M25.562, Y93.72

2. ICD-10 Codes: S71.111A, S71.011A, S31.119A, S51.811A, S41.011A, S01.81XA

3. ICD-10 Codes: B27.90

4. ICD-10 Code: J13

5. ICD-10 Codes: S20.219A, W52.XXXA, Y93.66, Y92.322, Y99.8

There's a Code for That 10.4

1. ICD-10 Code: I21.21

2. ICD-10 Codes: I21.02, I25.2

3. ICD-10 Codes: A41.02, R65.21, N17.9

4. ICD-10 Code: T22.692A, T22.691A, T23.691A, T23.692A, T31.30

5. ICD-10 Code: K35.32

There's a Code for That 10.5

1. CPT Codes: 99285, 74176
   ICD-10 Code: K35.80

2. CPT Codes: 99213-25, 94760, 94640, 90471, 90658, S9088, 99051
   ICD-10 Code: J45.41

3. CPT Code: 32551
   ICD-10 Codes: S27.0XXA, V57.0XXA

Chapter 11 Surgical Procedures

There's a Code for That 11.1

1. Code range: 61000–61070

2. Code range: 24800–24802

3. Code range: 55000

4. Code range: 53400–53520

5. Code range: 57452–57461

There's a Code for That 11.2

1. Modifier: -53

2. Modifier: -51

3. Modifier: -55

4. Modifier: -74

5. Modifier: -PB

6. Modifier: -66

There's a Code for That 11.3

1. CPT Code: 11643
   ICD-10 Code: C44.321

2. CPT Code: 11200
   ICD-10 Code: L91.8

3. CPT Code: 17110
   ICD-10 Code: B07.8

4. CPT Codes: 17263, 17262-51, 17261-51, 17260-51
   ICD-10 Codes: C43.61, C43.62
   (Each lesion destruction should be listed separately, with modifier -51 to indicate that they were multiple procedures all performed in the same surgical session. Diagnosis

code C43.61 supports the medical necessity for all three of the procedures performed on the right arm/shoulder, and it should only be reported once.)

5. CPT Code: 17311
ICD-10 Code: C44.319

There's a Code for That 11.4

1. CPT Code: 14000 (Note that lesion excision is included within the skin advancement code and is not coded separately.) ICD-10 Code: D23.5

2. CPT Code: 16025
ICD-10 Code: T24.202

3. CPT Code: 15935 (Note that the skin flap closure is included within the code description and is not coded separately.) ICD-10 Code: L89.154

There's a Code for That 11.5

1. CPT Code: 49500
ICD-10 Code: K42.9

2. CPT Code: 47562
ICD-10 Code: K80.00

3. CPT Code: 44970
ICC-10 Code: K35.3

Chapter 12 Anesthesia and Pain Management Services

There's a Code for That 12.1

1. 00402

2. 00406

3. CPT Code: 00211 (the base units for 00211 are 10, and the base units for 00215 are 9, so code 00211 would be reported, as it represents

the most work-the highest number of base units)

4. CPT Code: 00520

There's a Code for That 12.2

1. CPT Code: 01382-AA, -P1

2. CPT Code: 01742-P2, -QX

3. CPT Code: 01990-P6, QZ

4. CPT Codes: 00567-AA, -P3, 99100

There's a Code for That 12.3

1. CPT Code: 95869

2. CPT Code: 62321

3. CPT Codes: 64615, 95873

4. CPT Code: 63655

There's a Code for That 12.4

1. ICD-10 Codes: T88.3XXA, T41.0X5A

2. ICD-10 Code: S72.301B

3. ICD-10 Codes: G89.29, M45.5

4. ICD-10 Code: M51.14

5. ICD-10 Code: M60.112

There's a Code for That 12.5

1. CPT Codes: 22513, 22515 ICD-10 Code: S22.050A (chronic pain is not coded because the encounter is to treat the underlying condition

2. CPT Codes: 00620-P2-QZ, 99100 ICD-10 Code: S22.050A

3. CPT Code: 00580-P4 ICD-10 Code: D15.1, I50.9, I42

4. CPT Codes: 64490-50, 64491-50, 64492-50 ICD-10 Codes: G89.29, M54.2, M25.511, M25.512, M79.601, M79.602

Chapter 13 Radiology and Imaging Services

There's a Code for That 13.1

1. a. Technical
2. b. Professional
3. c. Global
4. b. Professional
5. c. Global

There's a Code for That 13.2

1. CPT Code: 74150 (the contrast material is not coded because it was not administered intravenously, intrathecally, or intra-articularly)

2. CPT Code: 74176

3. CPT Code: 71046

4. CPT Code: 72050

5. CPT Code: 73222
HCPCS Code: Q9966 × 100

6. CPT Codes: 73610-26, 73630-26

There's a Code for That 13.3

1. CPT Code: 76770
2. CPT Code: 78071
3. CPT Code: 76857
4. CPT Code: 77075
5. CPT Code: 77059
6. CPT Code: 78206

There's a Code for That 13.4

1. ICD-10 Code: R10.9
2. ICD-10 Code: E83.52
3. ICD-10 Codes: Z12.31, N63.20, Z80.3
4. ICD-10 Code: N20.2
5. ICD-10 Codes: J81.0, I50.9

There's a Code for That 13.5

1. CPT Code: 73630-LT
ICD-10 Code: M79.672

2. CPT Codes: 70553, A9585 × 500
   ICD-10 Codes: C72.41, H91.91

3. CPT Code: 74178
   ICD-10 Codes: R10.9, Z90.49

Chapter 14
Laboratory and Pathology Services

There's a Code for That 14.1

1. B. Quantitative (this information is contained in the guidelines paragraph directly above the code)

2. B. Quantitative (this code is within the same subsection of codes as the previous one, and so the guidelines still apply)

3. A. Qualitative

4. A. Qualitative

5. B. Quantitative

There's a Code for That 14.2

1. CPT Code: 80053

2. CPT Codes: 82040, 84075, 84155, 84460, 84450

3. CPT Codes: 80053, 80061, 80074

4. CPT Code: 82009

5. CPT Code: 82128

6. CPT Codes: 83718, 83719, 83721

There's a Code for That 14.3

1. CPT Code: 80305

2. CPT Code: 80307

3. CPT Code: 80325

4. CPT Code: 82075

5. CPT Code: 80186

6. CPT Code: 80171

7. CPT Code: 80346

There's a Code for That 14.4

1. CPT Code: 81211

2. CPT Code: 80415

3. CPT Code: 81025

4. CPT Code: 87086

5. CPT Code: 87660

There's a Code for That 14.5

1. CPT Code: 88304 × 2

2. CPT Code: 88305

3. CPT Codes: 88307, 88305 × 2

There's a Code for That 14.6

1. ICD-10 Codes: Z11.4, Z20.6, Z71.7, Z72.51

2. ICD-10 Code: A49.02

3. ICD-10 Code: A40.0

4. ICD-10 Codes: B20, C46.51

5. ICD-10 Code: J09.X2

6. ICD-10 Code: A56.19

7. ICD-10 Code: A02.0

There's a Code for That 14.7

1. CPT Codes: 88175, 87624
   ICD-10 Code: R87.619

2. CPT Codes: 87077, 87181
   ICD-10 Codes: L02.31, B95.62

Chapter 15
Orthopedic Services

There's a Code for That 15.1

1. CPT Codes: 27356, 27358

2. CPT Code: 24073

3. CPT Codes: 21045, 21215

4. CPT Code: 28041

There's a Code for That 15.2

1. CPT Code: 20606-50

2. CPT Code: 20610-RT

3. CPT Code:s 20612, 20612-59

4. CPT Code: 20611-RT
   HCPCS Code: J1040

There's a Code for That 15.3

1. CPT Code: 24505-RT

2. CPT Code: 28420

3. CPT Codes: 26605, 26605-59, 26605-59

4. CPT Codes: 26605, 26608
   CPT Codes: 73110, 29075 (Reporting the evaluation and management procedure for this encounter would be considered unbundling. The CPT code book states that additional E/M services should be reported only if they identify significant, further services, other than the application of the cast or strapping.)

There's a Code for That 15.4

1. CPT Codes: 22610, 22614 × 3

2. CPT Codes: 29827, 29824-51, 29828-59, 29826

3. CPT Code: 98926

4. ICD-10-CM Code: M79.7

5. CPT Codes: 22558, 22585, 22583, 22583, 20931

6. CPT Code: 27130-50

7. ICD-10-CM Code: M16.0

There's a Code for That 15.5

1. ICD-10 Code: S82.852A

2. ICD-10 Code: S82.852K

3. ICD-10 Code: S52.351B

4. ICD-10 Codes: S02.0XXA, S06.5X0A

5. ICD-10 Codes: S22.41XA, S62.101A

6. ICD-10 Codes: M13.152, S72.002S

7. ICD-10 Code: S42.432D

8. ICD-10 Code: M84.374G

9. ICD-10 Code: M84.521K, C79.51

There's a Code for That 15.6

1. ICD-10 Code: M25.361, S83.271S

2. ICD-10 Code: S83.222A

3. ICD-10 Code: S86.011A

4. ICD-10 Code: S83.512A

5. ICD-10 Code: M1A.3410

There's a Code for That 15.7

1. CPT Codes: 20610-RT, 73562-RT
   ICD-10 Codes: M65.161, E66.01, E11.9, F17.220

2. CPT Code: 27236-RT
   ICD-10 Codes: S72.031A, W01.0XXA, Y92.010

Chapter 16 Physical, Speech, and Occupational Therapy Services

There's a Code for That 16.1

1. CPT Code: 97010

2. CPT Code: 97018

3. CPT Code: 97110 × 2

4. CPT Code: 96001 (Gait training is bundled into the code for comprehensive gait and motion analysis procedures, and should not be reported separately)

5. CPT Code: 97140 × 3

6. CPT Codes: 97167, 97535

There's a Code for That 16.2

1. CPT Code: 92507

2. CPT Code: 92523

3. CPT Code: 97127 × 2

4. CPT Code: 92606

5. HCPCS Code: V5336

There's a Code for That 16.3

1. ICD-10 Code: G80.1

2. ICD-10 Code: G10

3. ICD-10 Codes: M25.661, M17.11, Z96.651

4. ICD-10 Codes: M54.2, G89.29

There's a Code for That 16.4

1. CPT Code: 97542 × 3
   ICD-10 Codes: G82.21, S24.114D

2. CPT Code: 92610
   ICD-10 Codes: I69.091, R13.12, I69.051, I69.020

3. CPT Code: 97537
   ICD-10 Code: Q90

Chapter 17 Obstetrics and Gynecology Services

There's a Code for That 17.1

1. CPT codes: 99212, 81025

2. CPT code: 56634-LT

3. CPT code: 56810

4. CPT code: 58544

5. CPT codes: 99213, 58300, J7298

6. CPT codes: 57455, 58110

7. CPT code: 99214

There's a Code for That 17.2

1. CPT code: 59320

2. CPT code: 59514

3. CPT code: A. 59425
             B. 59515

4. CPT code: 59400

5. CPT code: 59001

6. CPT code: 59830

There's a Code for That 17.3

1. ICD-10-CM Code: N92.2

2. ICD-10-CM Codes: Z31.69, E28.2

3. ICD-10-CM Code: R87.619

4. ICD-10-CM Codes: N95.1, G47.00, R51

5. ICD-10-CM Code: N76.0

6. ICD-10-CM Codes: A59.01, Z72.51

There's a Code for That 17.4

1. ICD-10-CM Codes: Z34.82, Z3A.16

2. ICD-10-CM Codes: T22.212A, Z33.1, Z3A.32

3. ICD-10-CM Codes: O98.712, Z21, Z3A.22

4. ICD-10-CM Codes: O24.415, Z79.84

5. ICD-10-CM Codes: O99.332, Z71.6, F17.210, Z3A.20

There's a Code for That 17.5

1. CPT Code: 58120
   ICD-10 Code: N80.0

2. CPT Code: 59612
   ICD-10 Code: O34.219, O70.1, Z37.0, Z3A.38

3. CPT Code: 99214
   ICD-10 Code: N83.201, N83.202

Chapter 18 Medical Specialist's Services, Part I

There's a Code for That 18.1

1. CPT codes: 57156, 77332

2. CPT code: 77290

3. CPT code: 77762

4. CPT code: 77261

5. CPT code: 77412

6. CPT codes: 96360, 96361

7. CPT code: 96402

8. CPT code: 96450

There's a Code for That 18.2

1. ICD-10-CM Code: D50.9

2. ICD-10-CM Codes: C25.9, D63.0

3. ICD-10-CM Code: C02.2

4. ICD-10-CM Codes: N63.11, Z80.3, Z15.01

5. ICD-10-CM Code: C78.02

6. ICD-10-CM Codes: Z51.11, C22.3

There's a Code for That 18.3

1. CPT code: 61253

2. CPT code: 61519

3. CPT code: 61690

4. CPT code: 62192

5. CPT code: 63015

6. CPT codes: 63077, 63078 × 2

There's a Code for That 18.4

1. ICD-10 Codes: G20, F02.81

2. ICD-10 Code: G11.0

3. ICD-10 Code: G21.4

4. ICD-10 Codes: G31.83, F02.80

5. ICD-10 Code: G35

6. ICD-10 Code: G40.A19

7. ICD-10 Code: G43.501

There's a Code for That 18.5

1. CPT code: 50070

2. CPT code: 50400

3. CPT code: 50590

4. CPT codes: 51728-51, 51741

5. CPT code: 54115

6. CPT code: 55650-50

7. CPT code: 55866

8. CPT code: 90961

9. CPT code: 90945

There's a Code for That 18.6

1. ICD-10 Codes: N18.6, Z99.2

2. ICD-10 Code: N32.81

3. ICD-10 Codes: E29.1, N52.1

4. ICD-10 Codes: N40.1, R39.16

5. ICD-10 Code: C61

6. ICD-10 Code: N39.46

There's a Code for That 18.7

1. CPT code: 99245
   ICD-10-CM Codes: C50.412, Z17.0, Z80.3

2. CPT Code: 27365
   ICD-10-CM Code: C40.22

3. CPT Code: 64858
   ICD-10-CM Code: S74.02XA

4. CPT Code: 99253
   ICD-10-CM Code: G40.301

Chapter 19 Medical Specialist's Services, Part II

There's a Code for That 19.1

1. CPT code: 45338

2. CPT code: 45300

3. CPT code: 43235

4. CPT code: 43100

5. CPT code: 43205

6. CPT code: 43282

7. CPT code: 43870

8. CPT codes: 44202, 44203

9. CPT code: 44390

10. CPT code: 43278

There's a Code for That 19.2

1. ICD-10-CM Codes: K21.0, F10.20

2. ICD-10-CM Codes: Z12.11, K63.5

3. ICD-10-CM Code: C19

4. ICD-10-CM Code: K25.2

5. ICD-10-CM Code: K50.112

6. ICD-10-CM Code: K58.0

7. ICD-10-CM Code: K91.2

There's a Code for That 19.3

1. CPT code: 33011

2. CPT code: 33391, 33141

3. CPT code: 33422

4. CPT codes: 33512, 35572-80

5. CPT codes: 33533, 33518

6. CPT codes: 35539, 35500

7. CPT code: 36415

8. CPT codes: 33249, 33225

9. CPT code: 75635

10. CPT codes: 75822, 36005

11. CPT codes: 92997, 92998

There's a Code for That 19.4

1. ICD-10 Code: I20.1

2. ICD-10 Code: I48.1

3. ICD-10 Code: I51.7

4. ICD-10 Code: I63.112

5. ICD-10 Codes: I70.442, L97.222

6. ICD-10 Code: I82.4Z2

7. ICD-10 Codes: I27.82, Z79.01

8. ICD-10 Code: I71.4

9. ICD-10 Codes: I83.11, I83.12, I83.813

There's a Code for That 19.5

1. CPT code: 43235
   ICD-10-CM Code: K22.710

2. CPT code: 43753
   ICD-10-CM Codes: R10.84, R11.10, R03.0, T62.1X1A

3. CPT code: 34846
   ICD-10-CM Codes: I71.3, I13.10, N18.3, F17.210

Chapter 20 Inpatient Hospital Services

There's a Code for That 20.1

1. ICD-10-CM Codes: O03.37, Z3A.08

2. ICD-10-CM Code: G03.9

3. ICD-10-CM Codes: C50.312, C78.02

4. ICD-10-CM Codes: I25.10, I13.10, I50.9, N18.4, I49.5

5. ICD-10-CM Codes: S36.539A, T81.530A

There's a Code for That 20.2

1. ICD-10-PCS Code: 0TY10Z0, Transplantation of Left Kidney, Allogeneic, Open Approach
ICD-10-CM Code: N18.6, End stage renal disease

2. ICD-10-PCS Code: 0W2BX0Z, Change Drainage Device in Left Pleural Cavity, External Approach
ICD-10-CM Code: J93.11, Primary spontaneous pneumothorax

3. ICD-10-PCS Code: 0DJ08ZZ, Inspection of Upper Intestinal Tract, Via Natural or Artificial Opening Endoscopic
ICD-10-CM Code: R10.13, Epigastric pain, R13.10, Dysphagia, unspecified

4. ICD-10-PCS Code: 0WQF0ZZ, Repair Abdominal Wall, Open Approach
ICD-10-CM Code: K42.9, Umbilical hernia without obstruction or gangrene

Glossary

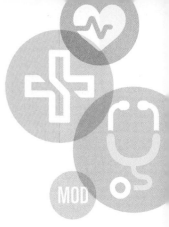

8-minute rule: When reporting time-based codes, for any time over 15 minutes, the additional time must be at least 8 minutes over the 15-minute unit to report an additional unit of the service; each additional 8 minutes over the last 15-minute mark equals one additional unit

Abdominal aortic aneurysm (AAA): An aneurysm located in the abdominal aorta, which can be life-threatening if it bursts

Ablation: A procedure that destroys tissue performed in several different ways including laser surgery, electrosurgery, cryosurgery, chemosurgery, surgical curettement, radiocautery, radiofrequency ablation, or tissue volume reduction; also called *destruction*

Abortion: Procedure performed to evacuate the uterus of the products of conception, or the remaining fetal and placental tissues after either a spontaneous miscarriage or elective pregnancy termination

Accidental intent: An unintentional effect of a substance that was either taken on accident or in excess

Accountable Care Organization (ACO): A legal entity that is recognized and authorized under applicable state, federal, or tribal law, is identified by a Taxpayer Identification Number (TIN), and is formed by one or more ACO participant(s) that is (are) defined at 425.102(a) and may also include any other ACO participants described at 425.102(b) (42 CFR 425.20 2011)

Accreditation: 1. An evaluative process in which a healthcare organization undergoes an examination of its policies, procedures, and performance by an external organization ("accrediting body") to ensure that it is meeting predetermined criteria. It usually involves both on- and off-site surveys (CMS 2006) **2.** The act of granting approval to a healthcare organization based on whether the organization has met a set of voluntary standards developed by an accreditation agency

Acquired condition: Condition that develops over the course of a person's life

Activity: What the patient was doing when the injury occurs

Acupuncture: An ancient method of treating a variety of ailments, that consists of inserting thin, flexible needles into specific areas of the body, to restore the body's balance and relieve discomfort

Acute condition: Severe and sudden onset of condition

Add-on code: A CPT/HCPCS code that describes a service that, excluding codes associated with the National Correct Coding Initiative (NCCI), is always performed in conjunction with another primary service (CMS 2019)

Administrative personnel: Individuals who handle the daily functions of the business side of the healthcare practice, such as sending claims and billing patients, as well as non-clinical patient services such as healthcare records requests, registering patients, scheduling appointments, and sending referrals to healthcare specialists

Administrative safeguards: Under HIPAA, administrative actions and policies and procedures to manage the selection, development, implementation, and maintenance of security measures to protect electronic protected health information and to manage the conduct of the covered entity's or business associate's workforce in relation to the protection of that information (45 CFR 164.304 2013)

Admitting provider: The provider that admitted the patient to the hospital

Advance beneficiary notice (ABN): A notice that a doctor or supplier should give a Medicare beneficiary when furnishing an item or service for which Medicare is expected to deny payment. If

(Continued on next page)

you do not get an ABN before you get the service from your doctor or supplier, and Medicare does not pay for it, then you probably do not have to pay for it (CMS 2006)

Advanced life support (ALS): A higher level of care used for patients with life-threatening illnesses, injuries, or other severe conditions, during transport to a facility that can provide them with full medical care that includes life-saving protocols to further support airway, breathing, and circulation

Adverse effect: An unintended effect caused by a substance that is correctly prescribed and correctly administered

Allograft: A skin graft from tissue from a donor

Allowable amount: The maximum amount of money that an insurance policy will agree to pay for a specific CPT (procedure) or HCPCS code

Alteration: Modifying the anatomic structure of a body part without affecting the function of the body part

Alzheimer's disease: A progressive form of dementia that causes loss of memories and cognitive abilities that interfere with activities of daily living

Ambulance modifier: Modifiers required on ambulance claims that identify the origin and destination for each transportation

Ambulance supplier: Those tasked with transporting a patient with a healthcare need to a provider or facility capable of treating that need usually in an emergency or urgent situation; the emergency responders must stabilize and provide a certain level of healthcare services to the patient until he or she can receive care from a healthcare provider

Ambulatory surgical center (ASC): Under Medicare, an outpatient surgical facility that has its own national identifier; is a separate entity with respect to its licensure, accreditation, governance, professional supervision, administrative functions, clinical services, recordkeeping, and financial and accounting systems; has as its sole purpose the provision of services in connection with surgical procedures that do not require inpatient hospitalization; and meets the conditions and requirements set forth in the Medicare Conditions of Participation; also called ambulatory surgical center

American Health Information Management Association (AHIMA): The professional membership organization for managers of health record services and healthcare information systems as well as coding services; provides accreditation, advocacy, certification, and educational services

Amputation: The complete removal of a body part, performed to remove dead, diseased, or damaged tissue, leaving only healthy and functional tissue behind

Amputee: The patient who has undergone an amputation

Amyotrophic lateral sclerosis (ALS): Also known as Lou Gehrig's Disease, a degenerative disease in which motor neurons slowly die, causing muscle weakness, stiffness, and twitching; and for which there is no cure

Analgesia: The inability to feel pain

Anemia: Occurs when a person has abnormally low red blood cells or hemoglobin in the blood

Anesthesia section: Section of the CPT code book that lists services performed by anesthesiologists, anesthesia assistants, or other healthcare providers

Anesthesia services: Procedures that create analgesia, the absence of pain, and are provided for a brief amount of time to facilitate a medical procedure, such as a surgery

Anesthesiology: The healthcare specialty of relieving patient pain before, during, and after surgery

Aneurysm: The bulging or ballooning of a small portion of an artery, caused by weakening or degeneration of the wall of the vessel

Angiography: The x-ray examination of blood vessels after the administration of a contrast material

Annual wellness visit: A visit in which a provider should develop and design a personalized prevention plan for the patient's chronic healthcare conditions and perform various health risk assessments; the initial AWV code may only be reported after the first 12 months of enrollment (ideally a year after the IPPE)

Antepartum: The period of pregnancy before childbirth

Anterior: Situated toward the front of the body (such as the face or the breasts)

Antero-posterior: Two projections during an imaging service consisting of two views that pass through the front to the back of the body

Anxiety disorders: Mental disorders that result in constant feelings of worry, fear, and panic when faced with everyday situations

Aphonia: Loss of voice

Appendectomy: Removal of the appendix

Appendicitis: Inflammation of the appendix that can be a life-threatening condition if the appendix ruptures, which can cause a systemic infection

Approach: Identifies the manner in which a provider accesses an area in order to perform a procedure

Arthritis: An inflammation of the joints

Arthrocentesis: The aspiration of a joint, a process that involves inserting a hollow needle into a joint or bursa to allow for the removal of fluid

Arthrodesis: The surgical fixation of a joint, performed to treat deformities of the bones and pain

Arthropathy: Any disease of the joints

Arthroplasty: Surgical repair of a joint

Arthroscopy: An endoscopically-assisted procedure of a joint

ASA crosswalk: A book that crosswalks all applicable CPT surgical and therapeutic procedure codes to the appropriate anesthesia codes

Assault: A toxic effect that occurs due to assault is one that was purposefully inflicted upon one person by another person, with the intent of hurting the recipient of the substance

Atherosclerosis: The hardening of fatty substances within the blood vessels, which leads to a buildup of plaque; this narrows the diameter of the blood vessel and reduces blood flow, and causes the formation of blood clots that can travel through the vessels and cause further obstruction of blood flow

Attention-deficit hyperactivity disorder: Disorder that typically appears in school-age children and impact a child's school and social functioning; symptoms include impulsivity, inattention, difficulty concentrating and following directions, difficulty completing tasks, too much energy and restlessness

Augmentative and alternative communication (AAC): Method used to communicate with other people that does not include oral communication; for example, hand gestures or facial expressions when speaking

Autograft: A skin graft from a different site from the patient's own body

Axial plane: A horizontal line, perpendicular to the long axis of the body that divides the body into superior and inferior portions (the top and the bottom halves); also known as the transverse plane

Bacteriology: The study of bacteria

Bariatric surgery: Surgery performed on the stomach or intestines to induce weight loss

Bartholin's glands: Greater vestibular glands that secrete mucus to lubricate the vagina

Base units: A set of numerical values created and maintained by the American Society of Anesthesiologists (ASA), that give each anesthesiology service a numerical relative value in relation to how complicated or risky a procedure is, and are used to set the relative cost of each procedures

Basic life support (BLS): A basic level of care that is used for patients with life-threatening illnesses, injuries, or other severe conditions, while they are being transported to a facility that can provide them with full medical care

Behavioral health services: A broad array of psychiatric services provided in acute, long-term, and ambulatory care settings; includes treatment of mental disorders, chemical dependency, mental retardation, and developmental disabilities, as well as cognitive rehabilitation services

Benign neoplasm: Non-cancerous growths of tissue that are not invasive and will not spread to other tissues

Benign prostatic hyperplasia (BPH): A condition in which the prostate gland is enlarged, which causes urinary frequency and urgency, nocturia (urinating at night), and urinary retention (among other symptoms)

Bilateral: Affecting both right and left sides

Billable code: A code that has been extended out to the full amount of required characters

Bipolar disorder: A mental disorder that affects a person's mood and behavior by switching from extreme highs (called mania) to extreme lows (called depression)

Birthing center: A facility that specializes in providing a comfortable setting for labor, delivery, postpartum care, and immediate newborn care

Block: Frozen specimen being examined by the surgeon

Body area: General area of the body, rather than specific organ systems, which may be examined during an evaluation and management encounter

Brachytherapy: A cancer treatment method in which small radioactive seeds, capsules, or elements are placed within or near a cancer or cancerous organ; also referred to as clinical brachytherapy

Burn codes: Codes for thermal burns that come from a heat source such as fire or hot appliance

Bursa: a fluid-filled sac beneath the skin that lies between tendons, ligaments, and bones, and assists in lubricating the joints

Business associates (BAs): 1. A person or organization other than a member of a covered entity's workforce that performs functions or activities on behalf of or affecting a covered entity that involve the use or disclosure of individually identifiable health information **2.** As amended by HITECH, with respect to a covered entity, a person who creates, receives, maintains, or transmits PHI for a function or activity regulated by HIPAA, including claims processing or administration, data analysis, processing or administration, utilization review, quality assurance, patient safety activities, billing, benefit management, practice management, and repricing or provides legal, actuarial, accounting, consulting, data aggregation, management, administrative, accreditation, or financial services (45 CFR 160.103 2013)

Bypass: Altering the route of passage of the contents of a tubular body part

Cadaver donor: Brain dead patient from whom organs are being harvested

Capitation: A specified amount of money paid to a health plan or doctor. This is used to cover the cost of a health plan member's healthcare services for a certain length of time (CMS 2006)

Carcinoma in situ: Neoplasms that are potentially cancerous growths of tissue

Cardiac electrophysiology: The study of the electrical system of the heart

Cardiologist: A healthcare provider who specializes in the diagnosis and treatment of the diseases of the heart, coronary vessels, and cardiovascular system

Cardiopulmonary bypass (CPB): A technique in which a machine takes over the function of the heart and lungs during surgery

Cardiopulmonary resuscitation (CPR): A medical procedure that involves the healthcare provider repeatedly compressing a patient's chest in an attempt to circulate the blood and restore breathing to a patient who has suffered cardiac arrest (a stopping of the heart)

Cardiothoracic surgery: Surgery that focuses on the surgical treatment of the heart and organs within the thorax (such as the lungs)

Care plan oversight (CPO): The monthly oversight of the healthcare plan for a patient in the home health, hospice, or skilled nursing facility settings, and includes healthcare provider time spent coordinating care, completing documentation, reviewing data, and discussions with other healthcare providers; care plan oversight codes identify the patient healthcare setting and the amount of time per month spent providing care plan oversight services

Category I code: The largest set of codes in the CPT code book, commonly referred to as simply CPT codes; these procedures have been approved by the Food and Drug Administration (FDA), are performed by physicians or other healthcare practitioners throughout the United States at a frequency consistent with their intended clinical use, are consistent with current clinical practice, and have a documented clinical efficacy for treating healthcare conditions

Category II code: Codes intended to facilitate data collection for performance measurement purposes; category II codes are supplemental tracking codes that report the performance of a test, evaluation, counseling service, or other procedure that is part of a facility's performance measurement program

Category III code: A set of temporary codes used to report emerging technology, services, procedures, and service paradigms, and the use of these codes is integral to the identification and establishment of new healthcare procedures and treatments

Catheterization: Procedure that involves the insertion of a catheter tube in through the urethra and into the bladder to drain urine

Centers for Medicare and Medicaid Services (CMS): The Department of Health and Human Services agency responsible for Medicare and parts of Medicaid. Historically, CMS has maintained the UB-92 institutional EMC format specifications, the professional EMC NSF specifications, and specifications for various certifications and authorizations used by the Medicare and Medicaid programs. CMS is responsible for the oversight of HIPAA administrative simplification transaction and code sets, health identifiers, and security standards. CMS also maintains the HCPCS medical code set and the Medicare Remittance Advice Remark Codes administrative code set (CMS 2006)

Central nervous system (CNS): Body system comprised of all of the nerves of the brain and the spinal cord

Central venous access devices (CVAD): Flexible tubes inserted in patients who require frequent access to the bloodstream; they can stay in place for up to a year

Cerclage: A stitch or band device that helps the cervix remain closed at the external os

Cerebrospinal fluid (CSF) shunt: A small one-way valve that is inserted in the ventricles of a patient's brain to allow for the drainage of cerebrospinal fluid from the brain and into the peritoneal cavity

Certificate of Medical Necessity (CMN): An official document completed by the physician and the DME supplier that details the patient's diagnosis, necessity for the DME supply, and other important patient demographics and information

Certified Coding Specialist (CCS): An AHIMA credential awarded to individuals who have demonstrated skill in classifying medical data from patient records, generally in the hospital setting, by passing a certification examination

Certified nurse midwife (CNM): A mid-level practitioner (as discussed in chapter 1) with an advanced degree as a registered nurse in midwifery, the study of assisting pregnant females in obstetric care and childbirth, including the postpartum period, female care, and birth control

Cervicalgia: Neck pain

Cervix uteri: Also known as the cervix, is the lowest part of the uterus, about two to three centimeters long and round in shape, and forms a canal from the upper portion of the vagina to the uterus

Cesarean delivery: A surgical procedure in which the provider incises the pregnant female's abdomen and uterus to remove the fetus; it is typically performed when a vaginal delivery would put the health of the pregnant female or the fetus at risk

Change: Removing a device from a body part and replacing it with an identical or similar device in or on the same body part without cutting or puncturing the skin or a mucous membrane

Character: Each of the individual numbers or letters within a code

Charge amount: A price assigned to a unit of medical or health service, such as a visit to a physician or a day in a hospital; may be unrelated to the actual cost of providing the service

Chemodenervation: The injection of botulinum toxin, a potent neurotoxin, to an affected nerve for

Chemotherapy: The use of a drug to treat a medical condition

Chief complaint (C/C): The principal problem a patient reports to a healthcare provider

Children's Health Insurance Program (CHIP): A program similar to Medicaid that covers children in low-income families but whose income is not low enough to qualify for Medicaid coverage

Chiropractor: a practitioner of manual spinal manipulation therapy through spinal subluxation techniques

Cholangiography: An examination of the bile ducts, used to identify an obstruction

Cholangitis: Inflammation of the bile ducts

Cholecystectomy: Removal of the gallbladder

Cholecystitis: Inflammation of the gallbladder

Choledocholithiasis: The presence of one of more gallstones within the common bile duct

Cholelithiasis: The presence of gallstones

Chronic care management (CCM): Services provided to patients with multiple chronic healthcare conditions, which necessitate the establishment, implementation, revision, or monitoring of a patient care plan

Chronic condition: A syndrome or condition that has been in development for a long period of time, and is a constant disease state

Chronic Obstructive Pulmonary Disease (COPD): A lung disease characterized by chronically poor airflow; symptoms include shortness of breath, chronic cough, and sputum production

Chronic pain: Constant or long-term sensation of pain that may be due to postoperative complications, past injuries, or nerve conditions

Circumcision: The surgical removal of the foreskin at the tip of the penis

Classification system: A clinical vocabulary, terminology, or nomenclature that lists words or phrases with their meanings, provides for the proper use of clinical words as names or symbols, and facilitates mapping standardized terms to broader classifications for administrative, regulatory, oversight, and fiscal requirements

CLIA-waived: Status that allows performance of certain in-office laboratory procedures, such as blood counts and bacterial cultures; CLIA-waived laboratory tests are simple and have low risk

Clinical modification (CM): The compilation of ICD codes used to report diagnoses

Clinical personnel: Individuals who are trained as healthcare providers or practitioners, such as doctors, nurse practitioners, and physician assistants, as well as personnel who are trained and qualified to provide assistive healthcare services, such as registered nurses, healthcare assistants, and clinical nursing assistants

Closed fracture: Fracture in which the broken bone does not penetrate the skin

Closed procedure: Procedure in which the skin is not opened to perform the procedure

Closed treatment: The site of the fracture is not surgically opened to perform the repair

CMS-1500: The uniform professional claim form (CMS 2006)

Code edit: An accuracy checkpoint in the claims-processing software that ensures all codes are valid and may be reported in conjunction with each other, and if any modifiers are necessary

Code first: Instructions that list conditions that should be coded *before* the code identified

Code linkage: Linking the diagnosis and procedure code together to identify the medical necessity for specific procedures

Code table: A table of all of the character options for PCS codes

Coding certification: Professional document of achievement given only to those coders who can demonstrate proficiency on a coding examination

Coding guidelines: The rules that specify what codes to use in which situations, how to sequence them, which modifiers to use, and how to combine them with other codes

Cognitive communication disorder: Disorder that includes difficulties for patients when organizing thoughts, remembering, paying attention, planning, and problem solving

Coinsurance: Cost sharing in which the policy or certificate holder pays a preestablished percentage of eligible expenses after the deductible has been met; the percentage may vary by type or site of service

Colonoscopy: The examination of the entire colon, from the rectum to the cecum at the end of the ascending colon, and may include an examination of the ileum

Colorectal surgery: Surgery of the colon, rectum, and anus

Combination code: Includes both the etiology and manifestation in one code

Commercial insurance: Insurance plans run by for-profit companies that are not government entities and require a monthly premium in return for healthcare coverage

Comminuted fracture: Fracture with more than two parts, usually with multiple broken pieces

Comorbid condition or comorbidity: 1. A medical condition that coexists with the primary cause for hospitalization and affects the patient's treatment and length of stay (IHS n.d.) **2.** Pre-existing condition that, because of its presence with a specific diagnosis, causes an increase in length of stay by at least one day in approximately 75 percent of the cases (as in complication and comorbidity [CC]) (HHS 2010, 23905)

Complication of care: A condition that occurs as a result of the medical care or surgery

Complication: 1. A medical condition that arises during an inpatient hospitalization (for example, a postoperative wound infection) (IHS n.d.) **2.** Condition that arises during the hospital stay that prolongs the length of stay at least one day in approximately 75 percent of the cases (as in complication and comorbidity [CC]) (HHS 2010, 23905)

Complication/comorbidity (CC): A condition that requires additional resources, affects treatment to the patient, or prolongs the patient's inpatient stay

Compound fracture: Fracture in which the bone penetrates the skin; otherwise known as an open fracture

Comprehensive ophthalmological services: Ophthalmological services that include a general evaluation of the complete ophthalmological system

Compression fracture: Fracture found in the spine that occurs when one or more vertebrae collapse under their own pressure

Computed tomography (CT): An imaging study that combines a number of x-ray images from different angles to produce a virtual cross-section of the area being studied; also known as computed axial tomography (CAT) scan

Computerized physician order entry (CPOE): Electronic systems that allow physicians to record medication or treatment orders, access electronic health records (EHR), and radiology, laboratory, and pharmacy applications electronically. These systems usually contain error prevention software that provides the user with prompts that warn against the possibility of drug interaction, allergy, or overdose and other relevant information condition; always reported as a secondary diagnosis conditions

Confidentiality agreement: A legal document signed by the employee after HIPAA training, which indicates that the employee has been trained in aspects of HIPAA compliance and agrees to abide by the healthcare facility's measures taken to ensure HIPAA compliance

Congenital condition: Condition that was present at or before birth

Conization: A procedure that uses either an electrical wire (LEEP), cold knife, or laser to remove a cone of tissue from the cervix, either for diagnostic purposes (biopsy) or to remove cancerous or pre-cancerous cells

Constant attendance code: Code reported according the length of time that the provider spent performing the service

Consultation: An evaluation and management encounter that is provided by one healthcare professional, often a healthcare specialist, at the request of another healthcare professional, such as a primary care provider

Continuing education unit (CEU): Unit of measurement used in continuing education programs—any type of industry-specific training that offers specific instruction on a topic within the professional's field of expertise; a certified coder must attain a certain number of CEUs each year in order to maintain his or her certification

Contralateral: The opposite side of the body (the right arm and the left arm)

Contrast material: A substance that is injected into the patient to enhance the contrast of certain structures within the body while performing x-rays and imaging procedures

Contributory factors: Counseling, coordination of care, and the nature of the presenting problem, which are used to help determine the level of the E/M service

Control: Stopping, or attempting to stop, postprocedural or other acute bleeding

Conversion factor (CF): The dollar amount per unit for the reimbursement of anesthesia services

Coordination of care: The cooperation between at least two healthcare practitioners to provide care to a patient

Copayment: Cost-sharing measure in which the policy or certificate holder pays a fixed dollar amount (flat fee) per service, supply, or procedure that is owed to the healthcare facility by the patient. The fixed amount that the policyholder pays may vary by type of service, such as $20 per prescription or $15 per physician office visit

Coronal plane: A vertical line that divides the body into anterior and posterior halves (front and back)

Coronary artery bypass grafts (CABG): Procedures in which a small piece of vein or artery is used to bypass a coronary artery

Coronary artery disease: Occurs when atherosclerotic changes are detected in the arteries of the heart

Corpora cavernosa: Erectile tissue

Corpora spongiosum: Tissue that lies under the corpora cavernosa and forms the internal shape of the penis, with a bulbous shape at the end of the penis, and helps to prevent urethral compression during erection

Corpus uteri: Also known as the uterus, is the body of the uterus above the internal os of the cervix and connects to the fallopian tubes at the fundus at the top of the uterus

Corrosion: Burns due to chemicals

Cortical cataract: Cataracts that begin on the peripheral edges of the lens and work their way inward toward the center

Counseling: The discussion between a healthcare provider and a patient and/or patient's family

Coverage limitations: The services that an insurance plan will pay for (cover) when they are provided by a healthcare practitioner, as well as what services will not be covered and classified as the patient's out-of-pocket charges

Covered entity: As amended by HITECH, (1) a health plan, (2) a healthcare clearinghouse, (3) a healthcare provider who transmits any health information in electronic form in connection with a transaction covered by this subchapter (45 CFR 160.103 2013)

Craniectomy: The removal of a portion of the skull

Craniotomy: An incision into the skull

Creation: Inserting biological or synthetic material to form a new body part that to the extent possible replicates the anatomic structure or function of an absent body part

Cross-reference: Instructs the coder to look elsewhere for a code

Current Procedural Terminology (CPT): A comprehensive, descriptive list of terms and associated numeric and alphanumeric codes used for reporting diagnostic and therapeutic procedures and other medical services performed by physicians; published and updated annually by the American Medical Association (AMA 2019a)

Cytopathology: Study that examines cells from a specimen to determine a cause or nature of a disease

Data analytics: The science of examining raw data with the purpose of drawing conclusions about that information. It includes data mining, machine language, development of models, and statistical measurements. Analytics can be descriptive, predictive, or prescriptive

Date of service: The date a test, procedure, or service was rendered

Debridement: The removal of dead, diseased, infected, or otherwise nonviable tissue from a wound to improve the healing ability of the area

Deductible: 1. The amount of cost, usually annual, that the policyholder must incur (and pay) before

(Continued on next page)

the insurance plan will assume liability for remaining covered expenses. **2.** Under Medicare, the amount a beneficiary must pay for healthcare before Medicare begins to pay, either for each benefit period for Part A, or each year for Part B, these amounts can change every year (CMS 2006)

Deep vein thrombosis (DVT): Blood clot that forms in the deep veins of the lower extremities

Definitive diagnosis: The condition or disease that has been confirmed to be the cause of the signs exhibited or symptoms experienced

De-identified documentation: 1. The act of removing from a health record or data set any information that could be used to identify the individual to whom the data apply in order to protect his or her confidentiality **2.** To remove the names of the principal investigator (PI), co-investigators, and affiliated organizations to allow reviewers to maintain objectivity

Delivery: Assisting the passage of the products of conception from the genital canal

Dementia: Loss of memory and mental abilities due to an underlying physical change in the brain

Depression: A mental disorder that affects a person's mood, thoughts, and actions

Destination: Location where the patient is taken by ambulance service

Destruction: 1. A procedure that destroys tissue performed in several different ways including laser surgery, electrosurgery, cryosurgery, chemosurgery, surgical curettement, radiocautery, radiofrequency ablation, or tissue volume reduction; also called *ablation*; **2.** Physical eradication of all or a portion of a body part by the direct use of energy, force, or a destructive agent

Detachment: Cutting off all of a portion of the upper or lower extremities

Device: Any material or appliance that remains after a procedure is performed

Diabetes mellitus: A condition in which the body does not control the amount of glucose (sugar) in the blood, and the kidneys excrete large amounts of urine

Diagnosis: A word or phrase used by a physician to identify a medical condition from which an individual patient suffers or a reason for which the patient needs, seeks, or receives healthcare

Diagnosis-related group (DRGs): 1. A unit of case-mix classification adopted by the federal government and some other payers as a prospective payment mechanism for hospital inpatients in which diseases are placed into

groups because related diseases and treatments tend to consume similar amounts of healthcare resources and incur similar amounts of cost; in the Medicare and Medicaid programs, one of more than 500 diagnostic classifications in which cases demonstrate similar resource consumption and length-of-stay patterns. Under the prospective payment system (PPS), hospitals are paid a set fee for treating patients in a single DRG category, regardless of the actual cost of care for the individual. **2.** A classification system that groups patients according to diagnosis, type of treatment, age, and other relevant criteria. Under the prospective payment system, hospitals are paid a set fee for treating patients in a single DRG category, regardless of the actual cost of care for the individual (CMS 2006)

Diagnostic and Statistical Manual of Mental Disorders (DSM-5): A nomenclature developed by the American Psychiatric Association to standardize the diagnostic process for patients with psychiatric disorders; the fifth edition is the product of more than 10 years of effort by hundreds of international experts in all aspects of mental health (APA 2019)

Diagnostic procedure: Procedure that is performed to determine a diagnosis

Dialysis: The process of filtering waste products from the blood, which replaces the function of the kidneys for patients with end-stage renal disease or renal failure

Diaphragm: 1. A barrier birth control method in which a small, cup-like device is placed over the cervix during intercourse, along with spermicide that is later removed; **2.** A muscle that lies underneath the thoracic cavity, separating the heart and lungs from the abdominal contents

Dilation: Expanding an orifice of the lumen of a tubular body part

Dislocation reduction: The act of relocating a joint to its original location, in the case of joint dislocation or subluxation (partial dislocation) dislodged and traveling into the lungs

Displaced fracture: Fracture in which the bone moves so the two ends of the bones are misaligned

Dissecting aneurysm: Aneurysm that contains a small tear in the inner lining of the arterial walls, in which blood is beginning to accumulate

Distal: Away from the body (the fingertips)

Diverticulitis: The inflammation of the diverticula small pockets lining the inside of the intestines

Diverticulosis: A condition in which diverticula begin forming within the intestines

Division: Cutting into a body part, without draining fluids or gases from the body part, to separate or transect a body part

Dominant side: The side of the body that the patient prefers when performing daily functions, such as writing with the right hand

Doppler ultrasound: A special technique that uses color-coded mapping during the ultrasound procedure, which allows the viewer to see oxygenated and de-oxygenated blood flow through body organs in real time

Dosimetry: Process performed to calculate the exact radiation dose amount

Drainage: Taking or letting out fluids or gases from a body part

Durable Medical Equipment (DME): Medical equipment designed for long-term use in the home, including eyeglasses, hearing aids, surgical appliances and supplies, orthotics and prostheses, and bulk and cylinder oxygen (CMS 2006)

Durable Medical Equipment, Prosthetics, Orthotics, and Supplies (DMEPOS): A category of durable medical equipment supplies that includes prosthetics and orthotics

Dyslexia: Difficulty reading

Dysphagia: Difficulty swallowing

Eating disorders: Disorders that affect the way a person eats or processes food and nutrition; there are two common types of eating disorders, anorexia nervosa and bulimia

Electrical stimulation: Therapeutic modality that causes one muscle or a group of muscles to contract, which helps to increase muscle strength and blood supply to the muscle, and decrease pain

Electrocardiogram (ECG/EKG): Procedure that records the heart's electrical activity as a line tracing on paper and can be used to evaluate heart rhythm and function

Electroconvulsive therapy (ECT): Involves the application of an electric current to a patient's brain to produce a seizure or series of seizures to alleviate mental illness

Electrodiagnostic studies: A way of measuring the electrical activity in muscles and nerves that can help diagnose the cause or specific area from which pain is originating

Electroencephalogram (EEG): A diagnostic study of the electrical impulses of the brain

Electromyography (EMG): Evaluates the condition of muscle and nerves to determine the cause of pain, such as a pinched nerve or a diseased muscle (Mount Sinai Hospital n.d.a)

Electronic brachytherapy: The use of a small, high-dose x-ray source, applied directly to the malignancy

Electronic Protected Health Information (e-PHI): Protected health information (PHI) that is stored in an electronic format. As amended by HITECH, means information that comes within paragraphs (1)(i) or (1)(ii) of this definition of protected health information as specified in this section which is (1)(i) information transmitted by electronic media, and (1)(ii) information maintained in electronic media (45 CFR 160.103)

Embolus: Thrombosis that dislodges from the vessel and begins to travel through the blood

Emergency department: Facility that provides same-day care for patients with healthcare emergencies or urgent healthcare needs and may be either a standalone facility or attached to a larger facility, such as a hospital

Emergency services: Services provided to patients in a life-threatening situation, when loss of life or limb is imminent

Emergency transportation: Ambulance service that responds immediately to the scene of an accident or incident to provide medical assistance and transport to a healthcare facility if necessary

Emergent: Life-threatening medical issues

Employer-sponsored insurance: An umbrella term used to describe health plans that are funded directly by employers to provide coverage for their employees exclusively in which employers establish accounts to cover their employees' medical expenses and retain control over the funds but bear the risk of paying claims greater than their estimates

Encounter: The face-to-face contact between a patient and a provider who has primary responsibility for assessing and treating the condition of the patient at a given time and who exercises independent judgment in the care of the patient

Encryption: The process of transforming text into an unintelligible string of characters that can be transmitted via communications media with a high degree of security and then decrypted when it reaches a secure destination

Endocervical curettage (ECC): Cervical tissue removal in which a curette is used to scrape cells off of the cervical canal

Endoscopic retrograde cholangiopancreatography (ERCP): A procedure performed to both diagnose and treat, when necessary, blockages of the pancreatic and bile ducts

Endoscopy: A procedure performed with the aid of an endoscope—a device with a small camera attached

Endotracheal intubation: Procedure performed to maintain an open airway, or to allow the administration of certain drugs, such as anesthesia (also called intubation)

Endovascular procedure: Procedure in which a catheter is inserted into the body to perform a procedure; literally, the procedure is performed "inside the vessel"

Enforcement Rule: Part of HIPAA that contains provisions that cover compliance to HIPAA rules and regulations, investigations into breaches in privacy, and the imposition of monetary penalties for HIPAA violations

Enthesopathy: An inflammation of the tendon or ligament at the site of attachment to the bone, which causes pain, tenderness, stiffness, and swelling

Entitlement health insurance: A type of insurance coverage for which individuals must be eligible, based on differing criteria

Enucleation: Removing the eyeball while leaving the orbital structures intact, including the extraocular muscles

Epididymis: A duct behind the testes, in which newly created sperm cells mature and then move into the vas deferens

Epidural steroid injection: A minimally invasive procedure that can treat pain in the neck, shoulders, arms, back, buttocks, and legs, resulting from irritation of spinal nerves due to conditions such as herniated discs, degenerative disc disease, and arthritis; it is an injection of long-lasting corticosteroid, which is an anti-inflammatory agent, and not an anesthetic substance

Epilepsy: A neurological condition that manifests in sensory disturbances, loss of consciousness, and seizures (convulsions) as a result of abnormal electrical activity in the brain

Episode of care: 1. In home health, all home care services and nonroutine medical supplies delivered to a patient during a 60-day period; the episode of care is the unit of payment under the home health prospective payment system (HHPPS) **2.** The healthcare services given during a certain period of time, usually during a hospital stay (CMS 2006)

Eponym: Coding convention in ICD-10-CM codes assigned to diseases or syndromes named for a person; listed in the alphabetic index as main terms in the Index

Esophagogastroduodenoscopy (EGD): A common type of endoscopic examination of the digestive system that is a complete examination from the esophagus to the duodenum at the end of the stomach

Essential modifier: In ICD-10-CM and ICD-10-PCS, they qualify the main term by listing alternative sites, etiology or clinical status. It is indented two spaces under the main term; also called subterms

Established patient: A patient who has received professional services from the physician or another physician of the same specialty in the same practice group within the past three years

Etiology: The cause of a disease

Evaluation and management (E/M) service: A patient encounter with a healthcare professional in which the patient receives assessment, counseling, or routine health services

Evaluation and management services section: The first section of Category I codes in the CPT code book; these codes describe patient encounters with healthcare and make up the majority of all codes reported for professional services in either the inpatient or outpatient setting

Evisceration: The removal of the contents of the globe of the eye, while leaving the remaining structures intact

Examination: The act of evaluating the body to determine the presence or absence of disease

Excised diameter: The size of the lesion in addition to the margins around the lesion that were removed

Excision: Cutting out or off a portion of a body part without replacement

Excludes 1: Under ICD-10-CM, a type 1 Excludes note is a pure excludes note. It means "not coded here." An Excludes 1 note indicates that the code excluded should never be used at the same time as the code above the note (NCHS 2019)

Excludes 2: A type 2 Excludes note represents "not included here." An Excludes 2 note indicates that the condition excluded is not a part of the condition represented by the code, but a patient may have both conditions at the same time (NCHS 2019)

Excludes notes: Identify conditions that are similar but independent of each other

Exenteration: [Of the orbit] the removal of the eye and ocular adnexa

External cause codes: Codes used to identify the circumstances surrounding an injury, poisoning, or adverse event, such as the activity that the patient was engaged in when the injury occurred, where the patient was when the injury took place, and the injury mechanism (how the injury happened)

External Causes of Injury Index: Location where codes identifying the external cause of an injury or illness are listed

External os: Lower end of the cervix

Extirpation: Taking or cutting out solid matter from a body part

Extracapsular cataract extraction (ECCE): In this procedure the lens is either broken up via phacoemulsification or it is surgically removed in one piece, leaving the lens capsule intact

Extracorporeal shock wave lithotripsy (ESWL): A procedure in which shock waves are sent through the patient's body to break up a nephrolithiasis into tiny fragments

Extraction: Pulling or stripping out or off all or a portion of a body part by the use of force

Facet joint injection: Injections made into the facet joint of the vertebra, used to treat pain coming from the small joints of the spine

Fallopian tubes: Oviducts resembling long tubes that are attached to the fundus of the uterus and end with small finger-like fimbriae, through which eggs released from the ovaries travel

Fascia: a sheet of connective tissue that encloses the structures of the muscles and other internal organs, and subfascial tissues are underneath the fascial layers, such as muscles

Fee schedule: A complete listing of fees used by health plans to pay doctors or other providers (CMS 2006)

Fee-for-service: A method of reimbursement through which providers retrospectively receive payment based on either billed charges for services provided or on annually updated fee schedules

Fibromyalgia: A myalgia characterized by chronic, full-body pain, with a sensitivity to pressure; also causes fatigue, problems sleeping, memory problems, restless leg syndrome, numbness or tingling, and other psychological factors, such as depression and anxiety

First-listed diagnosis: In outpatient coding, this is the first diagnosis code that is listed on a claim when more than one diagnosis code is applicable

Foreign body (FB): Any unnatural object that is present inside the body or organ structure

Fragmentation: Breaking solid matter in a body part into pieces

Frozen block: A frozen piece of a specimen

Frozen section: For procedures that need a pathological examination quickly, the specimen may be frozen rapidly into a frozen block (a frozen piece of a specimen), which is cut into small slices of the tissue (a frozen section), and visualized under a microscope

Fundoplasty: A procedure in which the fundus of the stomach (the top bulging part of the stomach) is wrapped around the lower end of the esophagus, underneath the diaphragm

Fusion: Joining together portions of an articular body part rendering the articular body part immobile

Gastric bypass: Also called a Roux-en-Y procedure, a procedure in which a small stomach pouch is created by dividing the top of the stomach from the rest of the stomach; the first portion of the small intestine is separated and attached to the top stomach pouch, in essence creating a small stomach out of the larger stomach

Gastroenterologist: A healthcare provider who specializes in the diagnosis and treatment of disorders of the digestive system, including but not limited to disorders of the esophagus, stomach, intestines, colon, and rectum and anus

Gastroesophageal reflux disease (GERD): A common condition that causes heartburn, indigestion, and chest pain in affected individuals

General anesthesia: The administration of a substance that results in a complete loss of consciousness in order to produce analgesia to facilitate a surgical or other healthcare procedure (Palmetto 2013)

Gestation: The time period between conception (the moment at which the egg is fertilized) and birth (when the fetus is delivered)

Gestational condition: Condition that is a direct result from pregnancy

Glaucoma: A buildup of intraocular pressure that causes damage to the eye's optic nerve over time, and may eventually lead to irreversible vision loss

Global period: Amount of time included in the surgical package

Global radiology service: The performance of both components of the procedure—professional and technical—by the same facility

Global surgical package: A set of services that are included within a single code that identify the surgery performed, other services that are integral

(Continued on next page)

to the procedure, and a certain amount of time after the surgery

Goniolens: An ophthalmic endoscope

Gout: A painful type of arthritis that results from a buildup of uric acid in the bloodstream, which forms needle-like crystals, causing swelling, redness, heat, and stiffness in the joints

Government-sponsored insurance: A type of entitlement health insurance coverage that is provided by the government and managed at either the state or the federal level or a combination thereof, depending on the type of insurance

Gravida: Pregnant female

Greenstick fracture: Fracture that occurs when a bone bends and cracks on one side

Gross examination: An examination of the physical characteristics of the specimen, including the size, weight, consistency, and visual features such as discoloring

Gustilo-Anderson classification: Classification used to identify the type of open fracture, which is included as part of the code description for open fractures

Gynecologists: Healthcare providers who specialize in the health of the female reproductive system including the vagina, uterus, and ovaries, as well as the breasts

Habilitative services: Services that help a patient keep, learn, or improve skills and functions of daily living

HCC coding: Coding that is specially focused on capturing all patient conditions that impact the hierarchical condition category, and which are fully supported by documentation in the health record

HCPCS Level I codes: Commonly referred to as CPT and developed, maintained, and copyrighted by the AMA, these codes represent the healthcare procedure, treatment, or service provided at the healthcare encounter

HCPCS Level II codes: Commonly referred to as CPT as simply HCPCS or Level II codes, are codes developed, maintained, and published by CMS that represent the supply, service, or other treatment provided to the patient; they also include ambulance services

Health insurance exchange: Government-run health insurance exchange that allows insurance companies to offer health insurance plans to individuals, who must pay premiums for coverage

Health Insurance Marketplace: The federal online health insurance exchange that allows individuals

to purchase insurance plans offered by commercial companies

Health Insurance Portability and Accountability Act (HIPAA): The federal legislation enacted to provide continuity of health coverage, control fraud and abuse in healthcare, reduce healthcare costs, and guarantee the security and privacy of health information; limits exclusion for pre-existing medical conditions, prohibits discrimination against employees and dependents based on health status, guarantees availability of health insurance to small employers, and guarantees renewability of insurance to all employees regardless of size; requires covered entities (most healthcare providers and organizations) to transmit healthcare claims in a specific format and to develop, implement, and comply with the standards of the Privacy Rule and the Security Rule; and mandates that covered entities apply for and utilize national identifiers in HIPAA transactions (Public Law 104-191 1996)

Healthcare billing: The practice of sending a coded healthcare claim to a third-party payer or insurance company for payment, described in full in Chapter 2, and then following that claim until it is paid in full

Healthcare codes: The numeric or alphanumeric translations of all the services, supplies, treatments, diagnoses, conditions, and other reasons for medical treatments

Healthcare coding: The practice of assigning numeric or alphanumeric codes to identify the treatment, services, or supplies provided to a patient during a healthcare encounter, also known as the procedure

Healthcare Common Procedure Coding System (HCPCS): A medical code set that identifies healthcare procedures, equipment, and supplies for claim submission purposes. It has been selected for use in the HIPAA transactions. HCPCS Level I contains numeric CPT codes which are maintained by the AMA. HCPCS Level II contains alphanumeric codes used to identify various items and services that are not included in the CPT medical code set (CMS 2006)

Healthcare operations: Includes various services provided by healthcare practitioners during which patient PHI may be accessed and used

Healthcare provider: Physician or other qualified healthcare professional who is qualified by education, training, licensure/regulation (when applicable), and facility privileging (when applicable) who performs a professional service within his/her scope of practice and independently reports that professional service (AMA 2019b, xiii)

Healthcare specialty: A branch of healthcare practice in which a provider specializes after completing his or her residency after medical school, typically divided among four possible characteristics—surgical or internal technique, body or organ system, diagnostic or therapeutic services, or the age of patients treated

Heart failure: A condition in which the heart cannot pump enough blood to meet the body's needs

Hematologist: A healthcare provider who specializes in the diagnosis, treatment, and prevention of diseases of the blood (hematology)

Hemodialysis: The process of filtering the blood of waste products, through the use of a dialyzer machine, which removes the waste products from the blood

Hemorrhoids: Inflamed or swollen veins located near the anus or lower rectum, inside the rectal canal; sometimes referred to as piles

Hemothorax: Blood in the pleural cavity

Hierarchical Condition Category (HCC): The practice of categorizing all patient diagnosis claims within groups of conditions, which are positioned strategically in order of risk from least to most risky

Histologic type: The specific type of microscopic structure of the growth such as carcinoma, myeloma, or sarcoma

History of present illness (HPI): A chronological description of the development of the patient's present illness from the first sign or symptom or from the previous encounter to the present

History: The pertinent information about the patient, including chief complaint, past and present illnesses, family history, social history, and review of body systems

Homograft: A skin graft taken from a donor of the same species

Hospital: A healthcare entity that has an organized medical staff and permanent facilities that include inpatient beds and continuous medical or nursing services and that provides diagnostic and therapeutic services for patients as well as overnight accommodations and nutritional services

Hospital-acquired condition (HAC): A condition that a patient acquires at a hospital that results in additional resources being required to care for that patient

Hubbard tank: A large tub in which the patient can be fully immersed, to allow patients to perform exercises while in the water

Hydration: The administration of fluids or electrolytes without the presence of drugs

Hydrocele: A fluid-filled sac that can cause pain and discomfort

Hypercholesterolemia: A condition in which there are high levels of cholesterol in the blood

Hyperlipidemia: A condition in which there are high levels of lipids, or fats, in the blood

Hypernasality: Excessive nasal tone to the voice

Hypertension: High blood pressure

Imaging services: An inclusive term used for the wide array of different types of techniques used to produce images of the inside of the body, including radiology services, ultrasounds, fluoroscopy, and nuclear imaging

Immune globulin: Serum globulins that are extracted from human blood, or recombinant immune globulin products created in a laboratory through genetic modification of human and/or animal proteins

Impacted fracture: Fracture in which the ends of a bone are pushed into each other

Implantable cardiac defibrillator (ICD): A small device similar to a pacemaker that monitors the heart rate and delivers a small shock to the heart when it detects heart-threatening arrhythmias

Incidental appendectomy: Performed in addition to a primary procedure within the abdomen

Incidental pregnancy: Pregnancy that in no way complicates the reason for the healthcare encounter

Incision and drainage (I&D): A procedure performed on an abscess or cyst that requires drainage and consists of cutting into the skin above the cyst or abscess to allow for drainage of the pustular material; a treatment performed for soft tissue abscesses, for which medical treatment alone is insufficient; the abscess is incised with a sharp blade and drained of material

Incision: A cut made on a body part or organ

Includes notes: Coding convention in ICD-10-CM; a note listed below certain tabular list categories to further define, clarify or provide examples

Inclusion terms: These terms work similarly to includes notes, but instead pertain to specific codes, rather than a category of codes; they may be synonyms for the condition, or may be a list of various conditions that are assigned to a specific code

Indented code: Codes indented beneath a standalone code that depend on the explanation of the procedure within the standalone (or parent) code to complete the description of the indented code

Independent laboratory: A facility that is recognized and accredited to test and evaluate patient specimens as an independent entity free from a hospital or private practice

Independent radiology and imaging center: An office that specializes in only radiology and imaging techniques

Index to Diseases and Injury: The main index to the ICD-10-CM code book, often referred to as the Main Index

Individual insurance: Insurance plan that is purchased by a single individual, who does not go through an employer to attain coverage

Inferior: Toward the bottom of the body (the feet)

Infusion: The administration of a diagnostic, prophylactic, or therapeutic fluid or drug, given over a period of time longer than 15 minutes

Initial encounter: This episode of care is used during the active treatment phase of a condition, or when the patient is still receiving active treatment for a condition

Initial Preventive Physical Examination (IPPE): Also known as the "Welcome to Medicare" visit, this is a once in a lifetime benefit provided to a Medicare recipient, the goal of which is health promotion, disease prevention, and detection; it is only allowed during this first 12-month period, after which the patient may not receive the benefit

Injection: Administration of a therapeutic substance given intramuscularly

Injury mechanism: The way an injury happens

Inpatient: A patient who is provided with room, board, and continuous general nursing services in an area of an acute care facility where patients generally stay at least overnight

Inpatient Prospective Payment System (IPPS): The prospective payment system used in the inpatient facility setting, in which the diagnosis code(s) and procedure code(s) are combined using diagnosis-related groups

Insertion: Putting a nonbiological appliance that monitors, assists, performs, or prevents a physiological function but does not physically take the place of a body part

Inspection: Visually or manually exploring a body part

Insurance policy: 1. A purchased contract (policy) according to which the purchaser (insured) is protected from loss by the insurer's agreeing to reimburse for such loss 2. Reduction of a person's (insured's) exposure to risk by having another party (insurer) assume the risk

Insured party: A holder of a health insurance policy

Integrative medicine: Consists of complementary and alternative therapies that may be used to treat chronic pain

Intensity Modulated Radiation Treatment Delivery (IMRT): A radiation treatment method that uses computer-based mapping to create dosing distributions delivered by a radiotherapy treatment machine

Intent: Intent of the toxic effect is the reason why the toxic effect happened

Intentional self-harm: A toxic effect resulting from intentional self-harm is due to a substance that is taken deliberately as an act of hurting one's self

Interactive complexity: A psychotherapy service that is provided to a patient with specific communication factors that complicate delivery of psychiatric procedures

Intermediate ophthalmological services: Ophthalmological services that include an evaluation of a new or existing condition complicated with a new diagnosis

Internal fixation device: A device that is inserted into or across a bone or set of bones to fix it into place

Internal medicine provider: Provider who establishes the diagnosis and treatment of patients without using surgical techniques

Internal os: The upper end of the cervix, which opens into the uterus

International Classification of Disease (ICD): Code set developed by the World Health Organization and revised for usage in the United States through a development committee composed of CMS, NCHS, AHA, and AHIMA

International Classification of Diseases, Eleventh Revision, ICD-11: Coding classification system currently in development, and is expected to be implemented after 2018

International Classification of Diseases, Ninth Revision, ICD-9: Code set composed of three volumes, all published in the same code book: Volumes one and two are the index and tabular listings for diagnosis codes, and volume three contains procedure codes and was replaced by the ICD-10-PCS code set, which is used in essentially the same manner, but has greatly expanded the specificity for reporting inpatient procedures

International Classification of Diseases, Tenth Revision, Clinical Modification ICD-10-CM: The coding classification system that replaced ICD-9-CM, Volumes 1 and 2, on October 1,

2015. ICD-10-CM is the United States' clinical modification of the WHO's ICD-10. ICD-10-CM has a total of 21 chapters and contains significantly more codes than ICD-9-CM, providing the ability to code with a greater level of specificity (CDC 2019)

International Classification of Diseases, Tenth Revision, Procedure Coding System ICD-10-PCS: The coding classification system that replaced ICD-9-CM, Volume 3, on October 1, 2015. ICD-10-PCS has 16 sections and contains significantly more procedure codes than ICD-9-CM, providing the ability to code procedures with a greater level of specificity (CDC 2019)

Interspace: The space between two vertebrae

Interstitial brachytherapy: Brachytherapy that involves placing the radioactive elements into a body cavity, such as the vagina or the bladder

Interventional pain procedures: A range of different procedures that use invasive interventions to treat the patient's pain, that include epidural injections, medial branch blocks and facet joint injections, radiofrequency nerve ablations, joint injections, occipital nerve blocks, and kyphoplasty

Intracapsular cataract extraction (ICCE): This procedure removes both the lens and the lens capsule, and is performed only in rare cases

Intracavitary brachytherapy: Brachytherapy that involves placing the radioactive elements directly into the tumor or organ

Intractable condition: Condition that does not respond to medical treatment

Intraocular pressure: The pressure inside the eyeball

Intrauterine device (IUD): A small, T-shaped device inserted into the uterus for birth control purposes

Introduction: The insertion of a device, object, or substance into a body part or organ

Introitus: The vagina orifice

Invalid code: A code that is not extended out to seven characters and may not be used for coding or billing purposes

Iontophoresis: A form of electrical stimulation that is used to push medication through the skin to the affected body area, muscle, tendon, or ligament

Ipsilateral: The same side of the body (the right upper and lower extremities)

Keratoplasty: A corneal transplant, or a procedure that replaces the cornea with a donor cornea graft

Kidney: Bean-shaped organ that functions to filter waste products from the blood and to control electrolyte balance and the body's balance of fluid

Kyphoplasty: A treatment for vertebral compression fractures and the pain they cause where a balloon is threaded through an incision in the back, to the site of the compression fracture, and slowly inflated to push the compressed bone back into place; once in place, cement is injected into the area to hold the bone in the proper position (Mount Sinai Hospital n.d.b)

Kyphosis: A condition in which the back rounds forward

Labia majora: The tissue that surrounds the labia minora and the clitoris

Labia minora: Skin that surrounds the vaginal vestibule and the external urethra

Laboratory and pathology services: Diagnostic analyses of bodily tissue samples, such as urine, blood, or tissue

Language disorder: Difficulty with understanding or producing oral speech

Laparoscopy: Procedure that uses a fiber-optic laparoscope inserted into the body through several small incisions to perform a diagnostic or therapeutic procedure

Large group practice: A practice that may have anywhere from six to dozens of providers

Last menstrual period (LMP): The first day of the patient's last period (start of menstruation)

Lateral: Away from the midline of the body (the sides)

Lateral (view): Two projections during an imaging service consisting of two views that pass from one side of the body to the other (for example, from the right to the left)

Laterality: Refers to the side on which a condition appears

Legacy system: A type of computer system that uses older technology but may still perform optimally

Lifestyle impairments: Descriptions of how the patient's eye condition has negatively impacted his or her lifestyle

Living donor: The organ being donated is one that can be harvested from a living patient

Local anesthesia: Anesthesia blocks a small amount of nerves using an injection or a topical cream or spray that numbs a specific amount of the body

Loop electrosurgical excision procedure (LEEP): Procedure in which a fine wire with an electrical charge is used to remove cervical tissue

Lower urinary tract symptoms (LUTS): The different symptoms that can be present with benign prostatic hyperplasia, such as urinary frequency, urinary retention, or urinary urgency

Lumbago: Low back pain

Lumbar puncture: A diagnostic procedure used to evaluate cerebrospinal fluid that surrounds the brain and spinal cord (also called a spinal tap)

Lund-Browder classification: Chart that divides the body's surface into differing percentages, depending on the age of the patient

Macular degeneration: A deterioration of the central portion of the retina, called the macula

Magnetic resonance imaging (MRI): A form of imaging that utilizes strong magnetic fields and radio waves to produce detailed images of the anatomy and physiology of the internal structures of a patient's body, and can be used to diagnose a range of medical conditions

Main term: The noun that describes the patient's diagnosis or reason for encounter

Major complication/comorbidity (MCC): A higher-severity complication/comorbidity that requires more resources, treatment, or prolonged inpatient stay

Malignant neoplasm: Commonly referred to as cancer, these neoplasms invade surrounding tissues and destroy them, and can be fatal

Malunion: Occurs when the bones have fused back together in the wrong position after a fracture

Mammography: An x-ray image of the breast used to diagnose breast conditions such as tumors or fibrocystic diseases

Manifestation: Coding convention in ICD-10-CM; a condition that occurs as the result of another

Manipulation: Manually moving one body part into its original location or into another location; the attempt to return a fractured bone to its original location with manually applied forces

Map: Locating the route of passage of electrical impulses or locating functional areas in a body part

Margin: The area around a lesion that is excised in addition to the lesion

Marsupialization: A procedure in which a cyst is incised along one edge to form an open pouch, and then sutured open to allow for continuous drainage

Maternal fetal medicine (MFM) specialist: A medical doctor who specializes in high-risk pregnancies and focuses on the health of the mother and fetus before, during, and after pregnancy

Maternity services: Procedure or condition is one that is performed on a pregnant woman or related to a woman's pregnancy, such as a delivery or complication of pregnancy

Medial: Toward the midline of the body (the belly button)

Mediastinum: The area within the thorax in-between the lungs

Medicaid: A joint federal and state program that helps with medical costs for some people with low incomes and limited resources. Medicaid programs vary from state to state, but most healthcare costs are covered if a patient qualifies for both Medicare and Medicaid (CMS 2006)

Medical decision-making (MDM): The portion of the evaluation and management encounter in which the healthcare provider makes a decision about the patient's diagnosis and care or treatment plan

Medical necessity: 1. The likelihood that a proposed healthcare service will have a reasonable beneficial effect on the patient's physical condition and quality of life at a specific point in his or her illness or lifetime **2.** The concept that procedures are only eligible for reimbursement as a covered benefit when they are performed for a specific diagnosis or specified frequency (42 CFR 405.500 1995)

Medicare: A federally funded health program established in 1965 to assist with the medical care costs of Americans 65 years of age and older as well as other individuals entitled to Social Security benefits owing to their disabilities (CMS 2006)

Medicine section: The last section of the Category I codes in the CPT code book; it is a miscellaneous grouping of all of the procedures, treatments, studies, and tests that can be performed on patients, which do not belong elsewhere in the book

Medigap: A supplemental insurance policy that is specifically for Medicare beneficiaries designed to "fill the gap" left by patient out-of-pocket expenses such as copayments, deductibles, and coinsurance amounts

Mental health: A person's emotional, psychological, and social well-being

Mental illness: A condition that affects a person's thinking, feeling, or mood, and affects a person's ability to perform major life activities and functions each day

Metastasis: Offshoots (spreading) of the original cancer

Methicillin-resistant *Staphylococcus aureus* (MRSA): A bacterium that can cause infections throughout the human body; it is resistant to certain antibiotics, making it especially hard to treat and cure

Microscopic examination: The examination of the specimen at a microscopic level, which allows the pathologist to visualize the cells of a specimen

Mid-level provider: In addition to physicians, healthcare providers who are also trained, qualified, and licensed to provide healthcare services

Minimum necessary: States that only the least amount of information needed for treatment, payment, and healthcare operations may be released from a patient's health record

Minor surgical procedure: Minimally invasive (meaning that they only break the skin or mucous membranes and connective tissues) procedures that do not require any general anesthesia or respiratory assistance during the procedure

Moderate (conscious) sedation: A drug-induced depression of consciousness that allows a patient to respond to commands and tactile stimulation during a medical or surgical procedure; a type of anesthesia given either orally or via an injection that allows the patient to be sedated but awake, so he or she can respond to commands if necessary

Modifier: A two-digit numeric code listed after a procedure code that indicates that a service was altered in some way from the stated CPT descriptor without changing the definition; also used to enhance a code narrative to describe the circumstances of each procedure or service and how it individually applies to a patient

Modifying factors: Factors similar to CPT modifiers, that add additional information to the anesthesia procedure description and describe an anesthesia procedure that was more complex than it would have been had it been performed on a normal, healthy patient, or that required additional skill to complete

Modifying term: Term that alters (or modifies) the main term; it is indented below the main term, and present different versions of the procedure

Mohs micrographic surgery: Surgery used for the removal of complex and ill-defined skin malignancies, and includes the examination of all the excised margins; the surgeon acts as both the surgeon and the pathologist

Monitored anesthesia care (MAC): An anesthesia service that is made up of a conscious sedation, control of patient anxiety, and pain control

Monoarthritis: Arthritis in a localized joint

Morphology: The science of structure and form of organisms without regard to function

Motor vehicle accident (MVA): Any type of accident that involves any type of motor vehicle

Multiaxial structure: A code structure in which each individual character within the code can represent a specific detail of the procedure performed

Multiple sclerosis (MS): A disease that affects the central nervous system and causes nerve deterioration and damage

Musculoskeletal system: The body system comprised of all the bones, joints, muscles, cartilage, tendons, and ligaments in the human body

Myalgia: Muscle pain, which may be a symptom of many healthcare conditions including overuse of the muscle, overstretching, infection, or disease process

Mycology: The study of fungi

Myocardial infarction: The death of a portion of the heart muscle due to lack of oxygen supply; otherwise known as a heart attack

Myositis: An inflammation of the muscle that can be caused by an infection, injury, medicine, or a chronic disease, and causes muscle weakness and pain, along with other symptoms

Narcosynthesis for psychiatric purposes: The administration of sodium amobarbitol, otherwise known as a truth serum, which hinders inhibitions so that a psychiatric interview can be conducted

Nasal packing: Procedure performed for uncontrollable hemorrhage from the nose (epistaxis or bloody nose)

National Correct Coding Initiative (NCCI): Program developed to promote national correct coding methodologies and to control improper coding leading to inappropriate payment in Part B claims (CMS 2019)

Nature of the presenting problem: The type of condition for which the patient is receiving the evaluation and management service

Neoplasm: An abnormal growth of tissue that can be fast-growing and invasive, such as malignant cancer, or a benign mass or tumor

Neoplasm of uncertain behavior: Neoplasms that have not yet been confirmed as any of the other three types (benign, malignant, or ca in situ) and require further evaluation and testing before their behavior can be determined

Nephrolithiasis: Kidney stones

Nephrolithotomy: Incision into the kidney for the removal of a kidney stone

Nephrologist: A medical doctor who focuses on the diagnosis and treatment of conditions of the kidneys

Nerve condition study (NCS): A test that activates nerves and gauges their responses as a way of determining if there is a problem with the functioning of the nerve

Neurologist: A medical doctor who specializes in the diagnosis and treatment of neurological disorders, including disorders of the nerves and the nervous system

Neuropsychiatry: The treatment of mental or behavioral disturbances as a result of neurological

Neurosurgery: Surgical treatment of disorders of the nerves and nervous system

Never events: A term coined in 2001 by Ken Kizer of the National Quality Forum (NCF) to identify serious errors in medical treatment that should never happen (AHRQ 2019)

New patient: An individual who has not received professional services from the physician, or any other physician of the same specialty in the same practice group before or within three years; an individual who has not received professional services from any provider of a organization/healthcare facility before or within three years

Non-ambulatory: Unable to walk about independently

Noncovered services: Services not reimbursable under a managed care plan

Non-displaced fracture: Fracture in which the bone itself is fractured, but the bone has not moved and is still properly aligned

Nonemergency transportation: Ambulance services typically scheduled in advance for patient transfers from one facility to another, or to transport non-ambulatory patients for healthcare

Nonessential modifier: Words located in parentheses next to the main term or a subterm within the Index that offer more information, but do not impact code selection

Non-obstetric: Refers to a procedure performed to treat or manage signs and symptoms, or other healthcare encounter for gynecological or genitourinary services, such as reproductive, urinary, and breast health

Non-pressure ulcer: An ulcer on the skin that was caused by anything other than pressure, such as one caused by atherosclerosis of the extremities (and loss of blood circulation), chronic venous hypertension, diabetes mellitus, postthrombotic syndrome, postphlebitic syndrome, or varicose veins

Non-ruptured aneurysms: Often symptom-less aneurysms that are typically found during a radiological imaging procedure

Nonspecific test: Tests for a quality, such as whether or not any type of drug from a drug class is present

Nonunion: Occurs when the bones have not fused back together after a fracture

Not elsewhere classifiable (NEC): In ICD-10-CM this abbreviation in the Alphabetic Index represents "other specified" when a specific code is not available for a condition (NCHS 2019)

Not otherwise specified (NOS): In ICD-10-CM this abbreviation is the equivalent of unspecified (NCHS 2019)

Notice of Privacy Practices: As amended by HITECH, a statement (mandated by the HIPAA Privacy Rule) issued by a healthcare organization that informs individuals of the uses and disclosures of patient-identifiable health information that may be made by the organization, as well as the individual's rights and the organization's legal duties with respect to that information (45 CFR 164.520 2013)

Nuchal cord: Umbilical cord around the neck

Nuclear cataract: Cataracts that form in the nucleus of the lens and are often associated with aging

Nuclear medicine: The practice of using small radioactive elements designed to travel to a specific organ or type of tissue, which are introduced into the patient through an intravenous injection

Nulligravida: Female who has never been pregnant

Nulliparous: Female who has never carried a pregnancy longer than 20 weeks

Oblique fracture: Travels diagonally across the bone

Oblique: Two projections during an imaging service consisting of two views that pass through the body at a diagonal angle

Obstetric: Refers to a procedure performed on a pregnant woman or condition related to a woman's pregnancy, such as a delivery or complication of pregnancy

Obstetricians: Healthcare providers who specialize in the health of a patient during pregnancy, childbirth, and the postpartum period

Obstetrics and gynecology services: Services focused on the gynecological and reproductive health of female patients, as well as providing services for pregnant patients and performing deliveries

Occipital nerve block: An injection directly into the greater and lesser occipital nerves, used to treat headaches and migraines (Mount Sinai Hospital n.d.b)

Occlusion: Completely closing an orifice or the lumen of a tubular body part

Occupational therapist (OT): A healthcare professional who uses constructive activities to help restore a patient's ability to perform essential activities of daily living (occupations) and improve or maintain functional ability

Occupational therapy services: Noninvasive procedures aimed at improving fine motor skills and functions

Ocular adnexa: The accessory structures of the eye, including the extraocular muscles, eyelids, lacrimal system, orbit, and optic nerve and pathways

Official Guidelines for Coding and Reporting (OGCR): The set of official guidelines for the use of the ICD-10-CM code set, published by the set of four organizations that make up the Cooperating Parties for ICD-10: AHA, AHIMA, CMS, and NCHS

Oncologist: A healthcare provider who specializes in the development, diagnosis, and treatment of malignant neoplasms and tumors (oncology)

Open fracture: Fracture in which the bone penetrates the skin

Open procedure: Procedure in which the skin is incised (or cut into) to perform the procedure

Open treatment: The fracture site has been surgically opened to visualize the fracture site or apply internal fixation devices

Ophthalmologist: Healthcare provider who specializes in pathology and diseases of the eyeball, and performs surgeries to correct eye problems

Ophthalmology: Practitioners in this field specialize in the anatomy, physiology, and pathology of diseases of the eyeball, and perform medical and surgical procedures on the eye

Optometrist: Healthcare specialist who examines the eyes for visual defects, such as myopia (nearsightedness), and prescribes lenses to correct the defect (either glasses or contact lenses)

Optometry: Practitioners in this field perform examinations of the ophthalmological system, as well as medical treatment and management of eye conditions

Orchiopexy: Surgical fixation of undescended testes in the scrotal sac

Organ system: Specific group of organs that may be examined during an evaluation and management encounter

Origin: Location where a patient is picked up for transportation service

Orthopedic services: Services that focus on the management and treatment of conditions affecting the musculoskeletal system, such as fractures, arthritis, joint sprains and strains, and osteoporosis

Orthopedist: A medical doctor who specializes in correcting congenital or acquired abnormalities of the bones and musculoskeletal system through the use of casting, bracing, and surgical techniques

Orthotics: Instruments used on the outside of the body to support, align, or correct deformities, or to improve the movements of joints, the spine, or the limbs

Osteoarthritis: A degenerative condition of the joints that results from wear and tear of the cartilage between joints, and causes pain, swelling, and problems with range of motion of the joint

Osteopathic manipulative treatments (OMT): Treatments that involve the application of pressure, stretching, and resistance to body structures to relieve pain and improve range of motion

Otitis: Ear infection

Outcome of delivery code: Code that identifies the number of births and if they were live or stillborn

Out-of-pocket expense: Healthcare costs that a patient must pay out of pocket because they are not covered by Medicare or other insurance (CMS 2006)

Outpatient hospital: A part of the hospital facility that is designed to treat patients who do not need a bed or to be admitted as an inpatient for overnight care

Outpatient: 1. A hospital patient who receives services in one or more of a hospital's facilities when he or she is not currently an inpatient or a home care patient; 2. A patient who receives ambulatory care services in a hospital-based clinic or department

Ovaries: The glands found on either side of the uterus, below and behind the fallopian tubes, anchored to the uterus with suspensory ligaments

Overcoding: The practice of assigning more codes than needed to describe a patient's condition. Some instances of overcoding may be contrary to the guidance provided in the Official Coding Guidelines

Oviducts: The ducts through which the ovaries travel; also known as the fallopian tubes

Oximetry: A noninvasive test that measures a patient's oxygen saturation level

Pacemaker: A small, battery-powered device that is implanted in the patient's chest or abdomen and helps maintain a normal heart rhythm

Pain management services: Services performed as a treatment for chronic pain in patients who are not undergoing any type of surgical procedure

Paired organs: Organs that are symmetrically placed on the body (for example, eyes)

Panel: A group of specific tests (from the chemistry section) that are commonly performed together, such as a lipid or comprehensive metabolic panel

Parasitology: The study of parasites

Parenthetical note: Instructions for use of the codes, presented in parentheses throughout the Tabular List that are intended to prevent errors and help coders report codes appropriately

Paring: The process of cutting or trimming away the outer edges of a skin growth to make it smaller, remove pressure points, or remove it completely

Parity (or para): The number of previous pregnancies

Parkinson's disease: A progressive disorder of the central nervous system that causes tremors rigidity, and postural problems

Partial hospitalization: A structured program of active treatment for psychiatric care that is more intense than the care a patient receives in a doctor or therapist's office (CMS 2006)

Pass-through billing: Occurs when a laboratory performs an ordered lab test and sends the ordering provider a bill for the services (instead of billing the insurance company themselves), and the ordering provider bills the patient's insurance on the lab's behalf

Past, family, social history (PFSH): The patient's past experience with illnesses, hospitalizations, operations, injuries, and treatments; a review of healthcare events in the patient's family, including diseases that may be hereditary or place the patient at risk; age-appropriate review of past and current activities

Pathological fracture: Fracture that occurs in a diseased bone, such as osteoporosis or neoplastic disease (bone cancer)

Pathology and Laboratory section: Section of the CPT code book that lists codes that represent diagnostic studies on human specimens and tissue samples

Patient status: Identifies the patient's status during an accident, and identifies if the patient's injury was related to employment, volunteer work, or military status

Patient-Centered Medical Home (PCMH): A program to provide comprehensive primary care that partners physicians with the patient and their family to allow better access to healthcare and improved outcomes

Payment: 1. The money that a healthcare practice or facility receives in return for providing a healthcare service to a patient. **2.** As amended by HITECH, the activities undertaken by a health plan to obtain premiums or to determine or fulfill its responsibility for coverage and provision of benefits under the health plan; or a healthcare provider or health plan to obtain or provide reimbursement for the provision of healthcare (45 CFR 164.501 2013)

Penetrating wound: Wound that results from a trauma that pierces the skin and goes into the body's deeper structures, such as a stab wound or gunshot wound

Penis: The main male reproductive organ

Per member per month (PMPM): Amount of money paid monthly for each individual enrolled in a capitation-based health insurance plan

Percutaneous: Through the skin

Percutaneous skeletal fixation: A type of fracture treatment in which fixation devices are placed across the fracture site, typically under x-ray imaging guidance

Percutaneous transluminal coronary angioplasty (PTCA): Procedure where a catheter is threaded into the body through an incision in the femoral artery in the groin, to the site of the angioplasty (usually an area clogged by atherosclerosis); then a small balloon at the tip of the catheter is slowly inflated, stretching the sides of the vessel and creating a wider opening through which blood can flow

Performance measures: A set of predefined quality outcomes that are used to determine the quality of care provided to patients

Performing provider: The provider performing the surgery or other service

Pericardium: The sac that holds the heart

Perinatal: Period that extends before and after childbirth and pertains to the health and medical services for the fetus (and later newborn); extends from 20 to 28 weeks before childbirth to up to six weeks post-delivery

Perinatal condition: Condition that occurs at or during childbirth and may occur up to 6 weeks post-delivery

Perinatologist: A medical doctor who specializes in high-risk pregnancies and focuses on the health of the mother and fetus before, during, and after pregnancy

Perineum: The area between the vagina and the anus

Peripartum: Period that pertains to the mother's health and healthcare services, and extends from about one month before childbirth to up to five months after childbirth

Peripheral nerve stimulation: Pain treatment procedure performed by placing small electrodes next to peripheral nerves to ensure that the correct nerves have been identified; once the nerves causing the pain are found, the trial leads are removed and a neurostimulator is placed, with permanent leads and a small battery pack, to continuously stimulate the nerves and relieve pain (Mount Sinai Hospital n.d.c)

Peripheral nervous system (PNS): Body system compised of all of the nerves throughout the body except the nerves of the brain and spinal cord (central nervous system)

Peritoneal dialysis: Dialysis that involves the placement of a dialyzing solution into the peritoneal cavity in the abdomen, where it removes waste products from the body and is then drained, removing extra fluid and waste products

Peritonitis: Infection within the peritoneal cavity

Permanent block: A specimen contained in a small mold and surrounded with paraffin wax and cooled

Permanent section: A permanent section procedure is similar to a frozen section, except that instead of freezing the block, it is placed in a fixative agent, which makes the cells fixed so that they will not change; it is then placed in a small mold and surrounded with paraffin wax and cooled so the specimen is contained in a permanent block that may be stored indefinitely for future evaluations

Pessary: A small device placed inside the vagina to support the internal structures of the female reproductive system such as the uterus, vagina, bladder, or rectum

Phacoemulsification: A technique used during extracapsular cataract excision that uses ultrasound vibrations to break up the cloudy lens and extract it through a small hollow tube

Physeal fracture: Fractures of the growth plate in long bones in children

Physical safeguards: As amended by HITECH, Security Rule measures such as locking doors to safeguard data and various media from unauthorized access and exposures; including facility access controls, workstation use, workstation security, and device and media controls (45 CFR 164.310 2013)

Physical status modifier: Modifiers that should be appended to the code for the anesthesia service

Physical therapist (PT): A licensed healthcare professional who focuses on noninvasive procedures that alleviate pain and improve and restore mobility

Physical therapy services: Noninvasive procedures and treatments that alleviate pain and improve and restore mobility to limbs and areas of the body

Physician: A medical doctor who has completed post-doctoral medical training in his or her chosen specialty

Physician's Desk Reference (PDR): A compilation of information for prescription drugs to ensure that the correct drug is selected for the service

Place of occurrence: Where the patient was when the injury occurred

Place of service (POS): Place of service or point of service

Placeholder X: In ICD-10-CM "X" is used to extend a code to the required number of characters so that a seventh character extension may be placed

Pleural effusion: A collection of fluid in the pleural space between the pleural sac, which lines the lung, and the lung itself; this fluid places pressure on the lung and does not allow it to expand completely, causing shortness of breath or chest pain

Pneumothorax: Collapsed lung

Polyarthritis: Arthritis that occurs in many different areas

Posterior: Situated toward the back of the body (such as the buttocks or heels)

Postero-anterior: Two projections during an imaging service consisting of two views that pass through the back to the front of the body

Postoperative diagnosis: The definitive medical condition of the patient either diagnosed or treated during the procedure

Postpartum: Post-pregnancy period that extends after childbirth to six weeks post-delivery

Premium: Amount of money that a policyholder or certificate holder must periodically pay an insurer in return for healthcare coverage

Preoperative diagnosis: The diagnosis that is given to the patient at the beginning of a procedure

Pressure ulcer: An ulcer that has occurred on the skin as a result of prolonged pressure on the skin; also known as a bedsore or decubitus ulcer

Preventive medicine services: Comprehensive health evaluations that involve a physical examination, including an age and gender appropriate history, counseling and anticipatory guidance and health

(Continued on next page)

risk factor reduction interventions, and the ordering of laboratory and diagnostic procedures

Primary care: A basic level of care usually given by doctors who work with general and family medicine, internal medicare, pregnant women, and children (CMS 2006)

Primary care provider (PCP): 1. Physician who provides, supervises, and coordinates the healthcare of a member and who manages referrals to other healthcare providers and utilization of healthcare services both inside and outside a managed care plan (CMS 2006) 2. The physician who makes the initial diagnosis of a patient's medication condition

Primary neoplasm: Location where the growth originated

Prior authorization (PA): Process of obtaining approval from a healthcare insurance company before receiving healthcare services

Privacy Rule: The federal regulations created to implement the privacy requirements of the simplification subtitle of the Health Insurance Portability and Accountability Act of 1996; effective in 2002; afforded patients certain rights to and about their protected health information

Procedural coding system (PCS): Compilation of ICD codes used to report hospital inpatient procedures

Procedure: An action of diagnosing or treating a medical condition by a healthcare professional

Proctosigmoidoscopy: The examination of the rectum and may include a portion of the sigmoid colon

Products of conception (POC): The remaining fetal and placental tissues after either a spontaneous miscarriage or elective pregnancy termination

Professional component (PC): 1. The portion of a healthcare procedure performed by a physician 2. A term generally used in reference to the elements of radiological procedures performed by a physician, which may include the supervision and interpretation of a technical service

Professional organization: An association of individuals that is committed to furthering the interests of a particular profession

Projection: The direction in which the imaging rays pass through the body

Prolonged services: Services where a healthcare provider may spend an inordinate amount of time with a patient, either face-to-face or without direct patient contact, to manage or treat the patient's condition

Prospective payment system (PPS): A type of reimbursement system that is based on preset payment levels rather than actual charges billed after the service has been provided; specifically, one of several Medicare reimbursement systems based on predetermined payment rates or periods and linked to the anticipated intensity of services delivered as well as the beneficiary's condition

Prostate: A gland only found in males that stores and assists in making seminal fluid, and sits under the urinary bladder surrounding part of the urethra

Prosthetics: Designed to replace all or part of an internal body organ (such as an artificial hip or knee replacement) or to replace an external appendage as an artificial limb (such as a lower leg prosthesis for an amputee)

Protected health information (PHI): 1. Health information that is individually identifiable, such as health records, laboratory reports, and patient healthcare history forms. PHI can be held on any type of media including paper, electronic, and orally transmitted information. 2. As amended by HITECH, individually identifiable health information: (1) Except as provided in paragraph (2) of this definition, that is: (i) transmitted by electronic media; (ii) maintained in electronic media; or (iii) transmitted or maintained in any other form or medium. (2) Protected health information excludes individually identifiable health information: (i) in education records covered by the Family Educational Rights and Privacy Act, as amended, 20 U.S.C. 1232g; (ii) in records described at 20 U.S.C. 1232g(a)(4)(B)(iv); (iii) in employment records held by a covered entity in its role as employer; and (iv) regarding a person who has been deceased for more than 50 years (45 CFR 160.103 2013)

Provider contracting: Occurs when the insurance company and the healthcare provider come into an agreement so that when the healthcare provider delivers healthcare services to patients, the insurance company will provide reimbursement for the healthcare services provided

Proximal: Toward the center of the body (the upper arm)

Pseudophakia: An intraocular lens prosthesis

Psychiatrist: Medical doctors who specialize in the diagnosis and treatment of mental illnesses and are both qualified and required to perform healthcare E/M services for their patients, as well as any necessary mental health services such as psychotherapy or group counseling services

Psychologist: A provider who is not a medical doctor, but has a terminal degree (such as a PhD) from an educational institution and has been been trained in the art of psychology; he or she may provide mental and behavioral health services to patients but are not qualified to perform medical procedures and examinations

Psychotherapy: The treatment of mental illness and behavioral disturbance in which the healthcare provider attempts to alleviate the emotional disturbances, reverse or change patterns of behavior, and encourage personality growth and development through discourse with the patient

Puerperium: From birth to six weeks after birth

Pulmonary edema: A fluid collection within the lungs themselves caused by heart failure, myocardial infarction, cardiac ischemia, and other heart problems, as well as sepsis and severe anemia

Pulmonary embolism: An embolus that has traveled to the lungs, and can be a result of a DVT becoming dislodged and traveling into the lungs

Push: The administration of a therapeutic, prophylactic, or diagnostic substance via an IV line

Qualifier: Identifies any additional attributes of why or how the procedure was performed

Qualifying circumstances CPT codes: Add-on codes that should be used in addition to the code for the anesthesia service (as well as any applicable physical status modifier)

Qualitative examination: An examination that studies the quality of a specimen

Quality improvement (QI): A set of activities that measures the quality of a service or product through systems or process evaluation and then implements revised processes that result in better healthcare outcomes for patients, based on standards of care

Quantitative examination: An examination that identifies the quantity of a specific substance found in a specimen

Radiation oncologist: Oncologists who specialize in the treatment of cancers via radiation treatments, also known as an interventional radiologist

Radiculopathy: A nerve-related pain

Radiofrequency nerve ablation: A procedure used to treat back and neck pain by using a controlled heat source to disable nerves that are responsible for causing pain; it is performed using a small needle with a heated tip placed near the nerve causing the pain, to disrupt the nerve's ability to send a pain signal (Mount Sinai Hospital 2017b)

Radiologic guidance: Procedure performed along with an invasive or minimally invasive procedure, to help guide the provider performing the procedure to the correct anatomical location

Radiological supervision and interpretation (S&I): The professional component of the study and includes the supervision of the radiology service as well as interpretation of the results

Radiologist: A medical doctor who specializes in the diagnosis and treatment of medical conditions using radiology and imaging techniques

Radiology section: Section of the CPT code book that lists all of the procedures that use radiant energy to diagnose and treat medical conditions, such as x-rays, MRIs, and ultrasounds

Radiology services: Services that use radiation to produce images of the inside of the body, such as bones and organs

Reattachment: All or a portion of a separated body part is put back in its normal location or other suitable location

Referral: A written approval from the primary care doctor for the patient to see a specialist or get certain services. In many Medicare Managed Care Plans, a patient needs a referral before he or she can get care from anyone except a primary care doctor. If a referral is not obtained first, the plan may not pay for the patient's care (CMS 2006)

Refraction: A test performed to determine if a patient has any abnormalities with his or her vision, and used to identify the appropriate prescription for eyeglasses or contact lenses

Refractive surgery: Surgery performed to reshape the cornea of the eye and improve eyesight

Regional anesthesia: Anesthesia that employs an injection to block a large amount of nerves to numb a more extensive body area and prepare the patient for a more extensive surgery or procedure

Rehabilitative serves: Services that help a patient keep, recover, or improve skills, functions, and activities of daily living after they have been lost or impaired due to illness, injury, or disability

Reimbursement: Compensation or repayment for healthcare services

Release: Freeing a body part from an abnormal physical constraint by cutting or by the use of force

Remission: Term used to identify that the condition is currently not an issue, such as a temporary recovery

Remote coding: Position in which the coder is not required to actually be present in the office or facility setting while completing his or her work

Removal: Taking out a device, object, or substance from a body part or area

Repair: A procedure performed to return an organ or body part to its original function, or to improve functioning or improve a cosmetic outcome; restoring a body part to its normal anatomic structure and function to the extent possible

Replacement: Inserting biological or synthetic material that physically takes the place or function of all or a portion of a body part

Reportable diagnoses: Diseases or medical conditions that are important to public health so medical offices are required to report any positive results for these diseases or conditions to the necessary state or federal agency (MedlinePlus 2019)

Reposition: Moving all or a portion of a body part to its normal location or other suitable location

Reproductive endocrinology and infertility (REI) specialist: A medical doctor with additional training and expertise in human reproduction, including the function of hormones in reproduction

Reproductive surgery: Specialty that focuses on surgical treatments to treat infertility

Resection: The removal of all or part of an organ, body tissue, or body part without replacement

Resequenced code: Codes that are not placed numerically within the Tabular List and are out of numerical sequence; they are identified with the # symbol

Restriction: Partially closing an orifice of the lumen of a tubular body part

Retinal detachment: Occurs when the retina, which is a layer of tissue at the back of the eye, detaches from the eye tissues

Review of systems (ROS): A uniform system of performing an inventory of body systems through a series of questions seeking to identify signs or symptoms the patient may be experiencing or has experienced

Revision: Correcting a portion of a malfunctioning device or the position of a displaced device to the extent possible

Rhinoplasty: The surgical repair or revision of the nose, either for cosmetic or functional or medical purposes

Risk adjustment: The way that payments to health plans are changed to take into account a person's health status (CMS 2006)

Risk analysis: The first step to risk management, includes assessing security threats, security vulnerabilities, and the likely impact should the system expose a vulnerability

Robot-assisted surgery: A type of laparoscopic surgery that is performed with the aid of a robot with miniature instruments controlled by the surgeon

Root operation: The type of surgery, operation, or procedure that was performed

Route of administration: The way in which the drug is administered to the patient

Rule of nines: Divides the body's surface into percentages based on the number nine, with the groin area making up the remaining one percent of body surface

Ruptured aneurysm: Aneurysm whose walls have burst causing hemorrhaging into the surrounding body cavity or tissues

Sagittal plane: A vertical line that divides the body into right and left halves

Salter-Harris classification: Classification that identifies the type of physeal fracture

Schizophrenia: A mental disorder which manifests in the symptoms of delusions, hallucinations, paranoia, confused speech, isolation, outbursts of anger, and catatonic behavior that persist for at least one month

Sciatica: A combination of pain, numbness, and weakness along the sciatic nerve from the lower back area, radiating to the buttocks and the leg; typically caused by a lower back problem putting pressure on the sciatic nerve

Scoliosis: A condition in which the spine curves sideways

Screening, Brief Intervention and Referral to Treatment (SBIRT): Behavior change interventions administered to patients with suspected alcohol or substance abuse

Scrotum: A pouch of skin where the testes are located

Secondary neoplasm: The site of the metastatic growth of a neoplasm

Security Rule: The federal regulations created to implement the security requirements of HIPAA

See also: Instructs the coder to look elsewhere for a code if the precise condition cannot be found in the current index entry

See condition: Instructs the coder to search for the code by looking up the condition, rather than the term that is currently located

Segment: Two vertebrae with the space between it

Segmental fracture: Fracture made up of at least two fracture lines, which isolate a larger section of bone

Seminal vesicles: Small male accessory sex glands that help to form the lubricating fluid of semen

Separate procedure: A procedure that is commonly part of another, more complex procedure, but which may be performed independently or be otherwise unrelated to the procedure

Sepsis: A complication of an infection outside of the bloodstream, such as a tooth abscess or skin infection; once a patient is deemed septic, the infectious organism has invaded the bloodstream and has been carried throughout the blood to other sites of the body (also referred to as septicemia or bacteremia)

Septic shock: A severe drop in blood pressure, caused by sepsis, that can lead to organ failure or death

Sequela: A condition that is the consequence of a previous disease or injury

Sequencing: Placing multiple diagnoses codes in the correct order

Sequencing priority: Assigning codes from one chapter *before* codes from other chapters; for example, codes from chapter 15 of the ICD-10-CM code book should be assigned before codes from other chapters

Service-based code: A code that describes a full service, such as a physical therapy evaluation, application of hot or cold packs, or the performance of electrical stimulation; these codes are untimed, and one code should be reported no matter how long the provider spent performing the service

Services: Identified by HCPCS codes, miscellaneous services that may be provided to patients in the healthcare setting; some of these services are also identified by CPT codes, whereas other services are only identified by codes found in the HCPCS code book

Seventh character extension: The last possible character in a code, which is in the seventh location

Sexually transmitted infection: An infection that usually presents with symptoms of the genitourinary system and whose primary mode of transmission is sexual intercourse

Shaving: The act of sharp removal by transverse incision or horizontal slicing

Sigmoidoscopy: The examination of the entire rectum and sigmoid colon, and may include an examination of the descending colon

Signs: Objective evidence of a disease that can be observed or detected by someone other than the individual affected by the condition

Skeletal traction: An invasive form of traction, in which a screw, pin, or wire is inserted into the bone, after which weights, ropes, and pulleys are used to pull the bone into the correct position

Skin lesion: Any abnormality in the skin; includes freckles and moles, precancerous and malignant areas, skin tags, and scrapes or cuts

Skin traction: Traction that employs straps, ropes, pulleys, and weights are applied externally to the skin to slowly stretch and realign bones into place until they can be set and casted until fully healed

Skin ulcer: An open wound on the skin that may be caused by infection, pressure, or venous problems

Slit lamp: A high-intensity light that can be focused into a thin sheet to shine into the eye

Small group practice: A practice that has from two to five healthcare providers, all of whom see patients each day

Smear: If the specimen is a liquid or submerged in a fluid substance, then it may be smeared onto the surface of a slide, then allowed to dry; it is then fixed with a fixative agent, and then stained to allow for the visualization of certain cells

SOAP note: A common format for health record documentation, SOAP stands for S, Subjective; O, Objective; A, Assessment; and P, Plan

Social communication disorder: Disorder that occurs when a patient has difficulty understanding social cues in verbal and nonverbal communication

Solo practice: A practice in which the physician is self-employed and legally the sole owner

Special report: Included with the reporting of an unlisted procedure or other procedure that is rarely provided, unusual, variable, or new, and should include a complete description of the procedure, including the nature of the procedure; extent of the procedure performed; need for the procedure (the medical necessity for the procedure); amount of time spent on the procedure; effort needed to complete the procedure; and equipment necessary to provide the service

Specific test: Test that evaluates a specimen for an identified substance

Specificity: Ability to detect the absence of a characteristic when the characteristic is absent

Specimen: A bodily tissue sample from the patient

Spectrum concept: This concept identifies that a specific condition may expand from minimal

(*Continued on next page*)

or least-disruptive stage to maximal or most-disruptive stage

Speech-language pathologist (SLP): A healthcare professional who provides speech therapy services

Speech therapy services: Services that help adults and children improve their speech, advance social and cognitive communication skills, and treat swallowing disorders

Spermatic cord: A cord-like structure made up of the vas deferens and surrounding tissues

Spinal cord stimulation (SCS): Pain treatment procedure that identifies the exact spinal nerves causing the paint and places a battery and lead wires on these nerves to alleviate pain; similar to peripheral nerve stimulation

Spiral fracture: Fracture that spirals around and extends down the length of the bone

Sprain: The stretching or tearing of a ligament

Stage: Each layer excised

Staghorn calculus: Large kidney stones that are too big to pass naturally through the urinary system and may require surgical treatment

Standalone code: Codes that include a full description and do not depend on a parent code to provide more information

Status asthmaticus: An extreme form of asthma exacerbation that does not respond to treatment and can result in hypoxia and ultimately respiratory failure

Status epilepticus: A type of epilepsy in which the seizures occur too close together for the patient to fully recover in-between seizures, or when a seizure lasts for a long period of time

Status migrainosus: Long-lasting migraines that can last 72 hours or more

Stereotactic body radiation treatment (SBRT): Whole-body stereotactic radiosurgery (SRS) treatment used on body tumors

Stereotactic radiosurgery (SRS): A type of radiation treatment used for intracranial lesions that delivers a precision dose of radiation

Strabismus: A misalignment of the eye muscles that can be surgically corrected by repositioning and strengthening the muscles of the eye

Strain: An injury to a muscle or tendon, which ranges from a simple stretching of the muscle or tendon to complete tear of the muscle and tendon

Subcapsular cataract: Cataracts that form at the back of the lens and are more common in individuals with diabetes mellitus or patients on high doses of steroids

Subsequent encounter: This episode of care is used when the patient is seen during the healing phase of the encounter and is no longer under active treatment for the condition

Substance abuse: The misuse of alcohol or drugs, which impairs a person's ability to meet daily responsibilities

Subterm: Terms that are indented under the main term to indicate that they pertain to the main term, and to identify different variations of the main term

Superior: Toward the top of the body (the head)

Supplement: Inserting biological or synthetic material that physically reinforces or augments the function of a portion of a body part

Supplemental insurance: Insurance policies that help patients pay the out-of-pocket expenses related to healthcare. Supplemental insurance policies differ depending on the type of insurance offered and the specifics of coverage, ranging from accident coverage, coverage for cancer treatments, coverage for disabilities only, or for coverage of a specific set of healthcare services or treatments. Supplemental insurance plans are typically low cost, and patients can pick and choose which type of coverage they prefer and tailor coverage to their specific needs. These plans act as an umbrella, in that they help cover the patient from the financial burdens for which he or she may be responsible in the case of a healthcare emergency or unplanned treatment

Supplies: Items provided to the patient in the healthcare setting, typically designed for long-term or multiple uses

Surgery section: The largest of all sections within the CPT code book; it lists all of the invasive procedures that may be performed to treat patients

Surgical procedure: Any single, separate, systematic process upon or within the body that can be complete in itself; is normally performed by a physician, dentist, or other licensed practitioner; can be performed either with or without instruments; and is performed to restore disunited or deficient parts, remove diseased or injured tissues, extract foreign matter, assist in obstetrical delivery, or aid in diagnosis

Surgical specialist: Provider who treats and diagnoses patients through major surgical techniques

Symptoms: Subjective evidence of a disease or a disease process experienced

Synonym: Word or phrase that means the same thing as another word or phrase

Systemic inflammatory response syndrome (SIRS): A noninfectious process, such as heatstroke or a traumatic injury

Table of Drugs and Chemicals: The third section of the ICD-10-CM book that lists the toxic effects of drugs, chemicals, and other substances

Table of Drugs: A reference tool in the HCPCS code book that helps coders find the appropriate HCPCS code for drugs and medications administered in the healthcare setting, organized by the name of the drug or medicinal, dosage or unit amount given, and the method of administration of the drug

Table of Neoplasms: An index that allows coders to identify codes for neoplastic conditions, such as malignant tumors and diseases, and benign growths

Tabular List: The structured list of ICD-10-CM codes, organized alphanumerically, and divided into chapters based on body system or condition

Technical component (TC): The portion of radiological and other procedures that is facility based or nonphysician based (for example, radiology films, equipment, overhead, endoscopic suites, and so on)

Technical safeguards: As amended by HITECH, the Security Rule means the technology and the policy and procedures for its use that protect electronic protected health information and control access to it (45 CFR 164.304 2013)

Telemedicine service: 1. Professional services given to a patient through an interactive telecommunications system by a practitioner at a distant site (CMS 2006) **2.** A telecommunications system that links healthcare organizations and patients from diverse geographic locations and transmits text and images for (medical) consultation and treatment

Testes: Glands of the reproductive and endocrine systems that produce and store sperm and male sex hormones

Therapeutic procedure: Procedure that is performed to treat a diagnosis

Therapy services: Treatments aimed at rehabilitating the patient to optimal bodily function

Third-party payer: An insurance company (for example, Blue Cross/Blue Shield) or healthcare program (for example, Medicare) that pays or reimburses healthcare providers (second party) or patients (first party) for the delivery of healthcare services

Thoracostomy: An opening created in the thoracic cavity, otherwise known as a chest tube that acts as a drain for the thoracic cavity to drain blood, fluid, or air from around your lungs, heart, or esophagus

Thrombosis: A formation of blood cells, fatty deposits, or other particles that form a clot within the blood vessel, otherwise known as a blood clot

Time units: Values for anesthesia services that take into account the duration of the procedure, from the beginning of the anesthesia service until the patient is released to a postoperative or post-anesthesia care unit

Time-based code: Code reported according the length of time that the provider spent performing the service to the end of a long, thin, lighted tube, inserted through a natural opening or stoma; the healthcare provider can maneuver the endoscope through a body passage, such as the gastrointestinal tract, to see inside the organ for diagnostic or therapeutic services

Tophus: A lump or nodule under the skin that is composed of the uric acid buildup

Torus fracture: Fracture that occurs in children, when only one part of the bone buckles

Toxic effect: The result of a toxin, such as a chemical, medicinal, or other substance on the body

Trabeculectomy: Procedure used as a treatment for glaucoma by lowering the intraocular pressure (the pressure inside the eyeball)

Tracheostomy: Connection that is established by the insertion of the tracheostomy tube

Tracheotomy: Procedure that cuts through the trachea to allow for the insertion of a tracheostomy tube, or trach tube

Traction: The use of mechanical devices and mechanisms to straighten bones or relieve pressure

Transcranial magnetic stimulation (TMS): A noninvasive procedure that utilizes magnetic fields to stimulate areas of the brain

Transfer: Moving, without taking out, all or a portion of a body part to another location to take over the function of all or a portion of a body part

Transient hypertension: A temporary elevated high blood pressure reading without the diagnosis of hypertension

Transitional care management (TCM): Services provided to patients during the transitional period from an inpatient facility to a home setting; these codes cover a month's worth of healthcare services directed toward a patient's care, after they have been discharged from an inpatient facility, such as a hospital follow-up visit

Transluminal procedure: Procedure that is performed within a vessel

Transplantation: Inserting all or a portion of a living body part taken from another individual or animal to physically take the place or function of all or a portion of a similar body part; procedure that removes a damaged, diseased, or otherwise nonfunctioning organ from the body and replaces it with a donated organ in its place

Transportation indicator: A two-character code used to identify why the transportation service was medically necessary

Transurethral resection of the prostate (TURP): Procedure that involves the insertion of a resectoscope through the male urethra, which is threaded to the area of the prostate tissue to be removed; an electrocautery knife is then used to cut away at the enlarged prostatic tissue

Transverse fracture: Fracture that travels horizontally across the bone

Transverse plane: A horizontal line, perpendicular to the long axis of the body that divides the body into superior and inferior portions (the top and the bottom halves); also known as the axial plane

Traumatic brain injury (TBI): Brain injury that requires invasive surgery and a lifetime of medical treatment and rehabilitative services

Traumatic fracture: Fracture that occurs as a result of some sort of traumatic injury

Treatment modality: A method of therapeutic treatment designed to treat or rehabilitate a specific patient condition

Treatment, payment, and healthcare operations (TPO): Standard of the Privacy Rule that allows the use of protected health information for the following: treatment or the provision, coordination, and management of a patient's healthcare and related services by that patient's healthcare providers; payment or the activities of the patient's health insurance plan to obtain premiums for health insurance, to determine coverage benefits, and to furnish payment for healthcare services delivered to a covered beneficiary; and healthcare operations including various services provided by healthcare practitioners

Treatment: As amended by HITECH, the provision, coordination, or management of healthcare and related services by one or more healthcare providers, including the coordination or management of healthcare by a healthcare provider with a third party; consultation between healthcare providers relating to a patient; or the referral of a patient for healthcare from one healthcare provider to another (45 CFR 164.501 2013)

TRICARE: A healthcare program for active duty and retired uniformed services members and their families, formerly referred to as CHAMPUS (CMS 2006)

Trimesters: Three, roughly three-month periods of time, into which the 40 weeks of pregnancy are grouped

Tunica vaginalis: A layer of tissue covering the testes in the shape of a pouch

UB-04: A uniform institutional provider hardcopy claim form suitable for use in billing multiple third-party payers. The UB-04 is the only hardcopy claim form that CMS accepts from institutional providers (CMS 2006)

Ultrasound: Imaging that uses high-frequency sound waves applied to the body via a transducer on a specific area of the body; the sound waves bounce off internal structures within the body, creating an image on a computer screen

Unbundling: The practice of using multiple codes to bill for the various individual steps in a single procedure rather than using a single code that includes all the steps of the comprehensive procedure

Undercoding: A form of incomplete documentation that results when diagnoses or procedures that should be coded are not assigned

Underdose: Occurs when a patient does not take the correctly prescribed amount of a medication

Underdosing: An underdosing occurs when a patient takes too little or a prescribed substance and suffers an unintended consequence

Undetermined intent: An undetermined intent of a toxic effect is used only when the intention of the toxic effect cannot be determined to be any of the other types: accidental, intentional, assault, adverse effect, or underdosing

Uniform Hospital Discharge Data Set (UHDDS): A data set created to "improve the uniformity and comparability of hospital discharge data" for the Medicare and Medicaid programs

Unlisted procedure codes: Codes available in each section of CPT to describe procedures that have no specific procedure code assigned because the procedure is new or unusual

Ureters: Two thin tubes that connect the kidneys to the urinary bladder

Urethra: Part of the urinary system through which urine passes during elimination from the bladder

Urgent care facility: Facility that provides same-day care for patients with healthcare emergencies or urgent healthcare needs and may be either a standalone facility or attached to a larger facility, such as a hospital

Urgent care: Services provided to patients who need healthcare for non–life-threatening situations, illnesses, or injuries

Urinary bladder: A hollow muscular organ that holds urine until it is emptied from the body through the urethra

Urodynamics: The study of the motion and flow of urine

Urologist: A medical doctor who specializes in the diagnosis and treatment of conditions of the urinary system, adrenal glands, and the male and female genital systems (AUA 2018)

Use additional code: Instructions that list conditions that should be coded *after* the code identified

Uterus: Organ in the female reproductive system where the fetus develops during gestation

Vaccine administration: The act of giving the patient a vaccine

Vaccine toxoid: The actual substance that is injected or given to a patient and that creates an immune response from the patient

Vagina: The lower portion of the birth canal, which serves as the conduit for the birth of a fetus, uterine secretions and menstrual flow, and as the receptacle for semen from a male during intercourse

Vaginal birth after cesarean (VBAC): Successful vaginal birth after a woman has previously given birth via cesarean section

Vaginectomy: Removal of all or part of the vagina

Varicose vein: Vein that is a result of an insufficiency in the valves of the lower veins to push blood upward toward the heart, causing a buildup of blood various reasons including pain management and to reduce muscle spasticity

Vas deferens: Duct made of smooth muscle located within the spermatic cord that transport sperm from the epididymis to the urethra, which is later ejaculated through the urethral orifice

Vasectomy: An outpatient procedure that is performed commonly for elective sterilization where a small section of the vas deferens are cut and removed, so that semen does not flow through the vas to the urethra during ejaculation

Vasopneumatic device: Device used on the external extremities (like the arms and legs) that applies external pressure to the soft tissues and decreases swelling

Virology: The study of viruses

Vision insurance: Insurance similar to health insurance, but that only covers services that are related to visual acuity assessments, refractions, and corrective lenses

Vulva: Female genitalia that consists of the labia (both labia majora and labia minora), the bulb of the vestibule, vestibule of the vagina, the greater vestibular glands (known as Bartholin's glands, they secrete mucus to lubricate the vagina), the lesser vestibular gland, and the vagina orifice, also known as the introitus

Workers' compensation insurance: Insurance that employers are required to have to cover employees who get sick or injured on the job (CMS 2006)

Xenograft: A skin graft made from a different species (commonly pig skin)

X-ray: A form of imaging that produces a beam of x-rays, a form of electromagnetic radiation, that pass through the body

References

42 CFR 405.500. 60 FR 63175, Dec. 9, 1995. http://www.ecfr.gov.

42 CFR 425.20. 76 FR 67973, Nov. 2, 2011. http://www.ecfr.gov.

45 CFR 160.103. 65 FR 82798, Dec. 28, 2000, as amended at 78 FR 5687, Jan. 25, 2013. http://www.ecfr.gov.

45 CFR 164.304. 68 FR 8376, Feb. 20, 2003, as amended at 78 FR 5693, Jan. 25, 2013. http://www.ecfr.gov.

45 CFR 164.310. 68 FR 8376, Feb. 20, 2003, as amended at 78 FR 5694, Jan. 25, 2013. http://www.ecfr.gov.

45 CFR 164.501. 65 FR 82802, Dec. 28, 2000, as amended at 78 FR 5695, Jan. 25, 2013. http://www.ecfr.gov.

45 CFR 164.520. 65 FR 82802, Dec. 28, 2000, as amended at 78 FR 5696, Jan. 25, 2013. http://www.ecfr.gov.

Agency for Healthcare Research and Quality (AHRQ). 2019 (September). Never Events. https://psnet.ahrq.gov/primers/primer/3/never-events.

American Health Information Management Association (AHIMA). 2017. *Pocket Glossary of Health Information Management and Technology*, 5th ed. Chicago: AHIMA.

American Medical Association (AMA). 2019a. http://www.ama-assn.org.

American Medical Association (AMA). 2019b. *CPT 2020 Professional Edition*. Chicago: AMA.

American Psychiatric Association (APA). 2019. https://www.psychiatry.org/psychiatrists/practice/dsm.

American Urological Association (AUA). 2018. Urology. https://www.auanet.org/guidelines/urology.

Centers for Disease Control and Prevention (CDC). 2019. http://www.cdc.gov.

Centers for Medicare and Medicaid Services. 2019 (December 4). National Correct Coding Initiative Edits. https://www.cms.gov/Medicare/Coding /NationalCorrectCodInitEd/index.html.

Centers for Medicare and Medicaid Services (CMS). 2006 (May 14). Glossary. https://www.cms.gov/apps /glossary/default.asp?Letter=ALL&Language=English.

Department of Health and Human Services (HHS). 2010. Medicare Program: Proposed Changes to the Hospital Inpatient Prospective Payment Systems for Acute Care Hospitals and the Long-Term Care Hospital Prospective Payment System and Proposed Fiscal Year 2011 Rates. Federal Register 75(88): 23851–24362.

Indian Health Service (IHS). n.d. Indian Health Manual. Accessed Dec. 13, 2019. https://www.ihs.gov/ihm /index.cfm/dsp_folder/doa/progdel/documents /org_charts/dsp_folder/pc/p6c1/documents /functionalstmts/index.cfm.

MedlinePlus. 2019 (December 2). Reportable Diseases. https://medlineplus.gov/ency/article/001929.htm.

Mount Sinai Hospital. n.d.a. Electromyography. Accessed Dec. 11, 2019. https://www.mountsinai.org/health -library/tests/electromyography.

Mount Sinai Hospital. n.d.b. Interventional Pain Procedures Under X-Ray Guidance. Accessed Dec. 11, 2019. http:// www.mountsinai.org/patient-care/service-areas /pain-management/pain-management-services /interventional-spinal-procedures-under-x-ray -guidance.

Mount Sinai Hospital. n.d.c. Peripheral Nerve Stimulation. Accessed Dec. 11, 2019. http://www.mountsinai.org /patient-care/service-areas/pain-management/pain -management-services/peripheral-nerve-stimulation.

National Centers for Health Statistics (NCHS). 2019 (December 5). https://www.cdc.gov/nchs/.

Palmetto GBA. 2013 (July). Anesthesia Billing Guide. https://engage.ahima.org/HigherLogic /System/DownloadDocumentFile. ashx?DocumentFileKey=9af2a07d-26e1-4694-b1de -a4c59d0dbc30.

Public Law 104-191. 1996. 110 Stat. 1936. Short title see 42 U.S.C. 201 note. http://uscode.house.gov/.

Index

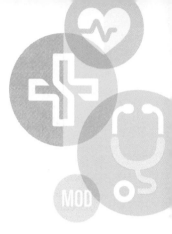